TOXICITY AND METABOLISM OF INDUSTRIAL SOLVENTS

TOXICITY AND METABOLISM
OF INDUSTRIAL SOLVENTS

BY

ETHEL BROWNING, M.D.

Formerly H.M. Medical Inspector of factories
Ministry of Labour and National Service
London

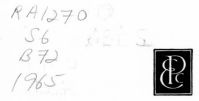

ELSEVIER PUBLISHING COMPANY
AMSTERDAM · LONDON · NEW YORK
1965

ELSEVIER PUBLISHING COMPANY
335 JAN VAN GALENSTRAAT, P.O. BOX 211, AMSTERDAM

AMERICAN ELSEVIER PUBLISHING COMPANY, INC.
52 VANDERBILT AVENUE, NEW YORK, N.Y. 10017

ELSEVIER PUBLISHING COMPANY LIMITED
12 B, RIPPLESIDE COMMERCIAL ESTATE
RIPPLEROAD, BARKING, ESSEX

LIBRARY OF CONGRESS CATALOG CARD NUMBER 65-13228

WITH 4 TABLES

PRINTED IN THE NETHERLANDS

Preface

It was with some trepidation, following notification that the 2nd Edition of my book 'The Toxicity of Industrial Organic Solvents' published by H.M.S.O. in 1953 was now out of print, that I embarked on the present publication. This does not represent a 3rd Edition of the former book; it is a completely new appraisal, though including some references to the work of earlier authors, of the present position of the principal industrial solvents now in use.

An entirely new feature is, wherever it has been possible, an account of the metabolism in the body of the individual solvents, a process which in the opinion of many authorities forms the real basis of their toxic effects.

It is with gratitude that I wish to express my thanks and indebtedness especially to the authors of two publications – those of Dr. F. A. Patty in his revised 2nd Edition of the second volume of 'Industrial Hygiene and Toxicology', published by Interscience Publishers, New York, and Dr. R. Tecwyn Williams, 'Detoxication Mechanisms', published by Chapman and Hall, London. Their innumerable references not only to published articles but also to their personal researches, have been invaluable in providing me with at least a starting point in my own researches into this vast subject.

Ethel Browning

Contents

Chapter 1

AROMATIC HYDROCARBONS

The term 'Aromatic Hydrocarbons' was originally applied to a group of vegetable products, such as balsams, resins and essential oils, distinguished by a characteristic pleasant aromatic perfume. It was many years before they were differentiated from the 'fatty compounds', now known as aliphatic hydrocarbons, by the fact, postulated by Kekulé in 1865, that the simplest aromatic substances contain at least 6 carbon atoms. Kekulé's formula for the structure of benzene, now generally represented by a hexagon with alternating double bounds

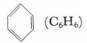 (C_6H_6)

is the foundation of the nomenclature and classification of the aromatic hydrocarbons.

Their present widespread use as solvents in industry can be traced back to 1784, when Lavoisier first demonstrated the true composition of organic substances, though it was not until 1817 that Berzelius postulated that organic compounds were subject to the ordinary laws of chemical combination. For the next twenty years new theories were constantly introduced and almost constantly disputed and rejected, but during these years "the foundation of the great edifice of aromatic chemistry was being laid" (Cohen, 1909).

Between 1830 and 1840 Mitscherlich had obtained benzene from benzoic acid by distillation with lime, and had formed nitrobenzene, chlorobenzene and other derivatives. The benzene so obtained was found to be identical with a hydrocarbon obtained by Faraday in 1825 from an 'Oil Gas' which was being manufactured and compressed into metal vessels for distribution to customers.

The real industrial use of the aromatic hydrocarbons, however, began about 1823, when coal tar naphtha made in the London gas plants was found to be an excellent solvent for rubber (Gerarde, 1960), and the demand for these substances has increased enormously both before and after the two World Wars. In 1957 the production in the U.S.A. of the principal industrial hydrocarbons (benzene, toluene, xylene, ethyl benzene, styrene and naphthalene) had reached a total of over 7500 million pounds (Katzen, 1958).

The chief sources of aromatic hydrocarbons are coal and petroleum. During the heating of coal at temperatures of 1000–3000 °F, without access to air, coke, coal gas and coal tar are produced. From the light oil fraction of coal gas are obtained benzene, toluene, xylene, crude coal tar naphtha and heavy solvent naphtha; from coke oven gas crude 'motor benzol' consisting chiefly of benzene and toluene; from coal tar, diphenyl, naphthalene, methylated naphthalenes, indene, acenaphthene, fluourene, chrysene and phenanthrene.

From petroleum, by various methods of fractional distillation or catalytic reforming, a wide variety of hydrocarbons are obtained. These include not only benzene, isolated from catalytically reformed light naphthas by distillation or solvent extraction, xylene, toluene and ethyl benzene, but also many other aromatic compounds less frequently encountered in industry. (For a detailed account see Gerarde, 1960.) They will be further described under their separate headings.

These aromatic hydrocarbons and their derivatives obtained from petroleum are known as 'petrochemicals', and the petrochemical industry is a rapidly growing source of the ever increasing demand of industry for aromatic hydrocarbons, with full knowledge of how to take full advantage of their enormous advantages with adequate precautions against their potential toxicity.

1. Benzene

Synonyms: benzol, phenyl hydride, coal naphtha, phene benzole, cyclohexatriene

1a. Pure benzene

Molecular weight: 78.11

Benzene, a coal tar product and petrochemical, has been until recently in Great Britain, and still is in many parts of the world, among the most widely used of all industrial solvents, partly on account of its excellent solvent capacity, partly because of its relatively low cost.

Of recent years the recognition of its great potential hazard of chronic poisoning from comparatively slight repeated exposure has led to considerable effort to substitute less toxic compounds.

The unfortunate similarity of the words 'benzene' and 'benzine' is also at last becoming generally recognised and the difference in chemical constitution and toxicity of these two solvents understood.

Benzine is not an aromatic hydrocarbon, nor even a chemical entity, but a volatile mixture of aliphatic hydrocarbons or 'petroleum ethers' derived from petroleum distillation, with a varying content of paraffins and cycloparaffins. Its chronic systemic toxicity is devoid of the haemopoietic effect characteristic of chronic benzene poisoning.

The danger of confusion between benzene and benzine has been exemplified by Heim de Balzac and Agasse Lafont (1933) in their report on a series of 36 cases of benzene poisoning, eight of them fatal, following the accidental substitution of crystallisable benzene for the benzine previously used as a rubber solvent.

Properties: a colourless liquid with a characteristic not unpleasant aromatic odour.

    boiling point: 80.1 °C at 760 mm Hg

    melting point: 5.4–5.5 °C

    vapour pressure: 74.6 at 20 °C

    vapour density (air = 1): 2.77

    specific gravity (liquid density): 0.884 at 15 °C

    flash point: 12 °F   *autoignition temperature:* 1000 °F

    conversion factors: 1 p.p.m. = 3.19 mg/m^3

                    1 mg/l   = 313 p.p.m. at 25 °C, 760 mm Hg

    solubility: in water, 1430 v/v; miscible with alcohol, chloroform, ether, CS_2, acetone, glacial acetic acid, CCl_4.

    maximum allowable concentration: 25 p.p.m. (see also p. 7)

1b. Commercial benzene

(sometimes called 'benzol')

(a) Commercial crystallisable – said to contain 99–100% benzene:
    boiling range: 80–81 °C
    specific gravity: 0.879 at 20 °C
(b) 'Benzol 90' (90% benzene) – contains toluene (13–15%), xylene (2–3%) and sometimes traces of olefins, paraffins, H_2S and other substances.
(c) 50% Benzol – a mixed product, 50% of whose constituents distil below 100 °C and 90% below 120 °C.

The term 'benzols' (plural) is sometimes applied to mixtures of benzene, toluene and xylene. That benzene may contain appreciable amounts of polycyclic aromatic hydrocarbons, some of them carcinogenic, has recently been demonstrated by Lynski and Raha (1961). Their analyses were made by adsorption and partition chromatography (Lynski, 1960), followed by spectroscopic analysis of the fraction.

The benzene samples were found to contain very low but identifiable concentrations of anthracene, benzanthracene, benzopyrene, pyridine, and other compounds, too low for identification.

ECONOMY, SOURCES AND USES

Production

As already mentioned, benzene is produced chiefly from the coal gas arising from the heating of coal at temperatures of from 1000 to 1300 °F. The coal gas is passed through tar and ammonia scrubbers and oil absorption tanks, with a resultant light oil fraction containing benzene, toluene, xylene, crude coal tar naphtha and heavy solvent naphtha. Crude 'motor benzol', consisting mainly of benzene and toluene, is obtained by scrubbing of coke oven gas (Gerarde, 1960).

Benzene is also produced from petroleum by the catalytic reforming (*i.e.* in the presence of molybdenum, chromium or precious metal oxide supported on alumina) of light naphthas from which it is isolated by distillation or solvent extraction.

Industrial uses

The applications of benzene are manifold and ubiquitous. In 1957 its production in Western Europe and the U.S.A. amounted to 2430 million pounds (U.S. Tariff Commission Report, 1958).

It is used not only as a solvent, a constituent of aviation and motor fuel and a degreasing agent, but also as the starting material for a wide variety of materials in the chemical industry. From this last application it makes its entry into a vast and sometimes unsuspected number of industrial processes. It is concerned in the manufacture of rubber, plastics, paints, lacquers, linoleum, artificial manure, glue and adhesives, rotogravure printing, extraction of oils and fats, floor waxes and polishes, etc. The rubber industry itself includes many aspects where the use of benzene might not at first sight appear prominent, *e.g.* the sealing of cans with rubber cement dissolved in benzene, the manufacture of straw hats, shoes, cameras, cardboard boxes, and even in the watchmaking industry for cleaning the separate parts. (In Sweden, according to Larssen and Thrysen, 1951, there have been many cases of benzene poisoning from this particular application.)

In addition to these processes, where benzene is used mainly as a solvent, there are also the 'closed systems', where it is handled in large quantities, as during its production from coal gas and in the blending of motorfuels.

SUBSTITUTES FOR BENZENE

It is becoming more and more widely realised that the individual susceptibility to a variation of exposure to benzene is so great that merely reducing its content in the working atmosphere is not the complete answer to the problem of reducing the incidence of benzene poisoning.

It is by no means an unusual experience when making blood examinations of a group of workers on an exactly similar benzene process to find a few showing relatively severe disturbance, while others show a normal blood picture. This inequality of reaction has been observed also with regard to the actual content of benzene in the blood. In 1949, Bernard, Braier and co-workers pointed out that some workers handling products with a high benzene content showed a low level of benzene in the blood, while others exposed to low concentrations had a high benzenemia. They attributed this variation to the differing capacity of individuals to eliminate benzene from the blood stream, normally a rapid process due primarily to exhalation of unchanged benzene from the lungs (Gerarde, 1960). Benzene has in fact in some cases of poisoning been detected in the blood several years after cessation of exposure (Fabre, 1946).

It is therefore of great importance to replace benzene wherever possible by a solvent which will be technically acceptable and at the same time, if not entirely innocuous, at least devoid of the specific haemopoietic effect.

Suggested substitutes

Among the solvents suggested as suitable replacements for benzene are toluene, xylene, isopropyl benzene, solvent naphtha, benzine, trichloroethylene, cyclohexane and heptane. None of them has been found completely ideal from either the toxicological or the technical aspect, and it has been emphasized (Fabre *et al.*,

Bibliography on p. 55

1955) that caution must be exercised in extrapolating to man the results of animal experiments on the relative innocuousness of the proposed substitutes; also that recommendation of any of these substitutes does not mean that they are entirely devoid of toxic effects, merely that they are less injurious to the health of workers than benzene itself.

Toluene, xylene and solvent naphtha, though devoid of the specific effect of benzene on the blood forming organs, have the disadvantage that the widely used commercial form contains a significant percentage of benzene.

Isopropyl benzene (Cumene) has been found to cause no significant variation of the blood picture in animals exposed to 500 p.p.m. 8 h a day, for 150 days (Fabre *et al.*, 1955), nor was the femoral marrow cell population diminished in rats given subcutaneous injections of 1 ml/kg body weight daily for two weeks (Gerarde, 1956). Hyperaemia of the lungs, liver and kidneys were, however, observed in Fabre's animals.

Cyclohexane has been chiefly recommended in France, where it is regarded as significantly less toxic than benzene. This view is supported by the experiments on animals of Treon *et al.* (1943) who found no symptoms of ill-effects or tissue damage from repeated exposure to 434 p.p.m., but minor degenerative changes in the liver and kidneys of rabbits exposed to 786 p.p.m.

Heptane. The most recent search for an acceptable substitute by Cirla (1960) had led him to recommend heptane, which in addition to presenting very slight systemic or haematological hazard to workers exposed to it, is also, according to the technologists, an adequate substitute from the point of view of solvent capacity. Earlier investigations on animals by Fuhner (1921) had shown it to be a narcotic in acute exposure (lethal in concentrations of 1.5–2%), but in human beings Baldi and Ricciardi-Polloni (1954) stated that it carried only a slight risk to workers using it and considered 300 p.p.m. as the maximum tolerable concentration. Slight variations of the blood picture were described by Nunziante and Granata in 1955.

In Cirla's investigation of 382 men and 149 women who had used heptane for 1–5 years in a rubber tyre process where the concentrations ranged from 0.75 up to 1000 p.p.m., the principal haematological variation was anaemia, which though slight, was present in fairly high percentage especially of the women; slight leucopenia (not less than 4100 /μl) was present in only 2%, and slight neutropenia in 9% of the men and 12% of the women. Clinical symptoms – headache, fatigue and dyspepsia – and positive liver function tests were also found but were not considered toxicologically significant. It was concluded that heptane does show a slight toxic effect similar to that of benzene, but in comparison it presents very little systemic or haematological hazard.

The 'Maximum Allowable Concentration' or 'Threshold Limit' for repeated exposure to benzene has been reduced from the original 100 p.p.m. postulated in 1939 by American Standards Association, to 35 p.p.m. from 1951 to 1957, to the level of 25 p.p.m. (0.08 mg/l) at the present time.

It has to be remembered that these threshold limit values are not intended as unalterable minimal levels. They are based on "various criteria of toxic effects or on marked discomfort; thus they should not be used as a common denominate of toxicity, nor should they be considered as the sole criterion in proving or disproving diagnoses of suspected occupation diseases" (Threshold Limit Values for 1962).

In Russia the limits proposed (Novikoff, 1957) are approximately 60 p.p.m. for a single exposure and 20 p.p.m. for 24-h level. They base these recommendations on the effects on the conditioned reflex activity of rats subjected to daily inhalations of benzene, and on the olfactory concentration in human beings; this was found to be about 75 p.p.m. for a sensitive person, and the imperceptible concentration about 60 p.p.m. (It may be noted that Gerarde, 1960, gives the olfactory threshold for benzene as 1500 parts per billion).

It may yet be found that a 'benzene effect' may be caused by concentrations even lower than 25 p.p.m. It has not always been possible to evaluate the concentrations in the air of workrooms where relatively slight, though definite signs of haematological disturbance characteristic of exposure to benzene have been detected by routine blood examination. It is always possible, as pointed out by Hamilton-Paterson and Browning (1944) that the general atmospheric concentration of benzene is not an entirely reliable criterion of benzene expousre, since workers may at some time be exposed to localised 'pockets' of high exposure. This was clearly brought out also by Graham (1958) in an investigation of a can-making process which was apparently very adequately enclosed and under good exhaust ventilation. Estimations of the air concentrations showed, however, considerable variation; even when they were generally low they showed 'surges' up to much higher levels. For example, while the general atmosphere away from the tanks showed usually a concentration of 28 to 42 p.p.m., there were surges of 55 p.p.m., and in the pump room during pumping the concentrations varied from 22 to 100 p.p.m.

BIOCHEMISTRY

Estimation

(1) In the atmosphere

The rapid method using formaldehyde and concentrated H_2SO_4, described in Leaflet no. 4 of the Department of Scientific and Industrial Research, (1939)

Bibliography on p. 55

has the disadvantage that the brown-violet reaction is interfered with by all homologues of benzene.

A reaction which is virtually specific for benzene in the presence of toluene, xylene and other homologues was described by Dolin in 1943. In this (the Butanone) method, a nitrating mixture (equal parts of concentrated H_2SO_4, and fuming nitric acid) is used as the absorption fluid. Butanone is added to the ether extract, diluted with ethyl alcohol, and the reading from a colorimeter compared with a calibration curve made by treating 50–500 g of benzene in the same way.

A modification of this method suggested by Zurlo and Metrico (1960) is the use of carbontetrachloride as the absorption fluid instead of the nitrating mixture.

Elkins (1959) describes an ultraviolet spectroscopic method for both benzene and toluene, using silica-gel apparatus with the addition of iso-octane. This method is based on that of Maffet et al. (1956).

(2) In blood and tissues

Several methods of estimating the amount of benzene in blood and tissues have been described, generally on the basis of colorimetric procedures (Yant et al., 1935; Pearce et al., 1936), or on ultraviolet spectroscopy (Mayer, 1938). The latter method has been used by Guertin and Gerarde (1959) for the blood content of benzene in a form modified to obviate the necessity for large samples of blood and of time consumed in two distillations. It depends on extraction of the benzene from the blood with cyclohexane. The blood is first haemolysed with 0.1 N HCl and the lower (aqueous) layer after shaking with cyclohexane removed. The cyclohexane layer is then centrifuged and its ultraviolet absorption spectrum compared with a previously prepared calibration curve.

(3) In urine

Since some of the metabolites of benzene (see p. 11) are excreted in the urine in conjugation with sulphuric acid as ethereal or organic sulphates, it follows that absorption of benzene is associated with an increase of these in proportion of the excretion of inorganic sulphates.

It was suggested by Yant et al. (1936) that determination of the ratio between them might serve as a method of diagnosis of early benzene poisoning. Owing to discrepancies in the results of many investigators of the relation between this proportional excretion and haematological evidence of benzene poisoning, it is now generally agreed that while the test may be accepted as a measure of the amount of exposure to benzene it is not to be regarded as an estimation of toxic effects.

The normal ratio of inorganic/organic urinary sulphates varies, according to several authorities, from 80/20 (Yant et al., 1936; Kammer et al., 1938) to 92.5/7.5 (Teisinger and Fiserova-Bergerova, 1955).

Discrepancies in the ratio in workers exposed to benzene are ascribed to the great individual variation in the absorption, metabolism and elimination of benzene, the proportion of metabolites excreted in conjugation with glucuronic or sulphuric acid, the time of exposure when the samples are taken and analysed (there is a tendency for the ratio to shift to the inorganic side on standing), and the atmospheric concentrations of benzene at the time. (Concentrations of approximately 35 p.p.m. have been stated by Elkins (1954), to lower the inorganic sulphates by about 15%, while Teisinger found 52 p.p.m. necessary to produce this decrease.)

With regard to the correlation with haematological changes, although animals exposed to 800 p.p.m. for one hour daily have been stated (Yant *et al.*, 1936) to show a decrease in inorganic sulphates in advance of these changes, there have been many records of haematological disturbance being present in human beings without significant alteration of the urinary sulphate ratio.

In a series of 17 women, examined by Hamilton-Paterson and Browning in 1944 for example, all the results of the urinary sulphate test were within normal limits, though these women were using a rubber solution and adhesive cements containing 5–20% of benzene, and all showed neutropenia. The lowest ratio recorded was 81/19. This result would appear to indicate that the results of animal experiments in this particular respect cannot be extrapolated to human beings so far as to provide an indication of damage in advance of the blood picture.

Some recent results obtained by Hammond and Herman (1960), however, do indicate how the test can be used as an evaluation of exposure if not necessarily of absorption. They found that in all cases where exposure was indicated by conformation with criteria which they had drawn up (see Table 1) a follow-up revealed that the employees involved had been lax in wearing protective equipment or had worked a double shift.

TABLE 1

Criteria of Significance of Urinary Sulphate Ratio
(after Hammond and Herman, 1960)

Inorganic Sulphate/Total	Exposure	Precautions recommended
80/95%	nil	none
70/80%	mild	vigilance
60/70%	dangerous	exposure controlled
0/60%	very dangerous	personnel removal

(a) *Test for urinary sulphate ratio.* – Tests for the urinary sulphate ratio based on gravimetric methods are described in various text books of physiological chemistry such as Peters and van Slyke (1932); Hawk and Bergeim (1927) or by Fiske (1921), the benzidine method.

The method described by Elkins (1959) using barium chloride and determining the ratio by comparing the weights of $BaSO_4$ in the unheated and heated portions of urine is widely used.

The test, whichever method is used, has certain possibilities of error. The organic sulphate metabolite excretion begins rapidly and stops abruptly, so that the specimen should be collected near the end of the work shift; the ratio changes with ageing, so that it is necessary to carry out the analysis shortly after taking the specimen.

(b) The phenol test. – It has been stated by several authorities that the amount of phenol in the urine is a more reliable evidence of benzene exposure than the urinary sulphate (Forssman and Frykholm, 1947; Walkley *et al.*, 1961; Pagnotto *et al.*, 1961), and of clinical damage. Pagnotto *et al.* regard an excess of 200 mg/l as indicating excessive exposure to benzene, while Timar suggests that values of 300–400 mg of phenol constantly present in a 24 h specimen of urine should be regarded as indicating definite intoxication.

According to Teisinger and Fiserova-Bergerova (1955) the average daily normal excretion of phenol in the urine is 8.2 mg, and they consider levels above 20 mg abnormal. Other estimates of the normal urinary phenol excretion are those of Deichmann and Schafer (1942), 11–42 mg; Porteous and Williams (1949), 5–10 mg; Walkley *et al.* (1961), an average of 30 mg/l. Porteous and Williams emphasize the fact that the result of the phenol test shows the content of phenol in the conjugated form; only traces of free phenol are excreted.

The same individual variabilities of retention, metabolism and elimination apply to the excretion of phenol as to that of organic sulphates, and it is not regarded as a completely accurate assessment of individual exposure, since it is affected by disorders such as intestinal, renal or hepatic disturbance which cause an increase of urinary phenol. It has however the advantage of serving as a collective test, in that the presence in one worker of a daily urinary phenol in excess of the normal suggests that the whole personnel may be working in a benzene concentration near the limit of the maximum allowable concentration.

The method of test described by Theis and Benedict (1924) has been used, with modifications, by Walkley *et al.* (1961), as follows:

The specific gravity of a 24 h sample is adjusted to 1.024. To a 10 ml aliquot is added 4 ml of 1:1 H_2SO_4 and steam distillation is carried out in a suitable apparatus. To a 10 ml aliquot of 100 ml of distillate is added 1 ml of 50% sodium acetate and 1 ml of *p*-nitroaniline reagent (0.75 g *p*-nitroaniline, 5–10 ml of distilled water and 20 ml conc. HCl diluted to 250 ml). After 1 min 2 ml of 20% sodium carbonate is added and the total volume made up to 20 ml. The colour is compared with a phenol standard, and with a 10 ml aliquot the result in micrograms is equivalent to mg/l of urine.

The most recent examinations of the phenol test by Walkley *et al.*, (1961) confirm the opinion of Teisinger and Fiserova-Bergerova that this test is more sensitive and reliable than the urinary sulphate test. Their results were obtained from persons working in the rubber-coating industry where the petroleum naphtha used may contain 1.5–9.3% of benzene by weight and where the average daily atmospheric content of benzene ranged from 5–68 p.p.m., with an occasional maximum of 125 p.p.m.

It was found that exposure to benzene in excess of the present maximum allowable concentration of 25 p.p.m. will be reflected in a urinary phenol concentration of more than 200 mg/l.

In the most recent investigation by Pagnotto et al (1961) the highest phenol excretion (917 mg/l) was found in a man employed as a saturator, i.e. in the process where additional solvent is added to the already prepared rubber stock and solvent mix, and where the atmospheric benzene may reach 125 p.p.m. Following the installation of local ventilation on the saturator and reduction of the benzene content of the naphtha to 3% the benzene exposure was reduced to about 7 p.p.m. and the urinary phenol to less than 70 mg/l. The next highest urinary level of phenol (450 mg/l) was present in a man in the churn room who showed a low haemoglobin and red cell level.

Examples of the correlation of benzene atmospheric concentrations in the various processes with the urinary phenol excretion are given in Table 2.

TABLE 2

Correlation of benzene concentrations and phenol excretion in urine
(after Pagnotto et al. 1961)

	Benzene in air (p.p.m.)	Urinary phenol (mg/l)
*Churn man	0.5–15	0.5–480
Spreaders	0.5–35	0.5–350
Saturators	0.5–125	51–917

*The unexpectedly low benzene-air content of the churn room compared with the high maximum phenol excretion is explained by the fact that some of the activities, including the high speed mixing, are done intermittently.

Metabolism

Great strides have been made in solving the problem of the specificity of the haemopoietic effect of benzene by means of studies of its fate in the organism.

The first step in the elucidation of this fate was taken in 1867 by Schultzen and Naunyn, who discovered that it was converted in the body to phenol. This was followed in 1880 by the detection by Nencki and Giocosa of quinol and catechol in the urine of animals exposed to benzene. The most intensive study of the route of its metabolic transformation and the metabolites produced is that of Professor R. T. Williams and his colleagues during the last ten years, and though

Bibliography on p. 55

Professor Williams (1959) emphasises that "the exact mechanism of the formation of these metabolites still remains to be studied in detail", enough is known to relate their attack on bodily enzymes to their toxic effect on the proliferating cells of the bone marrow.

(1) Absorption

In industrial practice absorption of benzene takes place almost exclusively by inhalation.

(a) Absorption by the skin is possible, and direct contact with the skin by leakage from apparatus, spillage or the practice of cleaning the hands with benzene does present a risk, though relatively remote in practice, of poisoning.

Animal experiments have demonstrated the possibility of this route of absorption. Lazarew et al. (1931) estimated the hydrocarbon content of the air exhaled by tracheotomised rabbits with one foot immersed in benzene and found that the total amount expired in the course of 115 min of immersion was 138 mg. The amount of benzene in the blood of the external jugular vein after immersion of the ear was shown to rise from 50–100 mg/kg of blood during 30 min. A more recent estimation of the capacity of benzene to penetrate the skin is that of Meyer and Kerk (1960), using benzene as a 'carrier' for eserine. A mixture of benzene and 2.5% of eserine was applied to the shaved skin of male mice and the time of appearance of an eserine effect on the jaw muscles was estimated. The initial effect appeared in 31 min with a further 10 min for its maximum, and a speed of absorption of 2.3 μl/ml/h.

(b) Absorption by mouth or by injection in doses of 1 g/kg is followed by exhalation of as much as 55–75% of the dose, most of it during the first twelve hours (Parke and Williams, 1950); very little in the urine unless a very large dose (3 ml) is administered (Drummond and Finar, 1938).

(c) By inhalation benzene is rapidly absorbed into the blood and rapidly eliminated, due primarily to exhalation, though more is retained in the body than when given by mouth or by injection. Of a concentration of 0.34 mg/l for 5 h, 46% is retained, but eventually 12% of this is exhaled again and very small amounts appear in the urine (Williams, 1959).

(2) Distribution in tissues

Because of its lipoid solubility benzene tends to accumulate in body tissues according to their fat content. The concentration of benzene in the fat and bone marrow of exposed animals has been found to be approximately 20 times that in the blood (Schrenk et al., 1941). The fat, acting as a reservoir, loses its benzene slowly; this applies especially to the bone marrow, though the amount of retention varies considerably in individual cases according to the amount of detoxication. Duvoir et al. (1946) reported two cases of fatal benzene poisoning arising 20 and 14 months after cessation of exposure in which at autopsy the bone marrow was found to contain 0.2 g/kg benzene, while in a third case 'of classic type' no benzene was demonstrated. This discrepancy was explained on the basis of the metabolism of benzene – if death occurs before complete oxidation, a toxic reserve will be found in the bone marrow, if detoxication is complete the results will be negative.

(3) Excretion

As already stated, most of the benzene ingested or inhaled is excreted by the lungs, partly as CO_2, and very little as such in the urine; most of the urinary excretion being in the form of its metabolites.

Estimation of the actual amounts of these excretory products has been much facilitated by the use of radioactive technique (Parke and Williams, 1953). The benzene labelled with ^{14}C contained about 100 μC of radioactivity. Following an oral dose to rabbits of 0.34 to 0.5 g/kg, about 45% of the dose was eliminated in the expired air in two days, of which 43% was unchanged benzene and about 1.5% CO_2. In the same time nearly 35% of the benzene was eliminated as metabolites in the urine: these consisted mainly of conjugated phenols, phenol accounting for about 23% of the dose, quinol for 4.8%, catechol 2.2%, hydroxyquinol 0.3%, phenylmercapturic acid 0.5%, and *trans-trans*-muconic acid 1.3%. Thus the respiratory and urinary excretions accounted for nearly 80% of the dose of benzene after two to three days; the remainder appears to remain in the body, to be eliminated slowly.

According to Teisinger *et al.* (1952), the excretion of phenol and catechol is highest in the first 24 h and complete within 48 h of exposure while that of quinol is slower.

The toxic effects of benzene are related to these phenol metabolites. When they are excreted in conjugation with ethereal sulphates or glucuronic acid they are 'detoxicated'. It is when the process of conjugation is inadequate or delayed that some of the phenols are left free to exert their toxic action.

The relation between excess phenol in the urine and the blood and the mitotic activity of the cells of the bone marrow has been studied in experimental animals by Rozera *et al.* (1960). The mitotic activity in the granuloblastic series showed some inhibition of proliferative activity; in the erythroblastic series complete inhibition of the metaphase in 60% of the animals but an increase in the remainder. These changes were most marked in advanced stages of intoxication, although at that time the levels of phenol in the blood and urine were not so high as in the early stages. It was suggested that the mitotic inhibition might be due to direct action of benzene itself which has accumulated in the bone marrow during the last phases of intoxication when oxidation and conjugation have become deficient.

Depletion of sulphydryl groups, brought about by the depletion of organic sulphur but the formation of sulpho-conjugates, is believed by some authorities to

Bibliography on p. 55

play some part in the production of benzene anaemia (Morelli, 1958; Paolino
et al., 1961). This, it is stated, may occur either by promoting haemolysis or by
altering the enzymatic processes which govern the incorporation of the iron of
protoporphyrin and the formation of folic acid. It was in fact shown by Parker
and Kracke in 1936 that the glutathione content of the blood and bone marrow
is reduced during benzene intoxication, and Duvoir and Derobert (1946) believe
that this important factor in the mechanism of cellular oxidation-reduction processes in essentially associated with the toxic action of benzene.

A change in protoporphyrin metabolism in chronic benzene poisoning, similar to that observed in lead poisoning, has recently been demonstrated by Bian-
caccio and Fermariello (1961). They found that rabbits subjected to repeated
inhalation of benzene showed a six-fold increase in the protoporphyrin content of
the erythrocytes and a two and a half times increase in the urinary coluropor-
phyrin.

(4) Enzymatic effects

It is now believed by most authorities that the fundamental toxic effect of
benzene is a disturbance of the enzymes which control the processes by which it
is oxidised in the body, especially peroxidase and catalase.

In 1947, De Franciscis and Marsico stated that both the peroxidase and
catalase activity of erythrocytes increased with the process of intoxication, and in
1959 Gabor found that the blood of rats exposed to varying concentrations of
benzene showed an initial increase of peroxidase followed by a fall, while catalase
showed a decrease from the beginning with temporary rises during recuperation.
This he interpreted as an indication of an initial functional disturbance, probably
a stimulative effect, by the free phenol metabolites on the production of peroxidase, and the ultimate fall as an exhaustion of the possibilities of detoxication and
the appearance of morphological changes.

Some idea of the nature of these morphological changes, particularly in the
reticulo-endothelial system, has been derived from some recent observations by
Wirtschafter and Bischel (1960) using what they call the 'imprint technique'
devised by Wirtschafter and De Meritt (1959). This technique consists in lightly
touching a series of slides with the blood or tissue and staining with Wright's
stain. The results, in rats given a minimal single subcutaneous injection of benzene,
showed an involvement of the reticulo-endothelial system in the form of an initial
increase of cells showing considerable deviation from normal morphology. The
bone marrow was highly cellular, with nucleated erythrocytes, neutrophils and
lymphocytes comprising the major series. Mitotic figures were double the upper
limit of normal 2 h after injection, but fell below the normal range at 16 h. Megakaryocytes were increased but with decreased thrombocyte production, and rare
foreign-body-type giant cells, 30 μ in size and of abnormal morphology, were
present. This reticulo-endothelial response reached a peak at 72 h.

There was also a marked proliferation of reticulo-endothelial cells of abnormal morphology in the lymph nodes, thymus and spleen, but no effect on the peripheral blood or the liver imprints. Cells of the macrophage type in the lymph nodes and thymus gradually diminished, returning to normal at the end of a week, but the remainder of the haemopoietic system was still not normal by that time.

(5) Effect on phosphatase activity

Phosphatase activity has also been stated to be altered. Ambrosio (1942) observed a reduced content of hepatic and renal phosphatase in animals poisoned with benzene, and Biondi (1956) a progressive reduction of alkaline phosphatase in the white corpuscles in subacute poisoning. More recently Rozera (1960) has examined the problem of phosphatase activity in the erythrocytes of rabbits given intramuscular injections of 0.5 ml/kg of a 30% oil emulsion of benzene.

The normal level for blood alkaline phosphatase, expressed in Bodansky units, was 1.90 and for acid phosphatase 11.12 units; for the serum 2.23 and 0.63 units respectively. After some days the blood phosphatases showed a definite diminution; the serum levels showed no variation and the blood phenol content increased. At 30–60 days the serum phosphatase levels had also fallen considerably, while the blood phenols, both total and conjugated, had nearly approached their initial level. This inhibition of phosphatase activity showed itself earlier and lasted longer in the erythrocytes than in the leucocytes, and Rozera and his colleagues suggest that it is due to the products of oxidation of benzene (the phenols) rather than to benzene itself.

TOXICOLOGY

Benzene, like practically all organic solvents, is in high dosage a narcotic, and can cause acute poisoning which may be fatal. It is best known, however, for its specific and characteristic form of chronic poisoning – its highly injurious effect on the haemopoietic system.

Chronic benzene poisoning was added in 1925 to the Schedule of Industrial Diseases of the Factory and Workshops Act of 1901–1920; in the present Schedule it is described as "Poisoning by Benzene or its Homologues or their effects in the process of handling benzene or its homologues or any process of manufacture or involving the use thereof". This is a fortunately wide description, since it includes the homologues of benzene, especially xylene and toluene, which while not, in the pure state, possessing the specific benzene capacity for injury of the bone marrow may, in the commercial form, contain up to 15% of benzene.

Bibliography on p. 55

Toxicity to animals

(1) Acute

In animals, acutely poisoned with benzene, Paterni (1958) and Dotta (1960) have noted that the adrenal cortex showed increased functional activity and that changes in the medulla indicated increased formation of hormone and its rapid release into the blood stream. Dotta also observed a marked and constant eosinopenia. These observations tend to support the view that physical exertion (Hamilton, 1925) and emotional excitement (Feil, 1933 and Dworetsky, 1914) increase the suspectibility to severe poisoning (Lewin, 1907) since the liberation of adrenalin and symphathin in these conditions sensitise the myocardium to the action of benzene (Nahum and Hoff, 1934) and increase the risk of death from ventricular fibrillation.

(2) Chronic

The early experiments of Santesson (1897), while demonstrating the fact that chronic benzene poisoning could follow absorption from the skin, clouded the issue to some extent by the confusion between benzene and benzine.

It was not then realised that the petroleum oil of Baku, where one worker had died with purpuric haemorrhages, haemoptysis and haematemesis, was rich in coal-tar benzene, and Santesson administered both the crude liquid (which he called 'crude liquid benzine') and the pure 'benzol', distilling at 80–85 °C. He found the former the more toxic.

A similar confusion in the substances used for prolonged inhalation by animals is observable in the work of Langlois and Desbouis (1907), whose findings have never been completely confirmed. They defined 'benzol' as a mixture of benzine and toluene, and used concentrations of 16 and 24 ml/m³ of air. In animals they noted a marked polycythaemia, returning to normal in 15 days, but failed to produce a notable leucopenia. The most stable early contribution to the toxicology of benzene was that of Selling (1910, 1916) whose emphasis on the co-existence of stimulation and destruction of the bone marrow has been the foundation stone of much of the present understanding of the varying clinical aspects of chronic benzene poisoning. Most of his experiments were carried out by subcutaneous injection of equal parts of benzene and olive oil, and the most important eventual result was leucopenia, preceded by an outpouring of normal and abnormal leucocytes. When death occurred the bone marrow was usually aplastic, but Selling believed that regeneration could occur after an advanced degree of aplasia. The leucotoxic action of benzene thus demonstrated by Selling became a stimulus to the therapeutic use of benzene in cases of leukaemia.

Further animal investigations, by inhalation, ingestion and subcutaneous injection were carried out by Secchi in 1914 and Brandino in 1922, the latter emphasising the initial stimulatory effect followed by depression and later by regenerative hyperplasia.

SYMPTOMS OF INTOXICATION

(1) Blood

(a) Erythropoiesis. – While Selling found a fall in the red cell count much less marked than that of the white cells, and others, such as Secchi (1914), Fontana (1921) and Mauro (1925) noted anaemia in experimental chronic benzene poisoning, Orzechowsli (1929) insisted that benzene does not attack the erythropoietic system and indeed postulated a polyglobulia, as also did Langlois and Desbouis (1907) and Beyer (1933). On the whole however anaemia appears to be the most frequent phenomenon in animals (Latta and Davies, 1941; Caldwell *et al.*, 1945).

The haemoglobin level is usually decreased (Secchi, 1914; Fontana, 1921; Mauro, 1925; Engelhardt, 1931) but less in proportion to the fall in number of erythrocytes, so that the anaemia tends to be hyperchromic (Caldwell *et al.*, 1945).

Reticulocytosis, suggesting bone marrow hyperactivity, has been recorded by some observers (Paul *et al.*, 1927; Robinson and Climenko, 1941).

(b) Thrombocytopenia. – The effect on the platelet count was likened by Duke in 1913 to that on the red cell count: he found that an initial rapid rise was followed by an equally rapid fall accompanied by severe anaemia, and Caldwell *et al.* (1945) observed in their animals a reduction to one-half the original value.

Truhaut *et al.* (1959) attribute these discrepancies in the effects on the erythropoietic system to the diversity of experimental conditions and individual susceptibility of the experimental animals. They themselves have investigated the erythropoietic modifications by the technique of radioactive iron given intravenously and have confirmed in animals the variability of effect observed also in human beings.

The animals were exposed to inhalation of benzene concentrations of 6 mg/l for 8 h a day, 6 days a week for 30–125 days. The radioactive iron ^{59}Fe, with an activity of approximately 1 mC per mg was given by intravenous injection in autologous plasma. The animal was killed 40 min after injection and the decrease of radioactivity in the plasma and the amount of ^{59}Fe taken up by the red corpuscles were estimated by means of a scintillation counter. The validity of the method rests essentially on the hypothesis that the radioactive iron represents the actual fate of the pre-existing endogenous iron.

The results showed that in some animals acceleration or retardation of haemoglobin synthesis and erythropoiesis indicated a hyperplasia or hypoplasia of the bone marrow – an observation which was confirmed by later histological examination. In other animals there was acceleration of iron metabolism while its incorporation in the red corpuscles remained normal, suggesting a pathological aspect of erythropoietic tissue – a defect leading to the formation of imperfect erythrocytes and a corresponding 'ineffective' haemoglobin, which is destroyed at the same time as the cells by which it is transported. That is to say, the bone marrow of animals poisoned by benzene may produce abnormal erythroblasts which are

Bibliography on p. 55

either destroyed immediately or in their turn give rise to abnormal erythrocytes which also undergo rapid destruction.

The contrast in the initial stages of benzene poisoning between the well-defined peripheral decrease in erythrocytes and the over-active bone marrow has also been attributed to an inhibitory action of the toxic substance on the process of maturation and the entry of immature red blood cells into the circulation (Villani *et al.*, 1960).

They also used ^{59}Fe to assess the time of disappearance of iron from the plasma, the amount of iron used for the synthesis of haemoglobin and the time of entry of erythrocytes into the circulation. They found no significant variation between the animal given benzene intramuscularly (1.2 ml/kg daily) and the controls with respect to the time of disappearance of iron from the plasma or that of entry of erythrocytes into the circulation, but did observe a definite reduction of the coefficient of utilisation of iron in the benzene-treated animals. They suggest that benzene inhibits the utilisation of iron by the erythroblasts of the bone marrow but does not affect the uptake by the reticular cells; these are present in normal or even slightly increased numbers in benzene poisoning; they represent the daily renewal of circulating erythrocytes and are capable of transporting the iron of the 'basophilic' erythroblasts.

(c) *Leucopoiesis.* – A final fall in total leucocytes, preceded by an initial rise, has been by far the most frequent phenomenon observed in animals. The finding by Duke (1913) of an initial rise from 6600–11,000, followed by a fall to 1000 before death in one animal was confirmed by the experiments of Caldwell *et al.* (1945). They found a primary rise of 200–5000 during the first few days of administration, followed by a cyclic fluctuation in periods of 2–4 days, the peaks becoming progressively lower until total counts of 2500 or less persisted. An example of these unpredictable fluctuations of the leucopoiesis of animals receiving doses of benzene which were eventually fatal has also been given by Woronow (1929).

Lymphocytes were also, in the experiments of Simonds and Jones (1915) and Silberberg (1928) affected, though not so severely as the leucocytes. Caldwell *et al.* (1945) found an initial rise to be followed, like the total white count, by a cyclic fluctuation. The relative percentage was increased after each rise, so that over a period of 10 days 80% of the animals developed granulocytopenia. Some of the lymphocytes were larger than normal and showed a bluish cytoplasm with azure granules.

(2) Effect on formation of antigens

Animal experiments have demonstrated that severe leucopenia is accompanied by an absence of antibacterial bodies and therefore with an increased susceptibility to infection. Simonds and Jones (1915) found a high death rate in animals given benzene subcutaneously; they succumbed readily to spontaneous infections and both agglutinins and opsonins were decreased.

Further light was shed by Hektoen (1916) on this association between benzene poisoning and lowering of resistance to infection by his finding of a marked reduction in the production of specific precipitin and lysin. He concluded that benzene may lower the resistance to infection in at least three ways – reduction of antibodies; reduction of number of leucocytes; reduction of the phagocytic action of these.

These conclusions were reinforced by studies on experimental pneumonia (Winternitz and Hirschfelder, 1913), tuberculosis (White and Gammon, 1914), and chemical inflammation (Camp and Baumgartner, 1915) in animals.

(3) Bone marrow

The bone marrow of animals poisoned by benzene reflects the diversity of findings in the peripheral blood. Selling (1916) had laid the foundations of modern recognition of the benzene-poisoned marrow as not only aplasic, though this is the predominant condition, but also showing a co-existing hyperplasia. Selling had noted that regeneration began after 3–4 days with the formation of groups and islands of cells, chiefly large lymphocytes, granulocytes or erythroblasts, and that in any given island, after cellular differentiation had once begun, the type of cell remained constant. These reparative changes have been described by many subsequent investigators, though they have not always agreed as to the kind of cell predominantly affected either by aplasia or hyperplasia; this disagreement may be partly due to the variation in the administration of benzene. Heitzmann (1931) and Schillowa (1933) for example, used subcutaneous injection and both found the characteristic result to be hyperplasia, but in Heitzmann's animals the leucocytic elements were particularly affected, in Schillowa's pseudo-eosinophils, megakaryocytes and erythroblasts. Pappenheim (1914), on the other hand, using high subcutaneous dosage, found the bone marrow almost devoid of cells, with only a few small lymphocytes and polyblasts visible, and Silberberg (1928) observed, in addition to atrophy with disappearance of myeloid cells, areas of hyperaemia.

It can only be said, in agreement with the remarks of Truhaut *et al.* (1959) (see p. 17) applied to the discrepancies in the effects of chronic benzene poisoning on the erythropoietic system of animals, that the varying aspects of the bone marrow are due mainly to varying experimental conditions. It is nevertheless indubitably established that the most frequently observed condition of aplasia of the bone marrow can co-exist with areas of hyperplasia.

CHANGES IN THE ORGANISM

(1) The spleen

Atrophy of the Malpighian corpuscles with deposition of pigment in the connective tissue have been the most frequently recorded changes in the spleen, but hyperplasia has also been observed. Myeloid metaplasia has been observed and

Bibliography on p. 55

regarded as a regenerative phenomenon by some authorities (Selling, 1916; Brandino, 1922) but was not present in the more acute forms of poisoning (Ferguson et al., 1933). A similar difference of opinion has existed with regard to the deposition of pigment and parenchymatous injury. Neumann (1915) noted marked hyperaemia and pigment deposition as also did Engelhardt (1931), while Ferguson et al. (1933) in their more acutely poisoned animals found no evidence of haemosiderin deposition in the spleen. Silberberg (1928) found congestion, with only slight damage of lymphoid tissue, and Lignac (1932) an increase of lymphoid tissue with a decrease of myeloid tissue, while Veit (1921) observed no parenchymatous injury.

Marked hyperplasia of the reticulo-endothelial elements was reported by Schillowa in 1933, in animals undergoing injections of benzene.

(2) The Liver

While some of the earlier authorities recorded lesions of the parenchyma in the form of hepatitis, fatty infiltration and even necrosis (Selling 1916; Pappenheim, 1914), others, including Monckeberg (1913), Neumann (1915), Veit (1921) and Silberberg (1928), denied these findings.

More recent investigators (Granati et al., 1958; Rozera et al., 1960) have come to the conclusion that though there is evidence of disturbance of liver function this is not accompanied by histological changes. Rozera et al. (1960), examining the hepatic function of rabbits at various stages of administration of benzene by intramuscular injection (1 ml/kg of a 30% solution in oil) found that disturbance of function, as estimated by the bromosulphthalein, Takata-Ara and Bufano (estimation of amino acids in the blood) tests, began only when the myelotoxic action of benzene was manifest in well-marked blood changes. They suggest that such changes are secondary to the haematological disturbance, and possibly also to the strain imposed on the liver by the oxidation processes of which its detoxicating capacity is a function.

(3) The Kidneys

These have usually been reported as escaping severe injury: only one group of investigators (McCord et al., 1932) state that nephritis, with the convoluted tubule as the special point of attack, is an outstanding characteristic, while Pappenheim (1914) also reported some injury. Batchelor (1927) observed cloudy swelling and casts only when the concentration inhaled reached 440 and 815 p.p.m.

(4) The endocrine glands

A series of investigations of the effect of repeated subcutaneous injection of benzene on the various endocrine glands of the rat has been carried out by Iannacone and Cachella from 1957 onwards and summarised by them in 1959. The dosage given was 1 ml/kg of a solution containing equal parts of benzene and olive oil, each day for 22 days.

(a) Anterior pituitary. – Changes in the cells believed to secrete some of the pituitary hormones, including ACTH, suggested an increased secretion and discharge of these hormones in the benzene-treated rats.

(b) Thyroid. – Changes in the follicular cells suggested an increased secretory thyroid activity.

(c) Parathyroid. – Changes were not significant.

(d) Thymus. – Changes suggested only a mild involutive process.

(e) Pancreas. – Changes in the form of very slight modifications of the cells of the islands of Langerhans suggested a somewhat increased functional activity.

(f) Adrenals. – The cortex showed increased functional activity but no degenerative change; changes in the medulla indicated increased formation of hormone and its rapid release into the blood stream.

Other investigators have also indicated that the adrenals are implicated in chronic benzene poisoning in animals. Paterni (1958) noted a three-fold increase in weight, a marked deposit of fat and an increase in cholesterol and ascorbic acid, both diminishing rapidly before death. Dotta (1960) has observed a marked and constant eosinopenia, a feature which was also prominent in rats which had had the adrenals removed before being given benzene.

(g) Testes. – The main effect was a retardation and depression of maturation of the germinal epithelium.

The intestinal mucosa was also examined for possible evidence of a direct antimitotic effect of benzene or its metabolite but no significant variation in mitotic acitivity was found.

Toxicity to human beings

(1) Acute

The severity of the symptoms of acute benzene poisoning and their possibly fatal outcome depend mainly on the amount and duration of exposure, though it is apparent from records of fatal cases that there is a marked variation in individual susceptiblility.

The lethal and toxic concentrations for human beings postulated by Flury and Zernik (1931) were as follows:

Lethal if inhaled for 5–10 min	20,000 p.p.m.	(64 mg/l)
½–1 h	7,500 p.p.m.	(24 mg/l)
Can be tolerated for ½–1 h	3,000 p.p.m.	(10 mg/l)

Bibliography on p. 55

(a) Fatal cases recorded have practically all occurred when benzene was inhaled in closed spaces such as tanks containing residues of benzene. Between 1941 and 1959 in Great Britain 13 fatal cases were reported to the Chief Inspector of Factories. The symptoms are those of unconsciousness preceded by convulsive movements and paralysis.

(b) Severe but non-fatal cases show similar symptoms but survive after a period of unconsiousness.

(c) Milder forms exhibit at first a state of euphoria followed by giddiness, headache, nausea and staggering gait and, if not removed from exposure, unconsciousness.

(d) Atypical forms have also been described (Feil, 1933; Harrington, 1917) in which a state of violent excitement and delirium precedes unconsciousness.

(e) Individual susceptibility, as shown by the fact that in some cases the rescuers of workmen lying unconscious in tanks have died while the original victims have survived, has been related by some authorities to an implication of the adrenals in benzene poisoning.

AUTOPSY FINDINGS

In 1906 Kobert classified benzene under the heading "Poisons which can kill without causing severe anatomical changes", and many of the earlier investigators who made *post-mortem* examinations in cases of acute fatal benzene poisoning emphasized chiefly the presence of petechial haemorrhages and abnormal fluidity of the blood.

A very detailed examination of a case in which death followed the cleaning with benzene of a cylinder containing residues of asphalt was made 20 h after death by Koppenhöfer (1935). His findings were:

(1) Petechial haemorrhages
In the brain, pleura, gastro-intestinal mucous membranes, kidneys, ureters and bladder. These confirmed similar observations made earlier by Sury-Bienz (1888) and Beinhauer (1896), while minute haemorrhages in the pancreas, brain, pericardium, lungs, subcutaneous fatty tissue and serious membranes had also been noted by Buchmann (1911), Heffter (1915), Binder (1921), Ziel (1925) and Floret (1926.)

(2) Fluidity of the blood
A dark or cherry red colour of the blood had been noted by many of the earlier authorities, including Heffter (1926) who remarked that though the blood remained for a long time after death there was no evidence of haemolysis. No methaemoglobin was found in a sample of blood tested by Martland (cited by Hamilton, 1931) but Koppenhöfer (1935), as well as Carter (1928), noted that oxyhaemoglobin was present.

(3) Hyperaemia or cyanosis of internal organs

Hyperaemia of all the internal organs and a fluid exudate in the liver and lungs were observed by Koppenhöfer; Floret (1926) and Ziel (1925) had described the condition as "all the organs being full of blood".

Cyanosis of the liver, spleen, kidneys and brain were described by Martland.

(4) Respiratory changes

In Koppenhöfer's case there was marked hyperaemia of the lungs with swelling and oedema of the alveolar epithelium. Oedema and interstitial emphysema, with redness and irritation of the bronchi and 'bloody mucus' in the air passages had been the chief findings in earlier investigations. In one case reported to the Home Office in 1925, in which exposure had included also traces of pyridine (0.5%) the lungs showed cyanosis and recent adhesions.

(5) Benzene in the tissues and internal organs

Detection by odour of benzene in the tissues and organs after death has been varyingly recorded. Martland, for example, noted a distinct odour from the lungs in one case but not in another, although autopsy was performed in the latter while the body was still warm. In the Home Office case (1925) on the other hand, the odour of benzene was perceptible from the trachea, larynx and liver. Koppenhöfer noted a strong characteristic aromatic odour from the body cavity and sectioned muscles, and distinctly from the brain and spinal cord.

He was also able to estimate the actual amount of benzene in the various organs and tissues, and although it had previously been assumed (Heffter, 1915; 1915; Joachimoglu, 1915) that owing to its affinity for lipoid tissue the greatest amount would be found in the brain and spinal cord, Koppenhöfer found the greatest amount in the blood – 14 mg per 100 g as compared with 7.5 mg in the brain and 12.6 in the spinal cord. He calculated that the whole blood in the body of this man weighing 72 kg would contain approximately 1 ml of benzene.

(6) In the urine

It has already been noted that in benzene absorption very little benzene as such is present in the urine, but that conjugated ethereal sulphates and phenol derivatives are increased. In acute fatal poisoning increased 'phenol bodies' (phenyl sulphuric acid in the case described by Heffter, 1915), have been noted by some early authorities (Beisele, 1912; Simonin, 1934) but, as Heffter observes, conjugation being slow in rapidly fatal cases, phenol derivatives are not likely to appear during acute intoxication.

AFTER-EFFECTS OF ACUTE BENZENE POISONING

The immediate after-effects of acute poisoning are not as a rule serious – only temporary symptoms of pain in the head, shortness of breath, giddiness and some

Bibliography on p. 55

digestive disturbance. One case was recorded in the Report of the Chief Inspector of Factories for 1918 in which relapse into unconsciousness and final coma occurred two nights after returning to work. Later sequelae and manifestations were recorded with some frequency in early publications, such as:

(a) Dizziness and uncertain gait lasting about 12 days (Genhard, 1910; Wyss, 1910);

(b) Respiratory catarrh and pleurisy (Kobert, 1906; Schaefer, 1909);

(c) Nervous disorders – exhaustion (Lewin, 1907); depression, insomnia, bad dreams (Wyss, 1910);

(d) Skin changes – yellowish pallor (Lewin, 1907); eruption on the back (Genhard, 1910);

(e) Cardiac distress lasting 4 weeks after recovery (Lewin, 1907; Cronin, 1924);

(f) Hepatorenal injury. Accidental ingestion of benzene appears to produce, in addition to narcosis, symptoms relating to a hepatorenal syndrome. In a case cited by Derot and Philbert (1956) due to ingestion of benzene, the hepatic and renal lesions were relatively slight, but elevation of the blood urea and slight modifications of hepatic function were observed. Coma lasted for 9 h after ingestion and leucocytosis and polyglobulia were present. In Derot's case the predominant initial symptoms were severe abdominal pain and vomiting with icterus and oliguria, bile salts and pigments and a few red corpuscles in the urine, slight albuminuria and a raised blood urea. Recovery was marked by intense polyuria, and two days later, following treatment with vitamins, methionine and intravenous glucose, the blood picture was normal.

It is stated by Elkins (1959), however, that serious after-effects are less probable with benzene than with most of the organic halogen compounds.

TREATMENT OF ACUTE BENZENE POISONING

Immediate removal from the contaminated atmosphere is essential. If breathing has ceased, artificial respiration is indicated, followed on resumption of breathing by the administration of oxygen.

In one case of accidental ingestion of benzene, successful treatment was reported by the administration by injection of 5 ml of a lecithin-oil emulsion (Nick, 1922). It was not decided whether the favourable effect of the lecithin was due to direct affinity of the ingested benzene for the lipoid or whether the lecithin had actually formed a combination with the benzene circulating in the blood.

(2) Chronic

The outstanding characteristic of chronic benzene poisoning is disturbance of the blood picture, which is often in its initial stages entirely disassociated from any complaint of ill-health which might arouse suspicion. It is for this reason that routine blood examinations are especially valuable in detecting signs of abosorption which, though not necessarily indicative of true poisoning, might be followed by severe injury to the bone marrow if exposure is continued.

Air estimations, urinary sulphate ratio and phenol tests are all valuable in assessing and controlling the amount of exposure, and clinical examinations may reveal mild symptoms, mainly subjective, but the one criterion which should lead to removal from exposure is a deterioration in the blood picture from that shown by a pre-employment examination.

INCIDENCE

The incidence of chronic benzene poisoning has declined substantially during recent years. There are several reasons for this fortunate decrease:

(1) It has been replaced to some extent by less toxic substitutes.

(2) The industrial public and Industrial Medical Officers have become more cognisant of its potential capacity for severe injury, and are more ready to take measures to detect early signs of poisoning by periodic clinical and blood examinations.

(3) Engineering devices have become more efficient in preventing the fume from reaching the worker.

(4) Working conditions generally, with shorter working hours, adequate holidays and a more adequate diet have improved the general health, especially of women and young persons, so that their haemopoietic system is less prone to anaemia from other causes and less liable to the instability which invites attack from a haemopoietic poison such as benzene.

In 1926 Greenburg recorded that between 1922 and 1924 there were 15 fatalities and 83 cases of illness due to benzene, and that this was probably an understatement.

In Great Britain, where chronic benzene poisoning is compulsorily notifiable to the Factory Department of the Ministry of Labour, the definition of such notifiable poisoning excludes cases where blood deviations are not associated with haemorrhages under the skin or bleeding from mucous membranes. Blood disturbances not accompanied by these features are notified under the term 'Toxic Anaemia', and there is no doubt that some of these cases have been due to benzene exposure.

In 1942, for example, 7 cases of toxic anaemia were notified, most of which were associated with the use of mixtures of solvents for rubber, which contained only a low proportion of benzene, one with aeroplane dope containing less than 15%; they all showed a blood picture characteristic of a benzene effect, but since the abnormality was mild and transient they were not classified as true benzene poisoning. One of the rubber solvent workers, however, eventually died of aplastic anaemia.

Bibliography on p. 55

Similarly in 1943, blood examinations of 193 workers at 24 factories using benzene showed 11 with fairly severe deviations from the normal and 13 with slighter findings of dyshaemopoietic anaemia; none of these were classified as 'chronic benzene poisoning'.

The number of fatal cases notified as chronic benzene poisoning during the last 18 years has been only 6, but 5 more were originally notified as toxic anaemia.

In Japan, Hirokawa (1960) reports that while there are no exact statistics of the incidence of chronic benzene poisoning, 50% or more of workers in small factories using benzene show alterations of the blood picture and that several cases of aplastic anaemia have been recorded.

In spite of the reduced incidence of recent years, cases of severe poisoning do still arise. In 1959 Elkins stated that 140 fatal cases have been recorded in the literature and no doubt others may have occurred which have not been reported.

Factors in the incidence

(1) Individual susceptibility

Apart from the widely held belief that women are more susceptible than men to chronic benzene poisoning, there is no doubt that both men and women vary markedly in their response to similar conditions of exposure. One instance of this, from personal observation, was a fatal case reported to the Factory Department in 1954. This was a young man aged 21, using benzene for laboratory tests, who eventually died of aplastic anaemia. His only exposure was due to the fact that on finishing his tests he poured the remaining benzene down the adjoining sink. About 12 other technicians were employed in the same laboratory, and on the development of recognisable symptoms of ill-health of their colleague (sudden weakness and collapse) all underwent blood examinations which revealed no abnormality.

This is by no means an isolated example of the apparently selective action of benzene. In 1955 Rejsek and Rejskova found that of 4538 persons working with benzene only 10 showed severe blood disorder; Pardon and Foerster (1959), examining 100 persons in a paint works in which the solvents were 'the higher homologues of benzene', found that only in 8 among 90 who showed deviations from the normal blood picture could these be attributed to their exposure; the remainder were suffering from clinical disorders which would account for the abnormalities observed. The cause of this variation in susceptibility is not completely understood, but the most probable explanation lies in innate differences in the potency of different individuals to carry out the metabolic detoxication of benzene.

A possible family susceptibility was suggested by Reifschneider in 1922. He recorded three cases in one family, two of them fatal.

(2) Age

The view that young persons, especially girls, are specially susceptible to benzene poisoning was held by many of the earlier observers, but appears to be less firmly held at present. Nevertheless, Hogan and Shrader (1923) recorded two cases in girls of 17 and 15 years respectively, who had had only short exposure before developing symptoms which included haemorrhage and marked anaemia – 6 weeks in one case and only 3 days in the other. The National Safety Council in 1926 thought that youth was a predisposing factor, but an enquiry by the New York State Department of Labor in 1927 found no evidence of this; in fact the youngest group examined showed a lower percentage of cases of poisoning than the oldest.

The only case of chronic benzene poisoning occurring in infancy is that recorded by Saita and Perini (1958). This child, aged 2, had been exposed to benzene through the home occupation of her mother, who used a glue dissolved in benzene for affixing feathers; an open bowl of benzene was placed on the table. The child was admitted to hospital with fever and severe anaemia; three months after her discharge she developed septic infection, and sternal puncture showed almost complete aplasia. She died a month later.

(3) Sex

The widespread belief that women are more susceptible than men has recently received some support from the observations of Hirokawa (1955, 1960). Among 20 men and 19 women employed in spraying wagons with a paint dissolved in 'a mixture of xylene and aliphatic hydrocarbons' which was stated to contain some benzene, a progressive diminution of red and white cells was more marked in the women than in the men and recovery on removal from exposure was longer delayed. Further support for this increased susceptibility in women was suggested by animal experiments.

Male rabbits injected daily with 0.2 ml of benzene dissolved in oil showed no significant diminution of red or white cells; both were significantly decreased in the females and castrated males. Examination of the metabolism of benzene in the liver of rats suggested that the capacity of oxidation of benzene, dependent on catalase and co-enzyme A, in the female was about half that of the male.

(4) Pregnancy and abortion

Cases in which pregnancy appears to act as a 'trigger' have been reported, notably two recent ones described by Lachnit and Reimer (1959).

One of the women in question, employed in the rubber industry, for 10 years, had a normal blood picture on relinquishing her employment on marriage. Two years later when pregnant she showed profound anaemia, leucopenia and thrombocytopenia and the bone marrow a typical 'panmyelophthisia'; transfusions and antibiotics failed to prevent a fatal outcome.

Bibliography on p. 55

The second, employed one year, using an adhesive containing commercial toluene and xylene, developed a fatal aplastic anaemia after the birth of a healthy child.

Abortion appeared to be the precipitating factor in a case recorded by Saita and Perini (1958), the mother of the child referred to above (p. 27). This woman, $3\frac{1}{2}$ years after the death of the child had an abortion which was followed by severe anaemia and thrombocytopenia and was finally discharged from hospital in a moribund condition.

(5) Infections

In some of the cases reported to the Chief Inspector of Factories a history of infection preceding the onset of symptoms has been given. It is the author's personal opinion, based on the examination of some such cases, that the damage inflicted on the bone marrow of persons exposed to benzene, though not at the time suffering from obvious chronic benzene poisoning, may produce a condition of inability to resist any further demand, such as that of infection – in fact a condition of 'overt failure'.

(6) Anaemia

That a pre-existing anaemia can induce a susceptibility to chronic benzene poisoning is emphasised by Saita and Moreo (1959) with regard to the variety of anaemia known as thalassemia. They described three cases of chronic benzene poisoning in men who were found on investigation to carry the traits of thalassemia. The anaemia was not typical of either benzene anaemia or thalassemia but presented features of both, but the fact there was a persistent leucopenia and neutropenia, together with hypochromia, macrocytosis, presence of target and stippled cells and changes in haemoglobin characteristic of thalassemia, led to the conclusion that certain blood disorders compatible with apparently good health may favour the onset of severe blood disturbance following occupational exposure to benzene.

(7) Other conditions of ill-health

Among the predisposing factors suggested in the Report of the National Safety Council's study of Benzol Poisoning in 1926 (surveyed by Winslow, 1927) were general lowering of vitality, respiratory diseases, especially tuberculosis, alcoholism, heart disease, nervous disorders, nephritis and obesity.

SYMPTOMS OF INTOXICATION

It must be emphasised again that the absence in the early stages of chronic benzene of recognisable symptoms which would lead to its diagnosis is one of its most unfortunate features. It is frequently not until the damage to the bone marrow is well advanced and the abnormality of the blood picture unmistakeable that complaints of ill-health arouse suspicion. Nevertheless there are certain symptoms which, even if mainly subjective, especially if they occur in a number of benzene workers, indicate the advisability of a careful blood examination of all of them.

(1) The skin

Owing to the fat-solvent action of benzene on the superficial layers of the skin, dryness, folliculitis, irritation and dermatitis of an exzematous nature have been frequently described (Landé and Kalinowski, 1928; Oppenheim, 1930; Engelhardt, 1931).The lesions in the case described by Gadrat et al. (see below) were small rounded nodules, painful on pressure and surrounded by a reddish 'halo', with no specific histocytologic features. This same case later developed a severe staphylococcic infection of the arm, with lymphangitis and enlarged axillary glands.

Purpuric spots on the arms, legs, body and sometimes on the mucous membrane of the mouth may be an early manifestation of chronic benzene poisoning, as in the classical cases described by Selling in 1910.

In other cases purpura may not appear until the bone marrow shows almost complete aplasia. Such was the case of a young woman employed on a rubber process, described by Flandin and Roberti in 1922; she died within three weeks of the onset of purpura.

(2) Digestive disturbances

Nausea, a burning sensation in the epigastrium, sometimes vomiting, are usually regarded as purely subjective, but in a case described by Gadrat et al. (1959), X-ray examination of the stomach and gastroscopy revealed the presence of gastritis and marked hyperacidity.

(3) Undue fatigue

Undue fatigue, that is to say, a degree of fatigue greater than would be expected from the conditions and hours of work. Questioning may elicit the fact, especially in women, that though they are so tired during the day that they could almost fall asleep at work they do not sleep well at night.

(4) Change in weight

According to Mallory et al. (1939) a tendency to overweight is more common than loss of weight. In the author's experience no definite change of weight has been observed.

(5) The blood

In spite of the great diversity in the abnormal blood picture in chronic benzene poisoning, the most frequently observed type still corresponds to the 'hypoplasic' variety first described by Selling (1910).

Selling laid the foundation of the conception that benzene is a poison acting

Bibliography on p. 55

selectively upon the leucocytes in the bone marrow, emphasising this action so strongly that two years later Von Koranyi introduced benzene as a therapeutic agent for leukaemia. The gradual realisation that, though benzene certainly reduced the leucocyte count, it could later have disastrous results finally led to its abandonment for this purpose. Nevertheless it is true that leucopenia is not invariably the most prominent abnormality, nor is a tendency to aplastic anaemia an invariable manifestation. The idea, firmly held until about 1927, that a total white cell and differential count, with a history of exposure, suffice to make the definite diagnosis of benzene chronic poisoning is no longer valid. The haematological picture is now known to be much more varied and complex and leucopenia alone is not an infallible diagnostic sign, especially in the early stages where there may even be a leucocytosis.

Macrocytosis has been believed by some authorities to be a valuable sign in the early diagnosis of chronic benzene poisoning, but a recent investigation by Kuhbeck and Lachnit (1962) has led them to conclude that it is not an infallible sign. They used as their criterion haematocrit estimations in a group of workers in the rubber industry, but found that the levels did not vary consistently from those of a non-exposed group, nor did they show correlation with the duration of exposure.

Leucopenia alone as the only manifestation of a dyshaemopoietic effect has been described in one unusual case of benzene exposure (Gadrat *et al.*, 1959). In this case the total white cell count fell at one time to 600/μl, and of these 40% were eosinophils. There was no anaemia. In spite of transfusion, vitamin B6 and nuclear extracts, the blood picture 4 years after his first examination was that of leucopenia of about the same level but still without anaemia.

CHANGES IN THE ORGANISM

(1) The circulatory system

An increase in capillary fragility, as estimated by the appearance of one or more petechiae on the forearm under a pressure midway between systolic and diastolic, maintained by an arm cuff for 5 min, has been stated to occur in 66% of cases exposed to benzene in the photogravure industry (Mallory *et al.* 1939). Of these 79% showed evidence of haematological injury. Litzner (1932) stated that this phenomenon, accompanied by a lengthening of the time of bleeding and a normal coagulation time, is evidence of capillary injury.

(6) Effect on the Liver

(a) *Liver insufficiency.* – Signs have been reported in some cases of chronic benzene poisoning though clinically these are seldom perceptible. Most authorities consider that the liver disorders are not a primary toxic effect of benzene but a secondary and variable effect of factors relating to the severity of the poisoning, the anaemia or a terminal infection. Roche and Bruel (1950) for example observed a great predominance of digestive disturbance in 30 men exposed to benzene in the use of paints and varnishes. The chief symptoms were gastric pain, a sensation of weight and swelling of the abdomen, flatulence, dyspepsia, and in some cases symptoms resembling those of peptic ulcer, though no ulcers were revealed by X-ray examination. Vomiting was rare but diarrhoea fairly frequent. There was some pain on pressure over the liver in 6 cases, but clinical examination was otherwise negative and the blood picture was practically normal. It was concluded that the symptoms were due to a neuro-vegetative disturbance of the liver.

(b) *Enlargement of the liver* was an unusual feature in a fatal case described by Savy *et al.* (1948) but there was no jaundice and again no clinical signs of hepatic insufficiency, unless the terminal coma could be interpreted as hepatic in origin.

(c) *Jaundice*, when it appears, is usually regarded as being haemolytic in origin, but Loeper (1941) believes that true hepatic jaundice may exist. He records an example of this variety in a man aged 41, exposed to benzene and somewhat anaemic, who had marked yellow discoloration of the skin for 20 days. Loeper was not certain, however, that the liver disorder was in fact due to benzene. He remarks that at autopsy the liver is usually pale and moderately fatty in chronic benzene poisoning, but that this is so in many cases of anaemia.

(d) *Fatty infiltration and degeneration* have been postulated, especially by French authorities, in some cases of severe poisoning.

Such a case was described by Rachet *et al.* (1944), and Loeper insists that fatty hepatitis can be a consequence of benzene intoxication; he describes one case with a blood picture of severe anaemia and leucopenia but no icterus or ascites, where autopsy revealed a liver with severe fatty infiltration, the proportion of fat to dried liver tissue being 11.7%.

(e) *Sclerosis or cirrhosis* of the liver has also been stated to be an occasional accompaniment of severe chronic benzene intoxication (Bousser *et al.*, 1952; Loeper, 1941). Loeper quotes a case from the earlier literature in support of this view. This man had worked on a vulcanising process for 12 years and finally died of cirrhosis of the liver; all other causes, including alcoholism, had apparently been excluded.

Loeper himself also describes two cases of cirrhosis, one, a painter and varnisher, with fatty degeneration, the other, a woman employed 14 years in a dyeing and cleaning establishment, with severe anaemia and slight leucopenia. Both suffered from ascites.

(f) *Centrilobular necrosis* has also been described by Mallory *et al.* (1939) and by Paterni (1953).

Bibliography on p. 55

Benzene in petrol

It is not always realised that petrol containing benzene may present a characteristic benzene hazard. As early as 1928 it was stated by Askey that though the percentage of benzene in the mixed gasoline of West California was never constant, it was always present and might be as high as 17 to 20%. He reported a case of aplastic anaemia in a man employed in washing metal plates with gasoline.

Fabre (1960) has also drawn attention to the presence of benzene in certain petrols in variable concentration and has remarked that its depressive action on the leucocytes is preceded by a short phase of leucocytosis due to the initial transitory excitation of the haemopoietic organs. He notes that the first phase of intoxication in animals is produced by 22 mg/l of benzene as compared with 40 mg/l of light petrol

On the other hand, Buffet and Tara (1960) find that though a well-known petrol mixture some years ago contained 15% of benzene, various kinds of petrol now investigated by them contain only 1.5–2.5%. The atmospheric content of benzene to which certain workmen could be exposed was therefore never greater than 0.01–0.02 mg/l (3–6 p.p.m.). Haematological examination of these particular workmen revealed no significant deviation of the blood picture as compared with that of 60 other employees who had never had any contact with petrol vapour.

In Australia, according to McLean (1960), the concentration of benzene in petrol can be 10%.

An example of the diversity of blood disorder which can be caused by benzene is seen in the account by McLean (1960) of six cases of poisoning in workers exposed to petrol containing benzene. Three of these developed fatal aplastic anaemia, one haemolytic anaemia and myelofibrosis, and one thrombocytopenic purpura. The sixth, who had accidentally aspirated a large quantity of petrol, developed aspiration pneumonia followed by slight chronic neutropenia.

Criteria of abnormal blood picture

Estimation of what constitutes an abnormal blood picture in workers exposed to benzene has differed considerably at the hands of different authorities.

The criterion of a normal total white cell count given by Hunter in 1939 for example was 6000–9000/μl, while the Benzol Poisoning Committee of the National Safety Council (1926) had placed the normal level at 5500, and Whitby and Britton (1939) state that "fluctuations in the number of leucocytes between the normal levels of 4000 to 10,000/μl are of no significance".

In the author's opinion, the criterion of abnormality in persons exposed to benzene should be based rather on changes observed during periodical blood examinations, including wherever possible the pre-employment blood picture, than on the individual level at any one examination. From this point of view the 'normal' and the 'deviations' from the normal indicative of chronic benzene poisoning are suggested in Table 3.

TABLE 3

	Normal	Deviations
R.B.C.	4.5–5 millions	below 4.5 millions
W.B.C.	5000–10,000	below 5000
Polymorphs	55–60%	below 50%
Lymphocytes	30–45%	above 45%
Total polymorphs	2500	below 2500
Eosinophils	2–5%	above 5%
Basophils	0.5–2%	above 2%
No primitive white cells or nucleated red cells		myelocytes, premyelocytes or nucleated red cells.
Large monocytes	up to 10%	above 10%
Haemoglobin	85–100%	below 85%
Colour Index	0.9–1	above 1

MILD OR EARLY POISONING

(1) White Corpuscles

(a) Leucopenia and neutropenia. – A relative lymphocytosis with a lowered total white cell count is one of the most significant early signs of an injurious effect of benzene exposure, especially in what has been called 'latent benzolism' (Lechelle *et al.*, 1940); in other words the early phase of chronic benzene poisoning, when neutropenia may occur with little or no anaemia and only slight leucopenia.

Neutropenia was an outstanding finding in a series of blood examinations (Hamilton-Paterson and Browning, 1944) of 200 women employed in 13 factories manufacturing self-sealing tanks, and involving the use of rubber solutions and adhesives containing benzene. The results were compared with the blood counts of 200 women who had never, so far as was known, been exposed to benzene. In the women working with the rubber solution neutropenia occurred 50 times, leucopenia 44 and anaemia 41. Eighteen women who showed gross leucopenia and neutropenia were removed from contact with benzene and re-examined after 3 months; by this time their blood picture was within normal limits. In three cases who then returned to their former work, blood examination 4 months later again showed deterioration.

A somewhat similar but more extensive investigation by Mme. Danysz in 1942 brought out the interesting possibility of sensitisation to benzene by a former exposure which had produced only transitory signs of poisoning. Two women returned to their former work some years after cessation of exposure. After $3\frac{1}{2}$ months in one case and 5 weeks in the other both showed anaemia, slight leuco-penia and neutropenia, with slightly prolonged bleeding and coagulation time, but no diminution of thrombocytes. On further cessation of work the blood pic-ture in one case returned to normal within 6 weeks. This sensitisation did not appear to occur in male workers.

Neutropenia as the earliest and most frequent abnormality was also the experience of Bernard-Pichon (1942) in an investigation of 350 benzene workers, but repeated examinations gave variable results, in some cases a return to nor-mality even while continuing at work.

(b) Eosinophilia has been considered a somewhat later sign of mild chronic poisoning. Heim de Balzac and Agasse Lafont (1910) stated that in such cases the total red cells, haemoglobin and total white cells may remain unaltered for a long time, as also the differential count, except for the presence of an almost constant, moderate and stationary eosinophilia, and Duvoir and Derobert (1942) have also recorded this abnormality.

Taking the lower limit of normal as 5%, Duvoir and Derobert observed an eosinophil count above this level in 21.8% of 555 cases, the incidence being slightly higher in women than men, and showing some correlation with the duration of exposure. Other investigators, including Heim de Balzac and Agasse-Lafont (1933), Emile-Weil, Perles and Aschkenazy (1938) have supported this pheno-menon, most of them noting a mild eosinophilia (4–8%) in about 30% of all cases, but higher values have also been recorded. Lechelle *et al.* (1940) observed one case with 24% and another with 15% of eosinophils, and Duvoir and Dero-bert (1942) a maximum of 18.1% in one woman employed for 5–10 years. In their series of 190 men and 365 women employed in many industries involving exposure to benzene, the eosinophilia was not always accompanied by leucopenia or neutropenia and they considered that no special significance is to be attached to it when it is an isolated phenomenon. Other observers, including Teleky and Weiner (1924) and the present author have failed to find eosinophilia in cases of chronic benzene poisoning.

(c) Basophilia. – An increase in basophil leucocytes was recorded by Smith (1928) but has not been confirmed by other authorities.

(d) Monocytosis and lymphocytosis. – An increase in large monocytes is a rather rare occurrence and it is doubtful if it is a direct result of benzene intoxication (Mazel *et al.*, 1944), but lymphocytosis and monocytosis not always accompanied by neutropenia have been observed. Bénard *et al.* (1942) recorded the case of a woman handling benzene who showed a lymphocytosis of 79% with a high total white cell count and similar cases have been recorded by Laignel Lavastine *et al.* (1928); Brindeau (1931) and Garnier and Cordier (1942).

(2) Red corpuscles

A slight reduction in the number of red cells often appears in the early stages of mild poisoning, but may be transitory, reappearing in a more significant degree only in the later and more severe cases.

(3) Haemoglobin level and colour index

In mild cases the haemoglobin level is slightly lowered, corresponding with the fall in total red cells, so that the colour index remains below 1. Slight anisocytosis and poikilocytosis occur relatively infrequently.

(4) Thrombocytopenia

Although a marked deficiency of thrombocytes is usually associated with the purpura of severe chronic poisoning, many authorities consider a decrease in thrombocytes one of the most reliable signs of early injury. Greenburg et al. (1939) found that among 107 persons exposed to benzene in the rotogravure printing industry 32.7% had platelet counts below 100,000. On the other hand Grazioli and Monteverde (1960) found that in a group of workers in the printing industry, most of whom showed both leucopenia and platelet deficiency, several had no thrombocytopenia even when blood coagulation was affected; they consider therefore that in many cases chronic benzene poisoning reveals itself as a thrombopathy without thrombopenia.

LATER, MORE SEVERE CASES

(1) White corpuscles

At a later stage of poisoning the above changes become more marked and progressive, with anaemia usually of the hyperchromic type.

A study by Lamy and Kissel (1942) of 9 women employed in the shoe industry exemplifies this picture of severe benzene poisoning; in 4 of the women it was ultimately fatal.

(a) *Leucopenia and neutropenia* were present in all 9, and anaemia had become severe, with a colour index above 1.

In the early literature very low total white cell counts were reported. In one of Selling's cases (1910) the number was $480/\mu$l; in one of Harrington's (1917) 500, and, lowest of all, of Hogan and Shrader (1923) 104. In the author's experience levels below $1500/\mu$l have only occurred in cases which eventually developed into frank aplastic anaemia.

(b) *Abnormal white corpuscles*, immature leucocytes, myelocytes and premyelocytes, appearing in large numbers in advanced poisoning, are to be considered as giving a bad prognosis.

(c) *The Pelger–Huet anomaly*, as a very rare abnormality associated with chronic benzene poisoning, has been described in one case by Paterni and Russo (1960).

Bibliography on p. 55

This anomaly, in which segmentation of the nuclei of granulocytes in the peripheral blood is inhibited so that the majority of granulocytes contain not more than two lobes, is generally regarded as a familial disorder, but in the case recorded by Paterni and Russo, which showed the typical finding of panhaemocytopenia associated with severe chronic benzene poisoning, no family tendency could be traced. The anomaly appeared only in the final stage of intoxication, one month before death.

(d) Leucosis (pre-leukaemic). A form of benzene chronic blood disorder, also designated as 'odo-leucosis' by Chevallier (1942), characterised not by a reduction but by an abnormal increase in leucocytes, without evolvement into true leukaemia, has been described by several observers. The occurrence of leucocytosis as an initial phenomenon in chronic exposure to benzene is well recognised. It is usually transient, sometimes not even a manifestation of a benzene effect. It may be due to a local infection – nasopharyngitis, bronchitis, furunculosis etc.

Bousser (1948) has emphasised the distinction between the transitory early leucosis and the polymorphonuclear leucosis appearing one month to two years or longer after the beginning of exposure. The transitory form is rarely accompanied by any disturbance of health and in its most frequently observed form is mild in degree, the total white cells reaching 10,000 to 15,000/μl with usually a predominance of polymorphonuclears. In the later form it may be more marked, the total white cells reaching, in some of Bousser's cases, from 15,000 to 19,600 with a differential formula varying from a preponderance of polymorphonuclears to one of mononuclears, or even with a normal proportion. It is sometimes associated with a very slight anaemia, but occasionally with polyglobulia. The polymorphonuclear leucosis persists as long as the exposure to benzene, remaining fairly constant when its maximum is reached and returning to normal when exposure ceases. Such cases may occur with the same exposure to which other workers react with the more usual leucopenia and neutropenia.

It is not suggested that all such cases should be regarded as 'preleukaemic', but a case such as that of Tolot *et al.* (1960), described on page 43 emphasises the necessity for repeating the blood examination of any benzene worker in whom a leucocytosis of more than 10,000/μl appears, and if it persists after three examinations immediate removal from exposure should be advised.

(2) Red corpuscles

Very low red cell counts have been recorded in the later stages of severe poisoning, and may be regarded as heralding the onset of aplastic anaemia. One of the lowest recorded is that of Brocher (1929), 630,000; others with very low levels by Hogan and Shrader (1923), 880,000; Hayhurst and Neiswander (1931), 900,000; and Hamilton (1928) and Landé and Kalinowsky (1928), 1,000,000/μl.

These low counts are generally associated with severe anisocytosis and poikilocytosis (Rohner *et al.*, 1926; Hayhurst and Neiswander, 1931) and with the appearance of nucleated red cells and punctate basophilia (Bowers, 1947; Hunter and Hanflig, 1927; and others).

Slight reticulocytosis has also been observed by Mitnik and Genkin (1931) and Pulford (1931).

(3) Haemoglobin level and colour index

(a) Macrocytic anaemia. – In severe poisoning the anaemia is nearly always macrocytic, with a colour index above 1. Dimmel (1932) for example found the colour index between 1.1 and 1.3 in his cases, and in two fatal cases reported to the Home Office in 1934 it was 1 and 1.06 respectively.

(b) Haemolytic anaemia has occasionally been reported as a consequence of chronic benzene exposure (Erf and Rhoads, 1939; André and Dreyfus, 1951). In a case recorded by the latter, a girl aged 16, working in a shoe factory, the haemolytic anaemia was severe and accompanied by haemorrhagic purpura and an enlarged spleen, removal of which was followed by improvement.

(4) Thrombocytopenia

Very low thrombocyte counts are usually accompanied by purpuric manifestations and haemorrhage from mucous membranes. Probably the earliest cases of this kind were those recorded by Selling (1910); very low levels have also been observed by Brocher (1929) and Mitnik and Genkin (1931).

Thrombocytopenic purpura due to benzene poisoning closely resembles that of the idiopathic variety, though it has been stated that oozing is more characteristic of benzene.

In 1944 Vaughn reported a case which he then diagnosed as thrombocytopenic purpura due to benzol poisoning, but later (1947) he concluded that it was in fact a case of idiopathic thrombocytopenia in which the part played by benzene exposure remained undetermined. The case was that of a woman aged 33 whose 16 years' exposure to benzene in the handling of shoe cements had ceased about 12 months before the appearance of a purpuric rash on the lower limbs. This was accompanied by bleeding from the nose, gums and vagina, but the blood picture showed only slight abnormality – anaemia, moderate leucopenia, occasional eosinophilia and a platelet count of 20,000. She showed a brief remission following treatment by methyl testosterone but relapsed two years later, with the appearance of an increase in megakaryocytes in the bone marrow. Splenectomy was followed by complete haematological recovery.

Reduction of thrombocytes is not invariably associated with bleeding. Nikulina and Titowa (1934) record a case with a thrombocyte count of 18,790 and no sign of bleeding.

In addition to the actual diminution of thrombocytes in chronic benzene poisoning, some authorities believe that they are functionally inefficient owing to a defect in agglutinability. The two defects are not necessarily always associated, but are generally so in severe cases.

Bibliography on p. 55

Saita and Sbertoli (1954) demonstrated this phenomenon in cases of chronic benzene poisoning in a rotogravure printing works in Italy. Of these cases, 3 were severe, with thrombocytes below 100,000 and marked anaemia and leucopenia, 14 of moderate severity, and 4, exposed for periods of 6 months and 3 years, with a normal blood picture.

They estimated the agglutinability of the thrombocytes by means of an 'agglutinogram' devised by Rovatti (1949), in which the number of groups of 2, 3 and 4 platelets are counted in 100 isolated elements. This gives a normal count of 33 groups of 2, 13 of 3, and 8 of 4 elements, with the resulting formula $33 \pm 2 - 13 \pm 2 - 8 \pm 2$.

On this basis they found 10 cases with hypoagglutinability and 10 with a normal formula. All those with a normal blood picture showed a normal agglutinogram, but in the affected persons the hypoagglutinability was not always comparable with the severity of the clinical or haematological findings. In one case there was a marked haemorrhagic diathesis and hypoagglutinability but not a conspicuous diminution in the number of thrombocytes. In all cases with definite hypoagglutinability the thrombocytes showed morphological abnormalities – basophilia, anisocytosis, vacuolation.

Blood coagulation may be normal or delayed. Rohner et al. (1923) estimated it at 9 min in a fatal case, but Dimmel (1933) found no delay in a series of 66 cases of varying severity, and Hayhurst and Neiswander (1931) recorded 4 min in a case with purpura and bleeding from mucous membranes. According to Simonin (1934) the clot may be irretractable.

Bleeding time is also variable but apparently more often normal than prolonged except in cases of extreme thrombocytopenia (Dimmel, 1933).

Qualitative alterations in the thrombocytes have been held responsible for a deficiency in thromboplastin leading to an increase in time of coagulation and therefore to a haemorrhagic syndrome (Faure-Gilly et al., 1948). Deficiency of thromboplastin, attributed in severe cases to lesions of the bone marrow caused by benzene, has also been advanced by Saita et al. (1954) as the cause of the deficiency of blood coagulation in cases of chronic benzene poisoning. On the evidence of their investigation of 14 rotogravure workers suffering from chronic benzene poisoning and using as their criteria platelet counts, recalcification time, prothrombin time and in some cases clot retraction and capillary resistance tests, they concluded that at least some part of the coagulation disorder must be due to a defect of the thromboplastic factor.

Benzene content of the blood in chronic poisoning

It was at one time suggested that the amount of benzene in the blood of workers exposed to benzene might be a diagnostic pointer to their degree of absorption or actual chronic intoxication (Bernard et al., 1949). Careful investigations of a large number of workpeople, some of them never having had any obvious exposure to benzene, have however revealed great discrepancy in the results of estimations of benzenemia, and still more in the relation between the amounts found and the signs and symptoms of chronic poisoning.

Bernard et al., (1949) gave as their outstanding result of an investigation of a series of workers with varying degrees of benzene hazard the fact that the presence of benzene in the blood is inconstant, and its amount variable even in comparable conditions of work.

They did, however, note that when the benzene level of the blood is greater than 1 mg/100, slight modifications of the blood picture, chiefly leucopenia, are usually present.

The discrepancies were even more marked in an investigation by Tara et al. (1953). Among 403 persons examined, including some with doubtful exposure, some who had been previously diagnosed as cases of chronic benzene poisoning, some exposed at the time of examination, and 104 controls, the highest amount of benzene in the blood (800 μ) was present in a man exposed at the time to inhalation of the heated vapour of fuel oil, but with a normal blood picture. In another case, a photogravure worker who had shown severe anaemia, leucopenia, neutropenia and thrombocytopenia with purpura, repeated estimations of the blood benzene at intervals up to 4 years after cessation of work revealed its presence on only one occasion – at an interval of 25 months. At 4 years none was present though the haemopoietic disturbance had increased and the prognosis was serious. Even among the 104 controls, who had at any rate no occupational exposure to benzene, the same discrepancy was found – 35% showed some benzene in the blood.

Some possible interpretations of these discrepancies have been suggested by Bernard et al (1949):

(1) Technical errors, including the possibility of benzene arising from the materials used in the estimation (alcohol, rubber, etc.).

(2) Benzene absorbed from non-occupational sources, which may include gas used for lighting, other solvents containing benzene, etc.

(3) Individual variation in the capacity to eliminate benzene from the blood.

Benzene in the bone marrow

From the few autoposies made in cases of fatal chronic benzene poisoning it appears that discrepancies similar to those of the blood benzene occur in estimations of the benzene in the bone marrow, and with similar suggested explanations.

Duvoir et al. (1946) examined the bone marrow of three persons, in two of whom death had occurred 20 and 14 months after cessation of exposure; in each of these the benzene in the bone marrow amounted to 0.2 g/kg. In the third case, 'of classic type', no benzene was demonstrated. Perrault et al. (1944) found an appreciable amount of benzene in a fatal case of benzene intoxication when the

Bibliography on p. 55

total leucocyte count had at that time fallen to 600 μl, but on the day preceding death, had risen to 2700.

The explanation of the discrepany in the cases of Duvoir and co-workers suggested by them is that during exposure to benzene small repeated subacute intoxications result in a small storage in the bone marrow, the greater part being metabolised, with excretion of the conjugated portions. When the capacity for oxidation is at length exhausted larger quantities must be left for storage in the bone marrow, but during a haematological crisis, as shown by the classical signs of chronic benzene poisoning, strenuous effort is made on the part of the organism to detoxicate this toxic reserve. If death occurs before this is complete, benzene will be present in the bone marrow; if it is complete, the analysis will be negative.

It is also to be remembered that recent studies on the metabolism of benzene have shown that it is the metabolic products (phenols) rather than benzene itself which are responsible for the injury to the bone marrow, and that it is the individual capacity, differing in different individuals, to eliminate these or to conjugate them into less toxic excretory compounds, more or less rapidly, which is the most significant source of discrepant results of estimations of benzene in the bone marrow.

FATAL CHRONIC POISONING

The classical cause of death in chronic benzene poisoning is aplastic anaemia, but there is undoubted evidence that the final fatal condition may, though much more rarely, be one of the various types of leukaemia, sometimes though not always supervening on a previously existing aplastic anaemia.

Aplastic anaemia

The aplastic anaemia due to benzene closely resembles the idiopathic variety.

It has already been mentioned that chronic benzene poisoning is regarded in the United Kingdom as a notifiable disease only when any symptoms or blood changes are associated with haemorrhages under the skin or bleeding from mucous membranes. These are usually late symptoms of chronic benzene poisoning, occurring only when the depression of the bone marrow has reached a pre-fatal stage. This is usually preceded by symptoms and signs of severe anaemia – pallor, weakness, fatigability, shortness of breath, palpitation, and a marked deterioration of the blood picture.

In the idiopathic variety, haemorrhagic tendencies may be the first manifestation of the disease, with profuse bleeding from the nose, gums, rectum and uterus.

In both types however the peripheral blood count at this stage is one of marked and progressive reduction of all the formed elements of the blood and of the haemoglobin level.

In some of the recorded cases following benzene exposure the erythrocytes have been as low as or lower than 1,000,000/μl and the leucocytes as low
as or lower than 1000, with the polymorphs lower than the lymphocytes. In a
typical case recorded by Hayhurst and Neiswander (1937) the erythrocyte count
was 900,000/μl, the total leucocytes 850, and the haemoglobin level 10%.

Reticulocytes and thrombocytes are extremely sparse, and as a corollary of
the latter, bleeding time is prolonged and the clot may be non-retractile (Askey,
1928).

In a few cases, however, it has happened that even when the bone marrow
has reached this low level of depression, areas representing attempts at compensatory regeneration are reflected in the peripheral blood by the appearance of
premature myelogenous cells, a change suggestive of the development of a pre-
leukaemic condition.

In two such cases (Browning, unpublished observation) diagnosed as aplastic anaemia due to benzene, this development took place in one case a few weeks,
in the other a few days, before death.

Susceptibility to infection of all types is marked, and sepsis especially at the
site of transfusions may be a troublesome feature, as in one of the two above
cases.

Necrotising lesions of the mouth and pharynx, similar to those of agranulocytosis, are also of common occurence.

The prognosis is poor, the duration of the disease from the appearance of
definitely diagnostic symptoms being usually not more than 12–18 months. The
bone marrow shows in most cases a marked diminution of all the cellular elements,
but frequently also 'islands' of regeneration, especially when premature cells of
the myeloid type and myeloblasts have appeared in the peripheral blood.

According to Rosenthal (1938) some cases of aplastic anaemia due to benzene may show a bone marrow with signs of fibrosis and calcification.

Leukaemia

Experimental leukaemia in animals

Attempts to produce leukaemia (or aplasia) in animals poisoned by benzene
have given conflicting results.

In 1932 Lignac claimed to have produced among 54 white mice given weekly
subcutaneous injections of 0,001 ml of benzene in 0.1 ml of olive oil 3 cases of
mediastinal lymphosarcoma, 3 of leukaemia (1 myeloid and 2 aleukaemic) and
2 of 'mast cell leucosis'. His results were partially confirmed by Hess (1935), and
regarded as 'factual' by Sabrazès and Bideau (1937), but were rejected in a recent
investigation by Amiel (1960). Amiel obtained entirely negative findings in respect
of both leukaemia and aplastic anaemia in 30 male mice of three groups of one
strain, receiving weekly subcutaneous injections of pure benzene in olive oil. In

Bibliography on p. 55

another group of another strain 16 died between 16 and 17 months with leucoses of the lymphoid type, and half of them of leukaemia, but these figures were in fact lower than those in the control group of the same strain. Amiel explains these results and their non-agreement with those of Lignac by the fact that certain strains of mice are highly susceptible to spontaneous leucoses and that Lignac's mice should have been compared with similarly susceptible controls.

Myelosis of an erythraemic type was, however, reported (Sabrazès et al., 1937) in guinea pigs exposed to benzene vapour, and in rats poisoned by benzene (Paterni et al., 1954) and an abnormal myelogram (Elmino et al., 1960), considered characteristic of an erythromyelosis, in rabbits after 30 days of intramuscular injections of benzene. This condition consisted of reticuloerythroblastic islands, atypical karyokinesis, numerous large polychromatic and basophilic erythroblasts and an increase of histiocytes and plasma cells.

Leukaemias in human beings

The association between benzene exposure and leukaemia, though relatively infrequent, is now recognised by most authorities as an established fact. Until 1931 very few cases had been recorded. In that year, in a review of 36 autopsies of benzene workers, Hamilton (1931) noted that though in human beings aplastic anaemia was the most characteristic effect of fatal chronic benzene poisoning, cases with a hyperplastic bone marrow did occur, and she instanced one case of true leukaemia.

By 1938, Penati and Vigliani were able to collect 10 cases from the literature, to which in the following year two more were added by Mallory et al. Since then the number of cases recorded has gradually increased. In 1943 Vigliani and Saita stated that 14 had now been described, and in 1950 Bernard and Braier collected 37, including 5 of their own. In most of these the exposure had lasted from 5 to 21 years but in two only 8 months and one year respectively.

There is as great a diversity in the type of leukaemia associated with benzene exposure as in the idiopathic variety (see Table 4). This is not surprising since, as remarked by Damashek (1960), "leukaemia is unfortunately the number one problem in haematology. It is concerned with white blood cells which are produced in white cell-forming tissues, the most important of which is the bone marrow, producing granulocytes. There are also the lymphoid system, the reticuloendothelial system and the system of plasma cells, which produce corresponding cells found in the blood".

Benzene leukaemia is frequently superimposed upon a condition of aplastic anaemia, but it can develop without a preceding peripheral blood picture characteristic of bone marrow aplasia. Such a transition from aplastic anaemia to leukaemia is not of course unknown in the idiopathic form of leukaemia. Several cases of this kind have recently been recorded by Dul'tsin et al. (1960) in which aplastic anaemia ultimately assumed the clinical features of aleukaemic reticulosis and haemocytoblastosis.

Chronic myeloid leukaemia has been the variety most frequently reported following benzene exposure but all varieties have occurred – acute myeloid, acute aleukaemic, 'haemorrhagic aleukaemia', acute and chronic lymphatic, acute monoblastic leucosis, and during recent years erythroleukaemic myelosis or Di Guglielmo's Disease.

(1) Chronic myeloid leukaemia

Among the 16 cases included in Table 4, that described by Tolot *et al.* (1960) is perhaps most closely illustrative of the development of leukaemia in a benzene worker without previous premonitory signs of a tendency to aplasia. This was a man employed in a photogravure process where the ink solvents consisted of 'benzine hydrocarbons'.

During 10 years in this work he had only one transient episode of slight anaemia and leucocytosis. Six years after this a significant deviation from the normal appeared in the form of a progressive rise of leucocytes; one year later this was accompanied by 4% of myelocytes, with no anaemia or thrombocytopenia. At this point the man was removed from exposure and during the next two years his blood picture was simply that of leucocytosis with some myelocytes. At the end of that time it was found that the total leucocytes had risen to 300,000/μl and there was now some anaemia.

In some cases of fatal chronic benzene poisoning changes in the peripheral blood and bone marrow have resembled the classical picture of myelogenous leukaemia but have differed from it in some details both of appearance and also of evolution. As Emil-Weil (1932) remarked, "this myelogenous leukaemia . . . remains in fact aleukaemic the greater part of the time, the extreme hyperleucocytosis has been only transitory and the leucosis accompanied or complicated by aplastic anaemia".

His case was that of a woman who had worked in rubber production for 15 years and who presented at her first examination the features of aplastic anaemia and aleukaemia, which was finally transformed into acute myelogenous anaemia.

Many of the early reports were not of indubitable diagnosis. Such was that of Le Noir and Claude (1897), said by some authorities to be the first recorded case of benzene leukaemia. Unfortunately no enumeration of the peripheral blood cells was made and at autopsy no examination of the bone marrow. The case presented with purpura with progressive symptoms of aplastic anaemia. The only features which might be considered diagnostic of a late super-imposition of leukaemia on aplastic anaemia were that on examination of blood smears the white cells were observed to be much more abundant than the red, and that at autopsy the liver showed a great abundance of leucocytes in its trabecular capillaries. Another doubtful feature was that the exposure was said to be to 'la ben-

Bibliography on p. 55

zine', but the exposure occurred during the manipulation of paints, and the well known cases of Santesson (1897), were also stated to be due to exposure to 'la benzine' – a common confusion between benzene and benzine in the early literature.

(2) Chronic myeloid leukaemia with haemolytic anaemia

Two unusual cases of chronic myeloid leukaemia associated with haemolytic anaemia were reported (Marchal and Duhamel, 1950). One of these had been employed 12 years in a printing works where benzol was used for cleaning. He presented with chronic myeloid leukaemia, with a total white cell count of 109,000/μl. Following transfusion and splenic radiotherapy this total was reduced to 7600, but icterus developed and a few weeks later the total red cells fell to 500,000 and the white to 1900. Sternal puncture did not however reveal aplasia, but myelogenous hyperplasia of the bone marrow. Globular fragility was greatly increased and returned to normal only after repeated blood transfusions, while the leucocyte level again rose to 62,400 with 10% myelocytes. Marchal and Duhamal consider that the radiotherapy initiated the haemolysis but did not affect haemopoiesis in the bone marrow.

The second case, described as one of 'occupational benzolism', presented with hypoplastic anaemia, leucopenia and haemolytic icterus, but after numerous transfusions the aplasia syndrome gradually evolved two months before death into acute 'cryptoleucosis' with a leucoblastic bone marrow and infiltration of the liver.

(3) Acute myeloid leukaemia

Among the cases diagnosed as acute myeloid leukaemia, that described by Raynaud et al in 1947, was not quite typical, in that its onset with a sudden attack of purpura was not preceded by other signs of disturbance, and that the purpura was followed in 6 months by multiple haemorrhages, anaemia and thrombocytopenia, with a white cell count of 50,000/μl of which 80% were myeloblasts. The bone marrow showed myeloblastic leukaemic infiltration and death occurred 8 months after the appearance of purpura. This case exemplifies the long latent period sometimes observed with benzene exposure. The man had been exposed for 10 years with no apparent ill-defect.

A case of acute myeloid leukaemia described in 1939 by Mallory et al., and previously recorded by Hunter in the same year, had the unusual feature at autopsy of a localised tumour nodule in the liver.

(4) Acute aleukaemia

Some authorities believe that the acute aleukaemic variety occurs more frequently in association with benzene exposure than has actually been reported, since the blood picture often closely resembles that of an aplasia with symptoms and characteristics of this condition and with no marked leucocytosis. It is only when the bone marrow is examined that it is found to be hyperplastic.

A typical case of this kind was recorded in 1938 (Perrin *et al.*). This was a woman aged 44, exposed to benzene for 11 years in a shoe factory where an adhesive containing 75% of benzol was used. For several months before her condition became acute she had complained of headache, dyspnoea and digestive trouble. Three weeks before her death she was intensely anaemic, and had widespread purpura and a high temperature. Het blood picture at this time showed anaemia (1,560,000 red blood corpuscles), leucopenia (1800 white blood corpuscles), with 16% of granulocytes and 17% of leucoblasts. The bone marrow at autopsy proved to be neither aplasic nor hypoplasic but in a state of active proliferation, the white cells being almost exclusively leucoblasts; the spleen was also completely devoid of granulocytes.

In another case, described by Mallory *et al.* (1939), a schoolboy of 12 who had used a paint remover containing benzene in his father's shop, there was also severe anaemia and a white cell count ranging from 5,000 to 12,000, but with lymphoblasts as the predominating immature cell. The diagnosis of acute aleukaemic leukaemia was confirmed by sternal puncture.

The term 'haemorrhagic aleukaemia' was applied by Merklen and Israel (1934) to seven of the cases investigated by Heim de Balzac and Agasse Lafont (1933). These were characterised by leucopenia, granulopenia, with myelocytes and sometimes myeloblasts in the peripheral blood, and some anaemia and thrombocytopenia with extensive purpuric haemorrhages. A more complex case has been described (Guasch *et al.*, 1959) in which the acute aleukaemic thrombocytopenic leukaemia appeared to have developed independently of a pre-existing aplasia, not superimposed upon it. The period of exposure to benzene had been 15 years, and a hyperchromic anaemia had existed for 6 years. On the basis of bone marrow findings during these 6 years it was concluded that this was neither a case of transformation of anaemia into leukaemia nor a leukaemia with an unusually long pre-leukaemic phase, but two different processes, both apparently due to benzene.

(a) Lymphatic leukaemia following exposure to benzene is much rarer than myeloid. Perhaps the earliest case of acute lymphatic leukaemia was described by Delore and Borgamano in 1928. In this case the onset was sudden, after a period of normal health during 5 years of exposure to benzene, with epigastric pain, vomiting of blood, petechial haemorrhages and ecchymoses, and ulcerative stomatitis. There were also numerous enlarged glands, and the blood picture showed a white cell count of 542,500/μl of which 80% were lymphoblasts. Death occurred 6 weeks after the first appearance of symptoms.

A case of fatal acute lymphatic leukaemia was also observed by Browning (unpublished observation) in 1955 in a man employed on the manufacture of artificial leather; another worker on this process had died of aplastic anaemia.

Bibliography on p. 55

At that time the man in question had a normal blood picture. Six months later a repeat examination revealed a high total of white cells of which 84% were lymphocytes or lymphoblasts.

A more unusual case of 'chronic lymphomatosis' in a benzene worker was described by Drouet, Perquin and Herbeval in 1947. This was a woman aged 68 who had been employed in the shoe industry for 12 years. During the first three years her exposure had been heavy and she had complained of excessive fatigue, headache and occasional expectoration of blood, but had no apparent anaemia, other haemorrhages or fever. During the next 8 years the amount of benzene in the adhesive was reduced and finally eliminated, but at the end of this time the woman developed enlarged cervical glands and her blood picture showed 55–85% of abnormal white cells described as young lymphocytes with nucleolated nuclei. The bone marrow was also rich in lymphocytes and immature mononuclear cells. The condition was diagnosed as "Probable lymphoid leukaemia due to benzene"·

(b) Acute monoblastic leucosis was the picture in a fatal case reported (Marchand, 1960) in a man aged 29 engaged in spray painting metal furniture with a paint containing benzene. His blood picture, repeated three times in one year, showed on the third occasion a fall of total white cells, previously 9400 and 12,000, to 3800, with only 38% polymorphonuclears, 18% mononuclears, one plasma cell, 2 metamyelocytes and one blast cell. Two months later, following a severe intestinal haemorrhage, the picture was that of acute monoblastic leucosis with 84% monoblasts and only 1% polymorphs. Death took place the next day.

Another recent case of 'acute lymphoblastosis' (Gaultier and Fournier, 1959) was a girl who had been exposed to benzene (nature and duration of exposure not described) and who left on account of fatigue. Some months later she had an episode of fever, during which she was found to have monocytosis and was than diagnosed as infective mononucleosis. She died ten days later of what was called 'lymphoblastosis'.

The case reported by Bousser *et al.* (1948) was described as 'aleukaemic lymphomatosis of lymphosarcomatous type'. This was a man in whom the presence of generalised enlarged lymphatic glands was found 3½ years after he had ceased work as a painter, the diagnosis being based on the adenogram and biopsy, since at that time there was no modification of the peripheral blood picture. Benzene was present in the blood, spleen and glands.

(5) Erythroleukaemic myelosis (acute erythraemic leukaemia; Di Guglielmo's disease)

This condition was originally described by Di Guglielmo (1923) and has come to be called Di Guglielmo's disease. Its characteristic features have been further elaborated by Di Guglielmo during the following 20 years and his observations have been confirmed by many other authorities, some of whom have described cases associated with exposure to benzene.

In its idiopathic from it has been regarded as a systemic irreversible disease of the reticulo-histiocytic tissues with an eventual evolution into neoplasm of erythraemic elements – a 'pure' disorder of erythropoietic tissue. Di Guglielmo himself has emphasised the resemblance and the difference between the acute form of this disease and acute leukaemia. Both diseases are characterised not only by the extreme proliferation of the respective cellular elements but also by their atypical forms.

In Di Guglielmo's disease these latter are represented by grossly atypical erythroblasts, though typical and intermediate forms may also be present. Unlike the most frequently observed enormous increase of mature cells of the myeloid series in myeloid leukaemia, there is usually a decrease of mature red cells in Di Guglielmo's disease, even at times a marked anaemia, mainly due to the fact that the erythroblasts, which vary in number from 3200 to 143,000/μl (Lazzaro, 1933), mature only sparsely, and the newly formed erythrocytes have a shorter life span.

The original description of the disease has now been somewhat modified by other authorities. Damashek and Baldwin (1958) suggest that in the Di Guglielmo syndrome the erythroblastic proliferation is only a first stage, the disease ending with an almost 'pure' myeloblastic proliferation (acute granulocytic leukaemia) – in other words, the first, intermediate and final stages could all be included in the designation 'erythroleukaemia'.

The clinical symptoms are sudden in onset, though sometimes preceded by a short period of general ill-health – weakness, loss of appetite, vague pains and headache. Irregular fever and intense anaemia are constant features, as also are haemorrhagic manifestations and enlargement of the spleen and liver, both of which show evidence of extreme proliferation of the reticulo-endothelial system. Necrosis of the buccal mucous membrane has not been observed, probably owing to the fact that neutropenia is not present, and there is consequently no lack of resistance to infection.

The bone marrow shows an enormous proliferation of reticulo-endothelial elements with some giant cells.

(a) Association with exposure to benzene. – During the last ten years several cases of erythraemic myelosis following exposure to benzene have been reported, though not all correspond exactly to Di Guglielmo's description of the disease.

In 1940, in a review of the cases published up to that time, Moeschlin concluded that only five conformed exactly to Di Guglielmo's criteria, and until 1958 all these cases had been designated 'acute' *i.e.* with a rapidly fatal course and the presence of immature erythroblasts in the bone marrow. Only one case corresponding to a chronic form of the disease has so far been recorded (Di Guglielmo and Ricci, 1958).

(b) Acute cases. – In 1950 Galavotti and Troisi described an acute erythroleukaemia superimposed on a myeloblastic leukaemia in a worker with 5 months' exposure to benzene in his work as a cycle merchant.

Bibliography on p. 55

A case reported by André and Dreyfus (1951), a man who had for many years manipulated products with a benzene base, and two similar cases by Marchal (1952) were regarded as a form of pure erythraemia, characterised by a marked increase of cells of the erythrocyte series with abnormalities of the size, shape, nucleus and cytoplasm. Benzene was present in the blood to the amount of 0.8 mg/l in one case and 1 mg/l in the other, the latter having 2.5 mg/l in the bone marrow.

Nissen and Soeberg (1953) emphasised in their case, which they regarded as due to benzene, the markedly atypical karyokinesis of the erythroblasts. This man had been, for about 6 months before the onset of his illness, working at the benzene plant of a gas works transporting 'tar acids' with a presumed content of about 1% of benzene, from the plant into a pool, with development of intense heat and flame.

A well-documented case is that of Di Guglielmo and Iannacone (1950). This was a man working in a rotogravure plant where the benzene concentration had been "higher than the maximum allowable value". His initial symptoms were severe and rapidly progressive with anaemia, and a high temperature. The peripheral blood showed a marked predominance of erythroblasts not only of abnormal size and appearance but also with evidence of inhibition of mitosis at the earliest stage of the metaphase and with degenerative changes in the nuclei resembling those caused by ionising radiation and radiomimetic poisons. Death occurred 5 weeks after the onset of symptoms and on the preceding day there was a sudden marked increase of haemocytoblasts in the bone marrow and peripheral blood and also an increase in the circulating white cells which reached a total of nearly $300,000/\mu l$.

Another acute case is that of Kuhlmann (1959), designated 'acute myeloid erythroleukaemia', in a man employed 9 years in a small shoe-making factory. During the first 7 years of his employment an adhesive used contained 63% of benzene, for the next 2 years 18%. His illness began with fatigue, pallor, loss of weight, weakness and prolonged bleeding from a cut wrist. His peripheral blood showed severe anaemia (1.6 million red blood corpuslcles) with 28% haemoglobin and thrombocytopenia, and there was a predominance of blast cells. Sternal puncture showed increased erythropoiesis with some gigantoblasts. Death occurred, in spite of treatment with prednisone, ACTH, vitamin B12, vitamin C and blood transfusion, 6 months after recognition of the anaemia.

(6) Chronic erythromyelosis

The case considered by Di Guglielmo and Ricci (1958) to belong to the chronic form of the disease had a slow clinical course and the myelogram was not typical with regard to evidence of immaturity or nuclear degeneration of the cells. The patient was a woman aged 63 who had for many years assisted her husband in shoe making, using an adhesive containing 15% of benzene. The disease

TABLE 4

Leukaemia and Benzene Exposure

Type: myeloid		
Author	Year	Number of cases
Acute		
Lenoir and Claude	1897	1 (doubtful)
Undritz	1938	1
Emile-Weil, Perles *et al.*	1938	1
Mallory, Gall and Brickley	1939	1
Loeper and Mallarme	1942	1
Saita and Dompé	1947	1
Raynaud *et al.*	1947	
Subacute		
Emil-Weil	1932	1
Chronic		
Sabrazès and Bideau	1937	1
Sabrazès, Bideau and Glaunès	1937	2
Erf and Rhoads	1939	1
Chevallier *et al.*	1942	2
Van Schoenhaven Van Buerden	1949	1
Marchal and Duhamel	1950	2
Bernard and Braier	1950	5
Bousser and Tara	1951	3
Revol, Millet and Thivollet	1954	3
Tolot, Neulat and Mallein	1960	1
Type: lymphatic		
Delore and Borgamano	1928	1
Falconer	1933	1
Bernard *et al.*	1942	1
Drouet, Pierquin *et al.*	1947	1
Bousser, Neydé and Fabre	1948	1
Gaultier and Fournier	1959	1
Marchand	1960	1 (monoblastic)
Type: aleukaemic		
Merklen and Israel	1934	7
Thompson, Richter and Edsall	1934	1
Tzanck, Dreyfus and Jais	1937	1
Perrin, Kissel and Pierquin	1937	1
Van Ravensteyn	1941	1
Binet, Conté and Bourlière	1945	1
Saita	1945	1
Guasch, Pelayo and Villespin	1959	1
Type: erythroleukaemic		
Hamilton	1931	2
Storti	1936	1
Vigliani and Saita	1943	1
DiGugleilmo and Innacone	1950	1
Galavotti and Troisi	1950	1
André and Dreyfus	1951	1
Marchal	1952	2
Nissen and Soeberg	1953	1
DiGuglielmo and Ricci	1958	1 *(chronic)*
Kuhlmann	1959	1

Bibliography on p. 55

presented with asthenia, anorexia and intense and progressive pallor. Blood examination revealed profound anaemia (1400,000 red blood corpuscles) with
nucleated cells and 68% of erythroblasts.

The diagnosis was confirmed by sternal puncture which showed an almost
total substitution of the normal parenchyma by erythraemic tissue. The erythroblasts were nearly all very large, showing no arrest of maturation; atypical cells
were rare and showed no evidence of nuclear degeneration as in the acute case
described by Di Guglielmo and Iannacone (1950), but morphologically the picture was undoubtedly one of erythraemia. Treatment with prednisone, repeated
blood transfusion and antibiotics was followed by a temporary improvement
(a rise in red blood corpuscles and a fall in nucleated cells and erythroblasts)
but after a relapse became ineffective and death occurred probably about two
years after the true inception of the disease.

TREATMENT

The treatment of chronic benzene poisoning has been approached from many
aspects – dietetic, antibiotic, blood transfusion, therapy with iron and liver, pentose nucleotide, cysteine, ACTH, vitamins, methionine, and even transplantation of spongy bone.

In late severe cases success has been far from unqualified, initial improvement being almost invariably followed by relapse with an ultimately fatal outcome. In early cases, showing only slight abnormality of the blood picture, some
successes have been reported, but removal from exposure is the first and essential
measure; this alone usually results in a return to normality. Even in such cases
further exposure should be forbidden, if possible permanently, if not, for at least
6–8 weeks after three blood examinations have proved normal.

Iron and liver extract, in cases where a return to normality is delayed after
removal from exposure and where anaemia is more pronounced than leucopenia,
has sometimes in the author's experience had a favourable effect.

Antibiotics are useful when, in the presence of leucopenia, various infections
such as staphylococcal abscesses arise or when during blood transfusions the site
of injection becomes infected.

Blood transfusion is the treatment almost invariably given when the bone
marrow has become aplasic, and is often temporarily effective, but when severe
aplasia has set in, the outcome is essentially unfavourable in spite of the transient
improvement after each transfusion. In some of the cases treated by Appuhn and
Goldeck (1957) frequent transfusions were followed by haemosiderosis. A combination of transfusion, penicillin and transplantation of spongy bone was attempted by Debray et al. (1950). This was a very severe case of chronic benzene poisoning, with marked anaemia, leucopenia and an aplastic bone marrow and with
a bad prognosis. Following experience of therapeutic failure with transfusion and
pentose nucleotides in 6 cases of fatal benzene poisoning in rubber workers, trans-

plantations of lamellae of spongy bone taken from three incisions into the iliac bone of a fifteen year old girl were made into the lower border of the right pectoral muscle of the affected worker. Two weeks later there was some general improvement (rise in total red cells from 1,950,000–4,050,000 and of white cells from 400–2800/μl) but a week later a lung infection necessitated treatment with penicillin and streptomycin, and transfusions were also given. A second transplantation of spongy bone into the left pectoral muscle was given two months after the first and was followed by some improvement in the blood picture but with variations in leucopenia and neutropenia. After 8 months there was no trace of the bony implants on palpation, they appeared to have been completely absorbed. After one year the general health was much better and the blood picture appeared to be gradually approximating to the normal. It is suggested that this improvement was not entirely attributable to the implants of spongy bone, since transfusions and antibiotics were also given.

Vitamins

Three factors of the vitamin B complex, and vitamin C have been stated by some authorities to have a favourable therapeutic effect.

Vitamin B4 (adenine)

Described by Reader (1929) and Kline *et al.* (1936), present in yeast and necessary to the growth of rats, it has been justified as a therapeutic measure in chronic benzene poisoning chiefly on the basis of its favourable effect in subacute poisoning in rabbits following intramuscular administration of 1 ml/kg of benzene in a 4.0% solution of olive oil every second day. In the animals given benzene until the number of leucocytes decreased to less than a third of the initial level, a daily injection of 6 mg of adenine had no obvious influence on the severe leucopenia, but with larger doses (30 mg daily) from the beginning the initial decrease was very slight and the neutrophils were maintained for a long time at about the initial level. When the adenine was given only after the leucopenia had become severe it did not produce any improvement. It had also been stated by De Rosa (1955) that adenine is effective in protecting and repairing a deficiency of blood platelets in animals poisoned by benzene.

Although there may be a clear difference in the bone marrow of human beings gradually damaged by chronic poisoning with benzene and that of animals severely damaged by large doses, some authorities such as Paolino and Vercillino (1960) consider that it may be worth while to test the effect of adenine on the leucopenia of chronic occupational benzene poisoning.

Bibliography on p. 55

Vitamin B6 (pyridoxine hydrochloride)

A number of observers have reported beneficial effects from the use of vitamin B6 especially in mild chronic cases of benzene poisoning. This efficacy was suggested chiefly by observations of its therapeutic value in cases of agranulocytic angina. In one of these cases, after sulphathiazole, pentnucleotide and a blood transfusion had had no beneficial effect, intravenous injection of 200 mg of pyridoxine produced a rapid rise in leucocytes and disappearance of symptoms.

The efficacy of vitamin B6 in mild chronic benzene poisoning was then demonstrated by Dubois-Ferrière (1951) and by Zorina (1960). In the 6 cases treated by Dubois-Ferrière the vitamin B6 was combined with folic acid, with a resultant increase in total leucocytes and granulocytes.

Zorina has found vitamin B6 efficacious when given by mouth in early cases of benzene poisoning of moderate severity but not in more severe cases of long duration. When administered by mouth his dosage was 50, 100, 200 and 300 mg daily; when by intramuscular or intravenous injection, 2.5 ml of a 5% solution. In nine patients with leucopenia varying from 3100–4000/μl and neutropenia from 1353 to 2730, he obtained rises of total white cells to 4200–7700 and of neutrophils up to 2872. In two others, as also with one reported by Moeschlin (1951), with more severe poisoning, no favourable effect on the blood picture was obtained. In those who had symptoms of excitation, irritability, perspiration, general weakness, headache, loss of appetite and sleep disturbance considerable improvement was observed. These symptoms were, as Zorina suggests, probably symptoms of vitamin B6 deficiency.

Temporary improvement during dosage, but not maintained when treatment with Vitamin B6 is discontinued has been observed by Browning (1961, unpublished observation) in an early slight case of chronic benzene poisoning following very slight exposure as a laboratory assistant. Her blood picture had for several years shown some leucopenia and neutropenia (on one occasion the total white cell count had fallen to 3500/μl). Slight leucopenia had persisted for several months after all exposure to benzene had ceased and in spite of treatment with iron and liver extract. At the time when it was decided to try vitamin B6 her total white cell count was 4100/μl and total polymorphs 1990. After one month's treatment with vitamin B6 her total white cells had risen to 4560, with total polymorphs 2166 and two premature leucocytes in the stained smear; the fatigue of which she had complained had disappeared. During the next three months the total white cells oscillated between 4100 and 4560 and total polymorphs between 2000 and 2200. At the end of that time her blood picture became normal and vitamin B6 treatment was stopped, but this was followed by a return to the original slight leucopenia and neutropenia. Renewal of the treatment was again followed by a return to a normal blood picture, which remained normal for 9 months without further treatment, but later again deteriorated slightly in the form of a slight neutropenia and a colour index above 1, only to become normal again on resumption of the vitamin B6 dosage. At the time of writing it is completely normal and has remained so for some months without further therapy. It has to be remembered that in some hypersensitive individuals whose blood picture has been normal for some time after cessation of exposure, with or without treatment, any disturbance of health, such as influenza or a 'gastric upset' may be accompanied by a fall in white cells and total polymorphs. In such cases a second or third course of vitamin B6 therapy may again bring about a return to normal.

Vitamin B12 (cobalcocyanamin, cyanocobalamin)

Isolated from an extract of liver (Rickes *et al.*, 1948)), this vitamin is believed to retain most of the pure antianaemic factor and contains about 4% of cobalt, which participates in erythropoiesis. Experiments on rabbits poisoned by benzene (Di Porto and Maymone, 1951), suggest that vitamin B12 has some therapeutic value, particularly due to its cobalt fraction, both on hepatic function and on normal haemopoiesis. The animals receiving benzene alone showed congestion and degenerative changes in the liver and spleen and a bone marrow approaching a picture of aplastic anaemia. In the animals receiving vitamin B12 before the administration of benzene, there were no changes in the liver or spleen but the bone marrow showed a deficiency of the cellular elements, especially of the myeloid series, and of the erythrocyte precursors. Thus its protective action was not complete, but it was potentiated, especially on coagulation time and thrombocyte formation, when supplemented by vitamins C and K. It is not at present certain whether this effect in animals can be achieved in human beings suffering from chronic benzene poisoning. According to Appuhn and Goldeck (1957) the urinary excretion of vitamin B12 was decreased in all the chronic benzene poisoning cases investigated by them, to as practically low a level as in pernicious anaemia, but in one case, designated as 'paraerythroblastosis' it remained at the lower limit of normal.

Vitamin C (ascorbic acid)

The rationale of therapeutic administration of vitamin C in chronic benzene poisoning is based partly on animal experiments indicating that benzene poisoning is associated with an increased consumption of vitamin C and has a possible detoxicating effect owing to its stimulating action on liver function (Frada, 1937; Fischbach and Terbruggen, 1938) and that human beings exposed to benzene show a decrease in the urinary excretion of ascorbic acid (Friemann, 1936; Meyer, 1937). It is stated by Johnstone (1948) that good results have been achieved in cases of chronic benzene poisoning by the administration of 200–400 mg daily until a normal urinary level of vitamin C is obtained. Seyfried (1942) believes that the therapeutic value of vitamin C can be attributed to its effect on the slight haemorrhagic diathesis which he states is present among benzene workers especially during a season of deficient vitamin C intake. Di Porto and Maymone

Bibliography on p. 55

(1957) have also stated that vitamin C is capable of influencing favourably those factors with an anti-haemorrhagic action.

Folic acid, when used alone, has given insignificant results (Dubois-Ferrière and others), but when combined with vitamin B6 was more successful.

Cysteine was stated to have a favourable effect on the anaemia and leuco-penia of benzolism which had proved resistant to liver and intravenous iron (Pollet *et al.*, 1946). It was given in a dosage of 1 g per day. Its mode of action remained undetermined – whether a direct haemopoietic effect, an indirect sti-mulation of the bone marrow, or an antitoxic action related to sulpho-conjuga-tion.

Methionine was investigated by Duvoir *et al.* (1946), with the idea that the disturbance of balance of organic and inorganic sulphates in the urine might indicate a possibly beneficial effect of administration of sulphur. Loeper had pre-viously (1941) stated that animals given sodium hyposulphite during benzene intoxication tended to survive in greater numbers than untreated animals. Duvoir *et al.* did not find sodium hyposulphite efficacious in human blood dyscrasias. They administered successively sodium hyposulphite, penicillin and methionine (2 g daily by mouth) to a man suffering from benzene agranulocytosis. No favour-able change in the blood picture was obtained from any of the three, though penicillin had the effect of ameliorating the bucco-pharyngeal infection and was followed by a slight increase in total red cells.

ACTH and cortisone

In experimental animals poisoned with benzene, ACTH and cortisone have given good results in the hands of Massei and Marinari (1958). In human beings suffering from chronic benzene poisoning several observers have obtained en-couraging results, though Savilahti (1956) stated that ACTH and cortisone had no definite influence on the blood picture.

In Finland, Kauppila and Setälä (1956) and in Italy, Paterni and Teodori (1956) recorded results which were in complete agreement. They observed an improvement in general health and a significant increase in neutrophil granulo-cytes, which disappeared when treatment was discontinued, but no effect on erythrocytes, thrombocytes or reticulocytes. On the bone marrow it had the effect of improving maturation of the erythro- and myeloblasts. Paolino and Ver-cellino (1960) have also reported good results from ACTH treatment and point out that cortisone and its derivatives are to be recommended because they are so valuable in hypoplastic haemopathies of different etiology. The satisfactory outcome in a case of 'panmyelopathy' in a man with heavy exposure to benzene in a rubber-asbestos factory was attributed by Appuhn and Goldeck (1957) chiefly to the administration of ACTH and cortisone immediately his abnormal blood picture was discovered.

High Altitude

A somewhat empirical therapeutic measure is the suggestion of Jordi (1948) that cases of chronic benzene intoxication can be favourably influenced by a prolonged stay at high altitudes. The number of cases so treated was only 15, but it appeared that at an altitude of 1800 meters above sea-level red cells neutrophils and haemo-globin level showed a rise, and that after a return to a low altitude, though in some cases the red cell count fell slightly, the state of well-being and energy was strikingly maintained.

BIBLIOGRAPHY

Ambrosio, L. (1942) Behaviour of Blood Enzymes in Poisoning by Solvents, *Biochim. Terap. Sper.*, 29:335.

Amiel, J. L. (1960) Negative Attempt at Induction of Leukaemia in Mice by Benzene, *Rev. Franc. Etudes Clin. Biol.*, 5:198.

André, R. and B. Dreyfus (1951) Anémie hémolytique grave. Rôle probable du Benzol, *Sang*, 22:57.

Appuhn, E. and H. Goldeck (1957) Früh- und Spätschäden der Blutbildung durch Benzol und seine Homologen, *Arch. Gewerbepathol. Gewerbehyg.*, 15:399.

Askey, J. M. (1928) Aplastic Anaemia due to Benzol Poisoning, *Calif. [West.] Med.*, 29:262.

Baldi,G. and R. Riccardi-Polloni (1954) Patologia professionale da Etere di Petrolio e da Benzina, *Rass., Med. indust.*, 23:77.

Batchelor, J. J. (1927) Relative Toxicity of Benzol and its higher Homologues, *Am. J. Hyg.*, 7:276.

Beinhauer, F. (1896) Über Benzolvergiftung, *Münch. Med. Wschr.*, 43:902.

Beisele, P. (1912) Ein Beitrag zur Kasuistik der Benzoldämpfvergiftung, *Münch. Med. Wschr.*, 49:2286.

Bénard, R., L. Derobert and C. Albahary (1942) Examen anatomopathologique d'un cas d'Anémie mortelle survenue 20 mois après la Cessation de Travail dans le Benzol, *Sang*, 15:355.

Bénard, R., M. Poumailloux and J. Tiret (1942) Un nouveau Cas d'Hémopathie benzolique tar-dée, *Sang*, 15:351.

Bernard, J. (1942) La Lymphocytose benzénique, *Sang*, 15:501.

Bernard, J. and L. Braier (1950) Les Leucoses benzéniques, *Proc. 3rd Intern. Congr. Soc. Haematol.* (Grune & Stratton).

Bernard, J., L. Braier, A. Basset and A. Bruyet (1949) La Prophylaxie du Benzolisme, *Semaine Hôp. Paris*, 25:1634.

Bernard-Pichon, A. (1942) Incertitudes et Difficultés de la Prévention du Benzolisme par la Sur-veillance hématologique systématique, *Sang*, 15:340.

Berzelius, J. (1817) *Treatise on Chemistry*, 2nd. ed. Louis Harman et Cie., Brussels.

Bessis, M. and J. Breton-Gorius (1956) Étude au Microscope électronique, *Compt. Rend. Acad. Sci.*, 243:36, 1235.

Beyer, G. (1933) Chronische Benzolvergiftung bei Kaninchen, *Z. Ges. Exptl. Med.*, 91:401.

Biancacchio, A. and V. Fermariello (1961) Protoforine libere eritrocitaire e Coproporforine urinaire nel'Intossicazione subcronica sperimentale da Benzolo, *Folia Med. Nap.*, 43:588.

Binder, A. (1921) Zur akuten tödlichen Vergiftung mit Benzoldämpfen, *Mschr. Unfallheilk.*, 28:202.

Binet, L., A. Conté and H. Bourlière (1945) Intoxication benzolique mortelle chez une Femme vendant des Sacs en Cuir synthétique, *Bull. Mém. Soc. Méd. Hôp. Paris*, 61:118.

Biondi, S. (1956) Il Comportamento della Catalasi e della Perossidase nei Conigli trattati con Ben-zolo, *Haematologica*, 41:721.

Bousser, J. (1948) La Polynucleose benzolique, tardive, *Sang*, 19:430.

Bousser, J., R. Neydé and R. Fabre (1948) Un Cas d'Hémopathie benzolique très retardée à type de Lymphosarcome, *Arch. Malad. Profess.*, 9:159.

Bousser, J. and S. Tara (1951) A propos de trois Cas de Leucémie myéloide provoquées par le Benzol, *Arch. Malad. Profess.*, 12:329.

Bousser, J., C. Albahary and S. Tara (1952) Aspects atypiques des Hémopathies benzoliques, *Arch. Malad. Profess.*, 13:20.

Bowers, V. H. (1947) Reaction of human Blood-forming Tissues to chronic Benzene Exposure, *Brit. J. Indust. Med.*, 4:87.

Brandino, G. (1922) Osservazione istologiche nel'Intossicazione acute e croniche da Benzolo, *Gazz. Med. Lombarda*, 81:141.

Brindeau, A. (1931) Deux Cas d'Anémie pernicieuse par Intoxication benzolique, *Ann. Hyg. publ. Paris*, N.S., 9:99.

Brocher, J. E. W. (1929) Beitrag zur Panmyelopathia atrophicans und zur Frage der Benzolintoxikation in Druckereien, *Zbl. Inn. Med.*, 5:1186.

Buchmann, E. (1911) Zur Frage der akuten Benzolvergiftungen, *Klin. Wschr.*, 48:936.

Buffet, A. and S. Tara (1960) L'Hématologie des Ouvriers du Pétrole, *Sang*, 31:791.

Caccuri, S. (1946) Su alcuni Casi di 'Benzolismo latente', *Rif. Med.*, 60:416.

Caldwell, J. E., R. H. Quidzes, J. D. Porsche and F. Fenger (1945) Recent Studies on yellow Bone Marrow Extracts, *Amer. J. Med. Sci.*, 209:717.

Camp, W. E. and E. A. Baumgartner (1915) Inflammatory Reaction in Rabbits with severe Leucopenia, *J. Ecptl. Med.*, 22:174.

Cantor, M. M. and J. W. Scott (1945) Agranulocytic Angina effectively treated with intravenous Pyridoxine (vitamin B6), *Canad. Med. Ass. J.*, 52:368.

Carter, G. (1928) Fatal Case of accidental Poisoning by Benzol Vapour, *Brit. Med. J.*, 11:794.

Chassevant, A. and L. Garnier (1903) Toxicité du Benzène et de quelques Hydrocarbures aromatiques homologues, *Compt. Rend. Soc. Biol.*, 55:1255.

Chevallier, P., M. Lamotte and R. Undenstock (1942) Trois cas d'Anémieleucose benzolique, *Sang*, 15:391.

Cirla, P. (1960) La Sostituzione dal Benzolo con Eptano, *Rass. Med. Indust.*, 29:276.

Cohen, J. B. (1909) *Organic Chemistry for advanced Students*, p.3. Edward Arnold, London.

Cronin, H. J. (1924) Benzol Poisoning in the Rubber Industry, *Boston Med. Surg. J.*, 191:1164.

Damashek, W. and M. Baldwin (1958) The Di Guglielmo Syndrome, *Blood*, 13:192.

Damashek, W. (1960) Leukaemia. Present Status, *Maryland Med. J.*, 9:244.

Danysz, Mme. (1942) Quelques Resultats hématologiques constatés chez des Ouvriers travaillant dans le Benzène, *Sang*, 15:348.

Debray, M., R. J. Huguier, Mlle. Provendier, D. Frileux and J. Vinces (1950) Un Cas d'Hémopathie benzolique traité par Transfusions sanguines, Penicilline et Transplant d'Os spongieux, *Bull. Mém. Soc. Méd. Hôp. Paris*, 66:1069.

Debray, M., R. Wattlebled and J. Bertrand (1950) Un Cas d'hémopathie benzolique traité par Transfusions sanguines, Penicilline et Transplants d'Os spongieux, *Bull. Mém. Soc. Méd. Hôp. Paris*, 66:1069.

De Franciscis, P. and F. Marsico (1947) Il Comportamento della Catalasi e della Perossidasi nei Conigli trattati con Benzolo, *Bull. Soc. Biol. Sper.*, 23:808.

Deichmann, W. and L. J. Schafer (1942) Phenol Studies, *Amer. J. Clin. Path.*, 12:129.

Deichmann, W. and J. R. Thomas (1943) Glucuronic Acid in Urine as a Maesure of Absorption of certain Organic Compounds, *J. Indust. Hyg. Toxicol.*, 25:286.

Delore, P. and J. Borgamano (1928) Leucémie aiguë au Cours de l'Intoxication benzénique, *J. Méd. Lyon*, 9:227.

Dept. Sci. Ind. Res. (1939) Methods for the Detection of Toxic Gases in Industry, *Leaflet no. 4.* H.M.S.O. London.

De Rosa, R. (1955) L'Azione dell'Adenina sul Mielogramma nella Intossicazione sperimentale da Benzolo, *Folia Med. Nap.*, 38:398.

Derot, M. (1956) Autre Cas d'Intoxication aiguë par Ingestion de Benzène; syndrome hépatorenale aiguë, *Bull. Mem. Soc. Méd. Hôp. Paris*, 72:1037.

Derot, M. and M. Philbert (1956) Aiguë par Ingestion de Benzène, *Bull. Mem. Soc. méd. Hôp. Paris*, 72:1035.

Di Guglielmo, G. (1923) Eritremia acute, *29th. Congr. Intern. Med. Rome*.

—(1928a) Le Eritremie, *Haematologica*, 9:301.

—(1928b) La Patologia et la Clinica del Sistema reticoloendotheliale, *Haematologica*, 9:349.

—(1938) Analogie e Differenza tra Eritremia e Leucemia acuta, *Haematologica*, 19:341.

Di Guglielmo, G. and Iannacone (1950) Inhibition of Mitosis and regressive Changes in Erythro-blasts in acute Erythropathy caused by occupational Benzene Poisoning, *Acta Haematol.*, 19: 144.

Di Guglielmo, G. and M. Ricci (1958) Prima Descrizione di un Caso du Mielosi eritremica da Benzolo nella sua Varieta cronica, *Settim. Med.*, 45:365.

Dimmel, H. (1932) Vergiftungen mit aromatischen Substanzen, *Wien. Med. Wschr.*, 82:526.

—(1933) Zur Klinik der chronischen Benzolvergiftung, *Arch. Gewerbepath. Gewerbehyg.*, 4:414.

Di Porto, A. and S. Maymone (1951) L'Azione della vitamine B 12 potenziata della vitamine C e vitamine K nel Intossicazione sperimentale da Benzolo, *Il Policlinico, Sez. Med.*, 58: 116, 172.

Dolin, B. H. (1943) Determination of Benzene in Presence of Toluene, Xylene and other substances. Industr. Hyg. Bull., 22:373. *Industr. Eng. Chem. Anal. Ed.*, 15:242.

Dotta, F. (1960) Studi sul Comportamento del Surrene nel Intossicazione benzolica sperimentale, *Folia Med. Nap.*, 42:872.

Drouet, P. L., L. Perquin and R. Herbeval (1947) Lymphomatose chronique chez un Benzolique, *Sang*, 18:246.

Drummond, J. C. and L. Finar (1938) Muconic Acid as a metabolic Product of Benzene, *Biochem., J.*, 32:79.

Dubois-Ferrière, H. (1951) Influence de la Vitamine B6 (Pyridoxine) et de l'Acide folique sur la Neutropénie benzolique, *Schweiz. Med. Wschr.*, 81:1235.

Duke, W. W. (1913) Causes of Variations in Platelet Counts, *Arch. Int. Med.*, 11:100.

Dul'tsin, M. S., N. S. Rosanova and F. E. Fainshtein (1960) On the Problem of the Relation of Aplastic Anaemia to Leucosis, *Probl. Gemat.*, 5:3.

Duvoir, M., R. Fabre and L. Derobert (1916) La Signification du Benzène dans la Moelle osseuse au Cours des Hémopathies benzoliques, *Arch. Malad. Profess.*, 7:77.

Duvoir, M. and L. Derobert (1942) L'Eosinophile des Benzèniques, *Arch. Malad. Profess.*, 15:241.

—(1942) Les Hémopathies benzoliques retardées, *Sang*, 15:267.

—(1946) Les Réactions hématologiques exceptionnelles du Benzolisme chronique, *Rec. Trav. Inst. Natl. Hyg.*, 2:350.

Duvoir, M., L. Derobert and C. Albahary (1942) Examen pathologique d'un Cas d'Anémie mor-telle survenue vingt Mois après la Cessation du Travail dans le Benzol, *Sang*, 15:356.

Duvoir, M., L. Pollet and M. Gaultier (1946) Remarques thérapeutiques sur l'Intoxication benzo-lique, *Arch. Malad. Profess.*, 7:230.

Dworetsky, A. (1914) Rätselhafte Massenvergiftungen in Russischen Fabriken, *Münch. Med. Wschr.*, 61:1306.

Elkins, H. B. (1954) Analysis of biological Materials as Indices of Exposure to organic Solvents. *Arch. Industr. Hyg.*, 9:210.

—(1959) *The Chemistry of Industrial Toxicology*, 2nd. ed., p. 410. Wiley & Sons, New York.

Elmino, O., G. Rozera and G. Colicchio (1960) Mielosi eritremica del Coniglio nell'Intossicazione da Benzolo, *Folia Med. Nap.*, 42: 1228.

Emil-Weil, P. (1932) La Leucémie post-benzolique, *Bull. Mém. Soc. Méd. Hôp. Paris*, 46:750.

—(1938) A propos de l'Intoxication benzolique, *Sang*, 12:519.

Emil-Weil, P., S. Perles and Aschkenazy (1938) Le Benzolisme latent, *Sang*, 12:151.

Engelhardt, W. E. (1931) Chronische gewerbliche Benzolvergiftung, *Samml. Vergiftungsf.*, 2:2306.

Erf, L. A. and C. P. Rhoads (1939) The haematological Effects of Benzene (Benzol) Poisoning, *J. Ind. Hyg. Toxicol.*, 21:421.

Fabre, R. (1946) Sur le Métabolisme des Hydrocarbures cycliques, *Bull. Soc. Chim. Biol.*, 28:762.

—(1960) Sur les Propriétés toxicologiques des Constituants des Pétroles, *Arch. Malad. Profess.*, 21:97.

Fabre, R., R. Truhaut, E. Vernier and J. Bernuchon (1952) Recherches toxicologiques sur les Sol-vants de Replacement de Benzène, Isopropyl Benzène, *Trans. 3rd Congr. Techn. Nat. Sécurité Hyg. Trav. Avignon.* [Abs. in *Arch. Indust. Hyg.*, 6 (1953) 441.]

Fabre, R., R. Truhaut, J. Bernuchon and F. Loisillier (1955) Recherches toxicologiques sur les Sol-vants de Remplacement de Benzène, *Arch. Malad. Profess.*, 16:288.

Falconer, E. H. (1933) Instance of Lymphatic Leukaemia following Benzol Poisoning, *Amer. J. Med. Sci.*, 186:353.

Faure-Gilly, J., S. Morel and M. Bruel (1948) Syndrome hémorrhagique benzolique avec simple Alteration morphologique des Plaquettes, *Arch. Malad. Profess.*, 9:274.

Feil, A. (1933) Le Benzolisme professionel, *Progr. Med.*, 41:129.

Ferguson, T., W. H. Harvey and T. D. Hamilton (1933) Enquiry into the relative Toxicity of Benzene and Toluene, *J. Hyg. (Lond.)*, 33:547.

Fischbach, H. and A. Terbruggen (1938) Über die Wirkung von Vitamin C, thyreotropem Hormon und Thyroxin auf das Leberglykogen und die Schilddrüse, *Virchow's Arch.*, 301:186.

Fiske, C. H. (1921) Determination of inorganic Sulphate, total Sulphate and total Sulphur in Urine by the Benzidine Method, *J. Biol. Chem.*, 47:59.

Flandin, C. and J. Roberti (1922) Purpura hemorrhagica mortel due à une Intoxication professionelle par les Vapeurs de Benzol, *Bull. Mém. Soc. Méd. Hôp. Paris*, 46:35, 58.

Floret, F. (1926) Neuere Beobachtungen über gewerbliche Schädigungen durch Kohlenwasserstoff, *Zbl. Gewerbehyg.*, 13:7.

Flury, F. and F. Zernik (1931) *Schädliche Gase, Dämpfe, Nebel, Rauch und Staubarten*, Springer, Berlin.

Fontana, G. (1921) Nuove Richerche sul Sangue e sugli Organi ematopoietici nell'Intossicazione benzolica, *G. Clin. Med.*, 2:93.

Forssman, S. and K. O. Frykholm (1947) Benzene Poisoning with Reference to Presence of Ester Sulphate, Muconic Acid, Urochrome and Polyphenols in Urine, *Acta Med. Scand.*, 128:256.

Frada, G. (1937) Azione dell'Acido Ascorbio sul Tasso glicemico del Coniglio, *Biochim. Terap. Sper.*, 24:125.

Friemann, A. (1936) Zur Diagnose der chronischen Benzolvergiftung, *Arch. Gewerbepath. Gewerbehyg.*, 7:278.

Fuhner, H. (1921) Die narkotische Wirkung des Benzins und seiner Bestandteile, *Biochem. Z.*, 115:235.

Gabor, S. (1959) Modificazioni degli Enzimi nel Benzolismo, *Med. Lavoro*, 50:257.

Gadrat, J., J. Quercy and R. Fedou (1959) Hémopathie atypique consecutive à une Intoxication benzolique chronique, *Arch. Malad. Profess.*, 20:121.

Galavotti, B. and F. M. Troisi (1950) Erythroleukaemic Myelosis in Benzene Poisoning, *Brit. J. Ind. Med.*, 7:79.

Garnier, J. and R. Cordier (1942) Sur deux Cas de Réaction lymphomonocytaire important chez des Ouvriers en Contact quotidien avec les Emanations benzoliques, *Sang*, 15:496.

Gaultier, M. and E. Fournier (1959) Hémopathies toxiques d'Origine mixte ou incertain, *Ann. Méd. Lég.*, 39:309.

Genhard, A. (1910) Über Benzolvergiftung, *Schweiz. Korresp. Bl. Arz.*, 4:387.

Gerarde, H. W. (1956) Toxicological Studies on Hydrocarbons. A Method for the quantitative Collection of femoral Marrow in small Laboratory Animals, *Arch. Ind. Hlth.*, 13:331.

—(1960) *Toxicology and Biochemistry of Aromatic Hydrocarbons*, Elsevier, Amsterdam.

Graham, J. C. (1958) Unsuspected Benzene Contamination in a Can-making Process, *Trans. Ass. Ind. Med. Off.*, p. 86.

Granati, A., D. Scavo and L. Sereno (1958) Il Recambio protidico nella Intossicazione benzolica sperimentale, *Fol. Med. Nap.*, 41:923.

Grazioli, G. and C. A. Monteverdi (1960) [cited by L. Resegotti] Survey of Italian Literature on Industrial Medicine, *Panminerva Medicine*, 2:142.

Greenburg, L. (1926) Benzol Poisoning as an Industrial Hazard, *U.S. Treas. Publ. Hlth. Rep.*, 41:1410.

Greenburg, L., M. R. Mayers, L. Goldwater and H. R. Smith (1939) Benzene Poisoning in the Rotogravure Industry in New York City, *Ind. Med. Toxicol.*, 21:395.

Guasch, J., E. Pelayo and J. Villespin (1959) Benzol Anaemia complicated by acute Leukaemia evolving after 6 years, *Sangre*, 4:129. [Abs. in *Leukaemia Abs.* 8 (1960) 5418].

Guertin, D. L. and H. W. Gerarde (1959) Toxicological Studies on Hydrocarbons. A method for the quantitative Determination of benzene and certain Alkyl Benzenes in Blood, *Arch. Ind. Hlth.*, 20:262.

Hamilton, A. (1925) *Industrial Poisons in the United States*, MacMillan, New York.

—(1928) Lessening menace of benzol poisoning in American Industry, *J. Ind. Hyg.*, 10:227.

—(1931) Benzene (Benzol) Poisoning, *Arch. Pathol. Lab. Med.*, 11:434, 601.

Hamilton-Paterson, J. and E. Browning (1944) Toxic Effects in Women exposed to industrial Rubber Solutions, *Brit. Med. J.*, 1:349.

Hammond, J. W. and E. R. Herman (1960) Industrial Hygiene Features of a Petrochemical Benzene Plant Design and Operation, *Amer. Ind. Hyg. Ass. J.*, 21:173.

Harrington, T. F. (1917) Industrial Benzol Poisoning in Massachusetts, *Boston Med. Surg. J.*, 177:203.

Hawk, P. B. and O. Bergeim (1927) *Practical Physiological Chemistry*, p. 770, Blakiston, Philadelphia.

Hayhurst, E. R. and B. E. Neiswander (1931) Care of chronic benzene poisoning, *J. Am. Med. Assoc.*, 96:269.

Heffter, A. (1915) Über die akute Vergiftung durch Benzoldampf, *Dtsch. Med. Wschr.*, 41:182.

Heilmeyer, H. L. (1942) Hypochrome Anemien und Eisenstoffwechsel, *Verhandl. Gesellsch. Inn. Med.*, 52:276.

Heim de Balzac, F. and E. Agasse Lafont (1910) Réactions hématiques du benzénisme professionel, *Ass. Franc. pour l'avancement des Sciences, Congrés de Toulouse.*

—(1933) Intoxications mortelles ou de Gravité variable, en Serie, par Emploi d'un Adhésive solubilisé par le Benzène, *Bull. Acad. Med. Paris*, 110:31.

Heitzmann, O. (1931) Vergleichende pathologische Anatomie der experimentellen Benzol- und Benzinvergiftung, *Arch. Gewerbepathol. Gewerbehyg.*, 2:515.

Hektoen, L. (1916) Effect of Benzene on Production of Antibodies, *J. Infect. Dis.*, 19:69.

Hess, W. (1935) Atmung und Gärung bei der experimentellen Benzolleukämie, *Frankf. Z. Pathol.*, 47:522.

Hirokawa, T. (1958) Studies on Poisoning by Benzol and its Homologues, *Jap. J. Med. Sci. Biol.*, 8:275.

—(1960) Quelques Observations sur l'Intoxication Benzénique, *Arch. Malad. Profess.*, 21:46.

Hogan, J. F. and J. H. Shrader (1923) Benzol Poisoning, *Amer. J. Publ. Hlth.*, 13:279.

Holleman, A. F. (1915) Vijftig Jaar Benzolonderzoek, *Mitt. Gesch. Med. Naturw.*, 14:258.

Hunter, F. T. and S. S. Hanflig (1927) Chronic Benzol Poisoning, *Boston Med. Surg. J.*, 197:292.

Hunter, F. T. (1939) Chronic Exposure to Benzene (Benzol), *J. Ind. Hyg. Toxicol.*, 21:331.

Iannacone, A. and G. Cachella (1959) Histochemical Alterations of the Endocrine Glands in experimental Benzene Poisoning, *Sci. Med. Ital. (Eng.)*, 8:59.

Joachimoglu (1915) Über den Nachweis des Benzols in Organen und seine Verteilung im Organismus, *Biochem. Z.*, 70:93.

Johnstone, R. T. (1948) *Occupational Medicine and Industrial Hygiene*, p. 203, Henry Kimpton, London.

Jordi, A. (1948) Le Traitement aux hautes Altitudes de l'Intoxication chronique par le Benzol, *Arch. Malad. Profess.*, 9:599.

Kammer, A. G., N. Isenberg and M. E. Berg (1938) Medical Supervision of Benzene Plant Workers, *J. Am. Med. Ass.*, 11:1452.

Katzen, R. (1958) Watch Petrochemicals grow in Europe, *Petroleum Refiner*, 37:171.

Kauppila, O. and A. Setälä (1956) Chronic Benzene Poisoning. Report of 5 Cases, *Ann. Med. Int. Fenn.*, 45:49.

Kekulé, A (1865) [cited by J. B. Cohen in] *Organic Chemistry for Advanced Students*, p. 434, Edward Arnold, London, 1909.

Kline, O., C. A. Elvehjem and E. B. Hart (1936) Further Evidence for the Existence of Vitamin B4, *Biochem. J.*, 30:780.

Kobert, R. (1906) *Lehrbuch der Intoxikationen*, 2nd. ed., Ferdinand Enke, Stuttgart.

Koeffler, H. (1960) On the Pathogenesis, clinical Aspects and symptomatic aplastic Forms of Anaemia with final Picture of Leucosis, *Med. Klin.*, 55:1394.

Koppenhöfer, G. F. (1935) Morphologische und chemische Untersuchungen bei einem Fall einer tödlichen akuten Benzolvergiftung, *Arch. Gewerbepathol. Gewerbehyg.*, 6:417.

Koranyi, A. von (1912) Die Beeinflüssung der Leukämie durch Benzol, *Berl. Klin. Wschr.*, 49:1357.

Kuhbeck, J. and V. Lachnit (1962) The Problem of early Diagnosis of Injury from Benzol and Toluol, *Arch. Gewerbepathol. Gewerbehyg.*, 19:149.

Kuhlman, D. (1959) Mitteilung einer tödlichen Benzolvergiftung aus der Schuhindustrie, *Zbl. Arbeitsschutz.*, 9:62.

Lachnit, V and E. E. Reimer (1959) Panmyelopathien durch Aromatische Lösungsmittel, *Wien. Klin. Wschr.*, 71:365.

Laignel-Lavastine, Lévy R. and H. Desoille (1928) Un Cas mortel d'Anémie aplastique hémorrhagique par Intoxication benzénique professionelle, *Bull. Mem. Soc. Méd. Hôp. Paris*, 52: 1264.

Lamy, M. and P. Kissel (1938) Étude clinique et hématologique de 9 Cas d'Intoxication professionelle par le Benzol, *Bull. Mem. Soc. Méd. Hôp. Paris*, 62: 1117.

Landé, K. and L. Kalinowsky (1928) Zur Klinik der gewerblichen Berufserkrankungen durch Benzol, *Med. Klin.*, 24: 655.

Langlois, J. P. and G. Desbouis (1907) Des Effets des Vapeurs hydrocarbonées sur le Sang, *J. Physiol. Pathol. Gen.*, 9: 253.

Larssen, A. and E. Thrysen (1951) Benzene Poisoning in Industries and its Prevention, *Arkiv Hig. Rada* [Abs. in *Arch. Industr. Hyg.*, 4: 512.]

Latta, J. S. and L. T. Davies (1941) Effects on Blood and haemopoietic Organs of albino Rats of repeated Administration of Benzene, *Arch. Pathol.*, 31: 55.

Lavarino, A. and A. Masoero (1955) Osservazioni ematologiche su alcuni Casi di Intossicazioen professionale da Benzolo, *Rass. Med. Ind.*, 24: 291.

Lavoisier, A. L. (1901) *Traité élementaire de Chimie*, 1: 303, Deterville, Paris.

Lazarew, N. W., A. J. Brussilowskaya, J. N. Lawrow and F. P. Lifschitz (1931) Über die Durchlässigkeit der Haut für Benzin und Benzol, *Arch. Hyg. Berl.*, 106: 112.

—(1931) Quantitive Untersuchungen über die Resorption einiger organischer Gifte durch die Haut ins Blut, *Arch. Gewerbepathol. Gewerbehyg.*, 2: 641.

Lazzaro, G. (1933) Mielosi eritremica acuta, *Haematologica*, 14: 483.

Lechelle, Coste, Thieffrey and Cuadrano (1940) Les Modalités de l'Intoxication benzolique, leur Prognostic, leur Prophylaxie, *Bull. Soc. Méd. Hôp. Paris*, 56: 353.

Legge, T. M. (1920) Chronic Benzol Poisoning, *J. Ind. Hyg.*, 1: 539.

LeNoir and Claude (1897) Sur un Cas de Purpura attribué à l'Intoxication par le Benzène, *Bull. Mém. Soc. Méd. Hôp. Paris*, 3me. sér., 14: 1251.

Lewin, L. (1907) Die akute tödlich Vergiftung durch Benzoldampf, *Münch. Med. Wschr.*, 54: 2377.

Lignac, G. O. E. (1932) Die Benzolleukämie bei Menschen und weissen Mausen, *Klin. Wschr.*, 12: 109.

Litzner, S. (1932) Erkrankungen durch Benzol und seine Homologen, *Ergebn. Ges. Med.*, 17: 67.

Loeper, M. M. (1941) Benzol et Foie, *Progr. Med.*, 69: 729.

Loeper, M. M., R. Fabre and Borreau (1946) Leucémie benzénique très tardive avec Persistance du Benzol dans le Sang et la Moelle Osseuse, *Bull. Acad. Med.*, 130: 706.

Loeper, M. M. and J. Mallarme (1942) Leucose aiguë chez un sujet anciennement intoxiqué par le Benzène et traité par les Rayons X, *Sang*, 15: 406.

Lynsky, W. (1960) Separation of Polycyclic Aromatic Hydrocarbons in complex Mixtures, *Anal. Chem.*, 32: 684.

Lynsky, W. and C. R. Raha (1961) Polycyclic Hydrocarbons in commercial Solvents, *Toxicol. Appl. Pharmacol.*, 3: 469.

McCord, C. P., N. Cox and C. O'Boyle (1932) New Investigation of the Toxicity of Benzene and Impurities, *Ind. Hlth. Cons. Labs., Cincinnatti.*

McLean, J. A. (1960) Blood Dyscrasia after Contact with Petrol containing Benzol, *Med. J. Australia*, 47: 485.

Maffet, P. A., T. F. Doherty and J. Monkman (1956) Collection and Determination of Microamounts of Benzene or Toluene in Air, *Ind. Hyg. Quart.*, 17: 186.

Mallory, T. B., E. A. Gall and W. J. Brickley (1939) Chronic Exposure to Benzene, *J. Ind. Hyg. Toxicol.*, 21: 355.

Marchal, G. (1952) A propos de la Communication de André et Dreyfus (q.v.) Maladie de Di Guglielmo, *Sang*, 23: 682.

Marchal, G. and G. Duhamel (1950) L'Anémie hémolytique dans les Leucémies, *Sang*, 21: 254.

Marchand, M. M. (1960) Un Cas mortel de Leucose benzolique, *Arch. Malad. Profess.*, 21: 576.

Massei, G. and A. Marinari (1958) Effetti del Cortisone e dell ACTH nella Emopatia benzolica sperimentale, *Arch. per le Sci. Med.*, 106.

Mauro, G. (1925) Avvelenamento sperimentale da Benzolo. Prima Sintomi, *Med. Lavoro*, 16: 168.

Mayer, F. Y. (1938) Determination of Benzene in Blood and Parts of Organs by special Analysis, *Mikrochemie*, 24: 29.

Mazel, P., D. Picard and J. Bourret (1944) La Mononucléose est elle une Forme 'actuelle' de la Myélotoxicose benzolique?, *Arch. Malad. Profess.*, 6: 18.

Merklen, P. and L. Israel (1934) L'Intoxication par le Benzol; Aleucie hémorrhagique, *Sang*, 8: 700.

Meyer, A. (1937) Chronische Benzolvergiftung und Vitamin C, *Z. Vitaminforsch.*, 6: 83.

Meyer, F. and L. Kerk (1960) Über die percutane Resorption von Eserin aus Benzol und einigen verwandten Lösungsmitteln, *Archiv. Toxikol.*, 18: 131.

Mitnik, P. and S. Genkin (1931) Zur Klinik der Benzolvergiftung, *Arch. Gewerbepathol. Gewerbehyg.*, 2: 457.

Mitscherlich, A. (1835) *Elements der Chimie*.

Moeschlin, S. (1940) Erythroblastosen, Erythroleukamien und Erythroblastamien, *Folia Haematol.*, 64: 262.

Moeschelin, S. (1951) Alquinos Resultades de la Punsión del Bozo en las Emfermedades de la Sangre, *Rev. clin. Espan.*, 42: 382.

Monckeberg, J. G. (1913) Beitrage zur akuten und chronischen Myelämie, *Verh. Dtsch. Pathol. Gesellsch.*, 16: 148.

Morelli, A. (1958) Il Problema dell'Emopatia Benzolica, *Lav. Umano*, 10: 337.

Nahum, L. H. and H. E. Hoff (1934) Mechanism of sudden Death in experimental acute Benzol Poisoning, *J. Pharmacol. Exptl. Therap.*, 50: 336.

National Safety Council (1926) Chemical and Rubber Sections. Final Report on Benzol, *Natl. Bur. of Casualty and Surety Underwriters*.

Nencki, M. and P. Giacosa (1880) Über die Oxydation der Aromatischen Kohlenwasserstoffe in Tierkörper, *Hoppe-Zeyler Z.*, 4: 325.

Neumann, W. (1915) Experimentelles zur Wirkung des Benzols, *Dtsch. Med. Wschr.*, 41: 394.

Nick, H. (1922) Erfolgreiche Behandlung einer schweren akuten Benzolvergiftung durch Lethicin-emulsion, *Klin. Wschr.*, 1: 68.

Nikulina, M. and A. Titowa (1934) Die Frage der Thrombopenie als einer der frühesten Symptome der chronischen Benzolintoxikationen, *Arch. Gewerbepathol. Gewerbehyg.*, 5: 201.

Nissen, N. L. and O. Soeberg (1953) Erythromyelosis. Review and Report of a Case in a Benzene (Benzol) Worker, *Acta Med. Scand.*, 145: 56.

Novikov, Y. V. (1957) Data on Basis of which to establish the permissible Limit of Benzol Concentration in the Atmosphere, Abst. in *Soviet Med.* 1959, Part B. 3: 318.

Nunziante, C. A. and A. Granata (1955) Ricerche di Ematochimica en Sangue periferico nelle Intossicazione professionale da Benzina e da Eptano, *Acta Istichimica*, 2: 88.

Oppenheim, M. (1930) Hautschädigungen durch einer Benzol-vergussmasse Lösung, *Wien. Klin. Wschr.*, 43: 249.

Orzechowski, G. (1929) Chronische Benzolvergiftung und Knochenmark, *Virchow's Arch. Pathol. Anat.*, 271: 191.

Pagnotto, L. D., H. B. Elkins, H. G. Brugsch and J. E. Walkley (1961) Industrial Benzene Exposure from Petroleum Naphtha, *J. Am. Ind. Hyg. Ass.*, 22: 417.

Paolino, W., L. Resegotti and S. Sartoris (1960) Radioisotope Study of experimental Intoxication by Benzene, *Minerva Med.*, 51: 33.

—(1961) Comportamento dei Sulfridili serici e tessutali nell'Intossicazione sperimentale da Benzolo, *Folia Med. Nap.*, 43: 763.

Paolino, W. and E. Vercellino (1960) Effects of Adenine on Blood Disease due to Benzene Poisoning, *Panminerva Med.*, 2: 5.

Pappenheim, A. (1914) Experimentelles zur Wirkung des Benzols, *Dtsch. Med. Wschr.*, 41: 394.

Pardon, N. and L. Foerster (1959) Note complémentaire sur l'Hématologie des Sujets exposés aux Solvants Benzoliques actuels, *Arch. Malad. Profess.*, 20: 752.

Parke, D. V. and R. T. Williams (1953) The Metabolism of Benzene, *Biochem. J.*, 46: 236.

Parker, F. P. and R. R. Kracke (1936) Further Studies on Granulopenia, *Am. J. Clin. Pathol.*, 6: 41.

Paterni, L. (1953) Emopatia Benzolica; Rivista; Contributo casistica, *Riv. Infort. Malad. Profess.*, 40: 217.

—(1958) Emopatia de Idrocarburi Benzenici, *Rass. Med. Ind.*, 27: 337.

Paterni, L., P. Gemini and I. Dotta (1954) Emopatia Benzolica nel Ratto; Mielosi Typo leucemico erythremico, *Haematologia*, 38: 283.

Paterni, L. and G. Russo (1960) Il primo Caso di Anomalia Pelgeriana nella Emopatia Benzenica, *Hematol. Arch.*, 45: 213.

Paterni, L. and S. Teodori (1956) Sulla Terapia dell'Emopatia Benzolica, trattamento con ACTH, *Med. Lavoro*, 47:221.

Paul, W. D., V. A. Friedlander and C. P. McCord (1927) Basophilic Material in Benzol Poisoning, *J. Ind. Hyg. Toxicol.*, 9:193.

Pearce, S. J., H. H. Schrenk and W. P. Yant (1936) Microcolorimetric Determination of Benzene in Blood and Urine, *U.S. Bureau Mines Dept. Invest. no. 3302.*

Peltzer, J. (1934) Determination of Benzene in Organs, *J. Pharmacol. Chem.*, 20:224.

Penati, F. and E. Vigliani (1938) Sul Problema delle Mielopatie aplastiche, pseudoaplastiche e leuchemiche da Benzolo, *Rass. Med. Ind.*, 9:345.

Perrault, M. (1946) [in Discussion by Duvoir, Pollet and Gaultier, 1946], *Arch. Malad. Profess.*, 7:230.

Perrault, M. and S. Cottet (1941) Les Réactions hépatiques devant l'Intoxication Benzolique, *Séance plénière de la Soc. Méd. Hôp. Paris*, p. 133.

Perrault, M., L. Derobert and Tiret (1944) Hémopathie Benzolique retardée. Dosage du Benzène dans la Moelle osseuse, *Arch. Malad. Profess.*, 15:239.

Perrin, M., P. Kissel and L. Perquin (1938) Leucose aiguë Benzolique, *Paris Med.*, 1:533.

Peters, J. P. and D. van Slyke (1932) *Quantitative Clinical Chemistry*, p. 892, Bailliere, Tindall & Cox, London.

Picard, D., J. Bourret and A. Lafontaine (1944) Anémies transitoires chez des Ouvrières exposées au Benzol, *Arch. Malad. Profess.*, 6:137.

Pollet, A., M. Gaultier and A. Lafontaine (1946) Action favorable de la Cystéine dans un Cas d'Anémie Benzolique rebelle, *Bull. Mém. Soc. Méd. Hôp. Paris*, p. 598.

Porteous, J. W. and R. T. Williams (1949) Metabolism of Benzene in Rabbits, *Biochem. J.*, 44:46.

Pulford, W. S. (1931) Benzol Poisoning. Report of a Case, *Calif. [West.] Med.*, 35:361.

Rachet, J., Lumière and L. Derobert (1944) Hémopathie benzolique. Dosage du Benzène dans la Moelle osseuse, *Arch. Malad. Profess.*, 6:316.

Rachner, H. (1944) Chloroleukämie als Folge einer Benzolvergiftung, *Dtsch. Med. Wschr.*, 70:219.

Raynaud, R., C. Imbert and J. R. d'Eshouges (1947) Hémopathie Benzolique avec Myéloblastose intense sans Manifestations cliniques, *Sang*, 18:418.

Reader, V. (1929) A second thermolabile water-soluble Accessory necessary for the Nutrition of the Rat, *Biochem. J.*, 23:689.

Reifschneider, C. A. (1922) Benzol Poisoning; its Occurrence and Prevention, *Natl. Safety Council 11th. Ann. Congr. Proc. Detroit*, p. 249.

Rejsek, K. and M. Rejskova (1955) Long term Observation of chronic Benzene Poisoning, *Acta Med. Scand.*, 152:71.

Revol, L., C. L. Millet and Thivollet (1954) A propos de l'Étiologie de la Leucose aiguë, *Sang*, 25:825.

Rickes, E., N. G. Brink and F. R. Koniusky (1948) Vitamin B12 : a Cobalt Complex, *Science*, 108: 134, 634.

Robinson, F. J. and D. R. Climenko (1941) Effects of Inhalation of Benzene Vapours on red blood Corpuscles of Rabbits, *J. Ind. Hyg. Toxicol.*, 23:232.

Roche, L. and M. Bruel (1950) Troubles digestifs à Type de Déséquilibre hépato-neuro végétatif chez les Ouvriers exposés au Benzol, *Arch. Malad. Profess.*, 11:61.

Rohner, F. J., C. W. Baldridge and G. H. Hansmann (1926) Chronic Benzol Poisoning; Report of a Case with Autopsy Findings, *Arch. Pathol. Lab. Med.*, 1:220.

Rosenthal, N. (1938) [in] *Handbook of Haematology*, Ed. H. Downey. Paul B. Hoeber Inc. New York.

Rovatti, B. (1949) L'Agglutinabilita piastrinica studiata con l'Agglutiogramma, *Bull. Soc. Chim. Biol.*, 31:519.

Rozera, G. (1960) Phosphatase Activity of Erythrocytes and Serum in chronic experimental Benzolism, *Folia Med. Nap.*, 42:1572.

Rozera, G., G. Colicchio and O. Elmino (1960) Sul Rapporti tra Attività mitotica Midollae e Fenoli nel Benzolismo sperimentale, *Folia Med. Nap.*, 42:1558.

Rozera, G., O. Elmino and G. Colicchio (1960) Studio sulla Crasi ematica, l'Emocoagulazione e la Funzione epatica nel Benzolismo sperimentale, *Folia Med. Nap.*, 42:1373.

Rusk, G. Y. (1914) Effect of Benzol Intoxication and consequent Leucopenia on Formation of artificial Haemolysins and Precipitins, *Univ. Calif. Publ. Pathol.*, 2:139.

Sabrazès, J. and J. Bideau (1937) Leucémie myéloide chronique chez un Graisseur de Machines, *Gaz. Hebd. Sci. Med.*, 58:339.

—(1937) Les Leucémies Benzoliques, *Gaz. Hebd. Sci. Med.*, 58:387.

Sabrazès, J., J. Bideau and P. Glaunès (1937) Nouveau Cas de Leucémie Benzolique, *Gaz. Hebd. Sci. Med.*, 58 :726.

—(1937) Leucémie myéloide Benzolique chez un Ouvrier travaillant dans une Miroiterie, *Gaz. Hebd. Sci. Med.*, 58:676.

Saita, G. (1945) Myélose aplastique provoquée par le Benzol, *Med. Lavoro*, 36: 143.

Saita, G. and M. Dompé (1947) Sur les Risques de Benzolisme dans les principaux Établissements de Gravure de Milan, *Med. Lavoro*, 38:269.

Saita, G. and L. Moreo (1959) Talassemia e Benzolismo cronico, *Med. Lavoro*, 50:25.

Saita, G. and A. Perini (1958) Duo Cas da Benzolismo nel Lavoro in Casa, *Med. Lavoro*, 49:442.

Saita, G., E. Sartorelli and F. Calaresi (1954) Il Processo di Coagulazione del Sangue nel Benzolismo cronico professionale, *Med. Lavoro*, 45:313.

Saita, G. and C. Sbertoli (1954) L'Agglutinogramma nell'Intossicazione cronica del Benzolo, *Med. Lavoro*, 45:250.

Santesson, C. G. (1897) Über chronische Vergiftungen mit Steinkohlenteerbenzin; vier Todesfälle, *Arch. Hyg. Berl.*, 31 : 336.

Savilahti, M. (1956) Mehr als 100 Vergiftungsfälle durch Benzol in einer Schuhfabrik, *Arch. Gewerbepathol. Gewerbehyg.*, 15: 147.

Savy, P., C. Kochler and P. Buffand (1948) Un Cas d'Intoxication mortelle par le Benzol chez une Ouvrière travaillant à Domicile, *Arch. Malad. Profess.*, 9:38.

Schaefer, F. (1909) Verwendung und schädliche Wirkung einiger Kohlenwasser- und anderen Kohlenstoffverbindungen, *Hamburg Gew. Insp. Arbeit Sonderber.*

Schiff, F. (1914) Einfluss des Benzols auf die aktive Anaphylaxie des Meerschweinchens, *Z. Immun. Forsch.*, 23:61.

Schillova, A. (1933) Veränderungen bei chronischer Benzolvergiftung, *Folia Haemat. Leipzig*, 49: 447.

Schrenk, H. H., W. P. Yant and R. R. Sayers (1936) New Procedure for the Control of Benzene Exposure, *J. Am. Med. Ass.*, 107:849.

Schrenk, H. H., W. P. Yant, S. J. Pearce, F. A. Patty and R. R. Sayers (1941) Absorption, Distribution and Elimination of Benzene by Body Tissues and Fluids of Dogs exposed to Benzene Vapour, *J. Ind. Hyg. Toxicol.*, 23: 20.

Schultzen, O. and B. Naunyn (1867) Über das Verhalten des Kohlenwasserstoffes im Organismus, *Arch. Anat. Pysiol.*, 349.

Secchi, P. (1914) Ricerche ematologiche nelle Intossicazione acute e chroniche da Benzolo, *Rif. Med.*, 30:995.

Selling, L. (1910) Preliminary Report of some Cases of Purpura Haemorrhagica due to Benzol Poisoning, *Bull. Johns Hopk. Hosp.*, 21:33.

—(1916) Benzol as a Leucotoxin, *Johns Hopk. Hosp. Rep.*, 17:83.

Seyfried, H. (1942) Über Benzolschäden, *Wien. Klin. Wschr.*, 55:399.

Silberberg, M. (1928) Das Verhalten des aleukocytären und vital gespeicherten Körpers gegenüber der septischen Allgemeininfektion als Beitrag zur Entzündungs- und Monocytenlehre, *Virchow's Arch.*, 267:483.

Simonds, J. P. and H. M. Jones (1915) Effects of Injections of Benzol upon the Production of Antibodies, *J. Med. Res.*, 33:197.

Simonin, C. (1934) Considérations toxicologiques et médicolégales sur le Benzolisme et le Pétrolisme professionels, *Paris Med.*, 11:408.

Smith, A. R. (1928) Chronic Benzol Poisoning among Women Industrial Workers, *J. Ind. Hyg. Toxicol.*, 10:73.

—(1945) Delayed Case of Benzol Poisoning, *J. Ind. Hyg. Toicol.*, 27:118.

Storti, E. (1936) Mielosi eritremica spenomegalica con Aplasia Mieloide, *Minerva Med.*, 1:177.

Sury-Bienz (1888) Tödliche Benzoldämpfvergiftung. *Vierteljahresschr, Gerichtl. Med.*, 49: 138.

Tara, S., Lamberton Truffert, Y. Delplace and A. Cavigneaux (1953) La Benzenémie; Étude Critique, *Sang*, 24: 1.

Tareev, E. M. and H. M. Nikulenko (1933) Etiology of Leukaemia, *Vrachebnoe Delo*, 16: 15.

Teisinger, J., B. Fiserova-Bergerova and J. Kudrna (1952) Metabolismus Benzeni u Cloveka, *Pracovni Lekar.*, 4: 175.

Teisinger, J., B. Fiserova-Bergerova (1955) Valeur comparée de la Détermination des Sulphates et du Phénol contenus dans l'Urine pour l'Évaluation de la Concentration du Benzène dans l'Air, *Arch. Malad. Profess.*, 16:221.

Teleky, L. and F. Weiner (1924) Über Benzolvergiftung, *Klin. Wschr.*, 3:226.

Theis, R. C. and S. R. Benedict (1924) The Determination of Phenol in the Blood, *J. Biol. Chem.*, 61:67.

Thompson, V. P., M. N. Richter and R. S. Edsall (1924) Analysis of so-called Aplastic Anaemia, *Am. J. Med. Sci.*, 187:77.

Threshold Limit Values (1962) *Am. Ind. Hyg. Ass. J.*, 23:419.

Tolot, F., G. Neulat and Mme. Mallein (1960) Une Observation de Leucose myéloide due aux Hydrocarbures Benzèniques, *Arch. Malad. Profess.*, 22:159.

Treon, J. F., W. E. Crutchfield and K. V. Kitzmiller (1943) Physiological Response of Rabbits to Cyclohexane, Methylcyclohexane and certain Derivatives of these compounds, *J. Ind. Hyg. Toxicol.*, 25:199, 323.

Truhaut, R. and C. Paoletti (1957) Généralités sur l'Utilisation des Isotopes en Toxicologie experimentale, *J. Méd. Bordeaux*, 134:735.

Truhaut, R., C. Paoletti, M. Boiron and M. Tubiana (1959) Études expérimentales sur la Toxicologie du Benzène, *Arch. Malad. Profess.*, 20:121.

Tsanck, A., A. Dreyfus and M. Jais (1937) Hémopathie post-benzolique et Leucoblastose médullaire, *Sang*, 11:550.

Undritz, E. (1938) Un Cas d'Intoxication professionelle par des Vapeurs de Benzène. Collophane et Huile de Lin, *Progr. Med.*, p. 569.

U.S. Tariff Commission (1958) Synthetic Chemicals, U.S. Production and Sales, 1957. *Rep. no. 203, 2nd Ser. U.S. Govt. Printing Office, Washington.*

Van Ravensteyn, A. H. (1941) Chronische Benzolvergiftiging en Leucamie, *Nederl. Tijdschr. Geneesk.*, 85:408.

Van Schoonhaven van Buerden, A. J. R. E. (1949) Benzolleucemie, *Nederl. Tijdschr. Geneesk.*, 93:2584.

Vaughn, W. T. (1944) Thrombocytopenic Purpura due to Benzol Poisoning, *J. Ind. Hyg. Toxicol.*, 26:274.

—(1947) Idiopathic Thrombocytopenic Purpura in Women with prolonged Exposure to Benzol, *J. Ind. Hyg. Toxicol.*, 29:227.

Veit, B. (1921) Entzündungsvorgange beim Kaninchen die durch Benzol aleukocytär gemacht werden, *Beitr. Pathol. Anat. Allg. Pathol.*, 68:425.

Vigliani, E. C. and G. Saita (1943) Leucémie hémocytoblastique du Benzol, *Med. Lavoro*, 34:182.

Villani, C., G. Massei and F. Giudicini (1960) Experimental Data concerning the Participation of the Spleen in Benzol Haemopathy, *Folia Med. Nap.*, 43:205.

Villani, C., G. Massei and R. Zanobi (1960) La Eritripoiesi nelle Emopatia Benzolica sperimentale, *Folia Med. Nap.*, 43:842.

Walkley, J. E., L. D. Pagnotto and H. B. Elkins (1961) The Measurement of Phenol in Urine as an Index of Benzol Exposure, *J. Am. Ind. Hyg. Ass.*, 22:362.

Warren, S. (1957) Factors in the Causation of Leukaemia, *Mount Sinai N.Y.J.*, 24:1331.

Whitby, L. E. H. and C. J. C. Britton (1939) *Disorders of the Blood*, Churchill Ltd., London.

White, W. C. and A. H. Gammon (1914) Influence of Benzol Inhalations on Experimental Pulmonary Tuberculosis in Rabbits, *Trans. Ass. Am. Phys.*, 29:332.

Williams, R. T. (1959) *Detoxication Mechanisms*, 2nd. ed. Chapman & Hall, London.

Winslow, C. E. A. (1927) Survey of the National Safety Council Study of Benzol Poisoning, *J. Ind. Hyg. Toxicol.*, 9:61.

Winternitz, M. C. and A. D. Hirschfelder (1913) Studies on Experimental Pneumonia in Rabbits, *J. Exptl. Med.*, 17:657, 666.

Wirschafter, Z. T. and M. G. Bischel (1960) Reticuloendothelial Response to Benzene, *Arch. Environ. Health*, 1:10.

Wirtschafter, Z. T. and M. G. De Meritt (1959) Reticuloendothelial Response to Benzene, *Arch. Pathol.*, 67:146.

Woronow, A. (1929) Über die morphologischen Veränderungen des Bluts und der bluterzeugenden Organe unter den Einflusse des Benzols und dessen Abkommlinge, *Virchow's Arch.*, 271:174.

Wyatt, J. P. and S. C. Somers (1950) Chronic Marrow Failure, Myelosclerosis and extramedullary Haemopoiesis, *Blood*, 5:329.

Wyss, M. O. (1910) Gesellschaft des Ärzte in Zürich; über Benzolvergiftung, *Korresp.bl. Schweiz. Ärz.*, 4:387.

Yant, W. P., H. H. Schrenk and P. H. Mantz (1935) Procedure for the Removal and Determination of small Amounts of Benzene in biological Material, *U.S. Bureau Mines Dept. Invest. Rep. no.* 2382.

Yant, W. P., H. H. Schrenk, R. R. Sayers, A. A. Howarth and W. A. Reinhart (1936) Urine Sulphate Determination as a Measure of Benzene Exposure, *J. Ind. Hyg. Toxicol.*, 18:69.

Ziel. (1925) Zur Benzolvergiftung, *Med. Klin.* 21:93.

Zorina, L. (1960) The Use of Vitamin B6 in chronic Benzene Poisoning, *Probl. Gemat.*, 5:31.

Zurlo, N. and L. Metrico (1960) Simple Methods for Microdetermination of industrial Toxins in Air, *Med. Lavoro*, 51:241.

Chapter 2

OTHER AROMATIC HYDROCARBONS

2. Toluene

Synonyms: toluol, methylbenzene, methylbenzol, phenylmethane

Structural formula:

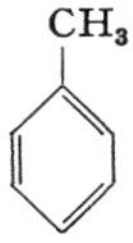

CH$_3$

Molecular formula: C$_7$H$_8$

Molecular weight: 92.13

2a. Pure Toluene

Properties
>   *boiling point:* 110.4 °C
>   *melting point:* −94.5 °C
>   *vapour pressure:* 36.7 mm Hg at 30 °C
>   *vapour density (air = 1):* 3.2
>   *specific gravity (liquid density):* 0.861
>   *flash point:* 40 °F
>   *conversion factors:* 1 p.p.m. = 3.76/m³
>   1 mg/l = 226 p.p.m.
>   *solubility:* 0.082 g/100 ml water at 22°C; miscible with ether, ethanol, chloroform, glacial acetic acid, CS$_2$, castor, linseed and other oils
>   *evaporation rate (ether = 1):* 6.1
>   *maximum allowable concentration:* 200 p.p.m. (USSR 25 p.p.m.)

2b. Commercial 'Toluol'

Commercial toluene may contain considerable amounts of benzene. In America, Wilson (1943) stated that commercial toluol contained 2–10%; in Germany, according to Humperdinck (1954) 15% and 10% xylol; and according to Bänfer (1961) it is only during the past 6 years that it has been possible to obtain 'pure' toluene containing traces (up to 0.3%) of benzene.

[66]

In Great Britain, a fatal case of leukaemia was reported to the Chief Inspector of Factories (1960) in a man using toluene which was eventually found to contain up to 6% of benzene.

ECONOMY, SOURCES AND USES

Production

(1) From petroleum, by dehydrogenation of cycloparaffin fractions, or by aromatisation of saturated aliphatic hydrocarbons.
(2) As a by-product, from the gases and coal tar, of the coke-oven industry.

Industrial uses

(1) As a solvent for gums, fats and resins.
(2) As a thinner for paints, varnishes, lacquers and enamels, and as a paint remover.
(3) As a starting material in the chemical industry.
(4) As a constituent of motor and aviation fuels.
(5) In fabric and paper coating.
(6) In the rubber industry, as a solvent for neoprene (Elkins, 1959).
(7) In the manufacture of artificial leather.

BIOCHEMISTRY

Estimation

(1) In the atmosphere
    (a) Ultraviolet spectrophotometry. – The procedure described by Maffet et al. (1956) depends on the use of silica gel, with the addition of iso-octane, followed by decanting the iso-octane layer into a spectrophotometer and reading the transmission at 268 mμ.
    (b) Microcolorimetric method. – A colorimetric method based on nitration and colour formation with H_2SO_4-formaldehyde mixture was described by Yant et al in 1936, using butanone as the extracting agent. A similar method, using methyl ethyl ketone, is described by Elkins (1959), the concentration being estimated by comparison with a standard colour transmission curve.

(2) In blood and tissues
    The ultraviolet spectrophotometric method described by Guertin and Gerarde (1959) for benzene and other alkyl benzenes including toluene and xylene,

Bibliography on p. 124

involves the extraction of the toluene from blood, haemolysed by 0.1 N hydro-chloric acid, with cyclohexane; the concentration is determined from a previously prepared calibration curve.

(3) In urine

The amount of toluene in urine is usually estimated in terms of its metabolite, hippuric acid. A modification of the test known as Quick's test (1926) for this substance, described by Von Oettingen *et al.* (1942), is described by Elkins (1959). It is carried out on a 200–300 ml sample of urine, which is acidified with acetic acid and concentrated to about half its original volume. To 100 ml of this are added 30 g of NaCl, and then 18 N H_2SO_4 drop by drop (2–6 ml) until no more precipitate forms. The precipitate, dissolved in hot water, is titrated with 0.2 N NaOH using a phenolphthalein indicator. Each ml of the NaOH is equivalent to 36 mg of hippuric acid. According to Von Oettingen's (1942) original calcula-tions, the degree of exposure to toluene can be correlated with the excretion of hippuric acid; an exposure of 200 p.p.m. would result in a hippuric acid concen-tration of about 3000–5000 mg/l in the 200–300 ml excreted during the last 4–5 h of exposure. Elkins considers that 1 g/l of hippuric acid in the urine indicates a harmful exposure to toluene, but there is, according to Von Oettingen, no cumu-lative increase; the excretion is practically complete 16 h after the exposure.

Metabolism

(1) Absorption and excretion

Toluene vapour is rapidly absorbed by inhalation, and the liquid from the gastro-intestinal tract, but poorly from the skin.

Part of the toluene absorbed is exhaled unchanged, 18% of the oral dose, according to Gerarde (1960), and following inhalation, excretion is at first rapid and later slow (Von Oettingen *et al.*, 1942) so that after 2 h only very small amounts are present in the blood.

The part not exhaled is metabolised by oxidation into its principal metabolite, benzoic acid, which is conjugated with glycine in the liver and excreted in the urine as the water-soluble hippuric acid.

As mentioned above, a concentration of 1 g/l of urine has been suggested as an indication of harmful exposure to toluene, and Teisinger and Srbova (1955) have used it as a test for such exposure, stating that 2.1 g in a 24-h sample indi-cates an exposure below 200 p.p.m. It is pointed out by Gerarde (1960) that the value of such a test is limited by the fact that hippuric acid, originating from a diet high in fruit and vegetables containing benzoic acid or its precursors (prunes, cranberries, plums and coffeebeans) is a normal constituent of the urine. Whether benzoic acid is itself a completely innocuous substance is discussed at length by

Fabre *et al.* (1955) with reference to its potential inhibition of certain enzyme systems, and of elimination of uric acid (Quick, 1931).

Even if such noxious effects are confirmed, they are much less harmful than those attributed to the phenolic metabolites of benzene, especially since they are not specifically directed towards the bone marrow.

(2) Distribution in tissues

In dogs subjected to inhalation of toluene, Fabre *et al.* (1955) found the highest concentration in the adrenals (20 μg/g), brain (19 μg/g in the cerebellum and 18 μg/g in the cerebrum) and the bone marrow (18 μg/g).

This distribution is similar to that of benzene observed by Fabre and Fabre (1948) and by Verain *et al.* (1949); the localisation in the central nervous system is correlated with the nervous symptoms noted by many observers in human cases of chronic toluene exposure.

TOXICOLOGY

Toluene is primarily a narcotic, even according to some observers, of greater potency than benzene; a few cases of unconsciousness, in one case fatal, have been recorded following severe exposure. It is also an irritant of skin and mucous membranes. Reliable records of prolonged exposure to non-narcotic concentrations of pure toluene are rare in the literature, since the commercial variety, which may contain benzene, is much more frequently used as an industrial solvent. It is now, however, generally believed to be much less toxic than benzene in chronic exposure, being devoid of the specific dyshaemopoietic activity of benzene. Evidence for an injurious effect on the liver has been advanced, but is not agreed upon by all observers.

Toxicity to animals

(1) Acute

(a) *The lethal dose.* – (i) *By inhalation* the lethal dose is believed by most recent authorities to lie between that of benzene and xylene. Exceptions to this order were given by Batchelor (1927), Lazarew (1929) and Svirbely *et al.* (1943) who all regarded toluene as more acutely toxic than benzene. Batchelor, for example, gave the lethal dose for rats as 1600 p.p.m. as compared with 2400 p.p.m. for benzene, Lazarew, for mice, 7800–9320 p.p.m. for toluene and 14,000 for benzene and Svirbely *et al.* 5300 p.p.m. for toluene, 10,400 for benzene and 11,500 for meta-xylene. For rabbits, the lethal dose of toluene observed by Carpenter *et al.* (1944) was much higher – 35,000 to 45,000 p.p.m. within 40 min. – (ii) *By intraperitoneal injection* the early investigations of Chassevant and Garnier (1903) also suggested a higher lethal toxicity for toluene than either benzene or xylene –

Bibliography on p. 124

toluene 0.50 ml/kg body weight, benzene 0.73 ml/kg and xylene 1.65 ml/kg and Winslow (1927) found toluene more toxic than benzene by this route.

A more recent investigation (1960) by Schumacher and Grandjean, places toluene between benzene and xylene – benzene 1.16 ml/kg, toluene 1.36 and xylene 1.85.

(b) The narcotic dose. – The narcotic effect of toluene, like that of benzene and xylene, is exerted in two phases – a preliminary narcosis followed by a stage of excitement, manifested by tremor, muscular cramps and disturbances of behaviour. The convulsive effect characteristic of benzene narcosis is apparently only relevant, however, to parenteral administration. Schuhmacher and Grandjean observed no such convulsive effect in rats subjected to inhalation of 15,000 p.p.m. of toluene. This stage of excitement, as an estimation of the acute narcotic effect of toluene, was produced by Mikiskowa (1960) by means of electrodes introduced by trephination over the frontal motor zone of guinea pigs injected intraperitoneally with benzol, toluol and xylol. In these experiments the effect of toluol was stated to be greater than that of benzol but less than that of xylol.

The earlier observers from Lehmann (1912) to Lazarew (1929) based their estimations of the narcotic potency of toluene on the concentrations which produced symptoms of varying severity, without taking into account the time of their appearance and the time of recovery; from this point of view they considered toluene more toxic than benzene, and their estimation of the narcotic concentration varied from 1250 p.p.m. (Batchelor, 1927; Smyth and Smyth, 1928) to 3200 p.p.m. (Lazarew, 1929).

Schuhmacher and Grandjean (1960) on the other hand estimate the narcotic potency in terms of affinity for the central nervous system, basing this on both the grade of severity and also on the time of recovery. They consider that solvents with a short time of appearance of deep narcosis and a short time of recovery have a high affinity for the central nervous system. From this point of view they found that toluene lies between benzene and xylene.

By intravenous injection. Braier and Francone (1959) also found toluene less acutely toxic than benzene.

(2) Chronic

Recent investigations on the effect of chronic exposure of animals to toluene have shown practically conclusively that this is much less injurious than to benzene, especially to the haemopoietic system, and have to a great extent resolved the controversy wich existed among the earlier observers on this aspect. The only point on which they were consistent was the degree, rather than the nature, of the blood changes caused by the two solvents, the severity being less with toluene. Some authors, (Batchelor, 1927; Engelhardt, 1935; Ferguson *et al.*, 1933; Smyth and Smyth, 1928) were among those who emphasised the similarity of leucopoietic injury inflicted by toluene to that of benzene, while Mgebrow (1930) stressed its effect in producing anaemia, which he regarded as haemolytic in character, and Bianchi (1915) claimed that repeated subcutaneous injections caused marrow hyperplasia with an increase of leucocytes and thrombocytes. It is more than possible that most of these discrepancies were due to the failure to realise that the toluene used was not pure, but contained amounts of benzene large enough to give rise to the varied blood changes characteristic of chronic benzene poisoning.

A more recent investigation by Fabre et al. (1955) was made in the most rigorous experimental conditions – pure toluene, its purity verified by ultraviolet spectography capable of detecting 0.1 % of benzene, rats and rabbits kept in conditions, including diet, identical with those of a number of controls, and verification of the constant concentration of the toluene content of the air inhaled.

These concentrations were 930–2128 p.p.m. for the rats, and 399–718 and 1755 p.p.m. for the rabbits.

The general condition of the animals showed no variation except in the case of the rabbits exposed to the higher concentrations. These showed some initial signs of agitation, and some dogs showed motor inco-ordination followed by slight paralysis of the hind quarters. There was no decrease in growth.

SYMPTOMS OF INTOXICATION

Blood examinations of all the animals confirmed the absence of significant variations postulated by some of the earlier investigators such as Hektoen (1916). They showed neither leucopenia nor anaemia in animals subjected to 900 and 2100 p.p.m. during periods up to 40 days.

The bone marrow, while showing some hypoplasia in one rabbit exposed to a low concentration (718 p.p.m.), was normal or even hyperplasic in others exposed to higher concentrations: this had also been noted by Bianchi in 1915.

The coagulability of the blood showed an increase in the time of coagulation, a phenomenon which admitted of no explanation in view of the fact that there was no notable variation in the level of calcium or prothrombin or in the number of thrombocytes.

CHANGES IN THE ORGANISM

(1) The liver

In the dogs examined by Fabre et al., congestion and haemorrhagic foci were present in the liver; these lesions were also present in goats examined by Sessa (1948) but he considered that the liver as a whole was not seriously damaged.

(2) The lungs

Congestion and some alveolar inflammation were present in Fabre's dogs and were the outstanding pathological manifestion in Sessa's goats.

Bibliography on p. 124

(3) The spleen

This showed some diminution of lymphoid follicles and plaques of haemo-siderosis.

(4) The kidneys

Like most of the earlier observers, Fabre *et al.* found some evidence of kidney injury – swelling of the glomeruli, cylinders and albumen in the urine in two of the dogs – but they note that the dogs were of a breed which frequently develops interstitial nephritis. Sessa, however, found both haemorrhagic and degenerative lesions in goats.

It is apparent from these careful investigations, that to animals at least, toluene is on the whole, and especially from the point of view of haemopoiesis, a much less hazardous solvent than benzene, but its effects on the central nervous system and on the kidneys indicate that it is not completely harmless.

Toxicity to human beings

(1) Acute

The narcotic effect of toluene in high concentrations can cause giddiness, lack of co-ordination and sometimes unconsciousness, but such a severe effect has rarely been reported in industry, and it is possible that individual suscepti-bility may play some part.

Contact of liquid toluene with the skin or mucous membranes may cause acute dermatitis, pneumonitis and pulmonary haemorrhage. Skin lesions have also been stated to be caused by the vapour (Zeman and Klatil, 1959).

Symptoms relating to the central nervous system. – A rare fatal case was reported to the Chief Inspector of Factories, U.K. (1957). This was a man who was over-come by the fumes from an overflow from a tank containing toluene. He became unconscious and was removed from his position over the manhole, but artificial respiration was not available and he died without regaining consciousness.

Another severe, but non-fatal case was similarly reported in 1954. This occur-red in an oil refinery; the man entered a pit containing a mixture of wax, methyl ethyl ketone, toluene and lubricating oil, in order to operate a steam-driven pump for emptying the sump. After 30–45 min he climbed out, and a few minutes later became unconscious. Following recovery he suffered severe headache, dizziness and weakness of the limbs, and since there was no irritation of the eyes or nose which might have been attributed to the methyl ethyl ketone, it was concluded that the narcotic action of toluene was the prime factor.

Intoxication described as 'acute' in a man cleaning the inside of a tank coated with an emulsion of D.D.T. and 45% pure toluene, was reported by Lurie (1949). The man became unconscious five minutes after beginning work in the tank, and on recovery showed symptoms of dyspnoea, excitation, disorientation, semi-coma, rapid pulse, high temperature, bronchial râles and blood-stained sputum; the urine contained blood and albumen and there was conjunctivitis and oedema of the eyelids.

Poisoning by D.D.T. was excluded on the ground that no case has been recorded where symptoms and signs of nervous involvement have shown themselves so soon after an attack of unconsciousness, and that the majority of investigators have concluded that D.D.T. in its insecticidal form is practically innocuous to man.

Several cases of 'drunkenness' or excitation followed by depression were reported by Christiansson and Karlsson (1947) in schoolboys who had purposely inhaled the vapour from a paint thinner which contained 35–70% of toluol, with 15–25% of ethyl and butyl alcohol and 10% of methyl isobutyl ketone. The immediate effect of inhalation was coughing; excitation reached its peak after 15–25 inhalations, and was succeeded by somnolence; in some cases there was nystagmus, a positive Romberg sign, and changes in the electrocardiogram. The only significant variation of the blood picture was punctate basophilia, but the bone marrow showed some increased haemopoiesis, with abnormal cells resembling myeloblasts. The authors attributed the intoxication to toluol.

(2) Chronic

It must be emphasised that although chronic exposure to toluene is not likely to produce severe narcosis, the conclusion of Von Oettingen *et al.* (1942) that "inhalation for 8 h of concentrations of 200 p.p.m. cause slight but definite impairment of co-ordination and reaction time, which may render persons thus affected more prone to accidents" is important from the industrial point of view. These observers found that exposure for 8 h to 800 p.p.m. resulted in severe nervousness, muscular fatigue, and insomnia lasting several days.

SYMPTOMS OF INTOXICATION

Wilson (1943) found that a number of employees exposed to concentrations varying from 50–1500 p.p.m. for periods of one to three weeks, suffered severely from nausea, headache, dizziness, anorexia, palpitation, extreme weakness, loss of co-ordination and impaired reaction time. Even with exposures from 200–500 p.p.m. similar symptoms were present, with the addition of momentary loss of memory, while in those exposed to less than 200 p.p.m. the chief complaints – headache, lassitude and anorexia – were so mild as to be considered non-pathologic.

Parmeggiani and Sassi (1954) examined two groups of workers in a varnishing process where the concentrations of toluol rose at times to between 300 and 580 p.p.m. During the process of washing tins the hand and forearms were in contact with toluol. At other stages of the work there was also exposure to butyl acetate, and here the concentrations of toluol ranged from 150–1800 p.p.m., and of butyl

Bibliography on p. 124

acetate from 150–2400. Symptoms included asthenia, general malaise, drowsiness, headache, epigastric discomfort, nausea, insomnia, irritation of mucosae, enlargement of the liver and nervous hyperexcitability; the last three occurred more frequently in the workers exposed to both solvents than to toluene alone.

CHANGES IN THE ORGANISM

(1) The liver

The most emphatic insistence on the importance of liver injury from exposure to toluene was given by Greenburg et al. (1942) following their investigation of painters in an airplane factory. The average exposures of the 106 men examined ranged from 100–1100 p.p.m., the majority (74.7%) being below 500 p.p.m. Of these 106 men, 30 had been previously exposed to benzene and 15 to other solvents of unknown nature. Except for dermatitis in a few of the men employed in hand-dipping, there were no clinical symptoms, but 30.2% had palpable enlargement of the liver, and of the 61 who had had exposure only to toluene the incidence of liver enlargement was 21.4% – three times the frequency of a control group. There was, however, no correlation between the enlarged liver and either clinical or laboratory evidence of disease, and it was suggested that the enlargement might be merely compensatory in nature.

The specificity of liver enlargement was not confirmed by Parmeggiani and Sassi (1954). They found that it was present in both exposed workers and also in non-exposed controls, and that none of the exposed workers showed any significant abnormality of functional liver tests, which included serum electrophoresis, colloidal lability reactions and galactosuria. A slight increase in gamma globulin in 5 cases, slight decrease in total blood protein in 2 and slight increase in galactosuria in 3 were regarded as non-pathogenic.

(2) The circulatory system

There has been much controversy in the past as to whether chronic exposure to toluene can produce a 'benzene-like' effect on the haemopoietic system, but from the evidence of fairly recent investigations (Fabre and Truhaut, 1954; Von Oettingen et al., 1942; Francone and Braier, 1954) it appears that it has an almost negligible effect on the bone marrow.

The chief protagonists of a possible severe effect are Ferguson et al. (1933) and Ravina et al. (1951) but in both the evidence is not indisputable. The only fatal case of blood dyscrasia attributed to toluene was that of Ferguson et al. This was a man in charge of the solvent recovery apparatus over the spreading tables of an indiarubber process, where the solvent was stated to contain 45% of toluene but no benzene. Following a fracture of the nose he developed nose bleeding and later purpuric spots on the tongue and bleeding from the gums. At this time his blood picture showed some anaemia and leucopenia (2200/μl); the white cell count rose, a few months later, to 5400, but shortly before his death from pneumonia some weeks later had fallen to 1200. With regard to the condition of the bone marrow at autopsy "one had the impression, that in spite of being truly a red marrow this was really a marrow in a state of aplasia and no longer manifestly haemopoietic". The diagnosis, in the presence of only 5.5% of polymorphs, was agranulocytic anaemia. The validity of evidence for a direct association of this blood disorder with exposure to toluene is in doubt from two points of view:

(a) No complete analysis of the solvent used is given, or of the freedom of the toluene from any content of benzene.

(b) The possibility that the anemia was idiopathic in origin and perhaps initiated by the trauma. Ferguson *et al.* themselves remark that the possibility that this might have been a case of a primary blood disease cannot be ruled out.

Similar doubt as to the actual nature of the exposure exists in the case presented by Ravina *et al.* (1951) This case, diagnosed as 'haemorrhagic agranulocytosis' was that of a girl aged 20 who had been employed for 6 months as a bobbin-winder; the bobbins were then soaked in a bath containing a mixture of toluene with an iron sulphide and rhodulin pigment. She was admitted to hospital semi-conscious, with double haemorrhagic retinitis and profound anaemia and leuco-penia. Sternal puncture showed an aplastic bone marrow. Daily transfusions of fresh blood were followed by a slight rise in red corpuscles but a further fall of white cells to $350/\mu$l. Complete clinical recovery, but with a slight residual anae-mia and leucopenia, was eventually achieved by transfusions of globular suspen-sions of red cells obtained from the combined blood of several donors. No analysis of the solvent or of its toluene constituent was made.

Slighter blood changes were recorded by Greenburg *et al.* (1942) – mild macrocytic anaemia and lymphocytosis without neutropenia; here again the con-stitution of the toluene was not given.

In the investigations of Von Oettingen *et al.* (1942) of human volunteers, inhalation for 8 h a day of concentrations varying from 50–800 p.p.m. caused no significant changes in the total or differential white cell count (erythrocyte counts were not made).

In a more recent investigation (Bänfer, 1961) of a large number of workers in rotogravure printing, the toluene used contained only 0.3% of benzene, and blood examinations were carried out every 3 months in young persons under 18, every 6 months in adults. The atmospheric concentration of toluene was less than 200 p.p.m. in one sample, 200 p.p.m. in one, and 400 p.p.m. in the third.

The results of blood examinations showed that only three times in all was the white cell count less than 4000, the polymorphs were never less than 2000, and there was no relative or absolute lymphocytosis; the erythrocyte and haemoglobin levels showed only occasional slight variations. Comparison with controls having at the time no contact with toluene showed a very similar blood picture, except for the fact that a higher proportion of the controls had a white cell count above

Bibliography on p. 124

8500. Bänfer declined to state categorically that pure toluene cannot have any injurious effect on the haemopoietic system, but considered that it is certainly much less toxic in this respect than benzene.

In the author's experience, based on a large number of blood examinations of persons exposed to toluene, no benzene-like effect on the blood picture has been observed except where the toluene was found to contain some benzene.

Perhaps the most unusual evidence of the relative non-toxicity of toluene to the haemopoietic system is that presented by Braier and Francone (1950). They administered toluene to patients suffering from leukaemia, with the object of comparing its possible leucopenic action with the known effect of benzol in reducing the total white cell count in the early trials of this remedy for leukaemia. Up to 10 g of toluol, in a capsule with olive oil, was given daily by mouth, up to a total of 130 g in three weeks. This was perfectly well tolerated, but had no clinical effect on the leukaemic process. Finally, the opinion of Gerarde (1960) based on a very extensive study of a number of alkyl derivatives of benzene, is that "the myelotoxicity of benzene is unique among hydrocarbons", and among these derivatives toluene is included.

3. Xylene

There are three isomers of xylene – *ortho*-, *meta*- and *para*-xylene. A mixture of these is frequently called xylol, which when derived from coal tar consists of 10–15% of the *ortho*-isomer, 45–70% of the *meta*- (53% according to Gerarde, 1960), about 23% of the *para*-, and 6–10% of ethylbenzene. A typical petrochemical commercial xylene consists of approximately 20% *ortho*-xylene, 44% *meta*-, 20% *para*-, and 15% ethylbenzene (Gerarde, 1960).

3a. Pure Xylene

Synonym: dimethylbenzene

Structural formulae:

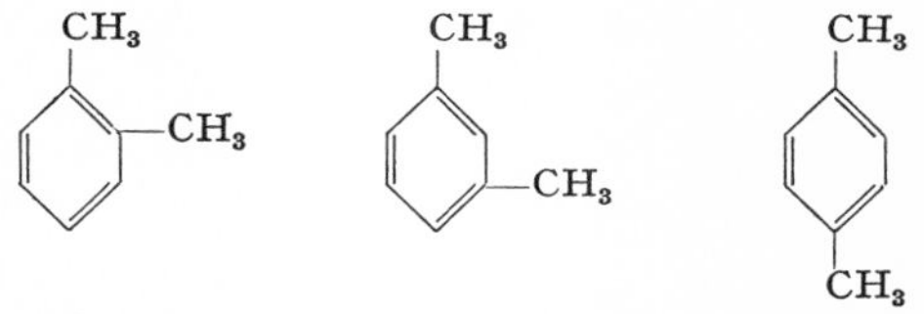

ortho   meta   para

Molecular formula: C_8H_{10}

Molecular weight: 106.16

Properties:

	ortho	meta	para
boiling point:	144.4 °C	139.1 °C	138.3 °C
melting point:	−13.3 °C	−54.2 °C	−55.9 °C
vapour pressure: 10 mm Hg	at 32.11 °C	at 28.26 °C	at 27.30 °C
vapour density (air = 1):	3.7	3.7	3.7
specific gravity (liquid density):	0.87583	0.85985	0.85666
flash point:	63 °F	77 °F	103 °F

conversion factors: 1 p.p.m. = 4.35 mg/m³
                1 mg/l = 230.9 p.p.m.

solubility: insoluble in water; soluble in ethyl alcohol and ether

maximum allowable concentration: 200 p.p.m. ACGIH 1965 revision 100 p.p.m.

3b. Commercial Xylene

Commercial xylene or 'xylol' is a colourless liquid with a characteristic aromatic odour; boiling point 129–150 °C (Fabre *et al.*, 1960).

Bibliography on p. 124　　　　　　[77]

ECONOMY, SOURCES AND USES

It is a solvent for some gums and resins, rubber, castor and linseed oils, and dibenzyl cellulose, but not for cellulose esters.

Industrial uses

(1) As a solvent especially in the paint industry (in a mixture with other solvents), in the printing, rubber and leather industries; in the manufacture of mirrors.
(2) As a cleaning agent and degreaser.
(3) As a constituent of aviation fuel.
(4) In the chemical industry as a starting material and intermediate for phthalic and terephthalic acids used in the manufacture of plastic materials and synthetic textile fabrics (Dacron, Terylene, Polyamides).
(5) In the manufacture of quartz crystal oscillators.
(6) In the coating and impregnation of fabric and paper.
(7) A recent use as a carrier in the production of epoxy resins has been described (Joyner and Pegues, 1961).

BIOCHEMISTRY

Estimation

(1) In the atmosphere

Spectophotometric methods, similar to those described by Luszczak (1935) and Maffet et al. (1956) for the determination of benzene and toluene, or colorimetric chemical methods based on nitration and colour formation with H_2SO_4-formaldehyde mixtures can be used for estimating the amount of xylene in the atmosphere; a sensitive method of the latter nature was described by Yant et al. (1936) for toluene, consisting of collecting the air sample in fuming nitric acid and subsequently extracting the nitrated toluene (or in this case xylene) with butanone. Elkins (1959) also describes a nitration method following extraction from silica gel with CCl_4. He states that the method is sufficiently sensitive to estimate about 10 mg of xylene, corresponding to 10 p.p.m. in a 25-l air sample if 1 ml of CCl_4 is nitrated and one fifth of the ether extract tested.

(2) In blood and tissues

Following separation of the xylene from the sample by distillation or extraction, estimation can be made by the colorimetric method described for its estimation in air.

A modification of the method described by Yant et al. (1936) was used by

Fabre *et al.* (1960) for xylene. The intensity of the colorimetric reaction was rendered more sensitive by the presence of potassium, and was measured by a Pulfrich colorimeter. By this method they were able to show that the main organs of accumulation in animals subjected to inhalation of xylene were the adrenals (148 μg/g), bone marrow (130 μg/g), spleen (115 μg/g) and brain (100 μg/g). The blood contained 91 μg/g.

Metabolism

The difference in the metabolism of xylene from that of benzene is generally held responsible for its relative lack of toxicity to the haemopoietic organs.

Part of the xylene absorbed by inhalation is exhaled unchanged, but according to Gerarde (1960) not so much as that so exhaled by benzene or toluene.

It is in the transformation of xylene within the body that the essential difference arises. As already described (see p. 11) benzene produces as its main metabolites phenols which have a potent toxic effect on the bone marrow. Xylene, by a process of oxidation of its methyl groups, produces mainly toluic acid. This process was first demonstrated in 1867 by Schultzen and Naunyn, being similar to the transformation of the CH_3 group of toluene into $COOH$, giving the resultant benzoic acid (see p. 11).

CH₃ → COOH

toluene   benzoic acid

xylene   toluic acid

These conversions differ from that of benzene in that the transformation of benzene is carried out by oxidation of its nucleus into phenol products (Truhaut, 1953).

At the same time, it was suggested by some early investigators such as Curci (1892) and Filippi (1914) that small amounts of phenolic compounds (xylenols and hydroxytoluic acids) were in fact formed, and more recent attempts have been made to ascertain which, if any, of the three isomers do indeed produce any phenolic metabolites. In the rabbit, Bray *et al.* (1950) have stated that 60% of ortho-xylene is transformed into toluic acid which is excreted in the urine, either free or conjugated as ortho-toluylglucuronide. In the case of the meta- and para-isomers the corresponding toluic acids are formed in greater proportion, as also are glucuronides. The early experimental results may owe their difference from the later to the fact that different experimental animals were used; it is pointed out

Bibliography on p. 124

by Fabre *et al.* that in the rabbit there is an inhibition of conjugation which does not exist in the dog (Quick, 1932).

Nevertheless it is now believed by Fabre *et al.* (1960) and by Williams (1959) that while the most important metabolic transformation of xylene is the conjugation of water-soluble metabolites with glycine, glucuronic acid or sulphuric acid (sulphoconjugates amount to 6% of the ingested dose of ortho-xylene), small amounts of phenolic products are formed by oxidation of the molecular nucleus. They have in fact been isolated in the urine of rats, rabbits and guinea pigs given all three isomers by mouth (Fabre *et al.*, 1960). On the basis of the results obtained by Bray *et al.* (1950) showing that the proportion of xylene transformed into toluic acid is least in the case of the ortho-isomer (60%), it is considered that only with this isomer is the production of phenolic products significant from the point of view of toxicity; this supports the view of Filippi (1914) that in the dog the chronic toxicity of ortho-xylene was greater than that of the other two isomers. It may be noted that Jost (1932) found no toluic acid in the urine of colour printers, a fact interpreted by Fabre *et al.* as indicating either a minimal absorption of xylene in this process or a difference in its metabolic transformation in human beings. It is on the basis of these metabolic investigations, showing that it is possible that xylene may form phenolic metabolites similar to those formed by benzene that the possibility of its having a similar haemopoietic effect, though remote, cannot be entirely disregarded. So far, fortunately, it has not been reported with indubitable evidence to have any such 'benzene-like' effect in its industrial application.

TOXICOLOGY

Liquid xylene is a skin irritant, causing erythema, dryness and defatting, and with prolonged contact, blistering. It is also an irritant to mucous membranes. As an acute poison by inhalation it is narcotic in high concentrations. With continued inhalation of non-narcotic concentrations it causes considerable gastro-intestinal disturbance, but does not produce the severe haematological changes characteristic of chronic benzene poisoning.

Toxicity to animals

(1) Acute

The acute toxicity of xylene to animals has been stated to be greater than that of either benzene or toluene, but the recent investigations of Schumacher and Grandjean (1960) do not confirm this view. They give the oral LD_{50} as 1.85 ml/kg, as compared with 1.36 for toluene and 1.16 for benzene.

(a) Lethal dose. – This differs in the three isomers, but again the order is differently placed by various authorities. Chassevant and Garnier (1903), on the basis of intraperitoneal injection, placed paraxylene first, followed by meta- and ortho-xylene, while Lazarew (1929), on the basis of inhalation, considered the meta-isomer the most toxic. He gave the lethal dosage by inhalation as 7000 ml/m³ for metaxylene, 10,350 for orthoxylene and 11,500 for paraxylene. These values were based predominantly on nervous symptoms.

(b) Narcotic dose. – By inhalation, given by Lazarew (1929) and Estler (1935) as 2100 to 3500 p.p.m. for the meta- and para-isomer, 3500 to 10,000 p.p.m. for ortho-xylene. Batchelor (1927) found that narcosis occurred only with concentrations higher than 1150 p.p.m.

According to Schumacher and Grandjean (1960), using concentrations of 15,000 p.p.m., xylene was slower in exerting an initial narcotic effect than either toluene or benzene but this effect was more severe in degree and slower to recover, When, however, the narcotic effect is judged by the rapidity of the first onset of paralysis, the time interval between this and complete loss of reflexes and the time of recovery, these authorities remark that the true criterion is that of affinity for the central nervous system, and that in spite of the more severe initial narcosis and the longer time of recovery xylene has a much lower affinity for the central nervous system, and therefore carries a lower risk of acute toxicity than either benzene or toluene.

The narcotic effect has been estimated by Mikisova (1960) by means of raising the threshold of excitability of the motor cortex. The method involves the use of epidural electrodes for alternating current, the skull being trephined. The threshold values are estimated from the level at which, with repeated stimulation, muscle contraction does not disappear (Mikiska and Mikiskova, 1960). The contraction of the fore-limbs was observed either visually or by an electric current recorder. Xylol (a commercial mixture of all three isomers) gave a greater contraction than benzene, but an earlier return to a normal level, and in a few animals clonic muscle contractions and tremor, as with benzene, were observed. These results indicated that the effect of acute xylene poisoning on the central nervous system occurs, like that of benzene and toluene, in two phases – an initial inhibition or narcosis of short duration, followed by increased excitability with a lowering of the cortical motor threshold, but the narcotic phase is longer with xylene than with benzene or toluene.

(2) Chronic

Using rats receiving inhalations of 609 p.p.m. and rabbits 1150 p.p.m. 8 h a day, 6 days a week, for periods of 40–130 days, Fabre *et al.* (1960) observed some somnolence, and in the terminal phase dyspnoea, disequilibrium and in some cases paralysis of the hind legs. At the higher concentrations, at the end of the first week, there was conjunctival irritation, anorexia and loss of weight.

Bibliography on p. 124

Narcosis, without the preliminary irritative phenomena characteristic of acute benzene poisoning, is the predominant symptom, and more complete and prolonged. Ataxia, developing into paralysis of the hind legs, was described by Estler (1935) with chattering of the teeth and redness of mucous membranes. Wocjiechowski (1910) also observed hypothermia.

(1) The eyes

Lesions in the form of fine vacuoles in the cornea of cats exposed to the vapour of commercial xylene, similar to the 'polishers' keratitis' observed in human beings following exposure to toluene and some acetates, observed by Schmid (1956).

(2) The blood

Among the earlier investigators using intraperitoneal or subcutaneous injections, only slight changes in the blood picture were recorded – slight diminution in red cells and haemoglobin (Winslow, 1927; Batchelor, 1927; Engelhardt, 1935), or an increase in white cells (Woronow, 1929; Engelhardt, 1935; Farber, 1933); transitory leucopenia and thrombopenia (Hultgren, 1926).

By inhalation, Batchelor found concentrations of 620 p.p.m. to produce only slight leucopenia, while Farber (1933) recorded some changes in both red and white cells, with slight hyperplasia of the bone marrow, and Engelhardt a slight reduction of red cells and haemoglobin and an initial leucocytosis with occasional degenerative changes in the cells.

In a more extensive investigation, Fabre and Truhaut (1954) exposed rats and rabbits to a concentration of 690 p.p.m. of mixed xylenes for 8 h a day for 130 days and found no significant abnormality of the blood picture. With higher concentrations (1150 p.p.m.) some changes, in the form of a decrease in both red and white cells were observed, but these changes were much less severe than with similar concentrations of benzene and were reversible following cessation of exposure. Still more recently, Fabre *et al.* (1960) have confirmed these findings. The bone marrow was hyperplasic with both concentrations, showing no tendency to aplasia and the slight anaemia was only transitory. Neither the differential count nor the coagulation time were affected.

Changes in the blood picture. – It is generally conceded that so far as the haemopoietic system is concerned chronic exposure of animals to xylene is much less injurious than to benzene or even to toluene, but it appears that xylene can exert some moderate effect.

Slight injury of the kindneys and liver and hyperplasia of the bone marrow following dosage by subcutaneous injection or inhalation, but no other characteristic lesions, were noted by Batchelor (1927), and Smyth (1928) observed some inflammation of the lungs following inhalation.

CHANGES IN THE ORGANISM

The most definite lesions in the animals studied by Fabre *et al.* (1960) were found in the kidneys, in the form of congestion, inflammation and some cellular des-quamation with some signs of commencing necrosis at the level of the convoluted tubules.

Similar lesions had already been reported by Smyth and Smyth (1928) and Rosenthal-Deussen (1931) and in Fabre's animals these were accompanied by an increase in blood urea and albumen and blood in the urine.

The amounts of xylene found in the various organs after 130 days (Fabre *et al.*) of 8 h daily inhalations were highest in the adrenals (148 μg), bone marrow (130 μg), spleen (115 μg) and central nervous system (100 μg). The kidneys contained only 86 and the blood 91 μg.

Toxicity to human beings

SYMPTOMS OF INTOXICATION

(1) Skin and mucous membranes

Dermatitis, eczema, irritation of the eyes and respiratory catarrh have been recorded as prominent symptoms of heavy exposure.

(2) Blood and bone marrow

In assessing the evidence for and against a severe haemopoietic effect of xylene similar to that of chronic exposure to benzene, the relatively rare use of pure xylene in industry must be considered one of the factors making such an assessment difficult. It is necessary to examine carefully the constitution of the xylene alleged to be the cause of such disturbance. Unfortunately this is often not stated in des-criptions of cases of aplastic anaemia attributed to xylene exposure, though some-times the statement is made, almost as an afterthought, that the xylene, or mixture of xylene and toluene, contained some benzene. This would appear to be the crucial factor in determining the role of xylene in severe cases of blood disturbance.

(i) Severe and fatal cases. – The above difficulty is exemplified in a case des-cribed by Lachnit and Reimer (1959). This was a 20 year old girl who had been employed one year in a textile factory, using an adhesive containing 27% of toluol and xylol with some esters and benzine. She complained, while at work, of head-ache and nausea which disappeared when she gave up her occupation. When she became pregnant she developed bleeding from the gums and was found to have severe anaemia, leucopenia and thrombocytopenia; the bone marrow was generally aplasic but with some reticular hyperplasia. In spite of intensive therapy by blood transfusions, prednisone and antibiotics she died six weeks after the birth of a healthy child. It was later found that air estimations during the early

days of her employment had shown the presence of 8 p.p.m. of benzene and 11.1 p.p.m. of toluol, though the label on the adhesive had stated that it was "free from benzol and chlorinated hydrocarbons".

A second fatal case of 'panmyelopathy' also described by Lachnit and Reimer was that of a man who had been employed as a printer for 30 years before he was involved in helping to put out a fire in which 40 l of xylol were burnt. After this incident his health deteriorated and he had some nose bleeding. A blood examination showed anaemia but a normal white cell and differential count. The anaemia became more severe and leucopenia and thrombocytopenia developed and the bone marrow now showed myeloid aplasia and reticular hyperplasia with a relatively normal erythropoiesis. It was concluded that the sudden exposure to xylol had 'triggered' a severe reaction in the already damaged haemopoietic tissues, but since the only reference to the xylol used is that of 'technical xylol', it is not impossible that it contained some percentage of benzene.

In a series of cases, some of them fatal, recorded by Appuhn and Goldeck (1957) and attributed to "benzol and its homologues", it is also clear that the predominant injurious agent was benzol, since the solvent used was stated to contain 40–60% of benzene.

A case reported in the Annual Report of the Chief Inspector of Factories in 1960 was that of a man who died of myeloid leukaemia following exposure to a mixture of toluene and xylene. It was later found that the toluene contained from 6 to 10% of benzene.

A more severe, ultimately fatal, case of an unusual form of anaemia alleged to be the result of exposure to xylene was described by Grammarinaro (1956), but here again no details of the composition or concentration of the xylol nor of the nature of the exposure were given. The condition was designated "osteosclerotic anaemia with aplastic myelosis". In the idiopathic form of this disease in adults, osteosclerosis is accompanied by aplasia of the bone marrow, which is attributed by some observers to constriction of the medullary spaces damaging the bone marrow function.

Grammarinaro's case was that of a man aged 46, employed since his youth as a typographer, in constant contact with xylene. He complained initially of gastrointestinal disturbance, with nausea, abdominal pain, diarrhoea and episodes of fever. Later symptoms included severe frontal headache, keratitis, redness, stiffness and swelling of the joints especially of the hands and feet. There was tenderness over the right hypochondrium and slight enlargement of the liver. The urine contained a trace of albumen and increased urobilin, some leucocytes, erythrocytes and hyaline cylinders. The serum bilirubin was 0.99 mg/100, the Hijmans-Van den Bergh direct reaction negative, the indirect weakly positive. The blood picture showed anaemia and leucopenia, with 1% of myelocytes and metamyelocytes, 2% of proerythroblasts and 1% of erythroblasts.

Death took place 9 months later, preceded by a rise in total white cells, polymorphs and reticulocytes, regarded as signs of regeneration and activity of extra-medullary foci of haematopoiesis. Autopsy revealed osteosclerosis of the sternum, ribs, iliac crest and femur. Grammarinaro considered the blood and bone disorders as two manifestations independent of each other but both allied to chronic intoxication by xylene. The possibility that this was an idiopathic form of the disease or alternatively that the xylene contained some benzene cannot be ruled out.

(ii) Less severe cases of blood abnormality. – Similar uncertainty exists in some of the alleged cases of slight injury to the bone marrow by chronic exposure to xylene. Such are those described by Lob in 1952. He regarded these as analogous to those reported from chronic exposure to benzene, but in his investigation of 17 men and 2 women in a printing works where toluol and xylol were used as solvents for the printing inks, the only information as to the constitution of the solvent is that it contained "minimal traces" of benzene; moreover, benzene was used in appreciable quantity during one month in 1947.

He found slight macrocytic anaemia in 11 of these workers, leucopenia in 3, granulocytopenia in 5. He also found a tendency to bone marrow aplasia in 6 cases and hyperplasia in 7. The condition of the bone marrow could not always be correlated with the peripheral blood picture or with the general health, a discrepancy which Lob suggested may have been due to the fact that either the injury to the bone marrow was not severe enough to prevent normal or subnormal haemopoiesis or that extra-medullary haemopoiesis supplemented the medullary deficiency.

Other cases of anaemia and/or leucopenia in colour printers are those recorded by Glibert (1935), but the composition of the xylol is described only as having "variability of composition", pseudo-xylol being stated to contain toluene with 15% of benzene. Only a few German authorities have suggested that xylene has an effect especially on erythropoiesis comparable to that of benzene. Hirsch (1932) for example found the red cell count below 5 millions in 15 out of 34 cases, and Adler-Herzmark (1933) believed that the red cell picture was more disturbed by xylene than by toluene. In a series of workers exposed to xylene examined by the author in 1945 (Browning, 1953) where the xylene used was of uncertain composition, the disturbance of the blood picture was greater than that of workers exposed to pure xylene but considerably less than in those exposed to benzene. Table 5 shows the difference in severity of the blood changes in a series of 44 xylene and 70 benzene workers.

It is at any rate clear that the great majority of observers consider that xylene, if it has any toxic effect on the haemopoietic organs, is much less injurious in this respect than benzene. Francone and Braier (1954) have said that its toxic effects are "minor" and could be regarded as almost negligible if xylene could be generally substituted for benzene. It must be noted however that recent metabolic investigations do sound a warning of a possible benzene-like action of xylene, in

Bibliography on p. 124

the finding that a certain amount of products of nuclear oxidation do appear in the urine of exposed animals, compounds of the same type as the anti-mitotic phenolic metabolites of benzene. (see p. 11).

TABLE 5

Camparative effect of benzene and xylene on the blood
(from E. Browning, 1953)

Solvent	Total number of cases	Red blood corpuscles		Haemo-globin	White blood corpuscles			Polymorph
		4–4.5 million cases (%)	<4 million cases (%)	<85% cases (%)	>10000 cases (%)	4000–5000 cases (%)	<4000 cases (%)	<50% cases (%)
Benzene	70	22 (31.5)	7 (10)	19 (27)	4 (5.5)	14 (20)	10 (14.5)	30 (43)
Xylene	44	7 (16)		3 (7)		3 (7)		7 (16)

(3) Urine

The evidence for an injurious effect of xylene on the kidneys comes chiefly from experience with the weather proof paint 'Inertol' (see above). It is not clear to which constituent of 'Inertol' the symptoms of poisoning were definitely attributed. But in most of the cases described by Stocke (1929 and 1931) and Rosenthal-Deussen (1931) the accompanying symptoms were said to resemble most closely those of acute xylol intoxication. They included the irritative manifestations of eczema, conjunctivitis, cough and severe gastro intestinal disturbance, and in several cases the narcotic effect was shown by drowsiness, giddiness and even unconsciousness. Injury to the kidneys was indicated by the appearance of dark brown or red urine containing some albumen and erythrocytes. These abnormalities disappeared rapidly on removal from exposure. The actual cause of death in the one fatal case remained obscure; it followed an operation for paralytic ileus, which Rosenthal-Deussen suggested was due to damage of the sympathetic nervous system caused by the benzol constituent. It is of interest to note that in one of Stocke's cases in which blood examination was carried out the blood picture was normal except for a slight deficiency of haemoglobin.

(4) Gastro-intestinal disturbances

Nausea, vomiting, heartburn and loss of appetite are among the most frequent complaints of workers exposed to xylene in concentrations above the maximum allowable concentration.

A typical case of this kind has been recently (1961) described by Glass in a man engaged in cleaning paint-mixing pots with a mixture of xylene, ethyl benzene, methylethyl benzene and trimethyl benzene. It is probable that the severe giddiness and vomiting from which the man suffered was due to a summation of the effects of these constituents, but is was later found that when the pots were hot following a hot caustic wash, the maximum concentration of xylene rose to 270 to 350 p.p.m.

(5) Neurological disturbances

As would be expected from the known effect of xylene on the central nervous system of animals, the most widely reported effect of heavy acute exposure on human beings is narcotic, with a more marked irritant effect than that of benzene. This is shown by dizziness, excitement, inco-ordination and a staggering gait. These effects are, however, rarely observed in industry, because, as Johnstone (1960) remarks, workers will not voluntarily stay in an atmosphere of the highly irritant vapour long enough to develop them.

No fatal cases from acute exposure to an atmosphere containing the vapour of xylene alone or even predominantly xylene have been recorded. One fatal case, described by Koelsch (cited by Stocke, 1931), was due to exposure to 'Inertol', a weatherproof paint widely used in Germany and consisting of 35% of benzol and its homologues with other unidentified solvents.

Complete unconsciousness is also rare, but two cases were reported to the Home Office in 1934, in which the solvent used in leather manufacture contained 30% of xylene as well as butyl and ethyl acetate and diamyl phthalate.

Later symptoms following recovery from the acute poisoning have also been referred to the nervous system. Rosenblatt (1902) described them as 'neurasthenic' in a man employed in the rubber industry, who complained of fatigue, giddiness, palpitation, burning in the head, a feeling of drunkenness, numbness of the hands and feet and anxiety. In the two Home Office cases mentioned above, there were also residual symptoms – excitement, headache, insomnia, nervousness and gastric pain, and in one of them tremor and 'pins and needles' of the hands and feet. Nausea and vomiting were also described by Rosenblatt and by Brezina (1921) as post-narcotic manifestations.

CHANGES IN THE ORGANISM

(1) The heart

The possibility that xylene may cause cardiac injury was suggested by Hirsch (1932). In workers in a printing office where xylene was the predominating constituent (64%) in the ink diluting fluid as well as 18% in other solvents, the remaining exposure being to benzene and toluene used for cleaning, radiography revealed abnormalities of size and form of the heart in 50%. In some the aorta was dilated and in others the blood pressure was lowered. Hirsch related these abnormalities to dilatation of the blood vessels by xylene.

(2) The liver

Acute injury of the liver has been recorded chiefly as the results of accidental ingestion of xylene. Ghislandi and Fabriani (1957) describe the case of a man employed in spraying metallic objects with a nitrocellulose varnish in which xylol was the most prominent constituent of the diluent. This was contained in a flask from which the man drank a small amount in mistake for water. He experienced

Bibliography on p. 124

immediate retro-sternal burning, heat and redness of the face and some dyspnoea. Aspiration by gastric sound and introduction of weak alkalies and emetics was followed by apparent recovery, but liver tests indicated the presence of toxic hepatosis. A positive bromsulphthalein test gradually decreased during the next three weeks from a retention of 20%–6.2% and recovery was then apparently complete.

In 18 out of 34 of the printing office workers mentioned above Hirsch (1932) noted an increase in the urine of urobilin and urobilinogen; this he regarded as an indication of liver injury.

(3) The kidneys

It has already been noted (see p. 85) that injury to the kidneys was postulated in the fatal case described by Rosenthal-Deussen and Stocke (1931) and that lesions of the kidney have been observed in animals subjected to repeated inhalation of xylene. In human beings such injury has rarely, if ever, been attributed definitely to chronic exposure to xylene.

A suggestion that xylene may have been the cause of slight kidney injury has come recently from the relatively new industry of epoxy resin compounds. This is an account by Joyner and Pegues (1961) of a somewhat frequent disorder of health occurring in men employed in the destructive removal of epoxy resin concrete which had been poured 18 months previously. The symptoms were headache, sore throat and dry cough, and urine examinations revealed small amounts of albumen and a few red and white cells. Two possible offending agents, the decomposition products of epichlorhydrin and free amines, were identified in the vapours from drilling, grinding or pyrolysing samples of the epoxy concrete, but in view of the fact that there had been a faint odour of xylene and that the presence of substantial amounts of xylene in the atmosphere were indicated by infra-red and spectrometer analyses, it was suggested that the operation produced a very fine dust mixed with the vapour of xylene and other unidentified vapours and that the xylene might be responsible for both the upper respiratory irritation and also for the slight nephrotoxic action. It is not at present possible to decide conclusively whether xylene was the actual cause of the trouble. An interesting point is that some of these men complained also of 'vague abdominal symptoms' which could be interpreted as liver involvement though no conclusive evidence of this was obtained.

(4) The nervous system

Drowsiness, giddiness, excessive fatigue, headache and a sensation of 'drunkenness' are common complaints in workpeople with no previous evidence of central nervous disability. That the same exposure which produces these symptoms in normal people can induce convulsions in those suffering from latent epilepsy is suggested by Goldie (1960) from his observation of such a case. This was a boy of 18 who had been employed for some months in spray painting gun towers with a paint containing 80% of xylene and 20% of methylglycol acetate. On reaching his home he had a convulsive seizure and became unconscious. He recovered consciousness after about twenty minutes but later had another slighter attack. His reflexes were normal, there were no pathological changes in the skull or the E.E.G. and the blood picture showed no abnormality. It transpired that at the age of 14 he had had what appeared to be an epileptic aura, with cramps but no loss of consciousness. Stocke also mentions a patient with latent epilepsy who complained of increasingly frequent seizures when exposed to xylene. Stocke also states that sensitivity to alcohol is increased by exposure to xylene.

Bibliography on p. 124

4. Ethylbenzene

Synonyms: phenylethane, ethylbenzol

Structural formula:

CH$_2$—CH$_3$

Molecular formula: C$_8$H$_{10}$

Molecular weight: 106.16

Properties: a clear colourless liquid with an aromatic odour.

    boiling point: 136.2 °C

    melting point: −94.95 °C

    vapour pressure: 10 mg Hg at 25.90 °C

    vapour density (air = 1): 3.7

    specific gravity (liquid density): 0.86258

    flash point: 63 °F

    conversions factors: 1 p.p.m. = 4.35 mg/m^3

                    1 mg/l = 230 p.p.m.

    solubility: hardly in water, miscible with ethanol and ether

    maximum allowable concentration: 100 p.p.m. ACGIH 1965 revision.

ECONOMY, SOURCES AND USES

Production

Chiefly by the alkylation of benzene (addition of ethylene in presence of a catalyst); also by dehydrogenation of cycloparaffins and by ultra-fractionation from a mixed xylene stream (Grearde, 1960).

Industrial uses

(1) As an intermediate in the production of styrene.

(2) As a constituent of solvents with properties similar to those of xylene.

(3) As a diluent in paints and lacquers.

(4) As a constituent of motor and aviation fuels, by virtue of its 'anti-knock' quality (Patty, 1949).

BIOCHEMISTRY

Estimation

(1) In the atmosphere
The same methods as used for xylene (see p. 77).

(2) In blood, tissues and urine
(a) By colorimetric or spectrophotometric methods following separation or distillation from the sample.
(b) In blood, by an ultraviolet-spectrophotometric method (Guertin and Gerarde, 1959).

Metabolism

The oxidation of ethylbenzene to methylphenylcarbinol in animals has been known since the observations of Neubauer (1901). The formation of this metabolite was confirmed by Smith *et al.* (1954), with the additional finding that both isomers of methyl phenyl carbinol (the + and − forms) in equal amounts are the result of its biological hydroxylation. It is suggested that the hydrogen group is abstracted from the α-methylene group by means of an enzyme, and that ethylbenzene does not undergo oxidation in the benzene ring in vivo.

Gerarde (1960) states that hippuric acid is produced in approximately the same amount, these two end-products accounting for 60–70% of the oral dose. Other minor metabolites are mandelic acid (2%) and phenaceturic acid (10–20%).

TOXICOLOGY

Ethylbenzene is primarily an irritant of skin and, less markedly, of mucous membranes. It is also a narcotic in high concentrations. Although there is some evidence that it may have some influence on the blood picture of animals, in the form of leucocytosis, there is none that it has any 'benzene-like' effect on the bone marrow. No systemic injury has been reported from its industrial use.

Toxicity to animals

(1) Acute
(a) Lethal dose. − *(i) By oral administration*, a lethal dose of 3.5 g/kg body weight (Wolf *et al.*, 1956) shows it to be, according to Gerarde (1960) the most acutely toxic for the rat of all the mono-*n*-alkyl derivatives of benzene. − *(ii) By inhalation*, in the experiments of Yant *et al.* (1930), 10.000 p.p.m. was fatal to guinea pigs in a few min, and 5000 p.p.m. dangerous to life in 30–60 min. Animals

Bibliography on p. 124

that died from exposure had intense congestion and oedema of lungs and generasised visceral hyperaemia.

(b) Narcotic dose. – Exposure to 2000 p.p.m. for up to 375 min caused in some of the animals of Yant *et al.*, motor ataxia and apparent unconsciousness; with 10,000 p.p.m. this stage was reached in 18 min. It was preceded by vertigo, unsteadiness and ataxia.

(2) Chronic

(i) By oral administration, repeated doses of 136 mg/kg body weight produced in female rats, no demonstrable injury (Wolf *et al.*, 1956). – *(ii) By subcutaneous injection* (1 ml/kg body weight daily for two weeks); the animals had a normal total marrow nucleated cell count, but developed a peripheral leucocytosis. – *(iii) By inhalation*, repeated exposure to concentrations ranging from 400 to 2000 p.p.m. for as long as six months had no other effect than a slight increase in the weight of the liver and kidneys of rats exposed to 400 p.p.m. for 186 days; none of these animals showed any abnormality of the haemopoietic system.

SYMPTOMS OF INTOXICATION

(1) The eyes

Instillation of undiluted ethylbenzene into the eyes of rabbits caused only slight conjunctival irritation and no corneal injury (Wolf *et al.*, 1956). This is in contrast to the results of Yant *et al.* (1930) in their inhalation studies on the acute toxicity of ethylbenzene. They found that exposure to 5000 and 10000 p.p.m. of the vapour in air produced immediate and intense irritation of the conjunctiva of guinea pigs, while 2000 p.p.m. caused moderate eye and nose irritation in one minute.

(2) The skin

Repeated application of undiluted ethylbenzene to the skin of rabbits caused, in the experiments of Wolf *et al.*, the type of response similar to that of benzene, its homologues and some of the alkylated benzenes, i.e. reddening and some exfoliation; ethylbenzene was one of those which caused actual blistering. Oettel (1936) had also found that ethylbenzene was the most severe skin irritant of the benzene series.

CHANGES IN THE ORGANISM

The lungs

It is pointed out by Gerarde (1960) that the aspiration of even a small amount of ethylbenzene may cause severe injury, since its low viscosity and surface tension will cause it to spread over a large surface of pulmonary tissue, causing oedema and haemorrhage.

Toxicity to human beings

Observations on six men by Yant *et al.* (1930) showed that exposure to 0.1%
(1000 p.p.m.) of the vapour in air caused severe irritation of the eyes, with profuse lacrimation, but after a minute or two tolerance appeared to be established.
Even 2000 p.p.m., while causing immediate lacrimation and nasal irritation, became less irritating on continued exposure, but this concentration caused dizziness,
and 5000 p.p.m. was so irritating as to make work in such an atmosphere impossible.

Bibliography on p. 124

5. Cumene

Synonyms: isopropylbenzene; 2-phenylpropane

Structural formula:

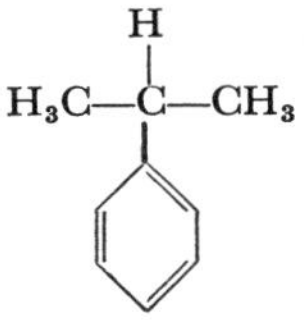

$$H_3C-\underset{\underset{\displaystyle \bigcirc}{|}}{\overset{\overset{\displaystyle H}{|}}{C}}-CH_3$$

Molecular formula: C_9H_{12}

Molecular weight: 120.19

Properties: a colourless mobile liquid with a strong, slightly irritant odour; less volatile than benzene, toluene or xylene; good solvent for fats and resins.
  boiling point: 152.5 °C
  melting point: −96.03 °C
  vapour pressure: 10 mm Hg at 38.33 °C
  vapour density (air = 1): 4.2
  specific gravity (liquid density): 0.85748 at 15 °C
  flash point: 102 °F
  conversions factors: 1 p.p.m. = 0.00492 mg/l
                1 mg/l = 203.5 p.p.m.
  solibility: very slightly in water; soluble in ethanol and ether.
  maximum allowable concentration: Gerarde (1960) suggests 50–100 p.p.m. ACGIH 1965 suggests 50 p.p.m.

ECONOMY, SOURCES AND USES

Production

Produced by fractional distillation of petroleum and by catalytic synthesis from benzene and propylene.

Industrial uses

(1) As a thinner for cellulose paints and lacquers.
(2) As a component of high octane aviation fuel.
(3) As a starting material for organic synthesis especially of phenol and acetone (Hock and Lang, 1944).
(4) In the production of styrene.

[94]

BIOCHEMISTRY

Estimation

(1) In the atmosphere

In the absence of other aromatic hydrocarbons cumene can be determined colorimetrically by nitration, or by treatment with sulphuric acid-formaldehyde mixture.

(2) In blood and tissues

(a) By nitration after preliminary separation by distillation (Fabre *et al.*, 1955).

(b) By ultraviolet spectrophotometry (Guertin and Gerarde, 1959).

Metabolism

(1) Absorption and excretion

Liquid cumene is absorbed through the intact skin rather slowly, but more rapidly than toluene, xylene or ethylbenzene (Vallette and Cavier, 1954). The vapour is readily absorbed into the blood stream and a small part (less than 5%, according to Gerarde, 1960) is exhaled unchanged. The greater part is converted in the liver to water-soluble metabolites-phenylpropanol and phenylpropionic acid, which are conjugated with glucuronic acid and glycine and excreted in the urine (Robinson *et al.*, 1955). The presence of small amounts of phenolic compounds in the urine of poisoned animals was postulated by Fabre *et al.* (1955), especially in the rat, where elimation is slower than in the rabbit.

(2) Distribution in tissues

Fabre *et al.* found amounts of cumene varying from 8 μg/g in the liver to 29 μg/g in the blood of rats 48 h after the last exposure (repeated for 2 months) to concentrations of 500 p.p.m.

The conclusion drawn from these experiments was that isopropylbenzene appears to be localised selectively and especially in the endocrine glands, the central nervous system, the spleen and the liver and that it disappears more rapidly in the rabbit than the rat, and that the blood retains a certain amount longer than the internal organs.

TOXICOLOGY

Cumene is a skin irritant and can be absorbed slowly from the intact skin. While it has the narcotic effect common to other homologues of benzene, it has no injurious haemopoietic effect. No ill effects to human beings have been reported

Bibliography on p. 124

from its industrial use, but animal experiments have suggested that it has a potential capacity for injury of the liver and kidneys (Werner *et al.*, 1944; Fabre *et al.*,
1955).

Toxicity to animals

(1) Acute

   (a) Lethal dose. – *(i) By intraperitonal injection*, according to the early observation of Chassevant and Garnier (1903) the minimum lethal dose was 1.310
g/kg, compared with 0.656 for benzene and 0.411 for toluene. – *(ii) By inhalation*,
the lower toxicity of isopropyl benzene compared with benzene and toluene was
observed by Rambousek in 1913; he found that exposure of dogs, cats and rabbits
to 60 mg/l (12200 p.p.m.) did not produce any signs of intoxication. Werner *et al.*
(1944) found the minimum lethal dose (MLD) for mice to be 10 mg/l (2000
p.p.m.) and on this basis it appeared to be more acutely toxic than either benzene
or toluene, but on the basis of their relative saturation concentrations the 'hazard
index' (saturation concentration divided by MLD) becomes: Cumene 4 – toluene 10 – benzene 12.

   (b) Narcotic dose. – In mice, by inhalation, Lazarew (1929) stated the narcotic dose to be between 20 and 25 mg/l (4000–5000 p.p.m.), representing a lower
toxicity in this respect than either benzene or toluene. According to Werner
et al. (1944) the narcotic effect of cumene is manifested much more slowly than
that of benzene or toluene but once established is much more persistent.

   In an attempt to reconcile the conflicting views on this question of relative
toxicity, Fabre *et al.* (1955) carried out a series of inhalation experiments on rats,
using concentrations of 6.5 mg/l (2000 p.p.m.) 8 h a day for 130–180 days. The
rat proved much more sensitive than the rabbit, showing at this concentration
symptoms of intoxication, followed by death after 6–16 h. Even 4 mg/l proved fatal
after 16 h, but at 2.5 mg/l (500 p.p.m.) no symptoms of disturbance of health were
observed.

(2) Chronic

   As already noted, Fabre *et al.* (1955) found that repeated inhalation of 2000
p.p.m. caused symptoms of intoxication in rabbits and rats. These included somnolence, motor disturbance, and loss of equilibrium.

SYMPTOMS OF INTOXICATION

The symptoms observed in mice were narcosis or slight inco-ordination, the narcosis developing more slowly and lasting longer than with benzene or toluene.
Werner *et al.* also noted dilatation of cutaneous blood vessels.

Blood and bone marrow

   Although certain changes in the peripheral blood picture and even in the bone marrow, similar to those stated to occur, with subcutaneous injection, with cymene (Woronow, 1929), an increase of immature white cells with a characteristic dark-blue staining of the protoplasm, a gradual rise in total white cells and an initial rise in erythrocytes followed by a slight fall at the end of the experiment, the bone marrow containing many of the characteristic white cells with blue proto-plasm, these changes were not present as the result of inhalation in the experi-ments of Fabre et al. (1955). They found no significant abnormality either of the peripheral blood or of the bone marrow in rats or rabbits exposed daily for 150 days to 2.5 mg/l (500 p.p.m.), and it is generally agreed that isopropylbenzene has no benzene-like effect on the haemopietic system.

CHANGES IN THE ORGANISM

Hyperaemia and congestion of the lungs, liver and kidneys have also been ob-served.

(1) The liver

Werner et al. (1944) found the liver injury to be more marked with lower concen-trations than those causing similar injuries with benzene, and about the same as with similar concentrations of toluene, and they suggested that slow elimination might be associated with a cumulative effect. Gerarde (1960) on the other hand, regards these changes as non-specific and common to the effects of exposure to many other solvents such as esters, ketones and esters.

(2) The kidneys

By gastric intubation to rats Wolf et al. (1956) found no evidence of injury after 139 doses of 154 mg/kg in 194 days. With an increased dosage there was an increase of weight in the kidneys. Kidney injury, in the form of epithelial nephri-tis, has also been postulated in inhalation experiments (Werner et al., 1944; Fabre et al., 1955).

Bibliography on p. 124

6. Styrene

Synonyms: vinylbenzene, phenylethylene, cinnamene

Structural formula:

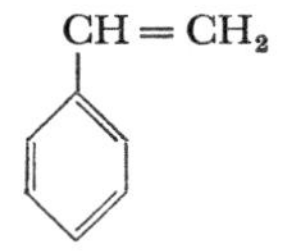

$$CH = CH_2$$

Molecular formula: C_8H_8

Molecular weight: 104.14

Properties: a clear colourless liquid with a characteristic pungent odour.
> *boiling point:* 145.2 °C
> *melting point:* −30.6 °C
> *vapour pressure:* 6.45 mm Hg at 25 °C
> *vapour density (air = 1):* 3.6
> *specific gravity (liquid density):* 0.902 at 25 °C
> *flash point:* 86 °F
> *conversion factors:* 1 p.p.m. = 0.00426 mg/l
> 1 mg/l = 235.5 p.p.m.
> *solubility:* little in water; miscible with ethanol and ether
> *maximum allowable concentration:* 100 p.p.m.

At the time of the investigations in 1952 the recommended M.A.C. was 200 p.p.m. but all the observers agreed that this level was too high for prolonged exposure. In 1957, following an analysis of air samples in the Plastics Industry by Rogers and Hooper, it was reduced to 100 p.p.m. During this investigation the dermatitis hazard was recognised as specially prominent, since styrene tends to degrease the skin, with resulting cracking and inflammation of the exposed areas; it was more widespread in fair-skinned individuals, who also complained most frequently of 'styrene sickness'.

With regard to the prevention of exposure to concentrations higher than the M.A.C. Rogers pointed out that the installation of 'duct systems, blowers and booths' would involve a large capital outlay and that dilution ventilation would be a more practical method of control. This was provided by stand fans to direct the vapours away from the breathing zone, supplemented by exhaust fans in the ceiling and an exhaust spray booth at one end of the room.

ECONOMY, SOURCES AND USES

Production

Stryrene is produced commercially by the dehydrogenation of ethylbenzene. It can also be obtained from benzaldehyde, and occurs naturally in the sap of styraceous trees (Gerarde, 1960).

Industrial uses

(1) In the plastics industry, as a solvent for synthetic rubber and resins (poly-styrene plastics).
(2) As a modifier or solvent for polyester resins.
(3) As a starting material in the manufacture of emulsifying agents.
(4) As an intermediate in chemical synthesis.
(5) In the manufacture of synthetic rubber.

BIOCHEMISTRY

Estimation

(1) In the atmosphere

(a) By ultra-violet and infra-red absorption (Rowe et al., 1943).

(b) Colorimetric method. – By a nitration process, suggested by Rowe *et al*, as the most suitable method for most laboratories.

(c) By interferometer or combustible gas indicator, with special calibration for styrene (Gerarde, 1960).

(2) In blood and tissues

By ultraviolet absorption, nitration or colorimetry, with a sulphuric acid-formaldehyde mixture, after separation by extraction or distillation.

Metabolism

(1) Absorption and excretion

Styrene can be absorbed by inhalation, oral administration, and slowly by the intact skin. Excretion is chiefly in the urine, in the form of its metabolites, of which benzoic and hippuric acid have been isolated and identified (Spencer *et al.*, 1942). Hippuric acid was found by Smith *et al.* (1954) to constitute about 40% of the dose, while an unidentified glucuronide to the amount of about 15% was also present.

Unlike ethylbenzene styrene is not converted to phenaceturic acid. Inhalation of 800 p.p.m. for 4 h by human subjects was found by Carpenter *et al.* (1944) to cause an added excretion of the glucuronide.

Bibliography on p. 124

An investigation by Danishefsky and Willhite (1954) using subcutaneous injections of radioactive styrene showed that it was rapidly metabolised, 85% of the radioactivity being excreted during the first 24 h; much the greatest part (about 71%) in the urine, 3% in the faeces, 12% as respiratory CO_2, and 3% unchanged by the lungs. Williams (1959) remarks that "it seems to be reasonably well established that styrene is partly split at the ethylene bond, the fragments appearing eventually as hippuric acid and carbondioxide, and partly hydrated to phenylglycol, which is further metabolised by conjugation with glucuronic acid and by oxidation to both mandelic acid and benzoic acid".

(2) Distribution in tissues

According to Danishefsky and Willhite (1954) retention after one hour is highest in the liver (4.62%) falling to 0.11% in 24 h; the next highest in the kidneys (1.82% falling to 0.01 in 24 h). In all the other organs the retention at 24 h is less than 0.02%, except for the adrenals (0.03%) and the small intestine (0.06)%. The blood retained only 0.02% after 24 h.

TOXICOLOGY

Styrene is principally an irritant of skin and mucous membranes, but in animals it has a toxic effect on the central nervous system, and neurological disturbances have also been described in human beings. It is not regarded as involving a serious systemic industrial hazard, since acute exposure causes such intolerable irritation that such exposure cannot continue. With chronic exposure to small doses no benzene-like action on the bone marrow has been observed.

Toxicity to animals

(1) Acute

Exposure to 5000 p.p.m., according to Spencer *et al.* (1942) produces irritation of the eyes and nose, followed by central nervous disturbance manifested by tremors, inco-ordination, loss of equilibrium and finally unconsciousness.

(2) Chronic

Repeated exposures to 650–1300 p.p.m. for periods up to 6 months caused, in the hands of Spencer *et al.* (1942), no significant changes indicating systemic poisoning and no abnormality of the tissues or peripheral blood, but they noted a marked rise of total benzoic acid in the urine of their animals. This has not been observed in human beings – see below (Barsotti, *et al.*, 1952).

According to Rylova (1955) repeated 3 h exposures to 1 mg/l (235 p.p.m.) caused some inco-ordination in young rats.

CHANGES IN THE ORGANISM

The degree of injury varies with the amount of exposure; as already mentioned Spencer and Irish found no significant changes with chronic exposure.

Acute deaths, according to Wilson *et al.* (1948), are due to injury of the central nervous system, and delayed deaths to pneumonia following initial lung irritation; the lungs show congestion, haemorrhage, oedema and exudation. The kidneys and liver also show congestion.

Toxicity to human beings

SYMPTOMS OF INTOXICATION

(1) Mucous membranes and eyes

A transient irritating effect on the eyes and mucous membranes appears at concentrations of 200–400 p.p.m. (Gerarde, 1960); at 500 p.p.m. irritation of the eyes and throat, with coughing, and at 800 p.p.m. immediate eye and throat irritation followed after termination of exposure by a metallic taste (Wolf *et al.*, 1956).

(2) The skin

Dermatitis has been reported from prolonged skin contact by Rogers and Hooper (1957). An investigation by Barsotti *et al.* (1952) of workers in a factory producing polystyrene resins, where the concentrations in workrooms where polymerisation was carried out reached 200 p.p.m., revealed, in addition to conjunctival and pharyngeal congestion, itching dermatitis in one case, and an erythematous papular dermatitis of the forearms in two others.

(3) Blood and urine

In no cases have any haematological disturbances been reported, and in Barsotti's series the urinary excretion of hippuric acid was normal. These observers conclude that hippuric acid excretion is of no practical interest in estimating the degree of exposure or the toxic effect.

(4) Neurological disturbances

Drowsiness, weakness, depression, inertia and unsteadiness were described by Carpenter *et al.* (1944), and a recent investigation by Klimkova-Deutschova (1962) which included examination by the electroencephalogram, has also emphasised the incidence of nervous disturbance, chiefly of a pseudo-neurasthenic nature.

Among 35 women employed in the plastic industry, where exposure included not only styrene, but also cyclohexyl peroxide, dibutyl phthalate, cobalt napthalate and trichloroethylene, the most frequent complaints were headache, fatigue, drowsiness, insomnia, loss or gain in weight, pain in the extremities, nervousness, forgetfulness and in a few cases a feeling of 'drunkenness'. Some women suffered also from menstrual irregularity and dysmenorrhoea. None of these symptoms were permanent; nausea, 'drunkenness' and giddiness disappeared when tolerance to exposure was established. The E.E.G. showed abnormalities in 38% of those tested, and were regarded as due partly to contact of the liquid with unprotected hands, partly to inhalation of the vapour affecting the reticular system of the medulla. The wearing of gloves, especially in spray processes, was recommended as a protective measure.

In the investigation by Rogers and Hooper (1957) it was stated that in cases where the dermatitis hazard was specially prominent, complaints of 'styrene sickness' were also noted, and Barsotti *et al.* (1952) observed an increased activity of deep reflexes in some of their subjects who showed dermatitis and mucous membrane irritation.

7. p-Cymene

Synonyms: cymene, p-isopropyltoluene, cymol, p-methylisopropylbenzene

Structural formula:

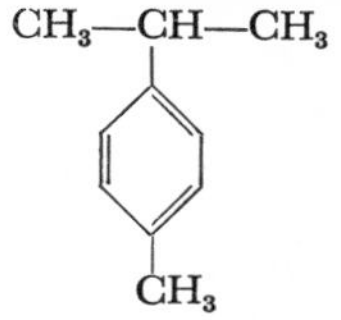

$$CH_3—CH—CH_3$$

CH_3

Molecular formula: $C_{10}H_{14}$

Molecular weight: 134.21

Properties: a clear colourless liquid with sweetish aromatic odour.

  boiling point: 176 °C

  melting point: −68.2 °C

  vapour pressure: 1 mm Hg at 17.3 °C

  vapour density (air = 1): 4.62

  specific gravity (liquid density): 0.86

  flash point: 117 °F

  conversion factors: 1 p.p.m. = 0.00548 mg/l

    1 mg/l = 182 p.p.m.

  solubility: insoluble in water; miscible with ethanol, ether

  maximum allowable concentration: not established; Gerarde (1960) suggests 50 p.p.m.

ECONOMY, SOURCES AND USES

Production

p-Cymene has the unusual feature of being obtainable from a natural source other than coal or petroleum. It is a constituent of many essential oils, including eucalyptus, and can be obtained commercially from stumps of pine trees and also by distillation from the fruit or seed of Cumin cyminium, a herb similar to caraway. It is also an important by-product in the sulphite process of making paper, and can be obtained by dehydration of camphor (Gerarde, 1960).

Industrial uses

In the paint industry as a thinner for lacquers and varnishes usually with other solvents, aromatic hydrocarbons or terpenes.

BIOCHEMISTRY

Estimation

(1) In the atmosphere

p-Cymene can be estimated by ultra-violet or infra-red absorption methods, or by the nitration or sulphuric acid formaldehyde process described for benzene or other aromatic hydrocarbons.

(2) In blood and tissues

Follows the methods for other aromatic hydrocarbons after preliminary separation of the cymene (Gerarde, 1960).

Metabolism

(1) Absorption and excretion

Absorption by the skin is more rapid than with toluene, p-xylene or ethyl-benzene (Valette and Cavier, 1954). By inhalation only a small part is excreted unchanged, the remainder being oxidised to water-soluble metabolites. As early as 1873 Ziegler suggested that the readily oxidised propyl side chain formed a COOH-group, and according to Gerarde (1960) the ultimate product, in the case of dogs and sheep, is cumic acid which is probably excreted as a conjugate with glycine.

In experiments on human beings given 3–4 g daily, Ziegler (1873) had suggested that the first oxidation product of cymene was toluylic acid, which would be combined with glycine, and the results of his investigation indicated that a number of oxidation products were excreted in the urine. It was found, however, that the cymol used was impure, containing a large percentage of pseudocumene. Further experiments, using a pure cymene, were therefore made, using dogs given 2 g by mouth daily. Ziegler then succeeded in isolating cumic acid and isopropylbenzoic acid, which did not conjugate with glycocollic acid. According to Williams (1959) there is apparently no hydroxylation of the ring.

(2) Distribution in tissues

No information.

TOXICOLOGY

p-Cymene is primarily an irritant of skin and mucous membranes, and when given by mouth causes headache, nausea and vomiting. In animals intravenous and subcutaneous injection has produced blood changes similar to those of xylene, but with the appearance of immature white cells. In man there has been only one case reported of severe blood dyscrasia, and the evidence for a direct association with exposure to cymene in this case is by no means indubitable.

Toxicity to animals

The lethal dose for guinea pigs by intraperitoneal administration is given by Chassevant and Garnier (1903) as 2.162 g/kg body weight. Dogs tolerated doses of 2 g daily with diarrhoea as the only adverse effect. Ziegler (1873) found it so innocuous to rabbits that he continued his investigations on human beings.

SYMPTOMS OF INTOXICATION

Blood and bone marrow

By subcutaneous injection of rabbits with 2 ml of cymene daily Miyamato (1938) observed a blood picture similar to that of xylol with regard to white cells, *i.e.* an initial slight fall followed by an increase; red cells and haemoglobin showed irregular changes with a tendency to fall. In similar conditions Woronow (1929) found the chief variation in the blood picture of rabbits to be the rapid appearance of immature white cells (shift to the left) followed by a blue coloration of the cytoplasm of practically all the neutrophils, with granulations which gave them an appearance similar to those seen in human myeloid leukaemia. There was no leucopenia; on the contrary, a steady rise of leucocytes from 4050 on the first day to 36 150 on the 17th; of these 1266 were myelocytes and 1085 Turk cells. The bone marrow also contained these characteristic large blue granulated cells, suggesting that they were formed in the bone marrow.

CHANGES IN THE ORGANISM

Woronow stated that the internal organs differed in no way from the changes observed with other substances containing a methyl group.

Toxicity to human beings

SYMPTOMS OF INTOXICATION

(1) Mucous membranes and skin

According to Gerarde (1960) *p*-cymene is a primary skin irritant which by contact with the liquid can develop erythema, dryness and defatting, the intensity depending on the dose and duration of contact.

(2) Blood and bone marrow

Only one case of severe blood dyscrasia has been attributed to the industrial use of cymene, and this case does not provide definite evidence of cause and effect. It was reported by Carlson in 1946. The man in question had been for twenty years manager of a pulp and paper company using the sulphite process, in which wood chips and calcium bisulphite are digested, and emerge as sulphite pulp. The relief liquor from the pulp mill contained an oil-soluble fraction representing about 4.5 parts in 12 000; of this about 90% was *p*-cymene. The other constituents were sulphur dioxide, acetaldehyde, acetone, methyl alcohol, acetic acid, formic acid and terpenes.

Symptoms possibly indicative of aplastic anaemia had been present for 18 months – weakness, lassitude, dyspnoea, epistaxis and easily produced ecchymoses, the last having apparently preceded the other symptoms. The blood picture showed severe anaemia (red blood corpuscles 1.6 millions, haemoglobin 4.5 g) leucopenia (1450 with only 34% polymorphs) and thrombocytopenia. Blood transfusions, liver extract, ferrous sulphate and yellow bone marrow failed to halt the progress of the disease, and death took place from cerebral haemorrhage. At autopsy the bone marrow contained normoblasts, erythroblasts and moderate numbers of myelocytes and granulocytes, but no fat, and a barely evident background of thin fibrous stroma. This case does not provide definite evidence that the aplastic anaemia was of occupational origin. No other case following exposure to cymene has ever been reported, and none of the other constituents are known to have a 'benzene-like' action on the bone marrow to which Carlson appears to attribute this case. It seems more probable that it was a case of the idiopathic variety of aplastic anaemia, but it should be on record in case of any further reports of this nature from the paper pulp industry.

CHANGES IN THE ORGANISM

The lungs

Extensive chemical pneumonitis may be caused by aspiration into the lungs of a small amount of liquid cymene, owing to its low surface tension and low viscosity (Gerarde, 1959).

8. *p-tert.*-Butyltoluene

Synonym: *p*-methyl-*tert.*-butylbenzene, TBT

Structural formula:

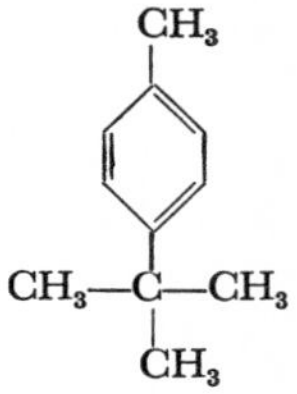

$$
\begin{array}{c}
\text{CH}_3 \\
| \\
\text{(benzene ring)} \\
| \\
\text{CH}_3-\overset{\displaystyle \text{CH}_3}{\underset{\displaystyle \text{CH}_3}{\text{C}}}-\text{CH}_3
\end{array}
$$

Molecular formula: $C_{11}H_{16}$

Molecular weight: 148.24

Properties: a clear colourless liquid with a distinct aromatic odour to which tolerance may be rapidly acquired (Hine *et al.*, 1954).

   boiling point: 192.8 °C
   melting point: —62.53 °C
   vapour pressure: 0.65 mm Hg at 25 °C
   vapour density (air = 1): 4.62
   specific gravity (liquid density): 0.8575
   flash point: 155 °F
   conversion factors: 1 p.p.m. = 0.00666 mg/l
                            1 mg/l = 150 p.p.m.
   solubility: insoluble in water; miscible with ethanol and ether.
   maximum allowable concentration: 10 p.p.m.

ECONOMY, SOURCES AND USES

Production

TBT is formed by the alkylation of toluene with isobutylene.

Industrial uses

(1) As a solvent for resins.
(2) As a primary intermediate in the chemical industry.

BIOCHEMISTRY

Estimation

(1) In the atmosphere

Gerarde (1960) states that methods used for the estimation of toluene, ethyl-benzene and cumene *(q.v.)* could be adapted and calibrated for TBT, while Hine *et al.* (1954) have used an ultra-violet spectrophotometric method by which concentrations of 2 p.p.m. could be detected in 1-litre samples.

(2) In blood and tissues

Extraction and distillation followed by estimation by colorimetric or ultra-violet spectrophotometric methods.

Metabolism

(1) Absorption and excretion

TBT is absorbed into the blood by inhalation of the vapour and by oral administration of the liquid. According to Gerarde (1960) it is probable that owing to its low vapour pressure only a small amount is exhaled unchanged, the major part being metabolised in the liver and excreted as water-soluble metabolites in the urine, as conjugates of alcohols or carboxylic acids with glucuronic acids or glycine.

(2) Distribution in tissues

No information.

TOXICOLOGY

TBT is predominantly a nerve poison with a potent injurious effect on the central nervous system. It is also an irritant of mucous membranes, and in animals by subcutaneous injection has caused liver damage. While it may cause some disturbance of the blood picture, this is transitory and is not regarded as a true benzene effect.

Toxicity to animals

Lethal dose. – In the investigations of Hine *et al.* it ranged from 165 p.p.m. after 8 h exposure to 934 p.p.m. after one hour.

SYMPTOMS OF INTOXICATION

With repeated short exposures (one hour) to 850 p.p.m., 30% of the animals showed clonic movements and tremor, and after two or three exposures flexor paralysis. In the 86% of animals dying after 10 exposures the most frequent cause of death was pulmonary oedema and pneumonia. With longer exposures (50 times to 25 p.p.m. or 25 times to 50 p.p.m.) there was no evidence of neurological injury, but some eye irritation. Of 3 animals exposed for 7 h daily to 50 p.p.m., however, one developed severe flexor spasticity of the fore legs.

(1) The eyes

Eye irritation resulted in purulent discharge.

(2) The skin

Skin irritation was only moderate in the intact skin, but subcutaneous injection was followed by extensive skin ulceration.

(3) Blood and bone marrow

The blood picture, in severely intoxicated animals, showed occasionally some decrease of red and white cells but no consistently uniform abnormality.

(4) Respiratory disturbances

Respiratory injury was reflected in dyspnoea, severe at concentrations of 135 p.p.m. and appearing 3–4 h after beginning of exposure.

(5) Neurological disturbances

Injury of the central nervous system was shown by paralysis of spastic and flaccid type, and moderate anaesthesia preceding death. Recurrent tremors, convulsions and epileptoid seizures were also observed, and those animals showing these disturbances, which survived 24 h, recovered only partially.

CHANGES IN THE ORGANISM

Animals exposed repeatedly to 25 p.p.m. showed practically no pathological changes; at 50 p.p.m. some showed moderate fatty change in the liver and patchy emphysema of the lungs.

The bone marrow showed some depression of erythropoiesis, but since similar abnormalities were found in the control animals, this was not regarded as significant.

The nervous system showed lesions which were regarded as essentially those of encephalomeningitis.

The results of these experiments, with regard to acute exposure, accord with the toxicological description of Hodge and Sterner (1943), who described the acute toxicity of TBT as "moderately toxic following exposure to vapour, slightly toxic following ingestion and practically non-toxic following skin absorption".

(1) The liver

Injury to the liver of animals receiving subcutaneous injection consisted of enlargement and yellowish discolouration, with fatty infiltration.

Bibliography on p. 124

(2) The kidneys

Some fatty deposits.

(3) The lungs

Oedema and haemorrhage were observed.

(4) The nervous system

Diffuse oedema and occasionally acute necrosis were shown, especially in the corpus callosum and the spinal cord. The nerve cells showed swelling, vacuolation and chromatolysis.

Toxicity to human beings

SYMPTOMS OF INTOXICATION

Sensory response studies (Hine *et al.*) with exposure for 5 min to concentrations varying from 5–160 p.p.m. elicited complaints of irritation of nose and throat, nausea and metallic taste; moderate eye irritation at 80 p.p.m., and giddiness and increased breathing effort at 160 p.p.m., but except at this level no real discomfort.

In industrial use subjective complaints from workers in experimental plants where TBT was used as a wash liquor in processes involving crystallisation and centrifugation of solid materials, were essentially those of nasal irritation, nausea, malaise, headache and weakness. Ten out of 33 operators showed decreased blood pressure and increased pulse rate, 4 showed tremor and anxiety, and 2 evidence of skin irritation from contact. There were some changes in the peripheral blood picture; in a few cases lowered haemoglobin and red cell levels, leucopenia, eosinophilia, prolonged clotting time and in two cases a raised icterus index.

All these deviations from the normal disappeared on removal from exposure, and while they were regarded as more nearly resembling those of benzene than of toluene, they were neither as constant nor severe.

9. Mesitylene

Synonyms: trimethylbenzene, 1,3,5-trimethylbenzol, TMB

Structural formula:

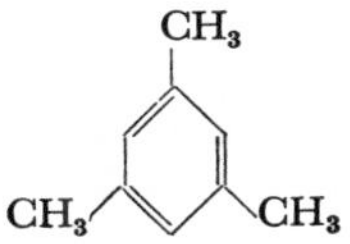

$$
\begin{array}{c}
\text{CH}_3 \\
\text{CH}_3 \quad \text{CH}_3
\end{array}
$$

Molecular formula: C_9H_{12}

Molecular weight: 120.19

Properties: A clear colourless liquid with a not unpleasant aromatic odour.
  boiling point: 164.6 °C
  melting point: −52.7 °C
  vapour pressure: 1.86 mm Hg at 20 °C
  vapour density (air = 1): 1.006 at 20 °C
  specific gravity (liquid density): 0.8634
  flash point: 122 °F
  conversion factors: 1 p.p.m. = 4.92 mg/m³
              1 mg/l = 203.5 p.p.m.
  solubility: slightly in water; miscible with ethanol, ether and benzene
  maximum allowable concentration: not yet established; Gerarde (1960) suggests 50 p.p.m. as a reasonable figure; Battig *et al.* (1958) suggest 35 p.p.m. for an 8 h working day.

ECONOMY, SOURCES AND USES

Production

(1) By fractionation of coal tar and petroleum distillates.
(2) By dehydrating acetone with H_2SO_4.

Industrial uses

(1) Chiefly as a constituent of paint thinners which usually contain also other isomers of trimethylbenzene – the 1,2,3- and 1,2,4-(pseudocumene).
  A solvent 'Fleet-X-DV 99' whose chief constituents are mesitylene and the 1,2,4-isomer has provided the only material for investigation of the effects of mesitylene on human beings.
(2) As a minor constituent of other aromatic solvents and motor fuels.

Bibliography on p. 124   [111]

BIOCHEMISTRY

Estimation

(1) In the atmosphere

By ultraviolet photometer, as for other aromatic hydrocarbons, with special calibration of the apparatus for mesitylene.

(2) In blood and tissues

By ultraviolet absorption, nitration or colorimetric methods, following distillation or extraction of the samples.

Metabolism

(1) Absorption and excretion

Absorption takes place most readily by inhalation of the vapour, but the liquid can be absorbed from the gastro-intestinal tract, and probably, though slowly, by the intact skin (Gerarde, 1960).

Only a small portion is excreted unchanged by the lungs; the greater part is oxidised to water-soluble metabolites, which are excreted by the urine, partly free, partly conjugated with glycine and mesitylenic acid.

Rossi and Grandjean (1957) have recorded an increase in urinary phenols, both free and bound, in rats subjected to inhalation of 200, 580 and 1700 p.p.m. of 'Fleet-X-DV-99'. This supports Gerarde's finding that a single subcutaneous injection of mesitylene (5 ml/kg body weight) increased the urinary excretion of organic sulphates, though not to the same extent as with benzene. Rossi and Grandjean state that the 'Fleet-X' on which their investigation was based contained 50% of 1,2,4-trimethylbenzol (pseudocumene) and 30% of the 1,3,5-isomer (mesitylene), with small amounts of the 1,2,3-isomer and of methylethylbenzol. They determined the free and total phenols in the 24 h specimens of urine of rats exposed for 42 to 46 days to concentrations of 1700 p.p.m., using a spectrophotometric method, and calculated that the difference between these two values represented the amount of conjugated phenols. Control animals were kept in the same conditions and on the same diet. The values found are given in Table 6.

Estimations made at 4, 8, 13 and 15-days' exposure, with the same concentration, showed, (a) that the excretion of the free phenols increased gradually, reaching a maximum after 13 days; (b) that total phenols had increased greatly at 4 days, reaching a maximum on the 8th day and tending to diminish thereafter, though remaining higher than the controls. On cessation of exposure the free phenols returned to normal more rapidly than the total and conjugated, which remained significantly higher than the controls after 9–10 days.

With concentrations of 580 p.p.m. the difference from the controls became significant only after 8 days, and on cessation of exposure only the total phenols showed a slight significant difference after 6 days. With 200 p.p.m. an increase in only the free and total phenols became significantly evident after 10 days.

Thus, the process of conjugation, representing the defences of the organism against toxic substances, appears to be most active in the early days of exposure and tends to diminish later, though still remaining at a higher level than normal.

Consequently, at the beginning of exposure, there is a greater elimination of total phenols, and at the end of that period free phenols predominate; the latter

TABLE 6

Correlation between free, total and conjugated phenols (mg/24h) in the urine of rats exposed to concentrations of 1700 p.p.m. of 'Fleet-X-DV-99'. (Spectrophotometric method, after Rossi and Grandjean, 1957).

Days	Treated Animals			Control Animals		
	Free	Total	Conjug.	Free	Total	Conjug.
42	5.96	7.49	1.53	4.54	5.41	0.87
46	5.67	7.20	1.53	4.38	5.19	0.87

return to normal rapidly either because absorption of trimethylbenzol is reduced or because the process of conjugation has increased in an effort to reduce the toxic effect. Rossi and Grandjean deduce from these results that the metabolism of trimethylbenzol varies according to the amount absorbed, and that some accumulates in the organism. From this point of view, as well as from the results of exposure of human beings (see below), it cannot be considered an entirely harmless substitute for benzene.

(2) Distribution in tissues
   No information.

TOXICOLOGY

Mesitylene – if judged from its presence in 'Fleet X' – is a central nervous depressant, a respiratory irritant and possibly a haemopoietic depressant, though not of a benzene-like nature.

Toxicity to animals

(1) Acute
   (a) Lethal dose. – (i) By intraperitoneal injection in the rat is, according to Spector (1956) 1.5–2 ml. For the guinea pig Gerarde (1960) found it to be 1.13 ml, and a single dose of 9–12 ml caused death within 24 h. – *(ii) By subcutaneous injection* rats given single injections of 12 ml/kg body weight survived (Cameron et al., 1938), while Hultgren (1926) stated that 8–10 ml/kg caused only leucocy-

Bibliography on p. 124

tosis. – *(iii) By mouth* Gerarde found that 5 ml/kg caused death in 1 out of 10 rats, compared with none with the same amount of benzene, and 3 with toluene. – *(iv) By inhalation,* even at 7000–9000 p.p.m., Lazarew (1929) noted only central nervous depression and loss of reflexes. According to Cameron *et al.* (1938) the lethal concentration for 4 out of 16 rats to a single continuous 24 h exposure was 2400 p.p.m.

(b) Narcotic dose. – No information.

(2) Chronic

Toleration of rats to 14 h daily exposures to 611 p.p.m. was observed by Cameron *et al.* (1938). In the investigations of Battig *et al.* (1956) on 'Fleet-X' no fatalities occurred with exposure for 4 months to concentrations of 1700 p.p.m. but there was some delay in growth during the first three weeks of exposure, and after this period a relative lymphopenia and neutrophilia.

SYMPTOMS OF INTOXICATION

The pre-lethal symptoms were those of central nervous depression and respiratory failure. Lazarew (1929) also noted a sedative effect at 5000–7000 p.p.m.

CHANGES IN THE ORGANISM

The only autopsy lesions were congestion of the lungs with acute poisoning. With chronic poisoning there was also evidence of central nervous depression. *Post mortem* there was some hyperaemia of the lungs, with thickening of the alveolar walls, and some fatty changes in the liver.

Toxicity to human beings

As already stated, the only account of the effect of mesitylene from the point of view of industry is based on its use as a component of the paint thinner known as 'Fleet-X' (Battig *et al.*, 1956). This thinner contained more than 80% of the two isomers of trimethylbenzol, and the results of investigations of the complaints of workers were related by these observers to trimethylbenzol; atmospheric concentrations of this substance were found to be 10–60 p.p.m. Those workers most severely exposed naturally showed the most definite symptoms.

SYMPTOMS OF INTOXICATION

(1) Blood and bone marrow

Disturbance of blood coagulation was evidenced by frequent bleeding from the gums, nose bleeding and a tendency to haematomata. In 40% of these cases coagulation time was delayed.

Decrease of the number of thrombocytes was found in some cases, but with no relation to the degree of exposure.

Decrease in erythrocytes was shown by half of the whole working population –
a total of less than 4.5 millions. Two of these workers had had little or no exposure.

(2) Respiratory disturbances

Bronchitis, of an asthmatic type, was also present in 70% of the severely
exposed group, in only a few of the remainder.

(3) Neurological disturbances

Headache, fatigue and drowsiness were present in 70% of the workers exposed
to the higher concentrations; in only 30% of the less severely exposed assistant
workers.

It is to be concluded that trimethylbenzol (whether pseudocumene or mesitylene
is the more responsible cannot be definitely judged from this unique investigation
of 'Fleet-X') can cause central nervous depression, respiratory irritation and possibly some haemopoietic disturbance, though not of a benzene-like nature.

Bibliography on p. 124

10. Pseudocumene

Synonyms: 1,2,4-trimethylbenzene, pseudocumol

Structural formula:

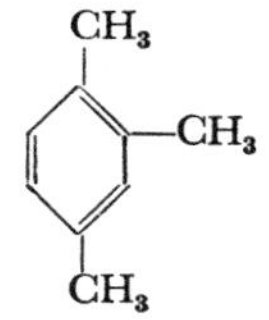

$$CH_3$$

Molecular formula: C_9H_{12}

Molecular weight: 120.19

Properties: A colourless liquid with an aromatic odour.
    boiling point: 169.4 °C
    melting point: −44 °C
    vapour pressure: 341 mm Hg at 140.1 °C
    vapour density (air = 1): 2.43 at 140.1 °C
    specific gravity (liquid density): 0.876 at 20 °C
    flash point: 112 °F
    conversion factors: 1 p.p.m. = 4.91 mg/m³
                    1 mg/l   = 204 p.p.m.
    solubility: insoluble in water; soluble in ethanol, ether and acetone
    maximum allowable concsntration: not established

ECONOMY, SOURCES AND USES

Production

Pseudocumene is produced by catalytic cracking of heavy oils and catalytic reforming of virgin naphtha (Gerarde, 1960), also by distillation of an aromatic hydrocarbon reformate fraction.

Industrial uses

(1) As a constituent of aromatic solvents and motor fuels.
(2) As a vermifuge (the technical variety) or as a 30% constituent of heavy coal tar naphtha.
(3) As a possible starting material for the synthesis of certain chemicals.

BIOCHEMISTRY

Estimation

(1) In the atmosphere
As for mesitylene (see p. 112).

(2) In blood and tissues
As for mesitylene (see p. 112).

Metabolism

(1) Absorption and excretion
The metabolism of pseudocumene resembles closely that of mesitylene. Absorption is chiefly through the lungs, but also, if swallowed, by the gastro-intestinal and slowly by the intact skin.

Like mesitylene, it is probably metabolised in the liver, with the formation of *p*-xylic acid which is excreted in the urine (Jacobsen, 1879; Williams, 1959). The fact that subcutaneous injection is followed by a slight increase in urinary sulphate excretion indicates that some hydroxylation of the benzene ring has occurred with formation of a phenolic compound (Williams, 1959).

(2) Distribution in tissues
No information.

TOXICOLOGY

Pseudocumene is toxicologically very similar to mesitylene, i.e. a central nervous depressant and respiratory irritant. Animal experiments have also suggested that it may have an injurious effect on the liver.

Toxicity to animals

The lethal dose. – *(i) By intraperitoneal injection,* 1.5–2 ml/kg body weight (Cameron *et al.* 1938), a slightly larger dose than that of mesitylene (1.13 ml according to Gerarde, 1960). – *(ii) By inhalation,* no deaths have been reported even at concentrations up to 8100 p.p.m. Cameron *et al* (1938) found no evidence of injury in rats exposed to 2000 p.p.m. for fourteen 8-h exposures, and Lazarew (1929) found that 8100 p.p.m. was followed only by loss of reflexes and narcosis. – *(iii)* Oral administration to rats was followed, in the experiments of Gerarde (1959) by generalised vaso-dilatation, hyperaemia of the gastro-intestinal tract and pulmonary haemorrhage, all reversible in animals which survived a dosage of 5 ml/kg.

Bibliography on p. 124

Gerarde (1960) states that aspiration of liquid pseudocumene will cause pneumonitis, oedema and haemorrhage of the lungs.

The results of the investigations of Bättig *et al.* (1956) into the toxic effects of 'Fleet-X', of which pseudocumene was a constituent, have already been described (see under mesitylene, p. 110)) and they do not distinguish between mesitylene and pseudocumene in this respect.

Blood changes described by Woronow (1929) in rabbits injected subcutaneously daily for 3 weeks with 2–3 g of pseudocumene were a moderate lowering of the red cell count and slight leucocytosis.

Toxicity to human beings

Since the only account of human exposure to pseudocumene is that of Bättig *et al.* (1956) in their investigation of 'Fleet-X', where mesitylene and pseudocumene were both involved, the possible toxic effect of pseudocumene can only be considered as the same as that of mesitylene.

11. Tetralin

Synonyms: tetrahydronaphthalene, tetranap

Structural formula:

Molecular formula: $C_{10}H_{12}$

Molecular weight: 132.20

Properties: A colourless liquid with an odour resembling that of naphthalene or turpentine.

    boiling point: 207.2 °C

    melting point: −30 °C

    vapour pressure: 1 mm Hg at 38 °C

    vapour density (air = 1): 4.6

    specific gravity (liquid density): 0.971

    flash point: 171 °F

    conversion factors: 1 p.p.m. = 5.41 mg/m³

                       1 mg/l   = 183 p.p.m.

    solubility: insoluble in water; very soluble in ehtanol and ether

    maximum allowable concentration: not established; Patty (1949) suggests that on account of its odour and irritative effects it should be less than 100 p.p.m. and Gerarde (1960) that a level of 25 p.p.m. appears to be a reasonable figure.

It is not highly inflammable but oxidises on exposure to air, leaving explosive resinous residues.

    It is a good solvent for fats, waxes, resins, camphor, sulphur and iodine. 'Essence of Tetralin' is a commercial mixture of tetralin and hexalin, a pale yellow liquid which is a better solvent of resins than tetralin alone (Gardani, 1942); B.P. 160 to 185 °C.

ECONOMY, SOURCES AND USES

Production

By the catalytic hydrogenation of naphthalene.

Industrial uses

(1) As a solvent for oils, fats, waxes, resins, asphalt and rubber.

(2) In shoe and floor polishes as a substitute for turpentine.

(3) In paint thinners, and, when mixed with decalin or white spirit, as a paint remover.

(4) As a degreaser.

(5) As a substitute for turpentine and petrol in Germany.

(6) As an insecticide for the clothes moth and a larvicide for mosquitoes (Coleman, 1935).

(7) As an addition to motor fuel (Koelsch, 1946).

BIOCHEMISTRY

Estimation

No specific method has been described for estimation in air, tissues and fluids, but interferometer, infrared and ultraviolet methods are applicable.

Metabolism

(1) Absorption and excretion

Only a small proportion of the tetralin absorbed into the blood was stated by Lehmann and Flury (1943) to be exhaled unchanged. Early observations by Pohl and Rawicz (1919) had suggested that it was excreted as dihydronaphthalene and naphthalene in the urine of rabbits, dogs and human beings, while Röckemann (1922) states that the metabolic processes differ in dogs and rabbits in the formation of different tetralyl glucuronides. It has been suggested that this species difference may account for some difference of opinion as to its capacity for cataract formation in animals. Bernhard (1939) found that while decalin was partly excreted by dogs as decahydronaphthol, and though tetralin had a similar behaviour, he had not succeeded in isolating pure tetrahydronaphthols. He found no conjugation with glucuronides.

According to Badinand *et al.* (1947) tetralin differs in its metabolic behaviour from naphthalene in that it does not produce naphthols in the urine, but they quote Bernhard and Muller (1938) as having shown that naphthalene causes a disturbance of intermediary hydrogen metabolism and suggest that the mechanism of cataractogenesis by tetralin may be due to a disturbance of oxidation-reduction processes. The oxidation processes in rats given tetralin, both pure and containing peroxides, by mouth and by subcutaneous and intravenous injection, were examined by Kanitz *et al.* (1935). They found that both caused an initial fall in body temperature followed by a rise, and that though tetralin scarcely altered oxygen consumption, it did cause an alteration in the respiratory quotient, the CO_2

elimination being decreased. They also observed an increase i n urinary nitrogen after prolonged administration of tetralin.

Williams (1959) concludes that while some of the suggested metabolites are artefacts the aromatic nucleus does not undergo transformation, the reduced ring being more readily metabolised. A decrease in the ratio of inorganic total sulphates in the urine of rats after a single subcutaneous dose of 5 ml/kg has been observed by Gerarde (1960) which suggests that hydroxylation of tetralin has occurred.

(2) Distribution in tissues
   No information.

TOXICOLOGY

Tetralin is an irritant to skin and mucous membranes, and has a characteristic effect of producing a green coloration of the urine without apparent injury to the kidneys. In animals it has been found to cause cataract in some species, and, in cats, methaemoglobin formation (Heubner, 1940).

Toxicity to animals

(1) Acute
   (a) Lethal dose. – The LD_{50} for rats following a single oral dose was given by Smyth *et al.* (1951) as 2.86 g/kg.
   (b) Narcotic dose. – This is apparently very high. In the experiments of Geppert (1926) with mice, it was administered on a mask; even when soaked this produced only semi-narcosis after an initial short period of excitation unless the mask was heated to increase the vapour. Its less severe acute toxicity compared with that of turpentine oil was shown by the fact that with a similar method of inhalation the animals exposed to turpentine died within a few minutes, while no fatalities occurred with the tetralin animals.

SYMPTOMS OF INTOXICATION

There is some difference of opinion between the investigations of Cardani (1942) and Badinand *et al.* (1947). The results of the former apparently indicate in most respects a more severe toxicity than those of the latter. Both were carried out on guinea pigs, so that in this regard species differences do not provide an explanation of the discrepancy. Cardani's experiments included dosage by mouth (0.25 ml. daily) cutaneous application (to 6 cm² of shaved skin) and inhalation (1.42 mgm/l for 8 h daily). Badinand *et al.* used only inhalation (no concentrations given) daily for 30 min in "a contaminated atmosphere".

In both investigations, loss of weight and tremors were noted, while Badinand observed also paralysis of the hind quarters and difficult respiration, and Cardani,

Bibliography on p. 124

after a week of apparent well-being, restlessness or apathy, roughening of the skin, anorexia and sometimes torpor. With oral administration there was intense diarrhoea and with skin application eczema.

(1) The eyes

Badinand *et al.* observed definite signs of cataract after 6 days of inhalation of tetralin vapour, actually more rapidly than with naphthalene. A similar observation in rabbits following oral administration was made by Basile in 1939, but Fitzhugh and Buschke (1949) were unable to produce cataracts in rats fed on a diet containing 2% of tetralin for 2 months.

(2) Blood and bone marrow

Changes in the blood picture were not, in Cardani's view, significant – slight normochromic anaemia, a tendency to leucopenia with long exposure, and relative lymphocytosis. Badinand *et al.* recorded an increase of polynuclear leucocytes and erythrocytes. Cesaro (1941) also observed anaemia, and suggested that it is associated with a diminution of resistance of the red cells owing to penetration of their lipoid surface layer by tetralin.

(3) Urine

In Cardani's experiments the urine of the animals receiving tetralin by mouth became scanty and dark coloured, with a greenish-brown tinge, but not a clear green. Kanitz *et al.* (1935) had found that a dark coloration of the urine was produced only after administration of several doses of pure tetralin, but after one dose of tetralin which contained peroxides.

The actual cause of the green colour has not been established. Heubner (1940) has pointed out that any of 18 to 25 urinary metabolites with differing molecular structure might be responsible.

CHANGES IN THE ORGANISM
(1) The liver

Cardani (1942) noted all stages of injury to the liver, from hyperaemia to fatty degeneration and centrilobular atrophy.

(2) The kidneys

Differences of opinion as to the amount of damage to the kidneys associated with the green urine also exist, but on the whole it does not appear to be as serious as that associated with the halogenated hydrocarbons. Kanitz *et al.* (1934) found no albuminuria in any of their animals by oral, subcutaneous or intravenous administration, and the only histological evidence of injury to the kidneys consisted of slight swelling and some yellow pigmentation of the peripheral layers. Cardani, on the other hand, stated that the kidneys showed all stages of a toxic effect, including severe necrotising nephrosis especially of the convoluted tubules, while according to Badinand *et al.* there was evidence of epithelial nephritis, and the urine contained albumen, cylinders and red blood cells.

(3) The lungs

Focal broncho-pneumonitis was present in some of Cardani's animals, but, as he remarks, this is a common lesion in the last stages of life in small rodents.

According to Gerarde (1960), however, direct contact of liquid tetralin with lung tissue by aspiration causes pulmonary oedema and haemorrhage at the site of contact.

Toxicity to human beings

Exposure to tetralin has been chiefly associated with green coloration of the urine not apparently connected with injury to the kidneys, but symptoms of systemic disturbance, as well as dermatitis and mucous membrane irritation have been recorded.

SYMPTOMS OF INTOXICATION

(1) The skin

A skin condition similar to turpentine dermatitis, eczematous in nature, was reported by Galewsky (1922) in four painters using tetralin or mixtures of tetralin with benzine or pine oil as a substitute for turpentine in oil paints. Two of the cases using the mixture were father and son, and Galewsky remarks that in view of the fact that dermatitis from the use of tetralin has been so rarely recorded, it is possible that hypersensitivity might have played some part in these cases.

(2) Urine

An early observation of the association of tetralin with a green colour of the urine was made by Pohl and Rawicz (1919), in a man who had ingested 5.7 g of a pigment called di-tetralin.

Among the first observations, from the industrial point of view, of what has been called 'tetralin urine' was that of Arnstein (1922). He described two cases in painters using varnishes containing tetralin in a badly ventilated bank vault. In addition to the green urine they had intense irritation of mucous membranes, profuse lacrimation, headache and stupor.

In 1926 Geppert noted an association of green urine with intense headache and asthenia in subjects sleeping in rooms which as described below had been recently waxed with a polish said to contain crude tetralin.

According to Arnstein 'tetralin urine' can be distinguished from 'phenol urine' by its chemical reactions. Tetralin urine gives a positive diazo reaction and a green colour with sodium nitrite and potassium ferrocyanide solution – tests which are negative for phenol – but no colour with ferric chloride and no precipitate with bromine water after heating – these tests are positive for phenol.

Bibliography on p. 124

(3) Neurological disturbances

Marked restlessness, headache, malaise, nausea and vomiting, and asthenia have been recorded by several observers. Röckemann (1922) noted that babies sleeping in a room recently treated with a varnish with a tetraline base showed restlessness to a marked degree and he attributed it to a direct action of tetralin on the central nervous system, Koelsch (1946) states that symptoms of headache, malaise and vomiting were so severe in a factory where tetralin was used that workers had to be completely removed from exposure, and Geppert (1926) also observed intense headache and asthenia in subjects sleeping in rooms which had been recently waxed with a polish later found, on centrifugation and distillation of the resulting oily fluid, to contain a substance corresponding in odour and properties to crude tetralin. Badinand *et al.* (1947) state that their attention was first drawn to the potential toxicity of tetralin when patients in a hospital at Saint Étienne complained of eye irritation, headache, nausea, diarrhoea and green urine, and it was found that the parquet floor of the ward had been wax polished by a polish with a tetraline base. All the windows had been closed on account of the cold weather.

BIBLIOGRAPHY

Adler-Herzmark, J. (1933) Periodische Untersuchungen von Wiener Arbeitern die mit Benzol-Toluol- und Xylolhältigen Materialen beschäftigt sind, *Arch. Gewerbepathol. Gewerbehyg.*, 4:486.
Appuhn, E. and H. Goldeck (1957) Früh- und Spätschäden der Blutbildung durch Benzol und seine Homologen, *Arch. Gewerbepathol. Gewerbehyg.*, 15:399.
Arnstein, A. (1922) Tetralinvergiftung, *Wien. Klin. Woch. Schr.*, 35:488.
Badinand, A., L. Paufique and J. Rodier (1947) Intoxication expérimentale par la Tétraline, *Arch. Malad. Profess.*, 8:124.
Bänfer, W. (1961) Untersuchungen über Einwirkung von Reintoluol auf das Blutbild von Drucker- und Hilfsarbeitern im Tiefdruck, *Zentr. Arbeitsmed. Arbeitsschutz*, 11:35.
Barsotti, M., L. Parmeggiani and C. Sassi (1952) Osservazioni di Patologia professionale in una Fabrica di Resine polystiroliche, *Med. Lavoro*, 43:418.
Basile, G. (1939) Sull Azione di alcuni prodotti di Idrogenazione della naftalina sul Cristallino e Membrane oculari profonde del coniglio, *Boll. Oculistica*, 18:95.
Batchelor, J. J. (1927) Relative Toxicity of Benzol and its higher Homologues, *Am. J. Hyg.*, 7:276.
Battig, K., E. Grandjean, L. Rossi and J. Rickenbacher (1958) Toxicologische Untersuchungen über Trimethyl benzol, *Arch. Gewerbepathol. Gewerbehyg.*, 16:555.
Battig, K., E. Grandjean and V. Turrian (1956) Gesundheitschäden nach langdauernder Trimethyl-benzol Exposition in einer Malerwerkstatt, *Z. prävent. Med.*, 1:389.
Battig, K., V. Turrian and E. Grandjean (1956) Toxicologische und arbeitsmedizinische Untersuchungen über Trimethylbenzol, *Z. Unfallmed. Berufskrankh.*, 49:265.
Bernhard, K. (1939) Stoffwechselversuche mit hydrierten Naphtalin und hydrierten Naphthalin-derivaten, *Z. Physiol. Chem.*, 257:54.
Bernhard, K. and L. Muller (1938) Stoffwechslungsversuche mit ω-cyclopentenyl und ω-cyclopen-tylsubstituenten Fettsäuren, *Z. Physiol. Chem.*, 256:85.
Bianchi, G. (1915) L'Azione sul Sangue e sugli Organi ematopoietici del Benzolo e dei suoi omolghi a Catena laterale satura, *Arch. Sci. Med.*, 39:1.
Braier, L. and M. P. Francone (1950) Phénomènes hémolytiques dus au Benzène et ses Homologues, *Arch. Malad. Profess.*, 11:367.

Bray, H. G., B. G. Humphris and W. V. Thorpe (1949) Metabolism of Derivatives of Toluene, *Biochem. J.*, 45:241.

Bray, H. G., B. G. Humphris and W. V. Thorpe (1950) Metabolism of Derivatives of Toluene, *Biochem J.*, 47:395.

Brezina, E. (1921) Internationale Übersicht über Gewerbekrankheiten, Springer, Berlin.

Browning, E. (1953) Toxicity of Industrial Organic Solvents, H.M.Stationary Office, London.

Cameron, G. R., J. L. H. Paterson, G. S. W. De Sarain and J. C. Thomas (1938) The toxicity of some methyl Derivatives of Benzene, with special reference to pseudocumene and heavy Coal tar Naphtha, *J. Pathol. Bacteriol.*, 46:95.

Cardani, A. (1942) Studio sperimentale sulla Tossicità della Tetralina e della Decalina, *Med. Lavoro*, 33:145.

Carlson G. W. (1946) Aplastic anaemia following exposure to products of the sulphite pulp industry, *Ann. Internal Med.*, 24:277.

Carpenter, C. P., C. B. Shaffer, C. S. Weil and H. F. Smyth Jr. (1944) Studies on the inhalation of 1:3 Butadiene with a comparison of its narcotic Effect ith wBenzol, Toluol and Styrene, *J. Ind. Hyg.*, 26:69.

Cesaro, A. N. (1941) La Resistanza globulare nell'Intossicazione sperimentale acuta da Tetralina, *Folia Med. (Naples)*, 27:65.

Chassevant, A. and M. Garnier (1903) Toxicité de Benzène et de quelques Hydrocarbures Aromatiques, *Compt. Rend. Soc. Biol.*, 55:1255.

Chief Inspector of Factories and Workshops. Annual Report, (1947) p.65, H.M.S.O., London.

Chief Inspector of Factories and Workshops. Annual Report, (1954) p.174, H.M.S.O., London.

Chief Inspector of Factories and Workshops. Annual Report, (1960), H.M.S.O., London.

Christiansson G. and B. Karlsson (1957) "Sniffung" – Berusnungstatt bland Barn, *Svenska Lakartidn.*, 54:33.

Coleman, W. (1935) Hydrogenated Naphthalene against Clothes Moths, *J. Econ. Entomol.*, 27:860.

Curci, A. (1892) Azione e Transformazioni dei Xileni nell'Organismo, *Ann. Chim. Farmacol.*, 6:3.

Danishefsky L. and M. Willhite (1954) Metabolism of Styrene in the Rat, *J. Biol.Chem.*, 211:549.

Elkins H. B. (1959) The Chemistry of Industrial Toxicology, Chapman and Hall Ltd., London.

Engelhardt W. E. (1935) Versuche über die akut-narkotische Wirkung alipatischer und aromatischer Kohlenwasserstoffe, *Arch. Hyg. Bakteriol.*, 114:249.

—(1931) Vergleichende Tierversuche über Blutwirkung von Benzin und Benzol, *Arch. Gewerbepath. Gewerbehyg.*, 2:479.

Estler W. (1935) Versuche über die akut-narkotischer Wirkung aliphatischer und aromatischer Kohlenwasserstoffe, *Arch. Hyg. Bakteriol.*, 114:261.

Fabre, R. and A. Fabre (1948) Sur le Dosage du Benzène et du Toluène dans l'Air des Ateliers et dans le Sang des Ouvriers, *Arch. Malad. Profess.*, 9:97.

Fabre, R. and R. Truhaut (1954) Le problème des Solvants de Remplacement de Benzène, XI Cong. Int. Méd. de Trav. de Naples, *Edit. Inst. Med. Trav. Naples*.

Fabre, R., R. Truhaut, J. Bernichon and F. Loisillier (1955) Recherches toxicologiques sur les Solvants de Remplacement de Benzène ou Cumène, *Arch. Malad. Profess.*, 16:285.

Fabre, R., R. Truhaut and S. Laham (1960) Recherches toxicologiques sur les Solvants de Remplacement de Benzène. Étude des Xylènes, *Arch. Malad. Profess.*, 21:301.

—(1960) Recherches sur le Métabolisme comparé des Xylènes ou Diméthylbenzènes, *Arch. Malad. Profess.*, 21:3194.

—(1960) Étude du Métabolisme des Xylènes ou Diméthylbenzènes chez le Rat, le Cobaye et le Lapin, *Compt. Rend.*, 250:2655.

Fabre, R., R. Truhaut, S. Laham and M. Peron (1955) Récherches toxicologiques sur les Solvants de Remplacement de Benzène, *Arch. Malad. Profess.*, 16:197.

Farber, M. (1933) Das Verhalten des Blutbildes unter den Einfluss von Xylol, *Beitr. Pathol. Anat.*, 91:554.

Ferguson, T., W. H. Harvey and T. D. Hamilton (1933) Enquiry into the relative Toxicity of Benzene and Toluene, *J. Hyg.*, 33:547.

Filippi, E. (1914) Azione fisiologica e Comportamento di alcuni Derivati del Benzene in confronto con quelli del Cicloesano, *Arch. Farmacol. Sper.*, 18:178.

Fitzhugh, O. G. and W. H. Buschke (1949) Production of Cataract in Rats by Tetralol and other Naphthalene Derivatives, *Arch. Ophthalmol.*, 41:572.

Francone, M. P. and L. Braier (1954) I Fondamenti della Sostituzione del Benzolo con i suoi omologhi superiori nell'Industria, *Med. Lavoro.*, 45:29.

Galewsky, S. (1922) Über Dermatitiden durch Terpentinersatz, *Dermatol. Wochschr.*, 74:273.

Geppert J. (1926) Zur Frage von gesundheitsschädlichen Bohnerwachs, *Deut. Med. Wochschr.*, 52:1080.

Gerarde, H. W. (1956) Toxicological Studies on Hydrocarbons. I and II. A method for the quantitative collection of femoral bone marrow in small laboratory animals, *Arch. Ind. Health*, 13:331; 14:387.

Gerarde, H. W. (1959) Toxicological Studies on Hydrocarbons. III. The biochemorphology of the phenylalkanes and phenylalkenes, *Arch. Ind. Health*, 19:403.

Gerarde, H. W. (1960) Toxicology and biochemistry of aromatic hydrocarbons, Elsevier, Amsterdam.

Ghislandi, E. and A. Fabriani (1957) Lesioni epatica da Ingestioni accidentale di Diluenti per Vernici alla Nitrocellulosa, *Med. avoro*, 48:577.

Glass, W. I. (1961) A case of suspected xylene Poisoning, *New Zealand Med.*, 60:113.

Glibert, D. (1935) Les Méfaits de l'Héliogravure, *Brux. Méd.*, 16:194.

Goldie, I. (1960) Can Xylene (Xylol) provoke convulsive Seizures? *Ind. Med. Surg.*, 29:33.

Grammarinaro, G. (1956) Mielosi aplastica globale con Osteosclerosi diffusa da Intossicazione cronica da Xilolo, *Osped. Maggiore*, 44:281.

Greenburg, L., M. R. Mayers, H. Heiman and S. Moskowitz (1942) The Effects of Exposure to Toluene in Industry, *J. Am. Med. Assoc.*, 118:573.

Guertin, G. L. and H. W. Gerarde (1959) Toxicological Studies on Hydrocarbons. A method for the quantitative determination of benzene and certain alkyl benzenes in blood, *Arch. Ind. Health*, 20:262.

Hektoen, L. (1916) Effect of Toluene on the Production of Antibodies, *J. Infect. Diseases*, 19:737.

Heubner, W. (1940) Methämoglobinbildender Gifte, *Ergeb. Physiol. Biol. Chem. Exptl. Pharmakol.*, 43:15.

Hine, C. H., Ungar, H. H. Anderson, J. K. Kodama, J. K. Critchlow and N. W. Jacobsen (1954) Toxicological Studies on p-tertiary Butyl Toluene, *Arch. Ind. Hyg.*, 9:227.

Hirsch, S. (1932) Über chronische Xylolvergiftung, *Verhandl. Deut. Ges. Inn. Med.*, 44:483.

Hock, H. and S. Lang (1944) Autoxydation von Kohlenwasserstoffe, *Ber. Deut. Chem. Ges.*, 76:169; 77B:257.

Hodge, H. C. and J. H. Sterner (1943) Tabulation of Toxicity Classes, *Am. Ind. Hyg. Assoc. Quart.*, 10:93.

Hultgren, G. (1926) Action du Benzol sur le Teneur du Sang en Thrombocytes, Leucocytes et Erythrocytes, *Compt. Rend. Soc. Biol.*, 95:1060.

Humperdinck, K. (1954) Besondere Form der Knochenmarkschädigung bei einem Tiefdrucker, *Berufs Genossensch.*, 89.

Jacobsen, O. (1879) Über das Verhalten des Cymols in Thierkörper, *Ber. Deut. Chem. Ges.*, 12:1512.

Johnstone, R. T. and S. E. Miller (1960) Occupational Diseases and Industrial Medicine, W. B. Saunders Co.

Jost, A. (1932) Harnuntersuchungen bei chronischer Schädigung durch Benzol und Benzolderivate, *Arch. Gewerbepath. Gewerbehyg.*, 3:791.

Joyner, R. E. and W. L. Pegues (1961) A Health Hazard associated with Epoxy-resin Concrete Dust, *J. Occupational Med.*, 3:211.

Kanitz, H. R., A. Lohmeyer and J. Scholz (1935) Über die Wirkungen von Tetralin, 5-Tetralol und 5-Tetralon auf Körpertemperatur und Stoffwechsel, *Arch. Hyg. Bakteriol.*, 113:234.

Klimkova-Deutschova, A. (1962) Neurologische Befunde in der Plastikindustrie bei Styrolarbeitern, *Arch. Gewerbepath. Gewerbehyg.*, 19:35.

Koelsch, F. (1946) Lehrbuch der Arbeitshygiene, vol I:294; vol II:405, Ferdinand Enkw., Stuttgart.

Kuhn, R. and J. Low (1939) Zur Kenntnis der Methyloxidation im Tierkorper, *Z. Physiol. Chem.*, 25:190.

Lachnit, V. and E. E. Reimer (1959) Panmyelopathien durch aromatische Lösungsmitteln, *Wien. Klin. Wochschr.*, 71:365.

Lazarew, N. W. (1929) Über die Giftigkeit verschiedener Kohlenwasserstoffdämpfe, *Arch. Exptl. Pathol. Pharmakol.*, 143:223.

Lehmann, K. B. (1912) Experimentelle Studien über den Einfluss technisch und hygienisch wichtiger Gäse und Dämpfe auf den Organismus, *Arch. Hyg. Bakteriol.*, 75:1.

Lehmann, K. B. and F. Flury (1943) Toxicology and Hygiene of Industrial Solvents, Williams and Wilkins, Baltimore.

Lob, M. (1952) L'Intoxication chronique au Toluol et au Xylol et ses Répercussions sur les Organes hémopoiétiques, *Schweiz. Med. Wochschr.*, 82:1125.

Lurie, J. B. (1949) Acute Toluene Poisoning, *S. African Med. J.*, 23:233.

Luszczak A. (1935) Die Bestimmung von Xylol und Xylol-Toluol-dämpfgemischen in der Raumluft, Abhandl. Gesamtgeb. Hyg., Urban und Schwarzenberg, Berlin.

Lüthy, F. (1940) Polyneurite due a une Intoxication par l'Inertol, *Z. Unfallmed. Berufskrankh.*, 34: 246.

Maffet, P. S., T. F. Doherty and J. L. Monkman (1956) A direct method for the Collection and Determination of micro-amounts of Benzene and Toluene in Air, *Am. Ind. Hyg. Assoc. Quart.*, 17:186.

Mgebrow, L. (1930) Materialen zum Studium der Wirkung einiger Destillations-produkte der Bakuer Naphtha auf den tierischen Organismus, *Virchow's Arch. Path. Anat. Physiol.*, 278:610.

Mikiska, A. and H. Mikiskova, (1960) Bestimmung der elektrischen Erregbarkeit der motorischen Grosshirnrinde, *Arch. Gewerbepath. Gewerbehyg.*, 18:286.

Mikiskova, H. (1960) Elektrische Erregbarkeit der motorischen Grosshirnrinde. Wirkung von Benzol, Toluol, und Xylol bei Meerschweinchen, *Arch. Gewerbepath. Gewerbehyg.*, 18:300.

Miyamato, Y. (1938) Über den Einfluss der Benzolderivate auf das Blutbild und verschiedene Organe, *Zentr. Gewerbehyg. Unfall.*, 25:70.

Neubauer, O. (1901) Über Glykuronsäurepaaring bei Stoffen der Fettreihe, *Arch. Exptl. Pathol. Pharmakol.*, 46:133.

Oettel, H. (1936) Einwirkung organische Flüssigkeiten auf die Haut, *Arch. Exptl. Pathol. Pharmakol.*, 183:641.

Parmeggiani, L. and C. Sassi (1954) Sul Rischio professionale da Toluolo, *Med. Lavoro*, 45:574.

Patty, F. A. (1949) Industrial Hygiene and Toxicology vol. II, Interscience, New York.

Pohl, J. and M. Rawicz (1919) Über das Schicksal des Tetrahydronaphthalins. (Tetralin) in Tierkorper, *Z. Physiol. Chem.*, 104:95.

Quick, A. J. (1926) Study of Benzoic Acid Conjugation in the Dog, with a direct quantitative method for Hippuric Acid, *J. Biol. Chem.*, 67:477.

—(1931) Conjugation of Benzoic Acid in Man, *J. Biol. Chem.*, 92:65.

—(1932) The Relationship between chemical Structure and physiological Response. The Conjugation of substituted Benzoic Acids, *J. Biol. Chem.*, 96:83.

Rambousek, J. (1913) Industrial Poisoning from Fumes, Gases and Poisons of Manufacturin Processes, T. M. Legge, Transl. and Ed., Arnold and Sons, London.

Ravina, A., B. Maupin, R. Claisse and H. Clumenes (1951) Traitement d'un Cas d'Aleuciehé orrhagique par Transfusions de Suspensions globulaires, *Presse Med.*, 59:1040.

Robinson, D., J. N. Smith and R. T. Williams (1955) Metabolism of Cumene, *Biochem. J.*, 59:153.

Röckemann, W. (1922) Über Tetralinharn, *Arch. Exptl. Pathol. Pharmakol.*, 92:52.

Rogers, J. C. and C. C. Hopper (1956) An industrial Problem in the Plastics Field, Ind. Health Rev. Sept. (Ind. Hyg. Sect., St. Louis Health Div.).

Rogers, J. C. and C. C. Hooper (1957) M. A. C. for Styrene, *Ind. Med. Surg.*, 26:32.

Rosenblatt, H. (1902) Neurasthenie herforgerufen durch Einatmung von Xyloldämpfen, *Aerzt., Sachverst. Ztg.*, 8:197.

Rosenthal-Deussen, E. (1931) Vergiftungen durch ein Anstrichmittel (Inertol), *Arch. Gewerbepathol. Gewerbehyg.*, 2:92.

Rossi, L. and E. Grandjean (1957) L'Eliminazione urinaria del Fenoli in animali esposti al Trimetilbenzolo, *Med. Lavoro*, 48:523.

Rowe, V. K., G. V. Atchison, E. A. Luce and E. M. Adams (1943) The Determination of Monomeric Styrene in Air, *J. Ind. Hyg.*, 25:348.

Rylova, N. J. (1955) Toxic action of styrene and a methylstyrene, cited by Klimkova-Deutschova 1962, *Gigiena i Sanit.*, 5:21; Arch. Gewerbepath. Gewerbehug., 19:35.

Schmid, E. (1956) Diseases of the Cornea in Furniture Polishers, *Arch. Gewerbepathol. Gewerbehyg.*, 15:37.

Schumacher, H. and E. Grandjean (1960) Narkotische Wirksamkeit und die akute Toxicität von neun Lösungsmitteln, *Arch. Gewerbepath. Gewerbehyg.*, 18:109.

Schultzen, O. and B. Naunyn (1867) Über das Verhalten des Kohlenwasserstoffes im Organismus, *Arch. Anat. Physiol.*, 3:349.

Seghini, C. (1941) Intossicazione di Toluolo, *Med. Lavoro*, 32:179.

Sessa, T. (1948) Relievi patologici nella Intossicazione cronica sperimentale da Toluolo, *Folia Med.*, 31:91.

Smith, J. N., R. H. Smithies and R. T. Williams (1954) Studies in Detoxication. LV. The Metabolism of Alkyl Benzenes. LVI. Stereochemical Aspects of biological hydroxylation of ethyl benzene to methyl phenyl carbinol, *Biochem. J.*, 56:320.

Smyth, H. F., C. P. Carpenter and C. S. Weil (1951) Range Finding Toxicity List, *Arch. Ind. Hyg.* 4:119.

Smyth, H. F. and H. F. Smyth Jr. (1928) Inhalation Experiments with certain Lacquer Solvents, *J. Ind. Hyg.*, 10:261.

Spencer, H. C., D. D. Irish, C. M. Adams and V. K. Rowe (1942) The Response of Laboratory Animals to Monomeric Styrene, *J. Ind. Hyg.*, 24:255.

Spector, W. S. (1956) Handbook of Toxicology, Saunders, Philadelphia.

Stocke, A. (1929) Akute Xylol- und Toluolvergiftungen beim Tiefdruckfähren, *Zentr. Gewerbehyg.*, 16:355.

Stocke, A. (1931) Gewerbemedizinische Erfahrungen mit dem Anstrichmittel "Inertol. 49", *Arch. Gewerbepathol. Gewerbehyg.*, 2:99.

Svirbely, J. L., R. C. Dunn and W. F. Von Oettingen (1943) The acute Toxicity of Vapours of certain Solvents containing appreciable Amounts of Benzene and Toluene, *J. Ind. Hyg.*, 25:366.

Teisinger, J. and J. Srbova (1955) L'Élimination de l'Acide Benzoic dans l'Urine et son Rapport avec la Concentration maximum torérable de Toluène dans l'Air, *Arch. Malad. Profess.*, 16:216.

Truhaut, R. (1953) Transformations métaboliques des Toxiques organiques, *Ann. Pharmacol. Franc.*, 11:46.

Valette, G. and R. Cavier (1954) Percutaneous Absorption and chemical Constitution. Hydrocarbons, Alcohols and Esters, *Arch. Intern. Pharmacodyn.*, 97:332.

Verain, M., J. Veltin and G. Noisette (1949) Le Dosage polarographique du Benzol en Biologie, *Arch. Malad. Profess.*, 10:600.

Von Oettingen, W. F., P. A. Neal and D. D. Donahue (1942) The Toxicity and potential dangers of Toluene, *J. Am. Med. Assoc.*, 118:579.

Von Oettingen, W. F., P. A. Neal, D. D. Donahue, J. L. Svirbely et al (1942) The Toxicity and potential Dangers of Toluene, *U.S. Publ. Health Serv. Publ. Health Bull.* no. 729.

Werner, H. W., R. C. Dunn and W. F. von Oettingen (1944) Acute Effects of Cumene Vapours in Mice, *J. Ind. Hyg.* 26:264.

Williams, R. T. (1959) Detoxication Mechanisms, Chapman and Hall, London.

Wilson, R. H. (1943) Toluene Poisoning, *J. Am. Med. Assoc.*, 123:1106.

Wilson, R. H., G. V. Hough and W. E. McCormick (1948) Medical Problems encountered in the Manufacture of American-made Rubber, *Ind. Med. Surg.* 17:199.

Winslow, C. E. A. (1927) Survey of the National Council Study of Benzol Poisoning, *J. Ind. Hyg.*, 9:61.

Wocjiechowski, A. (1910) Studien über die Giftigkeit verschiedener Handelssörten des Benzols in Gasform, Diss. Wurzburg.

Wolf, M. A., W. K. Rowe, D. D. McCollister, R. L. Hollingsworth and F. Oyen (1956) Toxicological Studies of certain Alkylated Benzenes and Benzene, *Arch. Ind. Health*, 14:387.

Woronow, A. (1929) Über die morphologische Veränderungen des Benzols und der Bluterzeugenden Organe unter den Einfluss des Benzols und dessen Abkömmlinge, *Virchow's Arch. Pathol. Anat. Physiol.*, 271:173.

Yant, W. P., S. J. Pearce and H. H. Schrenk (1936) A microcolorimetric Method for the Determination of Toluene, *U.S. Bur. Mines Rept. Invest.* no. 3323.

Yant, W. P., H. H. Schrenk, C. P. Waite and F. A. Patty (1930) Acute Response of Guinea pigs to vapors of some new commercial organic Compounds. – Ethyl Benzene, *U.S. Treas. Public Health Rept.*, 45: 1241.

Zeman, M. and M. Klatil (1959) Studies on Possibility of Skin Lesions in Workers exposed to Toluene Vapours, *Pracovni Lekar.*, 112: 315.

Ziegler, E. (1873) Über das Verhalten des Camphercymols im thierischen Organismus, Arch. Exp. Path. Pharmak., 1: 63.

Chapter 3

CYCLIC HYDROCARBONS

12. Cyclohexane

Synonyms: hexamethylene, hexahydrobenzol

Structural formula: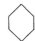

Molecular formula: C_6H_{12}

Molecular weight: 84.6

Properties: a colourless mobile liquid with an odour resembling that of benzene, but according to Gerarde (1960) with an 'olfactory threshold limit' much higher than that of benzene.

    boiling point: 80.3 °C
    melting point: 6.54
    vapour pressure: 103.67 mm at 26.3 °C
    vapour density (air = 1): 2.9
    specific gravity (liquid density): 0.7753
    flash point: 1 °F
    conversion factors: 1 p.p.m. = 0.0034 mg/l
                       1 mg/l   = 291 p.p.m.
    solubility: practically insoluble in water but miscible with alcohol, olive oil and most organic solvents; volatility about one-third that of ether at room temperature (Fairhall, 1957).
    maximum allowable concentration: 400 p.p.m.

ECONOMY, SOURCES AND USES

Production

Commercially, by the catalytic hydrogenation of benzene. It also occurs naturally as a constituent of Caucasian petroleum. The commercial variety may contain considerable amounts of benzene, up 0.3% according to Viola (1960).

[130]

Industrial uses

(1) As a synthetic rubber solvent, sometimes as a substitute for benzene and toluene.
(2) As an intermediate in the chemical industry.
(3) In the perfume industry as a solvent for fats, oils, waxes and resins.

BIOCHEMISTRY

Estimation

(1) In the atmosphere

There is no specific test for cyclohexane; the methods used for aromatic hydrocarbons already described are applicable. A combustible gas indicator was used by Treon *et al.* (1943) for concentrations from 0.95 to 2.65 mg/l of air, and is described in detail by Sallee and Guy (1962). Adsorption on activated charcoal had been described by Fieldner *et al.* in 1919.

(2) In blood and tissues

See above.

Metabolism

(1) Absorption and excretion

There have been many and varied opinions as to the fate of cyclohexane in the body, mainly owing to the lack of specific tests for cyclohexane itself and its metabolites. Bernhard (1937) presumed that in the dog it was totally oxidised, since he failed to find any metabolites in the urine except small amounts of oxalic acid, while Treon *et al.* (1943) found in rabbits an excretion of conjugated glucuronides corresponding to 50% of the dose.

One of the chief points of controversy was the possibility that cyclohexane might be metabolised with the formation of benzene. Pacault and Carpenter (1949) for example suggested that dehydrogenation of cyclohexane to form benzene could be carried out *in vitro* by a lyso-enzyme of vegetable origin (garlic).

Viola (1960) however, repeating these experiments, obtained completely negative results. None of the 'pseudo-solutions' of cyclohexane in water used for immersing the garlic bulbs contained any benzene as estimated spectrophotometrically. He suggests that the positive results of Pacault and Carpenter were attributable to the presence of benzene as an impurity in their cyclohexane.

It is interesting to note that in some of their experiments Elliott, Parke and Williams found small amounts of phenol in the urine, and that this proved to be due to the fact that the cyclo [^{14}C]hexane supplied contained small amounts of benzene. When a specially purified sample was used, no phenol was found in the urine, showing that cyclohexane is not aromatised and converted into phenol *in vivo*.

Fabre *et al.* (1952) denied that dehydrogenation was likely to take place in living tissue since they found no trace of benzene in pulped liver or kidneys treated with cyclohexane, though they demonstrated the presence of cyclohexane. They described the metabolic progress of cyclohexane in two phases – first, the transformation of one CH_2 group into CO, forming cyclohexane, then a second phase in which the nucleus of the cyclohexane is oxidised, giving adipic acid, which then undergoes partial combustion.

Many of these difficulties have been solved by the use by Elliott *et al.* (1959) of cyclohexane labelled with radioactive carbon [^{14}C]. By this method they were able to show that with a dose of 460 mg/kg body weight rabbits excreted about 30% of glucuronides, the primary metabolite being conjugated cyclohexanol, but also a small amount of trans-cyclohexane – 1,2-diolglucuronide. When the dose was 300–400 mg/kg, about 35 to 45% was eliminated in the expired air – 25–35% unchanged, 10% as CO_2, and about 50% in the urine as metabolites within 2 days. When the dose was very small, (0.3 mg/kg) only about 5% was expired and 90% excreted in the urine.

(2) Distribution in tissues
No information.

TOXICOLOGY

Cyclohexane is regarded as relatively non-toxic, especially with regard to any haemopoietic disturbance such as that caused by benzene. Animal experiments have shown that it can cause skin irritation, and with acute poisoning central nervous disturbance. Where haematological disturbances from its industrial use have been recorded it is probable that the commercial cyclohexane used contained some benzene.

Toxicity to animals

(1) Acute
(a) Lethal dose. – *(i) By oral administration* for the rabbit is stated by Treon *et al.* (1943) as between 5.5 and 6 mg/kg. – *(ii) By subcutaneous injection*, Launoy and Lévy-Bruhl (1920) gave the value of 3 ml/kg after 3–4 days, and by intravenous injection 0.6 ml/kg. – *(iii) By inhalation* the lethal dose has been given somewhat differing values by different investigators, but on the whole not varying widely except for the results of Henderson and Johnstone (1931), who give a much

higher lethal dose than any others. For mice, Lazarew (1929) postulated 60–70 mg/l for 2 h; for rabbits, Treon *et al.* (1943), 90 mg/l for 1 h. The results of Fabre *et al.* (1952) agree closely with these; Henderson and Johnstone's were much higher – 386 mg/l.

(*b*) *Narcotic dose.* – By inhalation, for mice 50 mg/l for 2 h (Lazarew, 1929); 62.5 mg/l for ½ h (Flury and Zernik, 1931), 132 mg/l (Henderson and Johnstone). Treon *et al.* were able to produce only lethargy and slight narcosis by exposure of mice to 25 mg/l for 60 h.

(2) Chronic

In the inhalation experiments of Treon *et al.*, deaths occurred as the result of repeated exposures (6–8 h per day, 5 days per week, for periods of 2–26 weeks) to concentrations of 25 mg/l or higher, with light narcosis and paresis of the legs. Loss of weight was a feature of exposure to concentrations which were ultimately fatal, but a gain was observed during sub-lethal concentrations.

Fabre *et al.* (1952) found no significant symptoms following exposure for 8 h a day to concentrations up to 22 mg/l.

SYMPTOMS OF INTOXICATION

(1) Neurological disturbances

Pre-mortal symptoms. Narcosis with loss of reflexes, diarrhoea (only with oral administration), prostration, but no convulsions even with inhalation of more than 150 mg/l, according to Lehmann and Flury (1938). Treon *et al.*, however, observed convulsions and, though rarely, opisthotonus, at concentrations of 89.6, 62.6 and 42.4 mg/l, and tremors with repeated exposure.

(2) Blood and bone marrow

Practically the only observers who have recorded changes in the blood picture of animals due to cyclohexane are Launoy and Lévy-Bruhl (1920) and Sato (1928). Launoy and Lévy-Bruhl noted a temporary hyperglobulia associated with the presence of normoblasts following subcutaneous injection of cyclohexane, and Sato recorded a transient leucocytosis followed by leucopenia and diminution of red cells and haemoglobin.

Neither by oral administration, application to the skin nor repeated inhalation did Treon *et al.* (1943) find any fluctuations in the blood picture other than those occurring among the controls. These findings were confirmed by Fabre *et al.* (1952) so far as regards any significant variations of the red and white cells or the leucocytic formula, but they did observe an increase in the coagulation time, unexplainable since it was not accompanied by thrombocytopenia or by diminution of prothrombin or calcium in the peripheral blood.

The bone marrow also showed no evidence of a toxic effect.

Bibliography on p. 140

CHANGES IN THE ORGANISM

No significant specific lesions of the liver or kidneys of rabbits were observed by Treon *et al.* after prolonged exposure to concentrations as high as 1.46 mg/l (424 p.p.m.) for 50 periods of 6 h each, and barely demonstrable microscopic changes at 2.65 mg/l (470 p.p.m.). Fabre *et al.* also found no lesions in these organs, or any others except the lungs, where there was congestion, but no oedema, with repeated exposure to 22 mg/l.

Toxicity to human beings

In 1953 Tara recorded three cases of haemopoietic injury in workers employed respectively in the rubber industry and in degreasing metal parts. In one of the former cases, though the solvent used for the last four years had been cyclohexane, for the preceding four years benzene had been used. In the worker employed in degreasing metal parts the solvent had contained 70% of commercial cyclohexane, 15% of ethyl acetate and 15% of ethyl alcohol. In the remaining rubber worker the only information as to the adhesive used was that it was a solution of cyclohexane. The first case showed hyperchromic anaemia, no leucopenia, and 8% eosinophils; the second, severe anaemia (1.14 million red blood corpuscles) and leucopenia (600 total leucocytes with 80% granulocytes) – a picture strongly suggestive of a benzene effect. In the third case the most marked feature was a persistent neutropenia.

Tara also mentioned that he had found appreciable amounts of benzene in the blood of 12 out of 14 workers using a cyclohexane adhesive. He raised the question of the possible metabolic liberation of benzene from cyclohexane, but this was stated by Truhaut (1953) to be an untenable hypothesis in the face of the results of his own investigations on the metabolism of cyclohexane. He was much more inclined to the opinion that the cyclohexane used in these three cases was of the commercial variety, which could contain significant amounts of benzene. In fact, he himself had found samples of cyclohexane used in adhesives which contained 1–3.6 g of benzene per 100 ml. He urged that all products bearing the name 'cyclohexane' should be strictly controlled for their benzene content.

13. Methylcyclohexane

Synonym: hexahydrotoluene

Structural formula:

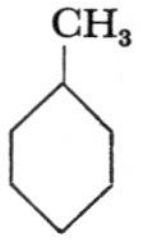

CH$_3$

Molecular formula: C$_7$H$_{14}$

Molecular weight: 98.18

Properties: – A colourless liquid.
    boiling point: 100.8 °C
    melting point: −126.3 °C
    vapour pressure: 43 mm at 25 °C
    vapour density (air = 1): 3.4
    specific gravity (liquid density): 0.7748
    flash point: 25 °F
    conversion factors: 1 p.p.m. = 4.02 mg/m³
                       1 mg/l = 249 p.p.m.
    solubility: insoluble in water, miscible with many organic solvents
    maximum allowable concentration: 500 p.p.m.

ECONOMY, SOURCES AND USES

Production

(1) By distillation from some Near East petroleums.
(2) By catalytic hydrogenation of toluene.
(3) By reaction between benzene and methane at high temperatures (Fairhall, 1957).

Industrial uses

(1) As a solvent particularly with other solvents, for cellulose.
(2) To some extent in organic synthesis.

Bibliography on p. 140   [135]

BIOCHEMISTRY

Estimation

(1) In the atmosphere

No specific method for the analysis of the atmospheric concentration of methylcyclohexane has been described, but a combustible gas indicator appears to be the most suitable instrument (Sallee and Guy, 1962).

(2) In blood and tissues

No information.

Metabolism

The methyl group in methylcyclohexane differs from that of toluene in that it is not oxidised to the corresponding acid, cyclohexylcarbonic acid, and is not aromatised in the animal body (Williams, 1959). It has been suggested that the primary reaction in its metabolism is complete oxidation by ring fission. Bernhard (1937) found neither unchanged compound nor any of its metabolites in the urine of the dog, and Treon *et al.* (1943) found only 4.5% of the dose to the rabbit excreted as conjugated glucuronic acid. This output was relatively slow but was related to the intensity of exposure. Williams remarks that it seems likely that much methylcyclohexane would be eliminated in the breath, but that this aspect of its metabolism has not been investigated.

TOXICOLOGY

Animal experiments indicate that, while methylcyclohexane has a stronger narcotic action than cyclohexane, it is less toxic with long exposure.

Elkins (1959) points out that while this relationship between narcotic and toxic effect of cyclohexane and methylcyclohexane is similar to that between benzene and toluene, this does not apply to the haematological effect, which is specific for benzene and completely absent in both cyclohexane and methylcyclohexane.

No toxic effects from industrial exposure have been reported.

Toxicity to animals

(1) Acute

(a) *Lethal dose.* – *(i) By oral administration*, the minimum lethal dose for rabbits was found by Treon *et al.* to lie between 4 and 4.5 g/kg body weight, as compared with 5.5 and 6 for cyclohexane. – *(ii) By inhalation* Lazarew (1929) gave the M.L.D. for mice as 40–50 mg/l (10,000 to 12,500 p.p.m.) as compared with

60–70 mg/l for cyclohexane. For repeated exposure Treon *et al.* found 28.75 mg/l (6150 p.p.m.) fatal.

(b) Narcotic dose. – Lazarew gave the narcotic dose for mice as 30–40 mg/l (7500–10,000 p.p.m.) as compared with 50 mg/l (12,500 p.p.m.) for cyclohexane.

Treon *et al.* were able to produce rapid narcosis by inhalation of 59.9 mg/l (15,227 p.p.m.) and light narcosis by 39.5 mg/l (10,054 p.p.m.).

(2) Chronic or subacute

No deaths followed inhalation by rabbits of 5600 p.p.m. for 4 weeks or 1162 p.p.m. for 10 weeks; but all the animals died following repeated exposure to 1000 p.p.m. 6 h daily for 2 weeks (Gerarde, 1963).

SYMPTOMS OF INTOXICATION

The outstanding symptom was, by oral administration as in the case of cyclohexane, diarrhoea, and by this route there was also evidence of widespread general vascular injury.

By inhalation of sublethal concentrations over 2 weeks, only slight lethargy was observed (Gerarde, 1963).

(1) Blood and bone marrow

Blood examinations revealed no changes in the peripheral blood picture at any of the concentrations used except for some fluctuations similar to those occurring in the non-exposed animals.

(2) Respiratory disturbances

By inhalation with high concentrations (10,000–15,000 p.p.m.) the narcosis was preceded by convulsions and accompanied by laboured breathing, salivation and conjunctival congestion.

(3) Neurological disturbances

At 5500–7000 p.p.m. there was some lethargy and incoordination of the limbs. No symptoms or signs of illness appeared after exposure for 90 h to 2886 p.p.m.

CHANGES IN THE ORGANISM

Treon *et al.* remark that damage to the heart, liver and kidneys was more extensive than with cyclohexane, but that this may have been in part due to intercurrent pulmonary infection.

Repeated inhalation of 3300 p.p.m. however was, according to Gerarde (1963) followed by only minor injury of liver and kidneys similar to that caused by cyclohexane.

Toxicity to human beings

No case of intoxication in human beings has been recorded.

Bibliography on p. 140

14. Decalin

Synonym: decahydronaphthalene

Structural formula:

Molecular formula: $C_{10}H_{18}$

Molecular weight: 138.25

Properties: Similar to those of tetralin though with a lower boiling point, a stronger odour and less solvent potency.

 boiling range: 183–192 °C

 vapour pressure: cis – 1 mm at 22.5 °C; *trans* – 10 mm at 472 °C (Gerarde, 1963)

 specific gravity (liquid density): 0.887–0.890

 flash point: 135 °F

 solubility: non-miscible with water or alcohol (unless anhydrous) but miscible with most organic solvents (Durrans, 1950).

 evaporation rate: slower than of turpentine, more rapid than of tetralin

 conversion factors: 1 p.p.m. = 5.65 mg/m³

       1 mg/l = 177 p.p.m.

 maximum allowable concentration: not established

ECONOMY, SOURCES AND USES

Production

By complete dehydrogenation of liquid naphthalene or tetralin at temperatures from 150 °C upwards.

Industrial uses

Good solvent for some gums and resins, but not for hard gums like kauri and copal. A thinner for paints and enamels (Heaton, 1923).

TOXICOLOGY

While no serious systemic intoxication from the industrial use of decalin has been

[138]

reported, it has been found to cause skin lesions, and animal experiments suggest that it has a toxic effect similar to that of tetralin (q.v.).

Toxicity to animals

SYMPTOMS OF INTOXICATION

According to Cardani (1942), judging from the shorter survival time, decalin is slightly more acutely toxic than tetralin while in the animals investigated by Badinand *et al.* (1947), though the symptoms of intoxication and lesions of internal organs were negligible, the cataractogenic potency of decalin was greater than that of tetralin.

(1) The eyes

Cataract formation, according to Badinand *et al.*, was more marked than with tetralin, both eyes showing cortical opacities and in one animal a diffuse milkiness of the whole lens.

(2) Blood and bone marrow

Blood changes, like those seen with exposure to tetralin, were not more significant than those commonly found in experimental animals.

(3) Urine

The urine also showed a change similar to that of tetralin, though, the coloration was more brownish than green in those animals given decalin by mouth.

CHANGES IN THE ORGANISM

In Cardani's experiments with guinea pigs, by oral administration, cutaneous application and inhalation, the effects of decalin were fundamentally the same as those of tetralin, especially with regard to the liver (atrophy) and kidneys (nephrosis); in one animal there was an unexplainable calcification of the kidney.

Toxicity to human beings

Eczema has been reported by Cardani (1942) and by Koelsch (1946). In the case described by Cardani, a man who was employed in cleaning paving stones with decalin and some detergents, vesicular eczema was present on the areas in closest contact with decalin – the forearms and the sacral region. It was accompanied by intense pruritus, and skin tests showed sensitivity to decalin but not to the detergents used.

The urine contained traces of albumen and urobilin, and a few leucocytes in the sediment, suggesting possible involvement of the kidneys.

Bibliography on p. 140

BIBLIOGRAPHY

Badinand, A., L. Paufique and J. Rodier (1947) Intoxication expérimentale par la Tetraline, *Arch. Malad. Profess.*, 8: 124.

Bernhard, K. (1937) Stoffwechselversuche zur Dehydrierung des Cyclohexanringes, *Z. Physiol. Chem.*, 248: 256.

Cardani, A. (1942) Studio Sperimentale sulla Tossicità della Tetralina e della Decalina, *Med. Lavoro*, 33: 145.

Elkins, H. B. (1959) The Chemistry of Industrial Toxicology, Chapman and Hall, London.

Elliot, T. H., D. V. Parke and R. T. Williams (1959) The Metabolism of Cyclo (14 C) hexane and its Derivatives, *Biochem. J.*, 72: 193.

Fabre, R., R. Truhaut and M. Peron (1952) Études toxicologiques des Solvants remplacents le Benzène, *Arch. Malad. Profess.*, 13: 437.

Fairhall, L. T. (1957) Industrial Toxicology, Williams and Wilkins, Baltimore.

Fieldner, A. C., G. G. Oberfel, M. C. Teague and J. N. Lawrence (1919) Methods of Testing Gasmasks and Absorbents, *Ind. Eng. Chem.*, 11: 519.

Flury, F. and F. Zernik (1931) Schädliche Gäse, Dämpfe, Nebel, Rauch- und Staubarten, Springer, Berlin.

Gerarde, H. W., (1960) Toxicology and Biochemistry of Aromatic Hydrocarbons, Elsevier, Amsterdam.

— (1963) The alicyclic Hydrocarbons. Patty F. A. Industrial Hygiene and Toxicology, Vol. 2, 2nd ed., Interscience, New York.

Heaton, N. (1923) Some Hydrogenation Products of Benzene and Naphthalene, *J. Oil Colour Chemists Assoc.*, 6: 93.

Henderson, V. E. and J. F. Johnstone (1931) Anaesthetic Potency in the Cyclohydrocarbon Series. *J. Pharmacol. Exptl. Therap.*, 43: 89.

Koelsch, F (1946) Vergiftungen. Aliphatische Verbindungen in Gottstein, *Handb. Soz. Hyg.*, 2: 390.

Launoy, L. and M. Lévy-Bruhl (1920) A Comparison of the Effects of Benzene and Cyclohexane on the Haemopoietic Organs. *Compt. Rend. Soc. Biol.*, 83: 215.

Lazarew, N. W. (1929) Über die Giftigkeit verschiedener Kohlenwasserstoffdämpfe, *Arch. Exptl. Pathol. Pharmakol.*, 143: 223.

Lehmann, K. B. and F. Flury (1938) Toxikologie und Hygiene der technische Lösungsmittel, Springer, Berlin.

Pacault, A. and S. Carpenter (1949) Déshydrogénation du Cyclohexane en Benzène à Froid par Action diastasique, *Compt. Rend.*, 22: 344.

Patty, F. A. (1949) Industrial Hygiene and Toxicology. Vol. Il, Interscience, New York.

Sallee, E. D. and A. C. Guy (1962) Combustible Gas Indicators. *Arch. Environ. Health*, 4: 306.

Sato, K. (1928) Über die pharmakologischen Wirkungen der hydroaromatischen Verbindungen; Cyclohexane, Cyclohexene and Cyclohexanol, *Japan. J. Med. Sci. Trans. Pharmacol.*, 3: 1.

Tara, M. S. (1953) Au Sujet de la Toxicité du Cyclohexane, *Arch. Malad. Profess.*, 14: 494.

Treon, J. F., W. E. Crutchfield and K. V. Kitzmiller (1943) The physiological Response of Rabbits to cyclohexane, methyl cyclohexane and certain Derivatives of these Compounds, *J. Ind. Hyg.*, 25: 199, 323.

Truhaut, R. (1953) Sur la Toxicité du Cyclohexane industriel. Rôle des Impuretés, *Arch. Malad. Profess.*, 14: 494.

Viola, P. L. (1960) Sulla Presenza deidrogenazione enzimatica del Cicloesano a Benzene, *Boll. Soc. Ital. Biol. Sper.*, 36: 1960.

Von Oettingen, W. F. (1940) Toxicology and potential Dangers of Aliphatic and Aromatic Hydrocarbons, *U.S. Treas. Public Health Bull.*, 225: 38.

Williams, R. T. (1959) Detoxication Mechanisms, Chapman and Hall, London.

Chapter 4

TECHNICAL HYDROCARBONS

15. Coal Tar Solvent Naphtha

Coal Tar Naphtha first became of industrial importance in 1823, when, as a product of gas plants in London, it was found to be an excellent solvent for rubber and was used in the manufacture of the first waterproof cloth.

Properties: Solvent naphtha is a colourless liquid with a characteristic odour. It may be divided into several grades, with different boiling ranges, specific gravities and flash points (Durrans, 1950).

a. Light Grade

Contains toluene, xylenes and cumene, and if it has a low boiling point, it may contain appreciable amounts of benzene.
  boiling range: 110–160 °C
  specific gravity (liquid density): 0.865–0.875
  flash point: 70 °F
  maximum allowable concentration: not established.

b. Heavy Grade

Contains 0.25% phenols; 0.25% pyridine (Durrans, 1950).
  boiling range: 160–190 °C
  specific gravity (liquid density): 0.860
  flash point: 90 °F
  maximum allowable concentration: 200 p.p.m.

ECONOMY, SOURCES AND USES

Production

During the refining of the gas from heated coal, its passage through oil-absorption plants results in the production of a light-oil fraction containing crude coal tar naphtha, heavy solvent naphtha as well as benzene, toluene and xylenes.

Industrial uses

Solvent naphtha is used in many industries similar to those using benzol, including (*a*) the rubber industry – waterproof cloth, shoe adhesives, rubber tyres etc., (*b*) the paint industry, for certain types of varnishes and especially in bituminous paints.

TOXICOLOGY

Coal tar naphtha is to be sharply distinguished, from the point of view of toxicology, from petroleum naphtha, which is a mixture of aliphatic hydrocarbons, though it may also contain some benzene. (Elkins and Pagnotto, 1956, found amounts varying from 0.6–7 in eight samples examined.)

Coal tar naphtha is primarily a narcotic, causing unconsciousness in high concentration, without the neuro-irritant phenomena characteristic of acute benzene poisoning. From the point of view of chronic toxicity, this appears to depend on its benzene content; *per se* it is regarded as relatively harmless (Gardner, 1925).

Toxicity to animals

(1) Acute

(a) Lethal dose. – (i) By intraperitoneal injection (for "Hiflash naphtha" with a B.P. of about 156 °C) was, according to Batchelor (1929) 2.5 ml/kg body weight. – *(ii) By inhalation* death did not occur with the highest concentrations available (567 p.p.m.).

(b) Narcotic dose. – (i) By intraperitoneal injection was very near the lethal dose. With doses up to 2.5 ml/kg there was profound depression with marked sluggishness and stupor, but no loss of reflexes or unconsciousness. With lower dosage (0.25 ml/kg) the animals showed instability, inco-ordination, weakness and paresis. – *(ii) By inhalation* no narcosis was produced by doses up to 567 p.p.m.

(2) Chronic

Prolonged exposure to 567 p.p.m. in Batchelor's experiments caused irritation of mucous membranes, with lachrymation, sneezing and coryza. There was also slight apathy, a possible tendency to instability and weakness and a loss of weight of 5–21 %.

SYMPTOMS OF INTOXICATION

(1) Blood

An abnormality of the blood picture noted by Gardner (1925), using solvent naphtha B.P. 160 °C and by Batchelor, using Hiflash naphtha, was slight anemia, but Batchelor also noted a mild leucocytosis after prolonged exposure to 567 p.p.m. and a slight late tendency to leucocytosis with the lower concentration of 312 p.p.m.

(2) Bone marrow

The bone marrow showed some hyperplasia with subcutaneous injection.

CHANGES IN THE ORGANISM

With subcutaneous injection (Batchelor, 1927) the kidneys showed changes varying with the amount injected from diffuse cloudy swelling to mild diffuse nephritis; the spleen some congestion and pigmentation, but less than with benzol, toluol or xylol, indicating probably less blood destruction. The liver showed only mild periportal focal necrosis.

With inhalation the only significant lesions were mild cloudy swelling of the kidneys and in one case slight congestion of the lungs and moderate pigmentation of the spleen. Batchelor concluded that Hiflash naphtha was practically devoid of the industrial hazards involved in the use of benzene.

Toxicity to human beings

(1) Acute

Cases of 'gassing' due to coal tar naphtha have been not infrequently recorded. Altogether, between 1938 and 1953 eight cases were reported in the Annual Reports of the Chief Inspector of Factories in Great Britain.

One 'doubtful' case in 1947 was said to be associated with exposure to bitumen paint and naphtha; the man suffered from giddiness and bleeding from the mouth. In another in 1953, a painter using a spray gun inside a garage, the paint containing white spirit and naphtha, became unconscious after the spray had accidentally discharged in his face; he suffered after recovery from nausea, dyspnoea and vertigo.

(2) Chronic

In 1944 (Annual Report of the Chief Inspector of Factories) a number of girls manufacturing tracing paper showed severe emotional disturbance (weeping and 'fainting') during a period of fog when ventilation was inadequate; they also complained of headache, lassitude and anorexia. None showed any significant disturbance of the blood picture, but one man working in the same atmosphere had nose bleeding and slight leucopenia, and one boy aged fifteen, employed in tending the machines, had more severe leucopenia and neutropenia. One other case of anemia, reported in 1950, was found to be associated with a cardiac disorder which was considered to be the cause of the anaemia.

In the only fatal case of aplastic anaemia reported in association with exposure to solvent naphtha (Annual Report of the Chief Inspector of Factories, 1945) it was found that although the naphtha had been stated to contain only about 1% of benzol the content was actually 5–6%.

Bibliography on p. 168

Coal Tar Solvent and Bitumen

A fatal case of poisoning by bitumen and coal tar solvent was reported by Saverin (1940) in a man painting the inside of a tank; he was found dead with his head lying in the paint.

Several cases of more or less severe acute poisoning have been reported from the use of 'Bitume-mastic', a black heavy liquid of complex chemical composition used largely for the protection of iron and steel against rust. It consists mostly of coal tar, the composition varying with the source of the tar, and may contain ammonia, pyridine, naphthalene, anthracene, fluoranthrene and phenols and cresols from 5–10%. Des Essarts (1932) describes three grades of poisoning from the use of this substance:

(1) Mild – similar to alcoholic intoxication, transient and with rapid recovery.

(2) Moderate – coma, with convulsions and syncope, followed by headache and nausea for some hours.

(3) Severe – coma, which may be fatal.

16. Petroleum Solvents

ECONOMY, SOURCES AND USES

Petroleum itself (*q.v.*) is a mixture of many hydrocarbons, including paraffins, cyclic paraffins and other cyclic hydrocarbons, olefines, acetylenes, and some aromatic hydrocarbons. These are separated by distillation, each fraction containing the major portion of all compounds having boiling points within the distillation range of the fraction.

The solvents among these distillate products include gasoline, petroleum ether, benzine, white spirit, etc., with boiling ranges below 450 °F.

TOXICOLOGY

As a class, the two predominant hazards of the petroleum solvents arise from their narcotic potency and their tendency to cause dermatitis, which tends to take the form of comedones, acne, folliculitis and photosensitivity rather than the eczematoid type of lesion. According to Klauder and Brill (1947) the dermatitis caused by petroleum solvents is regarded as "the expression of a non-specific sensitivity comparable to dermatitis from exposure to other eczematogenous noxae"; dry or senile skins are especially susceptible and this increased sensitivity is to be regarded as due to an anatomical or physiological defect of the skin rather than as an allergy. Schwarz *et al.* (1947) state that while their defatting action is less than that of solvents with a lower boiling point (unless they have a high content of aromatics) they have keratogenic and sensitising properties. Their photo-sensitising action has been described particularly by Dunn and Brackett (1948) with regard to methylated naphthalenes (see p. 14) and the rare manifestation of Schamberg's Disease (progressive pigmentary dermatosis) by Capellini and Parmeggiani (1948) with regard to benzine (see p. 159).

16a. Petroleum Naphtha

Petroleum naphtha is to be distinguished, especially from the toxicological point of view, from coal tar naphtha.

Properties: Petroleum naphtha is chiefly a mixture of paraffin hydrocarbons but may contain aromatic hydrocarbons in relatively small amount, including benzene and its derivatives and cyclo-paraffin aromatics. According to Gerarde (1960) the percentage of benzene in the total aromatic content is 0.121.

High aromatic petroleum solvent naphthas, for use with high temperatures, in certain paints, are also produced in different qualities with different characteristics *e.g.* (Durrans 1950).

	(1)	(2)
boiling range:	100–140 °C	130–180 °C
specific gravity (liquid density):	0.833	0.860
aromatic content:	73%	93%
maximum allowable concentration:	500 p.p.m.	(Elkins, 1959, suggests 1000 p.p.m.)

ECONOMY, SOURCES AND USES

Production

Heavy aromatic naphtha is a special fraction occurring in petroleum with a boiling range of 160–280 °C. It contains approximately 85% of aromatics by volume, but these are chiefly indanes, indenes, naphthalenes and diphenyls (Gerarde, 1960).

Industrial uses

(1) In the rubber industry.
(2) In the paint and varnish industry, especially as a lacquer diluent and thinner.
(3) Heavy aromatic naphtha is also used as a solvent for pesticides for fruit and vegetables.

TOXICOLOGY

From animal experiments it appears that both these varieties of naphtha have a lower toxicity than coal tar solvent naphtha. Fairhall (1957) remarks that their lower toxicity is due to the fact that they contain constituents which are far more toxicologically inert than those of coal tar naphtha.

In human beings nervous and gastro-intestinal symptoms; in the case of heavy aromatic naphtha no primary skin irritation has been observed, but some mild photosensitisation to ultraviolet light.

Toxicity to animals

Few experiments on animals appear to have been made, but Gerarde (1960) quotes Nelson and Fiero (1954) in stating that "a low order of toxicity was indicated by short-term intermittent vapor exposure tests" (low pressure aerosols of heavy aromatic naphtha).

Toxicity to human beings

Several cases of chronic poisoning by petroleum naphtha were reported by Hayhurst (1936) under the heading of 'Petroleum Distillates', in workers employed in cleaning metal trays with the naphtha, in a closed room without ventilation.

SYMPTOMS OF INTOXICATION

The case of one woman, more severely affected than the rest, was described in detail. She was exposed for five weeks, but noted headache, nausea and lassitude almost from the first day. Later, after a sickness absence of two days with acute sore throat, she complained of severe headache, weakness, nervousness, involuntary twitching and near collapse. Four months later she had lost 6 lbs in weight, and had vomiting of sticky mucus, marked anorexia and extreme nervousness. It was more than a year before she began to improve, but she then gained appetite, weight and strength, with no residual symptoms. It is to be noted that the other girls, whose symptoms, though similar, were not so marked, did not have their hands and forearms wet with the naphtha, while a young man who replaced the girl with the severe symptoms was equally badly affected after two weeks.

The skin

From the patch-testing results on 100 human subjects cited by Nelson and Fiero (1954) it appears that heavy aromatic naphtha causes no significant degree of primary skin irritation. They observed a mild photosensitising effect with exposure of the tested sites to ultraviolet light, in one subject the reaction persisting for 6 h, but considered that these reactions were not significantly more severe than with another pesticide solvent in frequent use which was used as control.

16b. Petrol – Gasoline

Petrol, or gasoline, is a mixture of paraffins, cycloparaffins and aromatic hydrocarbons, the relative amounts of the constituents varying with its origin.

Bibliography on p. 168

ECONOMY, SOURCES AND USES

Production

Crude petrol also contains sulphur derivatives which produce sulphuretted hydrogen and mercaptans with a highly disagreeable odour.

Borneo petroleum contains more aromatic hydrocarbons (benzene, toluene and xylene) than the petroleum of the U.S.A., though motor and aviation petrol produced by the recent method of catalytic reforming tends to be of a higher aromatic content than the former "straight-run gasoline" which, according to Machle (1941) contained more than 65% of paraffin hydrocarbons. Gerarde (1960) gives the total aromatic content of "catalytically cracked" gasoline as 23.98%, of which benzene represents 0.21%, toluene 2.32%, xylene 2.14%, ethyl benzene 1.07% and isopropyl benzene 0.18%.

Motor benzol is used as a component of motor petrol; it contains approximately 70% of benzene, also toluene and xylene.

In France, a distinction is made between "lighting petrol" (the non-distillable fraction of naphtha) and "essence", the automobile petrol, a much more volatile product (Castagnou, 1960) in much greater demand since 1925.

A good example of the varying content of various samples of petrol can be seen in the investigation of Davis *et al.* (1960). In assessing the effects of the vapour on human beings they found that of the three samples used, one contained 40%, another 20% and the third 65% of aromatics.

The addition of tetra-ethyl lead into automobile petrol has introduced an altogether separate hazard, as in the cases of poisoning described by Coste and Wolz (1935) and others.

Industrial uses

Petrol is used in industry as a substitute solvent for purposes similar to those of the aromatic hydrocarbons, *viz.*:

(1) In the rubber industry.
(2) In the paint and varnish industry. (When used as a thinner it is sometimes known as "mineral spirits" or "petroleum spirits" (Hayhurst, 1936).
(3) In the boot and shoe industry as a solvent for the rubber adhesive.
(4) As a degreaser and dry cleaner. Machle (1941) remarks that the use as a dry cleaner is particularly hazardous because in pressing clothes still damp with gasoline the high temperatures volatilise the more toxic heavier fractions.
(5) In the extraction of fat from bones and in the manufacture of glue.
(6) In the manufacture of waterproof plaster.
(7) In the petroleum industry itself.

BIOCHEMISTRY

Estimation

(1) In the atmosphere

In most of the cases observed in industrially exposed persons the concentration has not been recorded, since they have usually occurred in men entering tanks or wagons containing petrol (Chief Inspector of Factories, Annual Reports).

In some of these cases the petrol has contained benzene or benzine.

Statements in the Accident Prevention Manuals of the American Petroleum Institute (1942) implied that concentrations up to 2000 p.p.m. could be breathed without significant ill-effects, and Patty (1949) remarks that "it is not uncommon to find men working without respiratory protection in atmospheres approaching this level". Fieldner, Katz and Kenney (1921) had found that, even when mixed with a high concentration of oxygen in a breathing apparatus, 2–2.5% of gasoline vapour rendered a man dizzy and soon became intolerable, and Drinker *et al.* (1943) found giddiness and unsteadiness of gait produced by 7000 p.p.m. On the other hand some authorities believe that lower doses than these can cause acute intoxication, while others have noted no signs of intoxication at higher levels. Goodman and Gilman (1955) for example state that it is dangerous to life at 2000 p.p.m. and Sterner (1941) that it can cause acute symptoms at 300–500 p.p.m. It seems probable that this discrepancy is connected with the fact that the actual constituents of the petrol have not been taken into account; in one of the few investigations where the petrol used in a voluntary experiment was known to be uncontaminated by aromatic hydrocarbons (Davis *et al.*, 1960) concentrations of 1000 p.p.m. produced no significant symptoms other than eye irritation.

For continued exposure during an 8-h working day the 1962 Threshold Limit Value (for gasoline) is 500 p.p.m. This lowering of the value from that recommended by Bowditch *et al.* in 1940 (1000 p.p.m.) has no doubt been influenced by the possibility of benzene contamination. Smyth and Smyth (1928) noted that even with a benzene content of the petrol of 0.5%, the atmospheric level of benzene could exceed 100 p.p.m., and in Sterner's (1941) investigation of a workshop where gasoline was used as a paint solvent the actual atmospheric content of total aromatics ranged from 500 to 800 p.p.m.

(2) In blood and tissues

See benzene.

Metabolism

(1) Absorption and excretion

Absorption is chiefly through the respiratory tract, and if the concentration is high it may be very rapid, causing symptoms within a few minutes.

Absorption from the skin was not considered by most of the earlier observers

Bibliography on p. 168

except Friedeberg (1902) sufficient to cause intoxication; Lessar (1898) did report a fatality in a child following application to the skin as a remedy for scabies, but it is probable that inhalation was at least a contributory cause. Hayhurst (1936) however, reported that the most marked symptoms of chronic poisoning in his series of workers were in those who had their hands and forearms immersed in petroleum distillates, and Soprana (1941) described severe intoxication, followed by death within 3 days, in a woman who had applied a dressing soaked in petrol to her wrist for 11 h.

(2) Distribution in tissues
No information.

TOXICOLOGY

It should be mentioned that in many of the early descriptions of cases of intoxication listed under the heading of "gasoline", benzine has been regarded as synonymous with petrol or gasoline, and as recently as 1960 Fabre has drawn attention to the fact that "petroleum essence" with a B.P. of 45°–150 °C is still called "benzine" in some countries. Even in 1936 Hayhurst had remarked "the term benzine is archaic and should not be used" and this is true not only with regard to its confusion with petrol but also, even more seriously, with benzene. Cases of intoxication which obviously relate to benzine are here described under that heading (see p. 160).

The acute toxic effect of petrol itself is mainly that of narcosis, with loss of consciousness associated with a convulsive effect (Haggard, 1920) and sometimes fatal. Chronic exposure, if prolonged, can cause symptoms of nervous and digestive disorder, any significant change in the blood picture is usually due to the presence of benzene in the vapour. Skin contact can cause erythematous and vesicular dermatitis, and possibly a general sensitising or photosensitising effect.

Toxicity to animals

The results of most of the early investigations emphasise the fact that the hazard of inhalation is greater in animals than ingestion.

(1) Acute
(a) Lethal dose. – (i) By ingestion, Legludic and Turlais (1914) gave 20 ml/kg as the lethal dose for rabbits. – (ii) By intravenous ingestion, the same observers gave a lower toxicity (0.4 ml/kg) than Matsushita (1935) – 0.3 ml/kg. – (iii) By inhalation. The gap between the acute narcotic and the lethal concentration is narrow. According to Haggard (1920) using straight-run gasoline on dogs, death

occurred 4 min after full anaesthesia, which was obtained with a concentration of 25,000 p.p.m. Convulsions began in one dog at 8900 p.p.m. and in another at 10,200, but one dog subjected to 17,600 another to 19,600 p.p.m. were still conscious, and though they continued for some time to have clonic convulsions and were unable to walk, recovery was apparently complete a few days later.

It may be noted in passing, though it has no direct industrial application, that in the experiments of Kotin and Falk (1956), mice inhaling an atmosphere of ozonised gasoline exhibited a higher incidence of lung tumours than control animals inhaling washed air. It is not suggested that gasoline is *per se* carcinogenic, but that the eventual reaction of ozone with compounds produced by the primary ozonisation is to give diepoxides and peroxides which have already been shown to be carcinogenic (Fieser *et al.* 1955).

(b) Narcotic dose. – No information.

(2) Chronic

Inhalation of mixtures of petrol and air in concentrations similar to those found in industrial exposures and repeated at intervals, showed in dogs only slight disturbances of circulation and respiration; in rabbits some inco-ordination of movement and somnolence; in guinea pigs malaise, loss of appetite and weakness; all died within one to two years (Poincaré, 1885).

SYMPTOMS OF INTOXICATION

(1) General

Inhalation directly from a mask produced in the experiments of Poincaré (1885) agitation, then somnolence, loss of appetite, vomiting and intestinal haemorrhage, but such inhalations were not fatal. Lewin (1888) observed that inhalations of petrol were better tolerated than those of benzine.

Gastric or intravenous administration causes the symptoms of an acute narcotic poison with twitching, tonic or clonic convulsions, restlessness, tachycardia, dyspnoea and in some cases exophthalmus (Matsushita, 1935). Histological examination of the brain and spinal cord indicated that petroleum has a destructive action on the nerve cells of the brain, medulla, and spinal cord with dilation of the blood vessels of the brain and haemorrhages especially in the region of the ventricles.

(2) Blood and bone marrow

Effects on the blood picture of rabbits exposed to inhalation of 60 mg/l 8 h a day for 80 days indicated in the experiments of Salamone (1961) that a peripheral and later central effect was exerted especially on the red cells and platelets. The red cells showed poikilocytosis, basophilia, Heinz bodies and Cabot rings, a moderate initial erythroblastaemia, and reduction of globular resistance, with a diphasic Price-Jones curve due to the presence of microcytes and reticulo-cytes. Platelets were decreased in number and showed reduced agglutinability and adhesion. There was an initial leucocytosis followed by leucopenia, and neu-trophilia followed by neutropenia, with toxic granulation of the polymorphs.

The bone marrow showed an initial increased cellularity, but this decreased later.

Toxicity to human beings

(A) Acute, non-industrial intoxication

(a) By ingestion. In adults, ingestion of petroleum, has been generally assumed for many years to be practically innocuous. Siwe (1932) quotes Zangger (1927) as saying that pure petrol, as it is produced commercially to-day, has very little toxic action, and that several hundred grams can be ingested, usually without any severe effect. Nevertheless, many cases of intoxication, either accidental or by motorists attempting to siphon it from tanks, have been recorded.

In the cases reported by Nunn and Martin (1934) there was evidence that some of the petrol had also been aspirated. The single oral dose fatal to human beings is, according to Machle (1941), about 7.5 g/kg body weight, but this has been found elsewhere very variable.

One case, in a child, described by Siwe (1932) succumbed after as little as 10 g. Children are apparently more susceptible than adults, who are in any case warned by the unpleasant smell and taste. Relatively small doses can cause in children unconsciousness, convulsions or respiratory paralysis. That the con-stitution of the petrol also influences the degree of poisoning was pointed out by many of the early investigators. One of the earliest of such cases was recorded by Lesser (1898), a child who drank only a small quantity but at autopsy showed marked oedema of the glottis. A case described by Siwe (1932) was a boy only one year and eleven months old, who had picked up a can of petrol and drank an unknown quantity of it. He became blue in the face and vomited red mucus within a few minutes, was later restless and complained of pain in the abdomen and had several attacks of blueness of the face and dyspnoea; he recovered completely 11 days after the ingestion. Shallow and rapid respiration was a notable feature in this case, and dyspnoea and stertor in those of Johanssen (1896) and Conrads (1896). These early investigators reported that these symptoms were not apparent-ly accompanied by actual inflammatory lesions of the lungs, but were considered to be of central nervous origin. In a later investigation, however, Nunn and Mar-tin (1934) described seven cases of gasoline poisoning in children by ingestion, in which the mortality was 28%, and in all these there was definite clinical evidence of pathological changes in the lungs – moist râles, rapid shallow respiration and cyanosis, and in one case autopsy revealed oedema, the alveoli being filled with fibrin and serous exudate.

In non-fatal cases there were no complications or sequelae; the irritating effects on the lungs and gastro-intestinal tract disappeared within 48 h, and Nunn and Martin believed that in the cases showing pneumonitis the petroleum had been aspirated as well as ingested. In a fatal case described by Ainsworth (1960), a boy was trapped in an overturned car with his head in a pool of petrol. Autopsy revealed hyperaemia of the lungs, with oedema, some intra-alveolar haemorrhage and necrosis of the alveolar walls, and petrol was recovered from the lungs by distillation. A rise in temperature, when it occurs, is unconnected with any local source of infection, and the *post mortem* in Johanssen's case showed no pathological variations which could have been the cause of death, especially no sign of pneumonia.

(1) Mucous membranes

The digestive system, in some cases, shows abrasion of the mucous membranes (Siwe, 1932; Lesser, 1898).

(2) The skin

Skin lesions, excoriated areas with loose easily stripped epidermis, were present on the trunk and limbs in Ainsworth's (1960) case, and similar lesions were described by Aidan (1958) in a case where they were considered to be due to contact of petrol-soaked clothing with the skin. Apparently, however, such lesions can be caused by petrol vapour, for example, as in a case described by Stewart (1960) from a petrol lighter in conditions of high temperature and lowered pressure, as in air travel.

Some of the effects of inhalation of petrol fumes have been observed either in experiments on human volunteers, or in persons who have developed an addiction to petrol.

(i) Volunteers. – In two subjects investigated by Fieldner *et al.* (1921) inhalation for 18 minutes of air containing 300–700 p.p.m. of petrol failed to produce any symptoms; 14 min of exposure to 2800–7000 p.p.m. produced dizziness. In a more recent investigation (Davis *et al.*, 1960) the constitution of the petrol used was carefully controlled, especially for the absence of tetra-ethyl lead. Ten subjects were exposed for 30 min to the vapour of three different samples, in concentrations of 200, 500 and 1000 p.p.m.; control experiments with room air were also made. A questionnaire to each subject dealt with local irritation, headache, nausea and giddiness, and photographs of one eye of each subject were taken before and after the experiment. Very few symptoms were noted; the most significant effect of two of the samples being eye irritation. Nine out of the ten complained of itching or burning of the eyes at concentrations above 900 p.p.m.; this was verified by the increase in injection of the conjunctiva agreeing significantly with the subjective response.

(ii) Addiction. – Gasoline 'sniffing' by adolescents, for the purpose of pro-

Bibliography on p. 168

ducing mental stimulation and pleasant hallucinations has been reported by several observers in recent years, many of them in adolescents with psychopathic tendencies. Clinger and Johnson (1951) described two cases, one in a 16 year old negro boy regarded as schizophrenic, the other a white boy aged 13, who showed depression and anxiety and who had hallucinations of power. Another boy aged 11 also had hallucinations (Faucett and Jensen, 1952), while a 6 year old child who had been addicted to sniffing gasoline for 18 months became inebriated and unable to stand (Pruitt, 1959). Another case of 'sniffing', which had occurred periodically from the age of 6–17 was described by Edwards (1960). On many occasions of inhalation for 3–5 min he lost consciousness.

Similar cases have been described by Oldham (1961) and Lawton and Malinquist (1961). Oldham's case was that of a girl of 17 who had inhaled petrol from rags soaked in lighter petrol or car tanks as a substitute for trichloroethylene, to which she had previously been addicted. Although the immediate drowsiness, with pleasant "dreams" were followed by giddiness and nausea there were no objective toxic effects, but she was arrested for theft and larceny. In the three cases described by Lawton and Malinquist hallucinations were a prominent feature, and again, though there was no clinical or laboratory evidence of central nervous damage, all three were delinquents. Practically all such cases have in fact shown underlying emotional conflicts, and when these were treated and improved there were no organic sequelae.

(B) Acute, industrial intoxication

'Gassing' cases reported to the Chief Inspector of Factories are usually classified as 'due to petrol or benzine' so that it is not possible to attribute these exclusively to one or the other. Between 1939 and 1960 43 such cases were reported, of these 9 were fatal. In two cases the gassing occurred during the testing and repair of combustion engines (1944); in another (1945) while testing the level of the content of a petrol storage tank.

A recent fatal case has been recorded by Wang and Irons (1961). A man entered an aircraft tank which had not, as directives had required, been 'purged' of its gasoline. He was found unconscious 5 min later and in spite of artificial respiration died during transfer to hospital. Autopsy showed acute pulmonary oedema, exudative tracheobronchitis, congestion of liver and spleen and early acute haemorrhagic pancreatitis. The cause of death was stated to be respiratory arrest with irreversible cerebral damage.

Precautions against such accidents have been well summarised by Kehoe (1953): ". . . exposure to vapour in an enclosed space where liquid gasoline is present or has been spilled should never be permitted or indulged in. Entrance into such a space without the protection of respiratory equipment and assistance in supervision from without is a foolhardy adventure which invites death".

SYMPTOMS OF INTOXICATION

When symptoms of chronic poisoning by petrol are present they are usually vague and non-specific, though sometimes indicating an effect on the central nervous system, sometimes on the gastro-intestinal tract. It appears to be quite definitely agreed that petroleum (gasoline) does not carry the hazard of injury to the blood-forming organs from chronic occupational exposure unless it has a high aromatic content, especially of benzene.

(1) The skin

Prolonged contact can cause erythematous and vesicular dermatitis, and some authorities have postulated a general sensitising or photosensitising effect (Klauder and Brill, 1947; Dunn and Brackett, 1948). This latter effect Mir (1941) associated with a case of melanosis in a worker exposed to gasoline.

Recovery from symptoms of chronic gasoline intoxication is usually quite complete on removal from exposure − a fact which is helpful in making a definite diagnosis of their cause.

(2) Blood and bone marrow

Blood changes of a benzene-like character are only seen when benzene is present in the gasoline. Leucocytosis may be present where there is lung inflammation due to subacute exposure, or infections of the mouth and throat.

Some authorities have insisted on the prevalence of anaemia, (Hayhurst, 1936), but this may of course be secondary to the undernutrition observed in some gasoline workers (Amorati et al., 1952).

A rare case of aplastic anaemia in a gasoline worker was described by Askey in 1928, but the gasoline was later found to contain at least 17% of aromatic hydrocarbons, chiefly benzene. The man in question was employed in scrubbing old advertising panels with rags soaked in gasoline which was a mixture of Californian gasolines. His blood picture was that of bone marrow aplasia, and he had bleeding from the nose and gums, petechiae of the skin and haemorrhage of the retina. The bone marrow aplasia was finally attributed to the benzene content of the gasoline.

(3) Digestive disturbances

Digestive disturbance with nausea, abdominal pain, constipation or diarrhoea is fairly frequent, and loss of weight may be considerable. In Hayhurst's cases the loss amounted to 10–60% over a period of months.

(4) Neurological disturbances

Susceptibility to gasoline vapour varies considerably, and according to Machle (1941) habituation is a usual phenomenon. He notes that during observation of some 2300 refinery workers for periods of up to 10 or 12 years he found

Bibliography on p. 168

no definite cases of chronic gasoline intoxication. In a group of barrel fillers he did, however, find undernutrition, pallor and symptoms pointing to a central nervous effect. These included psychasthenic or neurasthenic manifestations, listlessness, mental confusion, loss of memory, depression, irritability, fatigue, vertigo and muscular weakness and cramps. Spencer (1922) had also noted headaches vertigo, drowsiness, conjunctival irritation, excitability and mild nervous symptoms in 22 persons exposed to gasoline vapours from coupon-cancelling machines.

In Hayhurst's (1936) series of cases, using petroleum as a paint thinner and degreaser, the initial symptoms, sometimes after 2–5 weeks of employment, were pre-eminently subjective – headache, dizziness, loss of appetite, dyspepsia, itching of the skin, pains in the back, legs and chest. Over a period of months and years, intercurrent mouth and throat infections were accompanied by a great variability of complaints which might lead to a diagnosis of extreme neurasthenia, but Hayhurst was convinced that the resulting disability, which might last for years, in fact might possibly be permanent, was due to the solvent effect of the gasoline upon the fat of the central nervous system, the medullary sheaths of the peripheral nerves and elsewhere in the body. He emphasised the special hazard of absorption through the skin, by immersing the hands and forearms – such cases, he stated, showed more marked symptoms even than the inhalation cases.

Machle also stresses the possibility of severe central nervous injury, with resulting ataxia, tremor, numbness, paraesthesia, neuritis and paralysis of cranial nerves. It should be noted that Machle does not always distinguish between petrol and benzine. He states, for example, that retrobulbar neuritis was reported by Peters in 1900, but Peters' own description is "retrobulbar neuritis from chronic benzine poisoning".

16c. White Spirit

Synonyms: White spirit sometimes known as 'light petrol', is one of the saturated or paraffin hydrocarbons (Simonin, 1934).

Structural formula (general): CH_3-CH_3

Molecular formula: C_nH_{2n+2}

Properties:
  boiling range: 150–190 °C
  flash point: 25 °C
  maximum allowable concentration: none at present established

It is a clear colourless fluid with a petrol-like odour. Its solvent properties vary with its source, the Rumanian product having the greatest general solvent potency and the least odour.

The British Standard Specification (1936, no 245) of white spirit used as a solvent for paint requires that it shall be neutral, free from grease and objectionable sulphur compounds.

ECONOMY, SOURCES AND USES

Production

White spirit is obtained from petroleum.

Industrial uses

(1) As a dry cleaning agent.
(2) As a paint solvent, especially as a substitute for turpentine.

TOXICOLOGY

Few examples of poisoning, other than occasional cases of gassing, have been reported, even more rarely of chronic poisoning. Most authorities, including Simonin (1934), consider that its only significant hazard is that of skin irritation, since, as Simonin says, 'it emits little vapour'.

Toxicity to animals

No experiments on animals with white spirit alone appear to have been made.

Toxicity to human beings

(1) Acute

(i) From ingestion. – During an investigation of the potential toxic properties of 'vaseline' (described as a 'heavy petrol' used as a substitute for fat in patisserie) and pronouncing it innocuous, Dubois (1885) mentioned a case of acute poisoning in a man who drank 'light petrol' from a wine bottle which had contained some. He became within a few minutes violently delirious, with clonic convulsions and a burning sensation in the throat and stomach. Administration of animal carbon was followed by vomiting; both the vomit and the expired air smelt strongly of petrol. He recovered rapidly, with only headache as a residual symptom. Dubois notes that 'other liquid hydrocarbons, such as benzine, are powerful anaesthetics

Bibliography on p. 168

and therefore violent poisons'. – *(ii) From inhalation.* – Two cases of 'gassing', one in a workman painting in a confined space with a paint containing oil of terebene and white spirit, the other in a dry cleaning establishment, were reported to the Factory Department of the Home Office in 1929. In the first case the man collapsed and became unconscious, the second suffered only from giddiness and vomiting.

(2) Chronic

No evidence of a toxic effect in men using white spirit alone or with turpentine as a paint thinner was revealed by an enquiry carried out by the Industrial Paints Committee in 1920, and though in one case, where the white spirit was used in painting radiators by dipping into a tank, a man complained of 'very strong fumes', there was no objective evidence of injury.

An interesting case of chronic poisoning, somewhat doubtfully attributed to white spirit, was that described by Hicguet (1930) – a painter, using lead paint with white spirit as the solvent, who developed 'nervous deafness', with violent tinnitus and some giddiness. He presented no evidence of lead poisoning, either clinical or haematological, and all the symptoms disappeared rapidly under treatment with potassium iodide. Hicguet was led to consider white spirit as the toxic agent because the painter himself remarked that his fellow-workers had complained of the same substance. It may be noted, as an example of the confusion which formerly existed between the aromatic and aliphatic hydrocarbons, (*e.g.* benzene and benzine) that Hicguet remarks that white spirit is 'a substance of the benzol series'.

SYMPTOMS OF INTOXICATION

Browning (unpublished observation) has made clinical and haematological examinations of a large number of workers in the dry-cleaning industry where white spirit was used, with a view to assessing the relative toxicity of various solvents used for dry cleaning. No significant abnormality of health or of the blood picture was found. Only one case of dermatititis of the wrists and forearms, in a worker using white spirit for 25 years, was reported to the Home Office in 1935. Some authorities, however, such as Farris and Sicca (1954) regard white spirit in the same category of sensitisers and irritants of the skin as other petroleum derivatives.

17. Benzine

Benzine is not a chemical entity but a mixture of hydrocarbons, containing, according to its mode of production and uses, pentane, hexane, octane and frequently some benzene.

Properties: benzine is a colourless liquid with a heavy vapour, three times as heavy as air (Russian benzine has a specific gravity ranging from 0.690–0.749). It has a time of volatilisation of 3.5 compared with ethyl ether 1.

A classification of the chief varieties of benzine according to their place of origin (Lazarew, 1929), shows the variation in constituents:

(1) From Pennsylvania and the Caucasus – contains paraffins (pentane, hexane, heptane).
(2) From Baku, Texas, California, Mexico, Japan and Galicia – contains cyclo-paraffins (cyclopentane, cyclohexane).
(3) From Rumania and some from Galicia and Borneo – contains aromatic hydrocarbons (benzene and its homologues).

Some varieties of 'crack' benzine also contain up to 20% of aromatic hydrocarbons together with olefines, acetylenes and terpenes.

Rectified benzine contains no benzene or aromatic hydrocarbons (Petrini, 1941). It distils at 55–85 °C; specific gravity: 0.70.

Benzine is explosive if mixed with air in a percentage of 1.4–7.5 (Baldi and Ricciardi-Pollini, 1954).

ECONOMY, SOURCES AND USES

Production

Benzine is generally produced by distillation of petrol, (light benzine at 60–110 °C, heavy at 100–150 °C), but during the last ten years it has been produced synthetically from lignite, carbon, tar, pitch or asphalt suspended in heavy oil and combined with hydrogen at a temperature of 450 °C; also from water gas in the presence of metal oxides or cobalt (Fischer *et al.*, 1951).

Industrial uses

The uses of benzine according to its variety were classified by Loewenberg (1932) as follows:

light benzine	– solvent for fat, resins and rubber; cleaning agent
motor benzine	– automobile fuel
middle benzine	– extraction and cleaning; filling for miner's lamps
heavy benzine	– lacquer industry; substitute for turpentine

BIOCHEMISTRY

Metabolism

Absorption and excretion

Absorption is mainly in vapour form, by inhalation. Absorption from the skin is practically without significance in human beings, but in animals some skin absorption, though less than that of benzene, has been indicated by the experiments of Lazarew *et al.* (1931). The air expired by dogs with one leg immersed in benzine was passed through silica-gel, the weight of which was found to be increased by $2\frac{1}{2}$–3 times as much as in control animals. The speed of absorption was estimated as not less than 0.01 mg/min/cm² of skin. Compared with benzene, the amount in the blood taken from the external jugular vein of rabbits after immersion of the ear was 10–12 mg/kg for benzine, 50–100 mg/kg for benzene.

Excretion, probably unchanged, is mainly through the lungs. Loewenberg (1932) states that it is never found in the urine even after massive ingestion.

TOXICOLOGY

Benzine is a narcotic, the degree of its narcotic effect varying with its constitution. Octane causes rapid deep narcosis; pentane and hexane are less powerful narcotics but both they and heptane exert a paralytic effect on the respiratory centre and the spinal cord (Holstein, 1958). The narcotic effect of benzine on the whole is less than that of benzene and its local irritative effect greater.

Acute poisoning, occurring in closed spaces, is initiated by irritation of the eyes, upper respiratory passages and lungs, and may progress to drunkenness, delirium and convulsions with cyanosis. Sequelae such as cardiac disorder, leucocytosis, albuminuria and erosions of the skin from contact, usually disappear soon after recovery from the narcotic effect.

Chronic poisoning is characterised chiefly by nervous and digestive disturbance (the nervous disturbance has been designated 'hystero-anaesthesia'). There may be some anaemia, but the severe blood disorder characteristic of benzene does not occur unless the benzine contains significant amounts of benzene.

Toxicity to animals

(1) Acute

(a) Lethal dose. – This varies with different varieties, the discrepancy arising from the difference in constitution, especially from the content of aromatic hydrocarbons. With Baku benzines, containing a relatively large amount of cycloparaffins, Lazarew (1929) found the lethal dose for mice between 40 and 80 mg/l.

With the Russian benzine known as 'Kalosche', with a content of aromatic hydrocarbons from 0.73–1.5%, Lestchinskaya (1933) found the minimum lethal dose for mice to be 74 mg/l, but different samples varied widely. For dogs, Babsky and Leites (1931) gave the lethal dose as 50–80 mg/l.

The rectified benzine used by Petrini (1941) was lethal to guinea pigs in a dosage of 71–91 mg/l. On the basis of this result, in which no benzene was present in the benzine, it appears that benzine is less lethal than benzene; 2.4–2.8 on the basis of varying concentration, 5–8.8 on the basis of time of action of the same concentrations.

(b) Narcotic dose. – Also estimated as showing less toxicity for benzine, but again varies in the hands of different investigators.

Bamesreiter (1932) gives the following comparative figures for cats:

Solvent	Inactivity	Light narcosis	Heavy narcosis
benzine	40 mg/l	60 mg/l	75 mg/l
benzol	22 mg/l	28 mg/l	50 mg/l

For German benzine, containing paraffins, especially the strongly narcotic hexane, Engelhardt (1931) observed complete narcosis with both benzene and benzine at 50 mg/l, but slightly more rapidly with benzene (12 min as compared with 15).

With rectified benzine, however, Petrini found the time of onset about the same for both, but the primary irritative action slightly more marked with benzine. This irritative effect has also been remarked especially with Russian benzine. Babsky and Leites (1931) observed restlessness, twitching, ataxia and convulsions in dogs inhaling 50–80 mg/l. This increased irritability has been attributed by Schachnowskaya (1935) to a toxic effect of benzine on the central nervous system membrane, increasing its permeability. Single inhalations of 50–70 mg/l were followed by the appearance in the cerebrospinal fluid of sodium ferrocyanide and trypan blue, to which the membrane is normally impermeable.

Bibliography on p. 168

Light benzine causes deep narcosis at 75 mg/l according to Bamesreiter (1932) and light narcosis at 60 mg/l – a much lower figure than that given earlier by Lehmann (1912) for light narcosis (250 mg/l).

Heavy benzine, from Lehmann's results, appears to be slightly more narcotic than light (200 mg/l for light narcosis).

The toxic effect rises with a rise of temperature of the air containing benzine (Lifschitz, 1935). The mortality of mice, with concentration of 50, 55 and 60 mg/l, was doubled as the temperature rose 3–4 deg. C above 17°, and with a further increase of three deg. trebled; above this limit a further rise gave no increase in mortality.

(2) Chronic

As in acute poisoning, the effects of chronic exposure of animals to benzine varies according to the variety used.

SYMPTOMS OF INTOXICATION

(1) Emaciation

Severe loss of weight, has been noted by some observers, notably Schustrow and Letawet (1927), who attributed it to the 'fat solvent' action of benzine. This view has not been confirmed by others, including Lazarew *et al.* (1931), though Briganti and Ambrosio (1941) did find that acute intoxication was accompanied by a loss of weight of about 20%.

(2) Blood and bone marrow

Anaemia has been observed in acute intoxication chiefly by Russian benzine with a high content of cycloparaffins. Reduction in red cells, beginning 2 h after a single acute exposure, and polychromasia, punctate basophilia, normoblasts and reticulocytosis with repeated exposures were noted by Schustrow and Salistowskaya (1926) and Brullowa *et al.* (1930); initial leucocytosis followed by leucopenia and lymphopenia was also a pronounced feature.

With American benzine, also consisting chiefly of cycloparaffins, a similar picture with regard to reduction of red cells, but with a high colour index and leucocytosis without a following leucopenia, was described by Engelhardt (1931). Haemolysis has also been stated to occur by some observers, and has been attributed to the solvent action of benzine on the erythrocytes, decreasing their resistance (Ambrosio, 1941).

Changes of the blood picture show the greatest discrepancy in the hands of various investigators; this is undoubtedly due to the presence or absence of benzene in the benzine used. The chief variation is shown by the leucocytes. In the case of benzine containing chiefly paraffins there is a leucocytosis (Engelhardt, 1931); this variety of benzine appears to cause proliferation rather than destruction of leucocytes. A transitory leucopenia has, however, been recorded following repeated inhalation of rectified benzine (Petrini) which he regards as due not to actual destruction of leucocytes but to their migration into various organs and tissues under the immediate toxic action of benzine.

With Russian benzine, hyperchromic and haemolytic anaemia has been noted (Schustrow and Salistowskaya, 1926; Schachnowskaya, 1935), the latter observed basophilic cells and normoblasts which she attributed to irritation of the bone marrow.

Benzine-benzol mixtures, as would be expected, show the most definite effect of a 'benzene-like' character. Schmidtmann (1930) found the initial leucocytosis followed by severe leucopenia and some anaemia.

A tendency to thrombosis and embolism from such mixtures was recorded by Kuntzen (1932).

(3) Neurological disturbances

Irritation, manifested by convulsions preceding narcosis, appears to be a characteristic feature of acute intoxication by benzine containing cycloparaffins. Lazarew (1929) remarks that it has a delayed action on the spinal cord, so that it is difficult to produce complete narcosis with loss of reflexes. The view of Schachnowskaya (1935) on the possible effect of increased permeability of the central nervous membrane has already been noted (see p. 160).

CHANGES IN THE ORGANISM

Acute hyperaemia, especially of the lungs and spleen (Lewin, 1932) has been regarded as a specific reaction of benzine on the reticulo-endothelial system, while Schwartz (1931), Briganti and Ambrosio (1941) believe that benzine has a selective effect on the walls of blood vessels, causing congestion and focal haemorrhages, and, according to Kolesnikow (1932), degenerative changes in the heart muscle.

Fatty infiltration of the liver and kidneys has also been observed in animals subjected to inhalation of high concentrations (Heitzmann, 1931; Lewin, 1932).

Acquired tolerance to inhalations of concentrations high enough to produce acute benzine poisoning has been postulated by Schustrow and Salistowskaya (1926) and Lazarew et al. (1931), while the latter have also reported a lowered resistance to tubercular and typhoid infection in guinea pigs and white mice.

(1) The lungs

Catarrhal bronchitis, progressing to pneumonia, has been the principal effect with motor-fuel and Russian benzine (Schmidtmann, 1930; Lewin, 1932). No such effect appears to occur with petroleum benzine containing chiefly hexane (Engelhardt, 1931). However, even with rectified benzine, Petrini (1941) found haemorrhagic extravasations in the lungs after inhalation of 39 and 12 mg/l for 6 h daily.

Bibliography on p. 168

(2) The nervous system

With concentrations of 40 mg/l some hours a day for 29 days, Penni and De Stefanis (1940) noted signs of irritation followed by depression of the central nervous system with somnolence and only slight reaction to stimuli, and at 51 mg/l paresis and torpor alternating with tonic-clonic spasms, but rapid recovery on cessation of exposure.

Toxicity to human beings

The effects of either ingestion or inhalation of large amounts of benzine are very similar to those of petrol (*q.v.*). In fact, much of the literature fails to distinguish between them in this respect. For example, Hamilton and Hardy (1949) refer to the sequelae of 'acute gasoline poisoning' described by Floret (1926) but in the same paragraph state that "both were exposed to benzine".

(1) Acute

Many of the cases of acute poisoning described by early observers occurred in children from ingestion. Loewenberg (1932) emphasised the individual predisposition especially in children, as well as in pregnant women, obese persons and alcoholics, in fact the symptoms could often be confused with alcoholic intoxication.

(i) Ingestion. – One of the earliest cases of poisoning in children from ingestion was that described by Falk (1892), a two-year old child who drank a mouthful and died in 10 min. Another fatal case was that of Racine (1901) also in a two-year old child, who drank 10–15 g, became immediately unconscious with cyanosis and convulsions which preceded death 2 h later. The autopsy report recorded death as due to suffocation; the lungs showed only occasional haemorrhage in both upper lobes, but the bronchi were swollen and red, and contained clear red mucus. Most of the organs, including the brain, showed congestion, and there was haemorrhage of the kidneys and of the peripheral cells of the liver; the gastro-intestinal tract showed follicular enteritis, with involvement of the lymphatic system. The blood, dark red and fluid, resembled that of carbon monoxide poisoning.

In a case described by Witthauer (1896), who believed that benzine was more narcotic than petroleum, the child recovered within a few days of regaining consciousness, having been treated by gastric lavage, immersion in a lukewarm bath, and an injection of ether. There had been a rise of temperature but not cough or signs of pneumonia. Witthauer attributed the raised temperature to acute gastritis, but Racine believed it to be due to the effect of benzine on the heat-regulating centre. He stated that slight cases differed from severe in that in the latter there is severe injury of the central nervous system leading to coma; in the former the chief manifestation is gastro-enteritis with only slight transient disturbance of consciousness.

(i) Inhalation. – Acute poisoning by inhalation of high concentrations of benzine is usually found in industrial workers who enter tanks or cylinders which have contained benzine. The unconsciousness so caused may last from 2 h to several days (Loewenberg, 1932). An early account of one such case was that of Foulerton (1886); a man found unconscious in a storage tank containing what Foulerton called "benzoline". On regaining consciousness, he was unable to stand, had muscular twitchings, a cold clammy skin, widely dilated pupils, and slow irregular respiration. He vomited, though he had not swallowed any of the benzine. Under treatment with ammonia and ether he improved after 2 h, though still with severe headache and profuse perspiration, and ultimately recovered completely.

Similar cases of acute intoxication in men entering tanks or cisterns have been reported by Helbling (1950) and others; in many cases the symptoms were headache, 'drunkenness', nausea, abdominal pain and diarrhoea. Loewenberg (1932) quotes the case of a worker repairing a benzine tank who was delirious for 24 h.

Helbling's (1950) case was apparently regarded as one of combined skin, lung and nerve injury. A boy of 16, after inhaling benzine from a reservoir, fell into it and remained for an hour and a half in clothes soaked with benzine. Half his body surface showed epidermolysis; he died three days later. Helbling concluded that the inhaled benzine had had an effect on the bronchiolar epithelium similar to that on the skin, causing an outpouring of lympho-plasma cells which blocked the alveoli; this combined severe toxic effect on skin and lungs was followed by paralysis of the central nervous system and myocardium.

Sequelae of acute poisoning

Most of the sequelae of acute poisoning are related to disorders of the nervous system – headache, giddiness, polyneuritis (Schwarz, 1933) and a peculiar feeling of a 'strange hand' (? neuritis, Zanger, 1933).

In one case Stiefler (1928) reported an epileptic attack 3–4 months after the initial attack.

One of the most detailed and graphic accounts of the aftermath of acute benzine poisoning is that of Dorner (1915). This was a man who fell into a tank and lay for 20 min immersed in benzine. He was completely unconscious for three days, but recovered. Two weeks later he complained of frequent attacks of giddiness, and after three weeks dyspnoea and profuse perspiration. This was followed 7 months later by increasing pain and weakness of the limbs, illegible handwriting and numbness in the right hand. The hands were bluish and cold with slight intention tremor, there was tremor of the eyelids, the left pupil was smaller than the right, and there was slight nystagmus. Perception of cold and heat was reduced in the ankles and feet, and of touch in the hands and feet. Romberg's sign was strongly positive and the Babinski reflex in both feet. The clinical picture was in

Bibliography on p. 168

fact very similar to that of multiple sclerosis but limited to the spinal cord and without cerebral involvement. Dorner considered benzine, especially crude benzine, a severe nerve poison. The blood picture and urine showed no abnormality. Helbling (1950) also mentions gastro-intestinal disturbance, hypochromic anaemia, polyneuritis and loss of weight, occurring some time after suction of a small quantity of benzine from a syphon; this did not at the time cause an obvious acute attack.

Local skin irritation, eczema and severe burns may remain after immersion in liquid benzine (Feil, 1932).

(2) Chronic

(a) *Addiction* to benzine has been observed, sometimes in chronic alcoholics as a substitute for alcohol, sometimes merely to produce the feeling of intoxication. Rosenthal (cited by Witthauer, 1896) recorded a case of the former in a man of 48, who suffered from insomnia, hallucinations, loss of appetite and tremor, while Peters (1900) described the addiction of a 14 year old child, who had for some years inhaled benzine used by his mother, a cleaner of gloves; this habit eventually resulted in amblyopia from retrobulbar neuritis.

The case described by Schwarz (1933) was not, strictly speaking, one of addiction, but small amounts of benzine had been ingested twice a day for five or six weeks by a man aged 28, in the belief that it was a cure for gonorrhoea. He developed such weakness of his arms and legs that he was unable to walk or stand unsupported. There was some atrophy of the muscles, and severe polyneuritis was diagnosed. Seven months later there was considerable improvement, only slight weakness of the leg muscles remaining.

(b) *Industrial exposure.* – Most of the cases of chronic industrial benzine poisoning have arisen in connection with the dry cleaning industry, especially the cleaning of gloves, but they are not numerous and the hazard should be fairly readily controllable by adequate ventilation.

SYMPTOMS OF INTOXICATION

(1) The skin

The possible carcinogenic effect attributed to some petroleum derivatives is not believed to be a property of benzine. Its most frequent effect is that of dermatitis with the features characteristic of other petroleum derivatives (see p. 145) *i.e.* dryness, irritative erythema, abrasions, fissures, and pustular lesions.

According to Farris and Sicca (1954) these are produced by the action of benzine on the sebaceous glands, but they describe some much more severe cases. In one of these, bullous lesions of the forearms and wrists and deep pigmentation of the face, neck and upper part of the thorax, resembling a pellagroid condition were present and patch tests indicated acute sensitivity to solar radiation.

A rare condition, similar to Schamberg's disease, has been attributed, at least in part, to chronic benzine exposure in two cases in Italy.

Schamberg's disease (progressive pigmentary dermatosis) is, even in idiopathic cases, a relatively rare affection and is confined almost exclusively to adult males. The lesions consist of numerous red, brown and, later, yellow spots, chiefly on the lower limbs; these may become confluent but may ultimately undergo slow spontaneous cure.

Of the two industrial cases associated with exposure to benzine, one was a woman employed for several months in the manufacture of rubber shoes (Quarelli and Midana, 1935). About a month before the appearance of the skin lesions she had complained of headache, giddiness, weakness and eye irritation. There were no eczematous lesions and the Schamberg-like dermatosis disappeared some months after cessation of exposure. The second case (Capellini and Parmeggiani, 1948) was a man, employed eleven years in the manufacture of gum boots. The skin lesions appeared at the end of ten years and extended slowly and with remissions, but finally became progressive and persistent with features typical of Schamberg's disease, over the whole surface of both lower limbs and slightly on the forearms.

(2) Blood and bone marrow

Slight anaemia, neutropenia and relative leucocytosis were noted by Frumina and Fainstein (1934), and similar slight haematological disturbance was observed by Aiello and Adrower (1955) in workers employed in the manufacture of rubber boots, but the erythropenia and slight leucopenia were attributed mainly to the small (not estimated) content of benzene in the benzine. Looft (1930) had also noted leucopenia, relative lymphocytosis and prolonged bleeding and coagulation time in two workers employed one year in a dry-cleaning establishment.

(3) Urine

In the case described by Capellini and Parmeggiani (1948) the urine was normal and the blood picture showed only slight hyperchromic anaemia, and there were no subjective or objective signs of chronic benzine poisoning either in this man or his fellow-workers. On the basis of the partial remission of the skin lesions during less intense work or complete suspension, and renewal with increased exposure, Capellini and Parmeggiani, while not attributing the skin affection entirely to benzine, consider that it was a contributory factor.

(4) Gastro-intestinal disturbances

Listed as a symptom of chronic benzine poisoning by most of the observers mentioned above.

(5) Neurological disturbances

Symptoms of chronic poisoning are especially focussed on the nervous system, are often purely subjective, and could easily be mistaken for those of chronic

Bibliography on p. 168

alcoholism – headache, nausea, giddiness, drowsiness, apathy, forgetfulness, euphoria, muscular tremors and weakness, loss of smell, and functional neuroses.

Symptoms of this kind were observed by Vigdortschik (1933) and Frumina and Fainstein (1934) in employees in a rubber factory, where the atmospheric concentrations of benzine were only 0.5–2 mg/l.

Chambovet (1922) had earlier noted signs of mild chronic intoxication in 6 women engaged in filling lamps with benzine – dyspnoea, rapid fatigue and a tendency to haemorrhage of the gums and uterus.

BIBLIOGRAPHY

Aiadin, R. (1958) Petrol Vapour Poisoning, *Brit. Med., J.* 2:369.
Aiello, G. and G. Adrower (1955) Benzol-benzinismo cronico, *Rass. Med. Ind.*, 24:384.
Ainsworth, R. W. (1960) Petrol Vapour Poisoning, *Brit. Med. J.*, 1:1547.
Ambrosio, L. (1941) La Resistenza globulare nell'intossicazione acuta e cronica da Benzina, *Folia Med. (Naples)*, 27:537.
Amorati, A., C. Cacciari and F. M. Troisi (1952) Research on chronic Effect from long Exposure to vapours of pure Gasoline, *Ind. Med. Surg.*, 21:466.
Askey, J. M. (1928) Aplastic Anaemia due to Benzol Poisoning, *Calif. West. Med.*, 29:262.
Babsky, E. and R. Leites (1931) Über die Bildung eines bedingten Reflexes bei Benzinvergiftung, *Arch. Exptl. Pathol. Pharmakol.*, 161:1.
Baldi, G. and R. Ricciardi-Pollini (1954) Patologia professionale da etere di petroli e da Benzina, *Rass. Med. Ind.*, 23:340.
Bamesreiter, O. (1932) Neue Versuche über die quantitative Giftigkeit von Benzol- und Benzindämpfen, *Arch. Hyg. Backteriol.*, 108:129.
Batchelor, J. J. (1927) Relative Toxicity of Benzol and its higher Homologues. Committee on Benzol of the National Safety Council, *Am. J. Hyg.*, 7:276.
Bowditch, M., C. K. Drinker, P. Drinker, H. H. Haggard and A. Hamilton (1940) Code for safe Concentrations of certain Common toxic Substances used in Industry, *J. Ind. Hyg.*, 22:251.
Briganti A. and L. Ambrosio (1941) Modificazioni anatomo-isopatologiche nelle intossicazione sperimentale da Benzina, *Rass. Med. Ind.*, 11:577.
Brullowa, L. F., A. D. Brussilowskaya, N. W. Lazarew *et al.* (1930) Das Blut bei der expirenmentellen Benzinvergiftung, *Arch. Hyg. Backteriol.*, 104:226.
Capellini, A. and L. Parmeggiani (1948) Su di un Caso di Dermatosi di Schamberg in un Operaio esposti a Vapori di Benzina, *Med. Lavoro*, 39:245.
Castagnou, M. R. (1960) Aperçu sur la Chémie du Pétrole, *Arch. Malad. Profess.*, 21:245.
Chambovet, L. (1922) Les petits Signes du Benzinisme. *J. Med. (Lyon)*, 69.
Chief Inspector of Factories and Workshops. Annual Reports (1944, 1945) H.M. Stationary Office, London.
Clinger, O. W. and N. A. Johnson (1951) Purposeful Inhalation of Gasoline Vapours, *Psychiatr. Quart.*, 25:557.
Conrads, H. (1896) Zur Casuistik der Petroleumvergiftungen bei Kindern, *Berl. Klin. Wochschr.*, 33:982.
Coste, F. and G. Wolz (1935) Deux Cas d'Intoxication par l'Essence, *Ann. Med. Leg.*, 15:909.
Davis, A., L. J. Schafer and Z. G. Bell (1960) The Effects on Human Volunteers of Exposure to Air containing Gasoline Vapours, *Arch. Environ. Health*, 1:548.
Des Essarts, J. Q. (1932) Notes sur quelques Cas d'Intoxication due a l'Emploi de Préparations dites Bitume-Mastic, *Arch. Méd. Pharm. Nav.*, 122:235.
Dorner, G. (1915) Akute Benzinvergiftung mit nachfolgender spinaler Erkrankung, *Deut. Z. Nervanheilk.*, 54:66.

Drinker, P., C. P. Yaglou and M. F. Warren (1943) The Threshold Toxicity of Gasoline Vapour, *J. Ind. Hyg.*, 25:225.

Dubois, R., (1885) Note sur la Vaseline, *Gaz. Hôp. (Paris)*, 58:1067.

Dunn, J. E. and F. S. Brackett (1948) Photosensitising Properties of some Petroleum Solvents, *Ind. Med. Surg.*, 17:303.

Durrans, T. H. (1950) Solvents, 6th Ed., Chapman and Hall, London.

Edwards, R. V. (1960) A Case Report of Gasoline Sniffing, *Am. J. Psychiatr.*, 117:555.

Elkins, H. B., (1959) The Chemistry of Industrial Toxicology, John Wiley and Sons, New York.

Elkins, H. B. and L. D. Pagnotto (1956) Benzene Content of Petroleum Solvents, *Arch. Ind. Health*, 13:51.

Engelhardt, W. (1931) Vergleichende Tierversuche über die Blutwirkung von Benzin und Benzol, *Arch. Gewerbepathol. Gewerbehyg.*, 2:479.

Fabre, R. (1960) Sur les Propriétés toxicologiques des Constituants des Pétroles, *Arch. Malad. Profess.*, 21:97.

Fairhall, L. T. (1957) Industrial Toxicology, Williams and Wilkins, Baltimore.

Falk, F. (1892) Tödliche Benzinvergiftung. *Vjschr. Gerichtl. Med.*, 3:399

Farris, G. and G. Sicca (1954) Dermatosi negli Operai dell' Industria dal Petrolio, *Rass. Med. Ind.*, 23:340.

Faucett, R. L. and R. A. Jensen (1952) Addiction to Inhalation of Gasoline Fumes in Child, *J. Pediatr.*, 41:364.

Feil, A. (1932) Les Intoxications professionelles par la Benzine et le Benzol, *Presse Méd.*, 40:1973.

Fieldner, A. C., S. H. Katz and S. P. Kinney (1921) Permeation of Oxygen Breathing Apparatus by Gases and Vapours, *U.S. Bureau of Mines. Technical Paper* 272.

Fieser, F., T. W. Green, F. F. Bischoff, G. Lopez and J. J. Rupp (1955) A carcinogenic Oxidation Product of Cholesterol, *J. Am. Chem. Soc.*, 77:3928.

Fischer, H. G. M., W. Priestley, L. T. Eby et al. (1951) Properties of high-boiling Petroleum Products, *Arch. Ind. Hyg.*, 4:315.

Floret, F. (1926) Neue Beobachtungen über gewerbliche Schädigungen durch Kohlenwasserstoffe, *Zentr. Gewerbehyg.*, 13:7.

Foulerton, A. G. R. (1886) Poisoning by Benzoline Vapour, *Lancet*, 2:865.

Friedeberg (1902) Intoxication by Petroleum, *Zentr. Inn. Med.*, 33:1042.

Frumina, L. M. and S. S. Fainstein (1934) Zur Benzintoxikologie, *Zentr. Gewerbehyg.*, 11:161.

Gardner, H. A. (1925) Physiological Effects of Vapours from a few Solvents used in Paints, Varnishes and Lacquers, *Paint Mfrs. Assoc. U.S Techn. Circ.*, 250

Gerarde, H. W. (1960) Toxicology and Biochemistry of Aromatic Hydrocarbons, Elsevier, Amsterdam.

Goodman, S. and A. Gilman (1955) Gasoline, the Pharmacological Basis of Therapeutics, 5th ed., Macmillan, New York.

Haggard, H. W. (1920) The anesthetic and convulsant Effects of Gasoline Vapour, *J. Pharmacol.*, 16:401.

Hamilton, A. and H. L. Hardy (1949) Industrial Toxicology, 2nd ed., p.324, Paul B. Hoeber Inc.

Hayhurst, E. R. (1936) Poisoning by Petroleum Distillates, *Ind. Med. Surg.*, 5:53.

Heitzmann, O. (1931) Vergleichende pathologische Anatomie der experimentellen Benzol- und Benzinvergiftung, *Arch. Gewerbepath. Gewerbehyg.*, 2:515.

Helbling, V. (1950) Über ein Fall von akuter tödlicher perkutaner und Inhalationsvergiftung mit Benzin, *Z. Unfallmed. Berufskrankh.*, 43:218.

Hicquet, G. (1930) Un Cas de Surdité nerveuse; toxi-névrite due au White Spirit. *J. Neurol. Psychiatr.*, 30:89.

Holstein, E. (1958) Grundriss der Arbeitsmedizin. 3rd ed. p.237, Johann Ambrosius Barth, Leipzig.

Industrial Paints Committee, (1920) Report of Departmental Committee appointed to examine danger of lead paints to workers, H.M. Stationary Office, 1923.

Jaffe, R. (1911) Über Benzinvergiftung nach Sektionsergebnisse und Tierversuche, *Münch. Med. Wochschr.*, 40:1220.

Johannssen, A. (1896) Ein Fall von tödlich verlaufende Petroleumvergiftung bei einem zweijährigen Mädchen. *Berlin. Klin. Wochschr.*, 317 and 349.

Kehoe, R. A. (1953) Aviation Toxicology, Blakiston, New York.

Klauder, J. V. and F. A. Brill (1947) Correlation of Boiling Ranges of some Petroleum Solvents with irritant Action on Skin, *Arch. Dermatol. Syphilis*, 56: 197.

Kolesnikow (1932) cited by I. E. Lewin (1932).

Kotin, P. and H. L. Falk (1956) Mouse Lung Tumours from ozonized Gasoline, *Cancer*, 9:910.

Kuntzen, H. (1932) Die Haufung der Thrombosen und Embolien und chronische Vergiftungen mit Autoabgäsen, *Ärtzl. Fortbild.*, 29: 663.

Lawton, J. J. and C. P. Malinquist (1961) Gasoline Addiction in Children, *Psychiatr. Quart.*, 35:555.

Lazarew, N. W. (1929) Zur Toxikologie des Benzins, *Arch. Hyg. Bakteriol.*, 102: 227.

Lazarew, N. W., L. P. Brullova, S. N. Kremnewa, L. T. Larionow, M. D. Lubimova and D. J. Stalskaya (1931) Experimentelle Untersuchungen über die Gewöhnung von Benzin, *Arch. Exptl. Pathol. Pharmakol.*, 159: 345.

Lazarew, N. W., A. J. Brussilowskaya, J. N. Lawrow and F. P. Lifschutz (1931) Über die Durchlässigkeit der Haut für Benzin und Benzol, *Arch. Hyg. Bakteriol.*, 106: 112.

Legludic, H. and C. Turlais (1914) Recherches sur la Toxicité du Pétrole et quelques unes de ses Actions physiologiques, *Ann. Hyg. Publ. Méd. Légale*, 21: 385.

Lehmann, K. B. (1912) Experimentelle Studien über den Einfluss technisch und hygienisch wichtiger Gäse und Dämpfe auf den Organismus. Die Kohlenwasserstoffe. Benzol, Toluol, Xylol, Leichtbenzin und Schwerbenzin, *Arch. Hyg. Bakteriol.*, 75: 1.

Lessar, A. (1898) Tödliche Glottisoedem durch Ingestion von Petroleum, *Vjschr. Gerichtl. Med.*, 16: 91.

Lestchinskaya, O. (1933) Zur relativer Giftigkeit verschiedener Benzine, *Arch. Gewerbepathol. Gewerbehyg.*, 4: 508.

Lewin, L. (1888) Über allgemeine- und Hautvergiftung durch Petroleum, *Virchow's Arch. Pathol. Anat. Physiol.*, 112: 35.

Lewin, I. E. (1932) Zur Frage der pathologischen Veränderungen und der Funktionsfähigkeit des Reticuloendothelsystems bei Vergiftung mit Benzindämpfen, *Arch. Gewerbepathol. Gewerbehyg.*, 3: 340.

Lifschitz, I. I. (1935) De l'Influence des Conditions de Température sur la Toxicité de la Benzine, *Méd. Trav.*, 7: 41.

Loewenberg, R. D. (1932) Die praktische Bedeutung des Benzins, Benzols, und ihrer Verbrennungsprodukte (Auspuffgäse) in Industrie, Gewerbe und Verkehr, *Fortsch. Med.*, 50: 394.

Looft, A. (1930) Blood Changes in Benzine Poisoning, *Med. Rev. (Bergen)*, 47: 1.

Machle, W. (1941) Gasoline Intoxication, *J. Am. Med. Assoc.*, 117: 1965.

Matshushita, K. (1935) Pathologische-histologische Studien über das Zentralnervensystem bei experimenteller Petroleumvergiftung, Abstr. in *Zentr. Gewerbehyg.*, 22: 190.

Mir, C. (1941) Melanosis de Riehl con hipersensibilidad cutanea a la Gasolina, *Actas Dermo-Sifiliog.*, 32: 821.

Nelson, F. C. and G. W. Fiero (1954) A selected aromatic Fraction naturally occurring in Petroleum as a Pesticide Solvent, *J. Agr. Food Chem.*, 2: 735.

Nunn, J. A. and F. M. Martin (1934) Gasolin (Petroläther)- und Kerosin (Petroleum)- Vergiftungen bei Kindern, *Samml. Vergiftungsf.*, 5: 183. A459.

Oldham, W. (1961) Deliberate Intoxication with Petrol Vapour, *Brit. Med. J.*, 2: 1687.

Patty, F. A. (1949) Industrial Hygiene and Toxicology, vol. 2, p.741, *Interscience*, New York.

Penni, G. and C. de Stefanis (1940) Ricerche sull'Intossicazione cronica de Vapori di Benzina, *Rass. Med. Lav. Indust.*, 11: 516.

Peters, (1900) Retrobulbar Neuritis from chronic Benzine Poisoning, *Deut. Med. Wochschr. (Suppl.)*, 26: 249.

Petrini, M. (1941) Intossicazione acuta e subacuta da Benzina e da Benzolo, *Rass. Med. Ind.*, 12: 453.

Poincaré, L. (1885) Recherches expérimentales sur les Effets d'un Air chargé de Vapeur de Pétrole, *Ann. Hyg. Publ. Méd. Légale*, 13: 312.

Pruitt, N. (1959) Bizarre Intoxications, *J. Am. Med. Assoc.*, 171: 2355.

Quarelli, G. and A. Midana (1935) Morbo di Schamberg in un caso di Intossicazione professionale, *Rass. Med. Ind.*, 6: 23.

Racine, (1901) Über den Tod durch Benzinvergiftung, *Vjschr. Gerichtl. Med.*, 22: 63.

Salamone, L. (1961) Haemopoietic Activity in Poisoning by Petrol Vapours, *Boll. Soc. Ital. Biol. Sper.*, 37:1190.

Saverin (1940) Tödlicher Unfall beim Streichen eines Wasserbehalters, *Reichsarbeitsblatt.* 20:224. Abstr. in *Zentr. Gewerbehyg.*, 28 (1941) 29.

Schachnowskaya, S. B. (1935) Über die Durchlässigkeit der Blutliquorschränke und Blutveränderungen bei experimenteller Benzinvergiftung, *Arch. Gewerbepathol. Gewerbehyg.*, 6:144.

Schmidtmann, M. (1930) Experimentelle Untersuchungen über die Wirkung von Einatmung kleiner Benzin- und Benzolmengen, *Klin. Wochschr.*, 9:2106.

Schustrow, N. and K. Letawet (1927) Die Bedeutung der Fettsubstanzen bei der Benzinintoxikation, *Deut. Arch. Klin. Med.*, 154:180.

Schustrow, N. and Salistowskaya (1926) Die Benzinangewöhnung, *Deut. Arch. Klin. Med.*, 150:277.

Schwartz, S. M. (1931) Über den Einfluss der akuten und chronischen Benzinvergiftungen auf der Tierversuche, *Fortsch. Med.*, 49:215.

Schwarz, H. G. (1932) Über chronischen Benzinvergiftungen auf der Tierversuche, *Fortsch. Med.* 49:215.

Schwarz, H. G. (1933) Bezin-vergiftung; chronische, medizinale, *Samml. Vergiftungsf.*, 4:247.

Schwarz, L., L. Tulipan and S. M. Peck (1947) Occupational Diseases of the Skin, Kimpton, London.

Simonin, C. (1934) Considérations toxicologiques et médico-légales sur le Benzolisme et le Pétrolisme professionels, *Paris Méd.*, 2:408.

Simonin, C. and E. Marcouse (1960) Accidental Submersion in crude Petroleum, *Ann. Hyg. Publ. Méd. Légale*, 40:55.

Siwe, S. A. (1932) Symptomen bei akuter Vergiftung mit flüssigen Kohlenwasserstoffe, *Monatschr. Kinderheilk.*, 55:146.

Smyth, H. F. and H. F. Smyth Jr. (1928) Inhalation Experiments with certain Lacquer Solvents, *J. Ind. Hyg.*, 10:261.

Soprana, C. (1941) Avvenalamente da Petrolia per Cure empiriche de guaritore, Atti Ist. Med. Leg. Univ. Padova.

Spencer, O. M. (1922) The Effect of Gasoline Fumes on Dispensary Attendance and Output in a Group of Workers, *U.S. Treas. Publ. Health Rept.*, 37:2291.

Sterner, J. H. (1941) Study of Hazards in Spray painting with Gasoline as Diluent, *J. Ind. Hyg.*, 23:437.

Stewart, I. (1960) Petrol Vapour Poisoning, *Brit. Med. J.*, 1:1739.

Stiefler, G. (1928) Epilepsie nach Benzinvergiftung, *Wien. Med. Wochschr.*, 78:938.

Threshold Limit Values for 1962 (Amer. Conf. of Governm. Ind. Hygienists), *Am. Ind. Hyg. Assoc. J.*, 23:419.

Vigdortschik, A. (1933) Zur Frage der chronischen Benzinwirkung auf den Organismus, *Zentr. Gewerbehyg.*, 10:219.

Von Oettingen, W. F. (1940) Toxicity and potential Dangers of Aliphatic and Aromatic Hydrocarbons, *U.S. Publ. Health Serv. Bull.*, 255.

Wang, C. C. and G. V. Irons (1961) Acute Gasoline Intoxication, *Arch. Environ. Health*, 2:714.

Witthauer (1896) Ein Fall der Benzinvergiftung, *Münch. Med. Wochschr.*, 43:915.

Zangger, H. (1927) Vergiftungen durch wenigflüchtige flüssige Kohlenwasserstoffe, Handb. Inn. Bergmann-Sachelm, 2nd ed., v.4:1649, Springer, Berlin.

Zangger, A. (1933) Arbeitsunfälle und Arbeitsgefährdung bei den Arbeit in Innern von geschlossenen Behältern, *Arch. Gewerbepathol. Gewerbehyg.*, 4:117.

Chapter 5

HALOGENATED HYDROCARBONS

The halogenated hydrocarbons comprise a large group of compounds which, as solvents, have an almost universal application in industry. One such potent solvent, carbon tetrachloride, has also obtained considerable recognition as a fire extinguisher; others, such as trichloroethylene, perchloroethylene and dichloroethane are specially valuable as cleaners and degreasers, and still others as constituents of paints, varnishes and paint removers. The toxic properties of the individual compounds differ considerably, particularly with regard to their effect on the liver and kidneys, but common to all is their narcotic action.

Many of them are highly volatile and are eliminated to a large extent unchanged, undergoing relatively little metabolic change in the body, but may react with specific enzymes in the liver and kidney, with the result that the functions on which perfect enzymatic organisation depends become completely disorganised.

The actual reaction of work people to each individual solvent may differ considerably, and the Maximum Acceptable Concentration, as defined by the American Conferences of Governmental Industrial Hygienists, represents only the average conditions in which the average worker can be exposed daily to any halogenated hydrocarbon without suffering any injury. It is very necessary to realise that peak concentrations of short duration, with levels much higher than those recommended, may occur, and that these levels may carry the hazard of acute, even fatal, poisoning.

18. Tetrachloromethane

Synonym: carbontetrachloride

Structural formula:

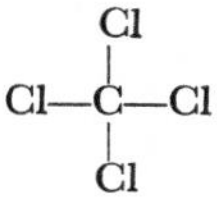

$$Cl-\underset{\underset{Cl}{|}}{\overset{\overset{Cl}{|}}{C}}-Cl$$

Molecular formula: CCl_4

Properties: A clear colourless liquid of heavy density with an odour somewhat resembling that of chloroform.

> *boiling point:* 76.8 °C
> *freezing point:* solidifies at -22.6 °C
> *vapour pressure:* 91 mm Hg at 20 °C; 143 mm Hg at 30 °C; increasing $\pm$ 100 mm Hg for every 10 deg. rise until boiling point (Fairhall, 1957)
> *vapour density (air = 1):* 1.5 for 'saturated air' (Patty, 1949).
> *specific gravity (liquid density):* 1.595
> *flash point:* non-inflammable
> *conversion factors:* 1 p.p.m. = 6.29 mg/m³ at 25 °C
> 1 mg/l = 159 p.p.m.
> *solubility:* slightly in water, readily in chloroform, alcohol, ether, and benzene
> *maximum allowable concentration:* 10 p.p.m. (Threshold Limit Values, 1962)

ECONOMY, SOURCES AND USES

Production

(1) By chlorination of methane.
(2) By direct chlorination of CS_2 or direct with sulphur chloride.

Liberation of phosgene

CCl_4 is decomposed to a certain extent by contact with an open flame or a hot surface with liberation of phosgene ($COCl_2$). Such liberation has been observed particularly in connection with the use of CCl_4 as a fire extinguisher, Fieldner *et al.* (1921) found that the gas produced from fire extinguishers in experimental conditions consisted of 15–80 p.p.m. of phosgene, 2000–5840 of CCl_4 and 60–236 of HCl, while Biesalski (1924) found that the greatest yield of phosgene came from CCl_4 at 250 °C in the presence of ferrous chloride. Comstock and Oberst (1952) stated that in the presence of a gasoline flash fire or prolonged gasoline fire original concentrations of 41 and 18 mg/l of CCl_4 can give rise to 0.4 and 0.0004 mg/l of phosgene respectively. The approximate lethal dose for rats of inhaling unde-composed CCl_4 is given by Fawcett (1952) as 29,000 p.p.m. as compared with 300 p.p.m. when it is decomposed at 800 °C.

It should be noted however, that Smyth and Smyth (1936), testing the phos-gene content of the air in a kitchen where home dry-cleaning was being done with a gas stove pilot light on, found no phosgene with CCl_4 concentrations up to 5000 p.p.m. and relative humidity of 70%. In order to lessen the risk of phosgene for-mation with the use of fire extinguishers Boye (1935) suggested that the CCl_4 should be used in combination with solid carbon dioxide or stabilised aqueous emulsions of CCl_4.

Presence of CS_2

In 1909, when a fatal case of CCl_4 poisoning from the use of a hair shampoo was reported, Veley found that the CCl_4 contained 1.5% of CS_2. This is apparently not the case with modern methods of production. Möller (1933) remarked that though even at the beginning of this century commercial CCl_4 contained more than 0.5% of CS_2, modern methods of production had reduced this contamination to a level unlikely to produce symptoms of CS_2 poisoning.

Industrial uses

(1) As a dry cleaner, on account of its rapid vaporisation, high degreasing ability and non-inflammability, also as a spotting agent especially for furs (Elkins, 1959). For these purposes it now tends to be replaced by the less toxic tetrachloroethylene (Hardin, 1954).

(2) As a fire extinguisher. Sometimes chloroform (freezing point − 70 °C) is added to the CCl_4 in order to depress its freezing point (Cameron, 1947). The resultant mixture, according to Fawcett (1952) may be even more hazardous to life than CCl_4 alone.

(3) As a fumigant for grain (Rager, 1945; Chiesura and Picotti, 1960). Chiesura and Picotti state that the most widely used parasiticide for plants and agricultural products in Italy is 'Granosan', of which 30% is CCl_4 and 70% dichloroethane, and that CCl_4 is the more active agent from the toxicological point of view.

(4) In the manufacture of the refrigerant Freon 12, and of D.D.T.

(5) In the extraction of oils and fats from plant and animal substances.

(6) As a degreaser of machine parts and electrical equipment.

(7) As a solvent in the rubber and paint industries.

(8) As a constituent of soap solutions in the textile industry.

(9) In the quartz crystal industry (Kazantzis and Bomford, 1960).

BIOCHEMISTRY

Estimation

(1) *In the atmosphere*

A method claimed to be free from the disadvantages of being cumbersome and time consuming, while maintaining accuracy together with simplicity and sensitivity is described by Elkins (1959). It is based on adsorption on silica-gel, followed by hydrolysis of the CCl_4 in isopropyl alcohol. Addition of pellets of KOH to 10 ml of the liquid is followed by that of one drop of phenolphthalein and 6 N acetic acid until the solution is just acid. After addition of 6 drops of 10% potassium chromate the solution is titrated with 0.1 N silver nitrate in yellow light. About 85% of the chlorine in the CCl_4 is recovered as inorganic chloride and the addition of 0.3 ml of silver nitrate corresponds to less than 2 p.p.m. in a 25-l air sample. Further details of the silica-gel method are given by Cralley *et al.* (1943), Pernell (1944) and Fahy (1948).

(2) *In blood and tissues*

A method of estimating by infra-red analysis the amount of CCl_4 in blood has been described by Stewart *et al.* (1960), based on infra-red spectrophotometry, CS_2 being used as the extracting solvent. A tracer method (^{14}C-labelled CCl_4) was also used in the preparation of the blood standard, since, CCl_4 being insoluble in blood, even distribution throughout the sample was difficult to ensure. The blood was obtained by cardiac puncture from rabbits exposed to 5000 and 2500 p.p.m. for 4 h. With 5000 p.p.m. the blood concentration at the end of this time was almost directly proportional to the vapour concentration at these two levels.

Metabolism

(1) *Absorption and excretion*

CCl_4 is metabolised in the body to only a slight extent (McCollister *et al.*, 1951). It is readily absorbed by the lungs and also by the intestinal tract (Robbins, 1929; Wells, 1925). Robbins found that the rate of absorption differed with the species, but when injected into the small intestine it appears in the expired air after a very few minutes, reaches a maximum concentration in approximately one hour, and then continues to be excreted at a slow rate for a considerable time. Using radioactive $^{14}CCl_4$, McCollister *et al.* (1951) found that monkeys inhaling 0.29 mg/l (46 p.p.m.) for various periods of time absorbed about 30%, half of this amount being exhaled unchanged within 1800 h after the end of the exposure. Radioactive carbon was present in the urea and carbonate of the urine and in the CO_2 of the expired air. About 95% of the radioactivity of the urine was in the form of an unidentified metabolite. When fed to rabbits at the level of 1 ml/kg Deichmann and Thomas (1943) found no detectable rise of glucuronide in the urine. According to Williams (1959) mice in which liver injury has been produced excrete as much as 26% through the lungs.

When given with fat, the concentration in the expired air increases decidedly, according to Robbins (1929) owing to the fact that the CCl_4 is carried into the general circulation with the fat up the thoracic duct and not passing through the liver, where it is usually retained. Alcohol also slightly increases the rate of absorption of CCl_4 (Wells, 1925) but the known effect of alcohol in increasing the toxicity of CCl_4 (see p. 178) was not believed by Robbins to be due to this increase in rate of absorption.

Excretion of ingested or injected CCl_4 is almost entirely by the lungs; none was found in the urine.

(2) Distribution in tissues

The highest concentration was found by Robbins in the bone marrow; in the liver, pancreas and brain it was about one fifth of this. McCollister *et al.* (1951) found that the highest concentration of radioactive CCl_4 was deposited in the fat.

Effect on the serum enzymes. – It has been shown that CCl_4 can increase the level of some serum enzymes and decrease that of others. In rats, according to Bell and Kay (1956) exposure to CCl_4 vapour decreases the serum esterase activity, while subcutaneous injection increases serum xanthine oxidase (Alfonso *et al.*, 1955; Block and Cornish, 1958).

Increase of the enzyme known as serum glutamic oxalacetic transaminase (SGOT) is however the most valuable indication of slight damage to liver cells not demonstrable by the usual tests for liver function; it is invariably present in severe liver damage. In a case described by Fry *et al.* (1959) the level rose from 58 units 3 h after exposure, to 900 two days later, falling to 580 the following day and to 44 a fortnight later. A study of the course of the SGOT during hepatic damage in a case of acute CCl_4 intoxication following accidental ingestion was recently made by Dawborn *et al.* (1961). On the third day after swallowing a mouthful of CCl_4 the SGOT level was 2120 units. This was associated, as shown by liver biopsy, with necrosis of one third to one half of every liver lobule in the sample. Two days later following treatment, which included choline hydrochloride and Benadryl, the SGOT level fell promptly to 520 units and continued to fall. Liver biopsy showed that this was accompanied by liver cell regeneration. It was suggested that the administration of choline and antihistamines might have contributed to the fall of SGOT by lessening the release of enzymes from the liver cell. Transaminases are widely present in animal tissues and in blood; they catalyse an amino-acid reaction, and when cells rich in these enzymes are injured increased quantities are released into the blood. This is especially the case with hepatic toxic agents such as CCl_4, and alteration of the serum transaminase level is therefore regarded by many observers as an index of the integrity or otherwise of the liver cells, especially with regard to injury by CCl_4. A single exposure of rats to a concentration of 250 p.p.m. raised the level to 103% of normal within 24 h (Wroblenski and La Due, 1955). An extremely careful and complex investigation by Beaufay *et al.* (1959) has revealed the interesting fact that the SGOT alterations may be present by as much as several hours before the typical microscopical appearance of liver necrosis can be detected. These enzymes are believed to be segregated in a group of particles in the cytoplasm which have been called "lysosomes", which can be distinguished from mitochondria. When their membrane, which is probably of a lipoprotein nature, is injured, they not only release these soluble hydrolytic enzymes but also allow the external substrates to penetrate into them.

The existence of two SGOT's has been established in animals but not with certainty in normal human serum (Fleisher *et al.*, 1960, 1961).

Estimation of SGOT. – A relatively simple method of spectrophotometric estimation of SGOT was described by Steinberg *et al.* in 1956. The principle of the reaction depends on the ability of the transaminase to catalyse the transfer of an amino group from aspartic acid to α-keto-glutamic acid. A phosphate buffer is mixed with the serum, and after 30 min, during which a certain amount of DPNH (reduced diphosphopyridine nucleotide) is oxidised, 0.2 ml of α-ketoglutarate and aspartic acid is added. The optical density of the assay tube is read at intervals from 2–15 min, and from the rate of change at 340 mμ the SGOT concentration is directly calculated, the rate of disappearance of DPNH being directly proportional to this, its curve of disappearance being strictly linear.

(3) Role of the sympathetic nervous system

A recent investigation by Calvert and Brody (1960) suggests that a predominant factor in the hepatoxicity of CCl_4 is an anoxia produced through the mediation of the sympathetic nervous system. This concept postulates that CCl_4 produces a long lasting effect on the sympathetic areas of the central nervous system, causing a constriction of the intra-hepatic blood vessels, with a decrease in flow which causes an anoxia beginning in the areas near the central vein, and resulting in centrilobular necrosis and later fatty infiltration of the parenchyma.

Release of epinephrine from the adrenal medulla under sympathetic stimulation is also suggested as a factor in the mechanism of fatty infiltration, but with this view not all authorities are in complete agreement.

TOXICOLOGY

In addition to its narcotic action in high concentrations, CCl_4 has a specific toxic effect on the liver and/or kidneys, usually delayed for some hours or even days after exposure. It has been widely believed that inhalation exposure is more closely associated with kidney damage and ingestion with liver injury, but in one recent case at least (Fry *et al.*, 1959) this view was not confirmed, inhalation being followed by severe liver injury with no effect on the kidneys. These toxic effects are increased by ingestion of alcohol. Chronic exposure is most frequently associated with disturbance of gastro-intestinal function. Injury to the blood-forming organs has rarely been observed. In three cases of aplastic anaemia described (Straus, 1954), the aetiology was doubtful.

Toxicity to animals

The effects of CCl_4 poisoning in animals differ from those in human beings chiefly in the fact that in animals damage to the liver is more prominent than to the kidneys (Clinton, 1947).

(1) Acute

   (a) Lethal dose. – The immediate lethal effects of inhalation depend to some extent on the size of the experimental animal. Mice, for example, were found by Lazarew (1929) to succumb to exposure to 65–70 mg/l (10,400–11,000 p.p.m.) while according to Reuss (1931) cats recovered from deep narcosis after inhalation for 70 min of 92.6 mg/l. Immediate death was due to respiratory paralysis but with some larger animals death was sometimes delayed for some days (Davies, 1934).

   (b) Narcotic dose, also differs with the species of animal and the length of exposure, the levels given by different observers varying from 6350–7500 p.p.m. for 2 h for mice (Lazarew, 1929), 14,300 p.p.m. for 4 h for cats (Lehmann 1911) and 21,000 p.p.m. for 9–13 min for dogs (Lamson *et al.*, 1924).

(2) Chronic or subacute

   The effects of repeated administration of CCl_4 to animals have been directed especially to the question of regeneration of the liver from the injury produced and to that of the ultimate production of cirrhosis.

   In the experiments of Cameron and Karunaratne (1936), the chronic effects were examined by means of subcutaneous injection of single doses of 0.5–0.1 ml and repeated doses (twice weekly) of 0.1, 0.25 and 0.0037 ml (the last just on the borderline of toxicity to the liver of rats). After a single dose of 0.1 ml there was so sign in the liver other than diffuse congestion until between the 5th and 24th hour, when hydropic and fatty degeneration appeared. With repeated dosage (3 injections of 0.25 ml) some rats showed microscopic areas of necrosis in both central and also peripheral parts of the lobules, and some peripheral haemorrhage. After 6 doses the picture resembled an early monolobular cirrhosis, after 10 doses an irregular fibrosis and with further increased dosage typical cirrhosis.

Severe narcosis is preceded by irritation of mucous membranes (conjunctivitis) and of the central nervous system – twitching and convulsions (Lehmann and Flury, 1943). Less severe narcosis may be continued for 1 h without fatal results, when restlessness, loss of equilibrium, excitement and tremor have been succeeded by quiet sleep with cessation of all voluntary and involuntary muscular movements (Lamson *et al.*, 1924).

In animals subjected to lethal or near lethal dosage of CCl_4 lesions of the liver, in the form of fatty degeneration, central necrosis and changes similar to acute yellow atrophy have been predominant (Lehmann, 1911; Davies, 1934; Landé and Dervillée, 1934).

Renal lesions have consisted of enlarged and fatty kidneys (Lehmann, 1911), cloudy swelling (Davies, 1934; Takahashi, 1929) but Lamson *et al.* found no injury of the kidneys even when liver necrosis had been produced.

The liver

Morphological alterations in the liver. – In animals given CCl_4 orally or by subcutaneous or intraperitoneal injection it is generally agreed that the lesions of the liver are central necrosis or fatty infiltration. In the mid-zonal region the cells became swollen and vacuolated and in the peripheral region may contain droplets of fat (Cameron and Karunaratne, 1936; Dixon and McCullagh, 1957; Hoffman *et al.*, 1955; McClosky and McGehee, 1959).

The mechanism of liver injury is not completely understood but is believed to be associated with injury of the mitochondrial enzyme systems. Swelling of the mitochondria in the livers of animals poisoned with CCl_4 has been demonstrated by Christie and Judah (1954), Dianzani (1954) and, using the electron microscope, by Dianzani and Bahr (1954), Oberling and Rouiller (1956) and Bassi (1960). Bassi succeeded in demonstrating the earliest alterations in the liver cells of rats following doses of 0.25, 0.50 and 0.75 ml/100 g body weight.

The first signs of damage – swelling and vesiculation of the endoplasmic reticulum – appeared 1 h after the subcutaneous injection of the lowest dose, and 'hydropic' cells after 6 h. After 24 h the three regions – central, midzonal and peripheral – show distinctly the changes described by the observers cited above. Thus the first result of CCl_4 poisoning appears, as already observed by Glynn and Himsworth (1948), to be an increased intake of water by the liver cells; this is followed by swelling of the mitochondria, and finally by deposition of fat, both in the mitochondria and also in the hyaloplasm. Recknagel and Anthony (1959) emphasised that the accumulation of fat in the liver occurs before mitochondrial injury and that the initial effect of CCl_4 on the liver occurs at about 3 h.

According to Rees *et al.* (1961), although the necrosis is associated with the escape of cellular enzymes and mitochondrial damage, fatty degeneration is a separate manifestation from the other hepatic changes. They examined the effects of various chemical compounds on the livers of rats poisoned by CCl_4, and found that while the administration of the antihistamine drug Phenergan lessened the necrosis, leakage of enzymes and mitochondrial damage, it did not affect the fatty degeneration. This indicated that the fatty degeneration is a separate manifestation, and that necrosis and mitochondrial damage are evidence of a fundamental disturbance of cell permeability. Phenergan, which has various effects on the respiratory chain of enzymes, could inhibit such a process. Adrenalectomy has a similar effect of inhibiting necrosis and mitochondrial injury without affecting fatty degeneration.

Regeneration of the liver. – After 6–10 doses the above changes disappeared rapidly on cessation and the liver returned to normal within 7–10 days; since a dose of 0.25 ml, which frequently produced fatal destruction of liver tissue, could be given subcutaneously at intervals of 10 days for 6 months or longer without producing liver damage, it was obvious that the time-spacing factor was important. But if cirrhosis is to be avoided, the time interval between successive doses must be long enough to allow complete recovery to take place, while the amount given must be larger than that known to be the minimal toxic dose for the liver. Small doses repeated at short intervals are apparently the conditions which produce permanent cirrhotic lesions.

Toxicity to human beings

(1) Acute

(i) *In rapid fatal cases* of acute intoxication by CCl_4 its initial effect is that of a narcotic. Patty (1959) gives the exposure immediately (or later) fatal for a half to one hour as 400–500 mg/l (64,000–80,000 p.p.m.), and according to Eddy (1945) fatal cases have occurred rapidly following exposure to high concentrations of the vapour.

Such cases, of almost immediate death, preceded by obvious signs of central nervous disturbance and unconsciousness, are now relatively rare, though they were reported with some frequency up to 1946 (Pagniez *et al.*, 1932; Leoncini, 1934; André and Feillard, 1946). In one case reported to the Home Office in 1934 autopsy showed the presence of cerebral haemorrhage and pulmonary oedema.

(ii) *Cases of unconsciousness (non-fatal)* are reported under the heading of 'gassing' in the Annual Reports of the Chief Inspector of Factories of Great Britain; 67 such cases were reported between 1945 and 1960.

(2) Chronic or subacute

Chronic poisoning by CCl_4 was for many years considered a slight, almost non-existent hazard. Smyth and Smyth (1936) for example found no significant disturbance of health or of liver or kidney injury in workers employed in 36 factories using CCl_4.

In more recent years, a certain amount of disturbance, chiefly of the digestive system, has been encountered.

Very few cases of a severe chronic toxic effect of CCl_4 have been reported, and of three fatal cases of aplastic anaemia described by Straus (1954), none shows an indubitably direct etiology; in all three there were other factors which might have been responsible. Nevertheless, these must be reported in some detail, in case they should ever be substantiated by others.

In the first case the work frequently involved the use for 2–6 h a week of sponges soaked in CCl_4 in a room without adequate ventilation. The initial symptoms were gastro-intestinal, with jaundice, but with no anaemia or leucopenia. A month later the haemoglobin, red cells and total white cells showed a decrease and blood platelets were low. As the liver symptoms subsided the blood abnormalities increased in severity and a year after the onset of the gastro-intestinal symptoms death occurred following a severe gastro-intestinal haemorrhage. At autopsy it was stated, without further details, that the clinical diagnosis of aplastic anaemia was confirmed. It is possible that in this case the manifest hepatic injury may have been the primary cause of the anemia.

In the second case, the patient's chief occupation for three years had been cleaning gun parts with kerosene and CCl_4; he had undergone, a year previously, splenectomy, following a diagnosis of thrombocytopenic purpura. He presented with fatigue, bruising and many nose bleeds and his blood picture was that of anaemia, leucopenia, neutropenia and thrombocytopenia. Biopsy of a pigmented area on the forearm showed haemosiderosis. Death in this case also followed gastro-intestinal haemorrhage and haematuria, and the autopsy stated that it was due to aplastic anaemia "probably secondary to CCl_4 poisoning". In this case it is possible that the previous splenectomy may have been carried out for some haemopoietic disturbance (possibly essential thrombocytopenia) which played at least some part in the etiology.

In the third case the exposure had been limited to cleaning tools and car upholstery in a garage once or twice a week. He had previously been treated for malaria with chloroquine and possibly primaquine. He presented with a purpuric rash, bleeding from the gums and epistaxis. His blood picture showed slight anaemia (red blood corpuscles 3.1 million) and leucopenia (4650) and platelet depression; the bone marrow was hypocellular. Thirty days later the white cell count fell to 550 with 100% lymphocytes.

At autopsy there was massive haemorrhage into the gastro-intestinal tract, and lesser haemorrhages in the pleural spaces, diaphragm and myocardium; the bone marrow was hypoplastic, with areas of fat, some immature erythrocytes and lymphocytes and no granulocytes. In this case there appear to have been two

Bibliography on p. 263

other possible etiological factors; the possibility of exposure to benzene also in the garage, and the unknown malaria therapy which may have been Atabrine, known to be injurious to the bone marrow. It is at all events difficult to judge whether these cases were directly due to CCl_4 exposure uncomplicated by other factors in the causation of aplastic anaemia.

SYMPTOMS OF INTOXICATION

Secondary severe injury

The predominant effects of severe, not immediately fatal, injury are those of a hepato-renal syndrome, occurring after a latent period of two to eight days. In some cases liver injury is the more obvious, in others renal insufficiency leading to anuria and uraemia. The immediate effects are narcosis and irritation of mucous membranes.

(1) Narcosis

A typical instance of a narcotic effect of moderate severity was described by Corcoran *et al.* (1943) in a welder who had sprayed CCl_4 into a gasoline tank in order to prevent an explosion – "he had to keep his car window down to keep awake on his two mile drive to his home".

(2) Mucous membranes

Irritation of mucous membranes, occurring 12–36 h after the exposure, may be manifested by conjunctivitis, vomiting and diarrhoea and cough.

(3) Blood and bone marrow

In acute intoxication by CCl_4 the most frequently observed change in the blood picture has been leucocytosis with a shift to the left.

In a case described by Fry *et al.* (1959) the leucocyte count, soon after consciousness was regained, was 24,850 per μl with 71% segmented and 15% unsegmented neutrophils, falling two days later to 10,050 with a normal differential count.

(4) Gastro-intestinal disturbances

One of the best known and most detailed descriptions of the effects of chronic exposure to CCl_4 is that of Stewart and Witts (1944), who found a high incidence of gastro-intestinal symptoms and metal hebetude. In the factory under investigation the process consisted of the chlorination of an aniline derivative in solution in CCl_4, and in wartime conditions difficulty of adequate ventilation and the possibility of spillage and leakage must have involved considerable exposure, though no actual figures for the concentrations were obtained.

The symptoms were predominantly of gastro-intestinal and nervous origin. Nausea, vomiting, colic and diarrhoea were severe, and occurred in repeated episodes, but without increasing severity and with relief during brief periods of absence from work. X-ray examination revealed hypertonicity, irregular peristalsis and spasmodic contractions of the stomach and intestines. Liver function tests (serum bilirubin, Takata Ara reaction and plasma proteins) did not support the view expressed by Elkins (1942) that the gastro-intestinal symptoms reflected an early stage of liver injury. Only one man showed enlargement of the liver, but he had no jaundice, and with recovery from an episode of vomiting and diarrhoea the liver became no longer palpable.

A somewhat similar experience of predominant gastrointestinal symptoms in a group of workers employed in the manufacture of quartz crystals for electronic equipment was recorded by Kazantzis and Bomford (1960), though diarrhoea was not prominent in this group. Of 17 workers examined, 15 complained of 'dyspepsia' – nausea, anorexia, vomiting, flatulence, epigastric discomfort or distension – as well as headache, giddiness, and depression. Atmospheric concentrations of CCl_4 ranged from 45–100 p.p.m. When these were reduced by covering the beakers containing CCl_4 and by discontinuing the cleaning of plates with cloths dipped in CCl_4, all the workers were symptom-free within a week, with no recurrences up to 6 months later.

Slight gastric symptoms in 17 workers employed in the degreasing of D.D.T. capsules were reported to the Chief Inspector of Factories, Great Britain, in 1945; all made a rapid recovery.

The predominant initial symptom suggesting liver injury is nausea, followed by vomiting, cramping pains in the abdomen and diarrhoea, and sometimes accompanied by dizzines and weakness. The certain diagnosis of liver injury appears when jaundice occurs and is verified by the results of liver function tests.

(5) Urine

A co-existing kidney injury is evidenced by oedema, oliguria and the presence in the urine of red blood cells, pus cells and casts. In such cases the outcome may be fatal within a few days, as in one of the cases described by Eddy (1945). In this case the exposure was due to accidental substitution of CCl_4 for solvent naphtha; the concentration of CCl_4, though not actually known, was estimated as probably more than 2000 p.p.m.

(6) Neurological disturbances

In Stewart and Witts' investigation (1944) loss of consciousness occurred in a few workers while attending to leaks or spills, followed by headache. Drowsiness, alternating with insomnia, and a loss of mental agility were common complaints, but disappeared rapidly with fresh air and exercise.

Bibliography on p. 263

Stewart and Witts concluded that the mental disturbance was due to the narcotic action of CCl_4 on the cerebral cortex, and the gastro-intestinal symptoms to stimulation of the parasympathetic and inhibition of the sympathetic centres in the hypothalamus.

CHANGES IN THE ORGANISM

(1) The heart

Cardiac complications, due to direct toxic action on the myocardium or secondary to renal insufficiency, are less frequent than renal injury alone. Dérobert (1954) states that myocardial congestion and degeneration are frequently found at autopsy on fatal cases of CCl_4 poisoning, and abnormal electrocardiograms have been observed by other authorities (Frada, 1952; Papparolli and Cati, 1956). In a subject poisoned by Granosan (a parasiticide containing 30% of CCl_4) there was an initial phase of hypotension and collapse (Gobbato and Sequi, 1960), during which signs of insufficiency, in the form of nocturnal crises of cardiac asthma, appeared, and the electrocardiogram indicated left ventricle insufficiency. This was followed by a hypertensive syndrome of nephrogenic origin.

(2) The liver

Maximum liver damage apparently occurs within 48 h of severe acute exposure. Patients who die whitin a week invariably show severe hepatic damage (Kirkpatrick and Sutherland, 1956) and many such cases have been reported. Jennings (1955) recorded four, three by ingestion and one by inhalation, and Moon (1950) two, both of which had renal as well as hepatic lesions.

Functional disturbance of the liver. – Tests for disturbance of liver function, without actual signs of clinical injury, have indicated that such disturbance is a constant and very early effect of CCl_4 poisoning (Chiesura and Picotti, 1960). These observers found this disturbance manifested by bilirubinaemia, and by the bromsulphthalein clearance test, which indicated a diminution of function of about 70% of the normal on the 5th day of intoxication, but with almost complete recovery on the 10th day. They point out, however, that recuperation and complete eventual cure of liver injury by CCl_4 is less probable in human beings than in animals and that even moderate damage may have pathological sequelae. They examined five out of six subjects who showed evidence of injury (in one the blood urea was 150–280 mg%). All except one of the five showed hepatomegaly, and one icterus. Re-examination 5 and 6 months later, and in the icterus case 4 years later, showed no urobilinuria, no bilirubinaemia above 0.6 mg% and a negative Takata Ara reaction, but slight enlargement of the liver was present in three cases with slight evidence of abnormality of function as shown by liver function tests. They concluded that on these findings it was possible that a certain residual inadequacy of liver function may remain permanently after CCl_4 intoxication even of mild degree.

Liver cirrhosis. – In spite of the opinion held by some authorities that chronic exposure to CCl_4 does not cause cirrhosis of the liver, other observations appear to contradict this view, though they are not always completely devoid of doubt. In a case described by Butsch (1932) for example, the solution responsible for the exposure contained 40 parts of benzene, while Hammes (1941) states that the air concentration of CCl_4 was "reported to be more than 10 times the so-called safe level at times". Faraone's (1956) case was "thought to be due" to CCl_4. Of the three most recently described cases (McDermott and Hardy, 1963) two give positive evidence of long-continued exposure to CCl_4, one during the cleaning of machines in conditions of inadequate ventilation, the other during immersion of dyed cloth in an open pail containing CCl_4. Both had all the signs and symptoms of liver disease and the first case, at autopsy, showed a small, shrunken cirrhotic liver. The second, following surgical removal of ascitic fluid, developed a neurological picture said to be consistent with 'hepatic' encephalopathy, but after further surgical treatment (exclusion of the colon by ileostomy) recovered completely.

In the third case the exposure was not so definitely established. The woman had worked in a small shoe factory, where she had used solvents, one of which was "probably CCl_4". She died in progressive hepatic failure and *post mortem* examination showed extensive cirrhosis of the liver. None of the three cases had any history of alcoholism, other hepatotoxin or viral hepatitis.

(3) The kidneys

Predominant renal injury. – A fatal case of uraemia was described by Ashe and Sailer in 1942, in which the total exposure to CCl_4 had been 4 h, when the man was occupied in cleaning machinery in an elevator shaft. On the following day he had pain in the abdomen and oliguria, four days later oedema of the feet, ankles and face, and two days later still pulmonary oedema. He died in coma on the 12th day. In this case it was suggested that in view of the absence of recognisable clinical symptoms of liver involvement, he was a susceptible individual from the renal aspect.

A less severe case was reported by Clinton in 1947, in a man who had been severely exposed for brief periods to CCl_4 vapour during the process of cleaning grease from machinery in open buckets of CCl_4. The clinical picture was dominated by anorexia, lethargy, hypertension, azotaemia and urinary findings of protein, red cells and occasional cellular casts. Therapy directed to the kidney injury (intravenous infusions of glucose, physiological saline and sodium bicarbonate) was followed by complete recovery 6 weeks after the exposure, with a return of the blood pressure to normal and of the non-protein nitrogen to 33 mg/100 ml. This case illustrates the progress to a more favourable prognosis in those with kidney involvement which has taken place in recent years. Death from acute uraemia or renal insufficiency was at one time said to occur in about 20% of cases (Smetana, 1939; Hamburger, 1958) but with modern methods of treatment,

Bibliography on p. 263

including the use of the artifical kidney, the frequency has fallen to less than 10%. In the less severe cases recovery of function usually takes place in 3 or 4 months, but according to Hamburger complete clinical recovery may take 18 to 26 months.

The uraemic syndrome is manifested by increase of non-coagulable protein in the blood and by alteration of the electrolytic balance.

Azotaemia increases with the intensity and duration of the oliguria. Among subjects examined by Gobbato and Sequi (1960) the highest level (2.80%) was present in two with oliguria of 100–200 ml for 8–9 days and 180–300 ml for 10 days respectively. The increase in blood urea is usually moderate. Dudley (1935) for example found the plasma urea to be 312 mg% after 10 days of anuria while in a case described by McGee (1949) there was a daily increase of 22 mg%; Hamburger (1958) noted more than 30 mg%, and Gobbato and Sequi (1960) in a severe case about 50 mg%. From this they concluded that it is probable that such increases occur only in the more severe cases and indicate an unfavourable prognosis.

Alterations in the electrolytic balance. – In the early stages of intoxication there is a loss of water and salt; during the anuric phase an increase of potassium in the blood and a moderate decrease of calcium. Chlorine follows the change in sodium, and phosphates and sulphates increase in proportion to the azotaemia. This loss of power of acid-base regulation causes acidosis with a fall in alkaline reserve (Gobbato and Sequi, 1960).

Mechanism of renal injury. – Factors in the production of injury of renal function include (a) ischaemia due to circulatory shock, (b) renal oedema, (c) diffuse tubular injury, (d) tubular occlusion by cylinders.

(a) Ischaemia. – In the first phase of acute CCl_4 poisoning hypertension and collapse have been observed (Partenheimer and Citron, 1952; McGee, 1949) accompanied by intense vasoconstriction of the renal blood vessels.

(b) Oedema. – This has been constantly observed in fatal CCl_4 poisoning (Allen, 1954; Woods, 1946; Bell, 1946 and others) and adds significantly to the occurrence of acute renal insufficiency (Corcoran, *et al.*, 1943).

(c) Tubular injury. – Swelling, granulation, vacuolation of the cells of the convoluted tubules, especially severe in the distal tubules, have been stated to diminish the capacity for tubular absorption and excretion and to cause a 'back diffusion' from the tubules with passive re-absorption of water and of glomerular filtrate. This causation of oliguria and anuria is regarded by many authorities as the most important factor in the renal insufficiency (Marshall and Hoffman, 1949; Sirota, 1949).

(d) Tubular occlusion. – The damage to the tubular epithelium favours the precipitation of organic materials in the distal convoluted tubules, where they form

occlusive cylinders; these rarely consist of haemoglobin since CCl_4 is not a haemolytic agent. Allen (1954) has demonstrated such cylinders in histological preparations.

Preventive effects of antioxidants

(1) Acute poisoning

Among the antioxidants which have been suggested as possible agents for preventing irreversible necrosis are *N*,*N*-diphenyl-phenylenediamine (D.P.P.D.) and Phenergan (Promethazine).

D.P.P.D. has been found to protect animals against the lethal effects of large doses of CCl_4, presumably, according to Gallagher (1961) by acting on a general permeability mechanism, thus preventing the loss of mitochondrial and cellular pyridine nucleotides which would otherwise result from the physical damage to the cell.

Phenergan has been suggested as a possible agent for preventing liberation of hepatic enzymes into the blood and therefore preventing irreversible necrosis, though it does not, according to Recknagel and Litteria (1960) have any effect on the fatty change. The rationale for this action suggested by Rees and Spector (1961) is that the Phenergan prevents the secondary disturbance (*e.g.* the entry of sodium and water into the cell) following the primary short-term irreversible but not immediately fatal damage, which continues in force until the vital constituents of the damaged system are re-synthesised about 48 h later.

(2) Chronic poisoning

It has been suggested by Fiume and Favelli (1961) that aminoacetonitrile may have an inhibitory effect on the development of cirrhosis in chronic exposure to CCl_4. They subjected rats to repeated inhalation of CCl_4, one group being given in addition daily subcutaneous injections of 20 mg of aminoacetonitrile hydrosulphate. Both groups showed a high mortality, but liver biopsies of the survivors showed a much smaller degree of newly formed collagen material in the group treated by aminoacetonitrile. Lathyrogenic compounds, of which aminoacetonitrile is one, are known to exert a delaying action on collagen formation, and Fiume and Favelli suggest that it may have in addition an inhibitory effect on the multiplication of fibroblasts.

Treatment of intoxication

Acute poisoning. – If unconscious, remove to fresh air, and, if indicated apply artificial respiration.

Later symptoms

Liver damage. – Liquid with a high fat content is definitely contraindicated. Administration of choline and antihistamines has been suggested by Dawborn *et al.* (1961) on the basis of a human case so treated.

Bibliography on p. 263

A liver preparation (a sterile protein-free water soluble fraction processed from fresh untreated cattle liver) is another suggestion, on the basis of animal experiments. Tanyol and Friedman (1961) found that it produced a reduction in the degree of fatty infiltration in the liver of cats poisoned by CCl_4. The nature of the lipotropic action of the extract is not explained; it did contain some vitamin B_{12}, choline and methionine, but these were apparently in amounts far below the minimum requirements.

Kidney damage. – If oliguria or anuria is present it is dangerous to force fluids to stimulate restoration of kidney function. Fluids, given best as 10% glucose, should be limited to about 800 ml/day. Hypertonic glucose or calcium gluconate given intravenously reduces hyperpotassaemia. In cases of severe renal damage artificial dialysis may be necessary. Sulphydryl compounds, methionine and cysteine have been reported as beneficial.

Stimulants such as epinephrine or ephedrine are contraindicated, since they may induce ventricular fibrillation (Arena, 1962).

19. Trichloroethylene

Synonyms: Trilene, Westrosol, Dukeron, Crawshawpol, Triol, Triklone, and in America names, giving no hint of its actual content, e.g. Blancosolv, Cincosolv, Flock Flip, etc.

Structural formula:

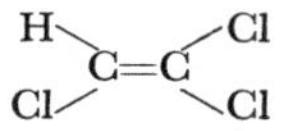

$$H \diagdown \diagup Cl$$
$$C=C$$
$$Cl \diagup \diagdown Cl$$

Molecular formula: C_2HCl_3

Molecular weight: 131.4

Properties

    boiling point: 87 °C

    melting point: -73 °C

    vapour pressure: 58 mm Hg at 20 °C

    vapour density (air = 1): 4.54

    specific gravity (liquid density): 1.455

    flash-point: non-inflammable

    conversion factors: 1 p.p.m. $= 5.38$ mg/m³ at 25 °C
                            1 mg/l $= 185.8$ p.p.m.

    solubility: insoluble in water but mixes freely with many organic solvents; relatively stable in air, but may decompose with formation of HCl under exposure to strong light or in presence of catalysts such as aluminium dust; in contact with naked flame may form phosgene.

    evaporation rate (ether = 1): 3.48

    maximum allowable concentration: 100 p.p.m. (Threshold Limit Values, 1962). Grandjean (1959) and Glass (1961) recommend 40 p.p.m.; Scandinavia 30 p.p.m.; U.S.S.R. 6 p.p.m.

Various reasons are advanced for these differing recommendations, including the possibility of national or individual idiosyncrasy, but the lowest values are considered unnecessary by U.S.A. authorities because of the lack of objective evidence of chronic injury (Ahlmark and Friberg, 1955).

ECONOMY, SOURCES AND USES

Trichloroethylene has many advantages as a solvent which account for its very wide use in industry. It carries for example no danger of explosion and very little fire risk compared with benzine and ether; it is a more rapid solvent than benzine for fats and resins, is rapidly volatilised and is relatively cheap.

Production

Obtained from pentachloroethane by thermal decomposition or by boiling with milk of lime.

Industrial uses

(1) As a dry cleaning agent, for textiles and furs.

(2) As a degreaser for metal parts, containers etc.

An investigation by Elkins (1959) of the concentrations of Tri vapour in degreasing units in Massachusetts showed that in over one-half the average level was below the M.A.C. and about one quarter below 200 p.p.m. When the degreasing is carried out in a pit or large tank the average exposure is much higher – 18,500 p.p.m. in the pit and 1270 inside the tank. Many of the cases of 'gassing' reported to the Chief Inspector of Factories in Great Britain have occurred during its use as a metal degreaser, some due to disregard of the requirements of the Factories Act, some to the fact that Tri may be trapped in pockets or held in sludge inside the plant, and some to failure or absence of the haemostatic control, which is regarded as an important safety measure in degreasing baths. Elkins also remarks that occasionally a mixture of Tri and ethylene dichloride is used as a degreasing solvent, a practice which he deplores owing to the greater toxicity of ethylene dichloride.

A recent survey of degreasing baths by Glass (1961) in New Zealand showed that, among 11 baths investigated, the average concentration at head height above the bath ranged from 20–500 p.p.m., the highest levels being over the baths which relied on manual removal of the articles.

(3) As a rubber solvent, especially for Neoprene (Greenburg and Moskowitz, 1945).

(4) In the paint industry, as a solvent for tar in the painting of casks, vats, etc.

(5) In extraction of oils and fats from vegetable products, corn, olives etc. and from bones, leather, wool and fish; in the recovery of fat-free glue in the residues from tanneries, and in recovery of wax and paraffin from refuse.

(6) In the boot and shoe industry as an adhesive mixed with rubber cement.

(7) In the artificial silk industry, for impregnation and dressing purposes.

(8) In the cleaning of films, photographic plates and optical lenses.

(9) In the chemical industry for many extraction processes.

(10) In gas purification, as a solvent of sulphur and phosphorus.

(11) As an addition to many other solvents bearing proprietary names.

(12) It is also used to some extent as a surgical and obstetrical anaesthetic.

BIOCHEMISTRY

Estimation

(1) In the atmosphere

   (a) Elkins' method (1959). – This method is similar to that used for carbon tetrachloride – absorption on silica-gel followed by hydrolysis of the CCl_4 in isopropyl alcohol (Fahy, 1948). Whereas with CCl_4 about 85% of the chlorine is recovered as inorganic chloride, almost half the chlorine content of Tri is recovered as KCl. The sensitivity of this method is stated to be about 5 p.p.m. in a 25-l air sample.

   (b) Zurlo and Metrico's method (1960). – This method is based on the Fujiwara (1914) reaction (formation of a red coloured compound with pyridine in an alkaline medium) modified by Truhaut (1951) for specificity for Tri. The original reaction applies also to CCl_4 and other substances containing 3 atoms of Cl on the same C atom. The modified procedure is suitable also for perchloroethylene and tetrachloroethane.

Procedure. – 10–15 l of the air to be tested are bubbled, at the rate of 0.5–1 l/min, through two Dreschel units arranged in series, each containing 20 ml of absolute ethyl alcohol. To 1 ml of this solution add 1 ml of a 50% aqueous solution of NaOH. Add 5 ml of pyridine. Stir, and keep in water bath at 70° for 3 min. Cool under running water, add 3 ml of water and shake. Read from a colorimeter with a 530 mμ filter 1$\frac{1}{2}$–3 min later. Calibrate by testing in the same way 20–200 μg of Tri in 5 ml of pyridine and 1 ml of ethyl alcohol. Calculation:

$$\text{Tri in mg/1000 l} = \frac{\mu\text{g of Tri} \times \text{ml of absorbing soln. used}}{\text{litres of air absorbed ml} \times \text{of absorbing soln. used}}.$$

   (c) Stack, Forrest and Wahl method (1961). – This method, also based on the Fujiwara reaction, is claimed to be capable of detecting 1 μg of Tri in the sample analysed and can be used to determine concentrations as low as 1 p.p.m. by volume, using a 250-ml air sample.

Procedure. – The Tri is extracted by toluene (2 ml added to a 250 ml gas sampling tube); to 1 ml of this is added 5 ml of dry pyridine and 0.35 ml of 1% ethanolic potassium hydroxide; after 5 min 9 ml of distilled water is added and the solution allowed to remain in the dark for 15 min. Addition of 3 ml of methanol is followed

30 sec later by measuring the optical density at 537 mμ. Calibration is achieved by preparing known solutions of Tri in toluene.

(2) In blood and tissues

Estimation of the arterial and venous blood content of Tri has also been based on the Fujiwara reaction, modified by Conway (1957). This method was used by Clayton and Parkhouse (1962) during anaesthesia of adult patients, when constant concentrations of Tri were delivered at a constant respiratory rate and volume. In this reaction the vapour diffuses into a toluene solution in the central chamber of a Conway Standard Cell (Conway and Byrne, 1933), the Tri-toluene solution then being subjected to the Fujiwara reaction. It was found that when 0.5% U/V Tri was given at the rate of about 10 l/min the Tri concentration in the arterial blood was about 6.7 mg/100 ml, with concentrations of 1% 12–17 mg/100 ml. In venous blood the amount in obese subjects was considerably less than in the arterial. In 1945 Habgood and Powell also had estimated the blood content of Tri. In Powell's (1945) investigation he estimated the amount resulting from inhalation of 2% for 1 h to be almost 10 mg/100 ml. The smaller content of Tri in venous than arterial blood is attributed to the fact that Tri, being a fat-soluble agent, is liable to be extracted from the blood by fatty tissue such as exists in the antecubital fossa; when taken from the back of the wrist the venous and arterial levels were much more comparable.

Metabolism

(1) Absorption and excretion

Tri is rapidly absorbed by the lungs by inhalation and a small amount is rapidly exhaled by the same route. Powell (1945) found very small amounts in the expired air and in the blood during the first one of two days. Conversion takes place in the body, by way of chloral hydrate (Uhl and Haag, 1958), to trichloracetic acid and trichlorethanol, both of which are excreted in the urine. Uhl and Haag describe the metabolic conversion as follows:

```
                                  trichloroacetic acid
                             ↗                          ↘
trichloroethylene ⟶ chloral hydrate ⟶ trichloroethanol ⟶ glucuronic acid ⟶ excretion in urine
```

Butler (1949) showed that the reaction resulting in the formation of chloral hydrate is very slow, but once it is produced it is converted rapidly into TCA and TCE, the latter, in the dog at any rate, in larger amounts than the former.

Trichloroacetic acid excretion – Barrett and Johnston (1939) noted that when the steam distillate of human urine of subjects exposed to Tri was tested in 20% alcohol (a standard solution for the determination of Tri vapour by a modification of the Fujiwara reaction), the colour was a distinct lemon-yellow instead of the orange solution of Tri itself. Further experiments on animals confirmed the conclusion that the halogen-containing material present in the urine was not Tri itself, and it was finally concluded that it was in fact trichloroacetic acid (TCA). According to Barrett *et al.* (1939) the trichloroacetic acid excreted by dogs during anaesthesia amounts to 5–8% of the Tri absorbed, while Teisinger (cited by Uhl and Haag, 1958) gives the amount as between 7 and 27%. Its excretion in the urine is very slow, in accordance with the slow rate of the whole metabolism of Tri, as shown by Hunold (1955). He found that it was a month after cessation of exposure before the Fujiwara reaction became negative. There is a short period of fairly high clearance from the serum; Abrahamson (1960) found that during the first two days human beings excreted 5.5–6.7 ml/min and after 14 days 2.2–2.9 ml/min while some was present in serum and urine after 53 days.

In two cases of acute oral poisoning mentioned by Uhl and Haag (1958) both of whom recovered, the trichloroacetic acid concentration in the urine was 80 mg/100 g and 92 mg/100 g respectively.

Attempts have been made by several observers to correlate the trichloroacetic acid excretion with either the degree of exposure or the occurrence of symptoms from such exposure to Tri, but without close agreement.

Grandjean *et al.* (1955) found little or no relationship between levels of exposure and levels of excretion, except when they included the relationship of time of exposure; here they found a variability of 1 : 20 to 1 : 2, which they explained on individual variation in metabolism and lack of precision in the estimation of atmospheric concentrations of Tri. Grandjean (1959) however recommended 96 mg/l as the maximum limit for trichloroacetic acid in urine.

In a survey of Tri degreasing baths in Auckland in 1961, Glass correlated the urinary TCA of operators with the concentration of Tri at various distances from the bath, the frequency of exposure and the time since the last exposure, and concluded: (a) that the time of exposure does not influence the level of TCA to a great extent; for example, in one case, exposed 6–8 h a day to 300 p.p.m. the level of TCA was 145 mg/l, while in another exposed for the same length of time to 400 p.p.m. the level was only 30 mg/l, and in a third, exposed only intermittently to 186 p.p.m. it was 180 p.p.m., (b) that the excretion of TCA is very slow; in one case it was still detectable 6 weeks after cessation of exposure, (c) that in all cases where exposure is heavy, the TCA excretion is high.

A similar wide variation in the correlation with the occurrence of symptoms of intoxication was found by Anderssen (1957). In one third of the cases examined excretion was less than 20 mg/l, in others up to 700 mg/l. The higher levels (76 to 150 mg/l) were shown by those complaining of shortness of breath and heart and digestive disorders, the purely neurasthenic cases showed lower levels, which did not increase with longer exposure to the same extent as those with heart symptoms and shortness of breath. This was explained by the fact that in those workers exposed to the lowest concentrations of Tri, neurasthenic symptoms must have had another etiology, such as social and domestic difficulties.

Bibliography on p. 263

Trichloroethanol (TCE). – TCE is believed to be the main metabolite of Tri, and according to Bartonicek and Teisinger (1962) it is much more toxic than TCA, loses its narcotic properties only after conjugation with glucuronic acid and is eliminated slowly. These observers therefore have attempted to diminish the toxicity of Tri by attacking the formation of TCE. Bartonicek (1962) tried to inhibit the oxidation of Tri into TCE at the chloral stage of metabolism by administering sodium lactate and fructose, while Forssman *et al.* (1955) reported that tetraethylthiuram disulphide (Disulfiram) greatly reduced the excretion of TCA in urine after administration of Tri or TCE to rats, an effect which they also ascribed to a suppression of the oxidation of chloral. In an attempt to verify their results Bartonicek and Teisinger (1962) examined the effect of giving Disulfiram to human subjects on the day before exposure to Tri, during single exposure for 5 h, and on the day following exposure. The results of a similar exposure without Disulfiram were used for comparison. In all the subjects the administration of Disulfiram decreased the excretion of both TCA and TCE. When the Disulfiram effect ended there was an increase in the level of both, indicating that this phenomenon is due to the release of a fraction of Tri from the fat depots in the organism, followed by their metabolism.

The elimination of Tri itself in the expired air was considerably increased, and for this reason it was believed that Disulfiram suppresses the oxidation of Tri, though it may also have an inhibitory effect on the enzymes (oxidases) which carry out the oxidation process and on the aldehyde dehydrogenases which convert chloral into TCA. It is interesting to note that whereas the enzymatic metabolism of many organic solvents can be regarded as 'detoxication' mechanisms, this is certainly not so in the case of the conversion of Tri to TCE, since TCE is the more toxic (Soucek and Vlachova, 1960; Mikiskova and Mikiska, 1960).

Other metabolites – monochloroacetic acid and chloroform – have been described (Soucek and Vlachova, 1954), but according to Bartonicek and Teisinger (1962) the production of these substances has not been confirmed.

The retention of the metabolites has been stated to amount to 56% of the Tri inhaled – 7–27% TCA, 22.2–22.5% TCE, free or conjugated, 22.5–45.5% urocholalic acid and small amounts, if any, of monochloroacetic acid and chloroform – but these amounts vary in individuals. Teisinger (1959) cites the case of a woman aged 51 who excreted more than 1 g of TCE in 24 h without showing any signs of disturbance of health.

Action on protein and fat metabolism. – According to Guyot-Jeannin and Van Steenkiste (1958) chronic exposure to Tri may cause a disturbance of protein and fat metabolism. They based their conclusion on the results of examination of 18 workers exposed for several years to an atmosphere "polluted with Tri vapour" (the actual concentrations were always below the M.A.C. but varied considerably with the different processes and the time of day from 5–19 p.p.m.). Electrophoretic and flocculation tests of serum protein fractions and estimations of total lipid content, lipid fractions and unsaturated fatty acid content were carried out.

(a) Protein metabolism. – The most constant abnormality was an increase in the β-globulin fraction (normal taken as 10–14%,) which showed an average of 16.39%, the highest level being 21.66% in one case.

(b) Lipid metabolism. – Total and esterified cholesterol and the relation between them was within normal limits in all but two cases, but there was an increase in nearly all cases of unsaturated fatty acids; this is often proportional to an increase in total lipids. In these cases the increase was represented by that of β-lipoproteins.

The question was raised whether this disturbance of lipid metabolism is reversible on cesssation of exposure – a question which has so far apparently remained unanswered.

(2) Distribution in blood and tissues

In 1945 Powell measured the blood concentration of Tri resulting from inhalation of 2% for an hour, and found it to be almost 10 mg/100 ml. A more recent investigation of the concentration of Tri in blood (and expired air) following exposure of human beings to concentrations of approximately 200 p.p.m. has been carried out by Stewart *et al.* (1962), using samples of venous blood and the method of CS_2 extraction and infra-red analysis (Stewart *et al.*, 1959, 1962). Tri was detectable in the blood of most of the subjects half an hour after the concentration had reached the desired level. It appeared to reach the maximum average blood level 2 h after the onset of exposure; at 3 h it had fallen to two thirds of this, and at 20 min after the end of exposure to one sixth. The amount in expired air also decreased rapidly – from 29–41 p.p.m. immediately after exposure to barely perceptible amounts 5 h later. This is in accordance with the view most generally held that a rather large percentage of the Tri retained is metabolised in the body to TCA and TCE, both of which are excreted in the urine. No appreciable quantity of unchanged Tri is excreted in the urine.

The fact that following inhalation of Tri the amount in venous blood is considerably less than in the arterial blood of obese subjects is attributed to the fact that since Tri is a fat-soluble agent (Clayton and Parkhouse, 1962), it is liable to be extracted from the blood by fatty tissue, such as exists in the antecubital fossa; when taken from the back of the wrist the venous and arterial levels were much more comparable.

It was noted by Helliwell and Hutton (1950) that Tri readily passes the placenta; they found higher concentrations in the foetal than the maternal blood; this they attribute to differences in the red blood cells.

Bibliography on p. 263

Action on the level of blood alcohol. – This problem may arise when workers exposed to Tri are accused of being "drunk in charge" of a car on the grounds that they have a high content of alcohol in the blood. Paulus (1951), in animal experiments, showed that inhalation of Tri, even when causing unconsciousness, did not cause any rise above 0.1% in the alcohol level of the blood, and did not increase the pre-inhalation level.

In a personal experiment Lob (1960) determined the curve of blood alcohol after ingestion of 1 decilitre of whiskey, and later of the same quantity 15 min after having inhaled 400 p.p.m. of Tri for 45 min. There was practically no effect on the curve.

In animals he estimated the blood alcohol following injection of 1.3 ml/kg of pure alcohol into the vein of the ear, and compared it with the level when this was preceded by injection of 10 mg/kg of Tri. Again the level was unaffected, as also when the injections were made simultaneously.

These results, while showing that 'acute' exposure to Tri does not influence the alcohol content of the blood, do not apply to the possible effect of long-continued inhalation, such as occurs in many industrial processes. Further investigation on this point is necessary for a definite opinion.

TOXICOLOGY

The predominant action of Tri is that of a narcotic, and inhalation of high concentrations causes complete unconsciousness, hence its use as a surgical anaesthetic, introduced by Striker *et al.* (1935). Opinions as to its complete harmlessness for this purpose have at times been conflicting. In 1936 the Council of Pharmacy and Chemistry of the American Medical Association suggested that further investigation was necessary, and after a further trial of its anaesthetic properties in London in 1940 a favourable report on cases investigated was given by Hewer (1941, 1942, 1943). Nevertheless, some authorities have maintained that cardiac arrest is a potential hazard (Bernstine, 1954; Norris and Stuart, 1957) and that acute necrosis of the liver can arise from prolonged anaesthesia (Dodds, 1945; Herdman, 1945), but later experiment has failed to establish a direct relationship between these injuries and Tri, if the Tri is pure and used with correct procedure (Atkinson, 1960). Its narcotic action has even been proposed as the basis of treatment of various nervous disorders, including trigeminal neuralgia (Glaser, 1931).

In industry an acute toxic syndrome was first noted following its use as a grease solvent (Plessner, 1915), and numerous cases of 'gassing' have been reported to the Chief Inspector of Factories in Great Britain, chiefly from entry into tanks or cleaning containers which have held Tri.

Chronic poisoning, as a specific syndrome apart from the depressant effect on the central nervous system common to all narcotics has also been widely discussed, and the question especially of possible liver and kidney injury is still not completely resolved, though the balance of opinion appears to be that Tri does not exert the effect so characteristic and specific of some other halogenated hydro-carbons, particularly carbon tetrachloride. Cases of liver and kidney injury follow-ing both acute and chronic exposure have been reported, but many authorities consider that these relatively rare cases tend to occur as conditions superimposed on previously susceptible liver or kidneys, or associated with other toxic factors.

In animals, although some of the earlier investigators recorded lesions of the liver and kidneys, the more recent results of investigations using pure Tri have failed to confirm the opinion that Tri is a specific liver or kidney poison.

Toxicity to animals

(1) Acute

(a) Lethal dose. – In their investigation of the effects of single exposures of monkeys, rats, rabbits, and guinea pigs to inhalation of varying concentrations of Tri, Adams *et al.* (1951) found that 20,000 p.p.m. represented 100% mortality in rats, while Bernardi *et al.* (1956) found that death occured in rabbits subjected to inhalation of 11,000 p.p.m. after 50 min and of 1800 p.p.m. after 20–30 days.

(b) Narcotic dose. – According to Adams *et al.* (1951) the anaesthetic effect of Tri occurred at 4800 p.p.m. but not immediately at 3000 p.p.m. Varying degrees of 'drunkenness', stupor and unconsciousness, with little initial stimulation were observed within 6 min at 6400 p.p.m. and within 12 min at 3000 p.p.m. Animals which survived recovered rapidly from the anaesthetic effects and showed no further external signs of illness.

Herzberg (1934) found that animals killed by an overdose also showed no toxic effects on the tissues, and no toxic effects from subcutaneous and intravenous injection were reported by Lehmann (1911), Joachimoglu (1921), Nowill *et al.* (1954) and Richards and Bachmann (1955).

(2) Chronic or subacute

As with acute toxicity, earlier investigators tended to the opinion that Tri resembled other chlorinated hydrocarbons in exerting a toxic effect on the liver and/or kidneys of animals (Meyer, 1929; Castellino, 1932; Germain and Marty, 1947), and among more recent authorities Mosinger and Fiorentini (1958).

SYMPTOMS OF INTOXICATION

Recent investigations (Adams *et al.*, 1951; Kylin *et al.*, 1962) however, appear to show that any hepatoxic effect, if it exists, is much less marked than with other chlorinated solvents, such as CCl_4, which are recognised as hepatotoxic agents. On the other hand, though repeated exposure to 3000 p.p.m. (27 exposures during 36 days) was found by Adams *et al.* (1951) to cause disturbances of equilibrium and co-ordination, and after the first week salivation, restlessness and hyper-

Bibliography on p. 263

excitability, they recovered rapidly when removed from exposure, and though the liver and kidneys showed an increase in weight, the only histological abnormality was that of a few small fat vacuoles in the liver of the female rats. With longer exposure (243 days) to lower concentrations (100–400 p.p.m.) similar results were obtained, and there was no alteration in blood protein nitrogen, urea nitrogen, serum phosphatase, plasma prothrombin clotting, total lipid, phospholipid, neutral fat or cholesterol in the liver, but there was some retardation of growth. For the different species of animals the concentrations which were tolerated over a long period without adverse effects were 400 p.p.m. for monkeys, 200 p.p.m. for rats and 100 p.p.m. for guinea pigs.

It was concluded that the responses of the rats at 3000 p.p.m. represented a functional disturbance of the nervous system, possibly of the autonomic nerves, analogous to the minimal response of human beings to chronic exposure to Tri – fatigue, headache, anorexia and gastro-intestinal disturbance.

CHANGES IN THE ORGANISM

(1) The liver

The investigations of Mosinger and Fiorentini (1958) were carried out on cats and guinea pigs exposed to 1000 p.p.m. daily for $1\frac{1}{2}$ h, for periods ranging from 10 days to 10 months, according to the time when the animals showed the first signs of intoxication (desequilibrium, muscular spasms). In those animals killed during the first month the liver was stated to show a fatty hepatitis, with a distension of interlobular veins; in those which survived several months, cirrhosis and biliary hyperplasia, the latter progressing in some animals to a proliferative 'biliary adenomatosis'.

In the experiments of Adams *et al* (1951) only minor changes were found in the liver – a slight increase in weight with slight cloudy swelling, but no fat globules; there was a slight increase in the total lipid content of the liver of the most severely exposed animals. A comparison of the effects on the liver of inhalation by mice of varying concentrations of Tri for single 4 h periods with those of tetrachloroethylene and chloroform (Kylin *et al.*, 1962) showed that Tri inflicted none of the injury found with the other two substances. At concentrations of 800–6400 p.p.m. Tri produced no histologically detectable fatty infiltration of the liver, whereas tetrachloroethylene and chloroform induced this effect at 400 and 200 p.p.m. respectively. Nor was any significant increase in extractable liver fat found in the animals exposed to Tri, while increasing concentrations of both the other compounds caused an increase.

(2) The spleen

The spleen was also stated to show an unusual toxic effect in the form of splenomegaly with haemorrhage of the pulp and hypertrophy of the Malpighian bodies.

(3) The kidneys

These showed glomerular and tubular lesions – dilatation and eosinophilic and lymphocytic infiltration.

(4) The lungs

These showed emphysematous and inflammatory changes (chronic bronchopneumonia).

(5) The nervous system

(a) The central nervous system. – According to Mosinger and Fiorentini, there was oedema, with areas of necrosis and degenerative changes. In the experiments of Bernardi *et al.* (1956) prolonged inhalation of 1800 p.p.m. produced some regressive changes in the ganglion cells, as well as non-specific changes similar to those in which anoxia has been caused by barbiturates or carbon monoxide.

With fairly high dosage Ricci (1956) found marked degenerative changes in the nervous tissues of rabbits and guinea pigs.

(b) The brain. – In animals with heavy acute poisoning, Bernardi *et al.* (1956) observed hyperaemia, oedema and small haemorrhages especially in the cerebrum and the marginal regions of the cerebellum.

Effects of admixture of other solvents with Tri

The toxicity of Tri has been stated to be notably augmented by the addition of some other solvents, especially methyl alcohol (Viallier and Brune, 1958). They investigated the effect also of white spirit, petrol, ethyl acetate, acetone and cyclohexane by exposing guinea pigs to Tri alone and to a mixture of equal parts of Tri and the solvent under investigation. Intoxication was estimated by loss of consciousness, inability to stand and twitching of the limbs. In most of the animals this condition was easily reversed when exposure ceased. None of the solvents except methyl alcohol increased the time of onset or the severity of the intoxication. They explain this action by the suggestion that the increase in toxicity is a property of the methyl alcohol itself, not of the mixture.

Transyl, an anti-rust agent, containing 3% of nitrobenzene, 95% of mineral oil and a chlorinated solvent assumed to be Tri, was reported by Hadengue *et al.* (1959) to have caused severe poisoning by its accidental ingestion through lack of suitable labelling. The chief symptoms were violent headache followed by unconsciousness with cyanosis, which yielded to treatment with methylene blue, and anaemia. There was no involvement of liver and kidneys. It would seem probable that in this case, as in that of the mixture with methyl alcohol, the symptoms not usually those of acute poisoning by Tri – anaemia and cyanosis – were due to the nitrobenzene constituent of the Transyl.

Bibliography on p. 263

Enzyme reactions

The results of many investigations on the association between an increase in serum transaminase (serum glutamic oxalacetic acid, SGOT) and the liver injury due to poisoning by carbon tetrachloride (see p.000) have led to similar investigations on Tri, with a view to helping to resolve the controversy as to whether Tri has in fact a hepatotoxic action. While SGOT is believed to regulate the equilibrium between aspartic acid and γ-keto glutaric acid, and also between glutamic and oxalacetic acid, another enzyme, aldolase, catalyses the splitting of fructose and di-phosphate. Animal experiments have shown (Agress *et al.*, 1955) that an increase of activity of both in the serum is an indication of necrosis of tissue. SGOT in particular has been studied in human beings (see p. 209) as a criterion of actual or potential damage to the liver by Tri.

Still another enzyme, serum ornithine carbamyl transferase (SOCT) has been studied from the same point of view – that of an indication of liver injury by Tri. In mice exposed to varying concentrations of Tri vapour for single 4 h periods, Kylin *et al.* (1962) attempted to establish the extent of toxic liver effect by determination of the presence of liver fat as well as of an increase of SOCT. They found no significant increase of either with concentrations of 800 to 6400 p.p.m. of Tri, whereas 2 groups of animals exposed to 200 and 800 p.p.m. respectively of chloroform showed fatty infiltration and necrosis as well as an increase in SOCT activity and extractable liver fat.

Toxicity to human beings

(1) Acute

(i) By ingestion. – Acute poisoning from ingestion of Tri, or mixtures of Tri with other solvents, is sometimes fatal, but cases of great severity have been known to recover with suitable treatment and without sequelae.

One such case of exceptional gravity was described by Calvet *et al.* (1959). This woman attempted suicide by drinking a glassful of Tri and water (25% Tri). She was found in a state of complete coma, with cardiovascular collapse and with abundant liquid diarrhoea streaked with blood. There was also evidence of renal injury in the form of albuminuria with many epithelial cells, granular cylinders, leucocytes and red corpuscles. These abnormalities disappeared within 8 days and there were no manifestations of hepatic injury. Two months later her general condition was satisfactory.

Five cases of acute intoxication from ingestion were recorded by Roche *et al.* (1958), two of them suicidal and three accidental, all making an eventual recovery and showing no signs of renal or hepatic injury. Another case of accidental ingestion of a cleaning fluid, later found to be Tri, described by Uhl and Haag (1958) in which severe vomiting was followed by collapse and prolonged unconsciousness also showed complete recovery after treatment by cardiazol, coramine and administration of oxygen/CO_2 mixture. The most notable abnormality observed was a decrease in thromboplastin time, but unacccompanied by bleeding. The ECG raised suspicions of a circumscribed myocarditis, but although 5 months later some ventricular and superventricular extra systoles were observed, it was thought that these were probably functional in origin. There was no evidence of liver or kidney injury. The presence of Tri was demonstrated in the vomit and of trichloroacetic acid (7.5 mg%) in the urine.

In two other cases of oral poisoning mentioned by Uhl and Haag, one was a suicidal attempt, the other a mistake for 'Schnapps' (about 100-200 ml). Both recovered; the urinari trichloroacetic acid concentration was 80 mg% in the first and 92 mg% in the second. Fatal poisoning from pure Tri is much rarer than that from cleaning materials containing it. Among the earliest reports of intoxication with pure Tri is that of Froboese (1943). This was a Russian aged 24 who drank about 200–300 ml of pure Tri. Death took place without recovery of consciousness 6–7 h later. At autopsy the liver showed only slight fatty infiltration of the liver cells, but fat droplets were presents in the Kupfer cells and there was acute congestion with accumulation of lymphocytes in the Glisson capsules. The brain also showed fat droplets in the glia, adventitial and endothelial cells and in the blood plasma of the leptomeningeal and intracerebral vessels.

The four cases described by Schoenemann (1944) were also Russians, who had made Tri the basis of the punch which they drank. One died, and the others all showed a similar syndrome – leucocytosis with a shift to the left, increase in residual nitrogen and in urinary urea. The autopsy report on the fatal case mentioned "acute liver atrophy" but without giving further details. In the survivors, the central nervous symptoms (increased unilateral muscle tension and abnormal reflexes) were slow to resolve.

Graber's (1950) cases were divided into two groups. In the first (3 men), the Tri was presumably pure; it was drunk by three postmen who mistook it for 'Schnapps'. All died, after 3, 4½ and 9 h respectively. The two who survived longest had vomiting and diarrhoea, cyanosis and cardiac collapse uninfluenced by coramine, strychnine and strophantin.

In the second series of 5 cases, one of which was fatal, it was not certain that the liquid drunk was pure Tri, but the toxic syndrome was very similar to that of the other three. Detailed descriptions of the autopsy findings were given by Graber; on the whole they agree closely with those of Froboese (1943), the characteristic injuries being present in the brain, liver, lungs and intestinal tract. The central nervous injury was held chiefly responsible for the fatal outcome.

Among the cases described by Roche et al. (1958) two were attempted suicides. In one, the chief injury resulting from ingestion of 150 ml of a cleaning fluid with a Tri base, was somnolence leading to coma lasting 5 days, burns of the skin and gastric mucous membrane and a lung infection; in the other similarly from cleaning fluid (50 ml) there was vomiting, somnolence and shock. Neither showed

Bibliography on p. 263

any manifestation of renal or hepatic injury, nor did two accidental cases, caused by drinking from bottles which had contained Tri. Their symptoms were similar to those of the suicidal cases, but in one the gastro-intestinal disturbance persisted for some days after recovery from the comatose condition.

A review of the cases, severe or fatal, from ingestion of Tri supports the view of many observers, including Forssman and Ahlmark (1945), Anderssen (1957) and Abrahamson (1960) that oral intoxication by Tri has no such toxic effect on the liver as that produced by CCl_4. Even in the severe case investigated by Abrahamson, liver function tests, including thymol, alkaline phosphatase, and total protein, with albumen and globulin, were normal, as also were those in the case with cardiac and renal symptoms described by Calvet *et al.* (1959).

Treatment.–When ingestion has occurred, gastric lavage is indicated; for coma, oxygen and cardiac stimulants (Calvet *et al.*, 1959, recommend noradrenaline in a blood transfusion); to prevent lung infection, antibiotics.

(ii) By inhalation. – Between 1941 and 1961, from the industrial use of Tri, 414 cases of 'gassing', most of them due to the entry into tanks which had contained it and 33 of them fatal, were reported to the Chief Inspector of Factories, Ministry of Labour, U.K.

One of the most detailed investigations of the pathogenesis of the severe effects of inhalation of Tri is that of Koch (1931) of a 19 year old worker who, through careless handling of a Tri apparatus inhaled a concentration which caused his death 5 h later. Autopsy showed severe blistering of the skin of the left side of the face, and less severe lesions of the forehead, shoulder, chest and left knee; inflammatory redness of the respiratory tract; areas of haemorrhage in the lungs and pericardium; acute dilation of the heart, with much blood in the cavities and large blood vessels; congestion of liver, spleen and kidneys; slight reddening of the gastric mucous membrane, congestion of the blood vessels of the brain cortex and ventricles, with an odour of aromatic nature from the brain. Histologically, the lungs showed areas of oedema, with fatty infiltration of the alveolar epithelium; the bronchi, leucocytosis in the subepithelial and submucosal blood vessels; the liver, a loose structure with brown pigment in the cells of the central zone with occasional fat granules; the brain, much fatty deposit in the endothelium of the vessels, especially of the corpus striatum.

Hepatonephritis. – In spite of the statement by Hunter (1962), referring to the use of Tri as an anaesthetic, that "Tri is incapable of producing liver damage in any ordinary circumstances", cases of hepatonephritis have been reported in fatal poisoning by inhalation of Tri (Germain and Marty, 1947; Piedelièvre *et al.*, 1943; Derobert, 1951; and others). The two cases described by Derobert are perhaps the most striking and the most closely investigated of the occurrence of liver and kidney injury due to prolonged inhalation of high concentrations of Tri.

The first, a woman aged 20 who had spent a half day in cleaning 40 articles in a badly ventilated room, with a solvent later stated to be "almost pure Tri", presented with dyspnoea, cyanosis, abundant red-tinged expectoration and anuria. Later, she showed abolition of reflexes and pulmonary oedema. The urine, removed by catheter, contained some albumen, and when centrifuged, epithelial cells, leucocytes, cylinders and a few red cells. She died 21 days after the original exposure. Autopsy revealed pleural and pericardial inflammation, and pulmonary oedema with zones of hepatisation. There was intense dilation of all the blood vessels. The liver, which was pale yellowish, also showed a moderate vasodilatation and lymphocytic infiltration of the perivascular areas with some haemorrhage, and fatty degeneration especially round the portal spaces. The kidneys also showed vasodilatation and haemorrhages in the pyramidal area, and the tubules lymphocytic infiltration. The organs contained amounts of "a volatile trihalogen derivative" which were calculated in terms of Tri, the brain having the greatest content (14 mg/kg), followed by the liver (11 mg/kg), with only 0.6 mg/kg in the kidney.

The second case was that of a man aged 36 engaged for $3\frac{1}{2}$ h in removing paint by Tri. On leaving work he felt 'drunk' and later complained of headache and gastric pain; during the night he vomited. Four days later he developed oliguria, followed after a week by anuria and haemoptysis which led to his death 13 days after the exposure. Autopsy showed pulmonary oedema, hypertrophy of the heart, hepatomegaly with congestion and slight fatty degeneration, renal hypertrophy with pyramidal congestion and discoloration of the cortex, and slight meningeal oedema.

Among the fatal cases reported to the Chief Inspector of Factories between 1941 and 1961 toxic changes in the liver were found in only one case, and renal damage in two.

Although renal and hepatic injury are much less frequent factors in a fatal outcome of acute inhalation toxicity, a picture of severe hepatonephritis has occasionally been reported (Léchelle et al., 1958; Germain and Marty, 1947; Derobert et al., 1952; Grisler and Gallina, 1956). In a few cases the renal injury was the actual cause of death from anuria, the liver injury consisting only of lymphocytic infiltration of the perivascular zone and some steatosis. Hepatic injury alone is variable in its clinical and pathological features, ranging from transient subicterus to severe, even fatal jaundice, and from simple steatosis to acute yellow atrophy (Vallée and Leclercq, 1935; etc.). Whether such injuries are the direct consequence of Tri intoxication is not certain; some authorities, including Roche et al. (1958) incline to the opinion that most of the relatively rare cases tend to occur as conditions superimposed on previously susceptible kidneys or liver or associated with other toxic factors.

Bibliography on p. 263

Other causes of death

Cardiac failure. – Most of the cases of sudden cardiac arrest have been report-ed in connection with anaesthesia by Tri, though not all these have been attri-buted directly to Tri itself. Of 20 cases reviewed by Ostlere in 1953, in only three was the evidence for a toxic effect of Tri considered definite. In 1957, Norris and Stuart recorded 7 cases in which 3 were considered due to Tri, and 3 cases were described by Hewer in 1958 in which, out of a series of 60,000 anaesthetics by Tri, it was considered responsible for cardiac arrest. Changes in the ECG during Tri anaesthesia have been reported (Hewer and Hadfield, 1941; Waters *et al.*, 1943; Hunter, 1944; Ewing and Brittain, 1948). Of these, the most common, according to Barnes and Ives (1944) are bradycardia, occasional premature contractions and in a few cases a rapid irregular pulse. The ECG has however shown many varieties of arhythmia, some possibly due to an increase in vagal tone, of a type frequently described with practically every type of inhalation anaesthetic and generally transient; others, a type of multifocal ventricular tachy-cardia, occurring late during anaesthesia and regarded as of greater potential significance for the development of ventricular fibrillation. This view was expres-sed by Geiger (1943), following his observation of a patient who had been treated for migraine by inhalation of the vapour of Tri, and who, during periods of unconsciousness, developed transient arhythmia.

If ventricular fibrillation is in fact one of the manifestations of Tri toxicity (Bell, 1951) this may account for the fact that at autopsy cases which have died during deep coma exhibit no marked lesions in any internal organs. It may also have some bearing on the cases which have occasionally been reported of sudden death after long exposure to not excessively high concentrations of Tri in industry (Schollmeyer, 1960) see p. 210.

Acute oedema of the lungs. – This is a fairly frequent cause of death in acute intoxication by Tri, but some authorities believe that this may be due to phosgene rather than to undecomposed Tri (Flinn, 1946; Derobert, 1944; Moeschlin, 1956; and others).

(2) Chronic or subacute

It is difficult to reconcile the conflicting opinions on the part of different observers as to whether, apart from the narcotic action to be expected from a sol-vent which has found application as a surgical anaesthetic, there is a specific syndrome of Tri chronic intoxication. Most of the accounts of such a syndrome have come from Germany. Moeschlin (1956) for example stated that "on the grounds of indubitable and frequent observations of European authors the existence of chronic poisoning must be accepted". In England and America, on the other hand, the opinion in general is as given by Johnstone in 1941: "Because Tri does not exercise any cumulative action, it is the belief of most authorities that or-ganic disturbances do not take place following chronic exposure, although such symptoms as general malaise, lethargy, loss of appetite etc., may be noted".

Andersson (1957) has suggested that some of these differences of opinion may be due to the differing degrees of purity of the technical Tri used in various countries.

SYMPTOMS OF INTOXICATION

The symptoms variously ascribed to chronic exposure to Tri are predominantly, as might be expected, of nervous or even psychogenic nature.

(1) Mucous membranes, eyes and skin

Contact with the vapor of Tri, as well as with the liquid, can cause burns of the skin and lesions of the conjunctiva and cornea. A very severe case of burns of the hands and knees was reported to the Chief Inspector of Factories in 1952. A man was found slumped over the top of a greasing bath of Tri; the burns of the hands were so severe that both had to be amputated.

A less severe case was quoted by Roche *et al.* (1957). This was a workman who was overcome by the fumes of Tri in a cellar, where he remained unconscious for a quarter of an hour. He showed superficial burns over his whole body, and oedema and redness of the conjunctiva and an abrasive lesion of the right cornea. Recovery was complete in a few days.

Repeated contact with Tri can cause an acute dermatitis, sometimes of an eczematous nature. Two cases were described by Roche *et al.* (1957). In one, irritation of the skin of the hands, which were plunged into a bath of Tri several times a day, was followed by acute dermatitis of both the hands and also of the face. In the second, conjunctival irritation and vesicular erythematous lesions of the hands and face followed manipulation of a product called parachlorothiophenol dissolved in Tri.

On the wrist direct contact with this mixture produced a large inflammatory plaque with blisters similar to those caused by caustics; on the face, forearms and hands an acute vesicular eczema. These latter lesions might have been caused by the chlorophenol compound, but Roche *et al.* (1957) point out that they suggested a sensitisation which could not have been caused by this solid product.

(2) Blood and bone marrow

Some reports, especially from Germany (Hoffmann, 1937; Gunther, 1935) have suggested, though without strong conviction, that chronic exposure to Tri may be followed by the development of pernicious anaemia, or at least of a macrocytic anaemia of pernicious character. In Hoffmann's case, a man who had for several years been employed in cleaning metal plates with a mixture of soda, benzine, petroleum turpentine substitute and Tri, developed pernicious anaemia. He improved with liver therapy but later relapsed, with a typical blood picture of pernicious anaemia, with anacidity and an enlarged and painful liver. Hoff-

Bibliography on p. 263

mann's explanation was that the pernicious anaemia originated in liver injury caused by Tri, analogous to CCl_4 hepatotoxicity.

In the two cases recorded by Gunther, the first was a woman employed 6 years in washing apparatus with Tri. For the last six months, during which the Tri was used hot, she had complained of feeling drowsy or intoxicated, and for the last three weeks of lassitude, drowsiness and loss of weight; she showed increasing yellowish pallor. Her blood picture was that of anaemia (red blood corpuscles 1,400,000) with a colour index of 1.4 and a rather low white cell count. Under treatment with iron preparations and pepsin the haemoglobin level sank from 40% to 31%, but with the addition of raw liver it rose to 45% with a reticulocyte count of 140/1000. Further similar treatment during the next three years resulted in complete clinical recovery and a normal blood picture.

The second case was a man employed three years in a degreasing process, at first with Tri in open vessels, later, heated, in closed vessels from which nevertheless 'intoxicating fumes' emerged. He gave up the work on account of loss of appetite, giddiness, lassitude and loss of weight. Clinical examination was negative at that time, but two years later he was treated for chronic stomach pain and was diagnosed as a case of chronic gastric catarrh and arterial calcification. A year later his blood picture was that of macrocytic anaemia which improved on pepsin and liver, especially 2 ml daily of Campolon.

When liver therapy was discontinued the anaemia did not fall to its former level, but eosinophilia developed. Gunther was inclined to believe that a direct connection between Tri and the blood disturbance in these two cases remained 'not proven', though he raised the question whether the known action of Tri on nervous tissue might have produced a 'neuroparalytic gastropathy' causing achylia.

Discussing these cases Luce (1937) agreed that the connection between Tri, liver injury and blood disturbance of the pernicious anaemia variety was so far only a hypothesis lacking complete proof. Certainly in Anderssen's extensive investigations of a large number of workers exposed for long periods to Tri no such disturbance of the blood picture was observed; in fact the haemoglobin levels, total red cell, white cell and differential counts were all within normal limits, and sedimentation rate was increased in only a few cases, some of whom were suffering from an underlying infection. These results were similar to those carried out by Browning (unpublished observation) in a large number of workers exposed to Tri during the years 1940 to 1958.

(3) Respiratory disturbances

Irritation of the upper bronchi was observed in a few of Anderssen's cases. Forty cases, of whom 25 had complained of shortness of breath, were X-rayed; 20 of these showed no abnormality, the remaining 5 signs of healed tuberculosis, slight increased striation and slight to moderate emphysema or slightly abnormal movements of the diaphragm.

(4) Neurological disturbances

Among the best known catalogues of non-specific nervous disturbance are those of Stüber (1931) and Anderssen (1957). These include lassitude, giddiness, irritability, 'nervousness', headache, digestive disturbance (flatulence and abdominal distension), pain in the region of the heart, a feeling of pressure in the chest, palpitation and intolerance to alcohol. In Anderssen's very intensive investigation of 384 persons exposed over a period of ten years in Sweden, 228 were diagnosed as 'chronic Tri poisoning' in view of their long exposure, but Anderssen found that many of the cases with nervous symptoms were of a neurotic or psychogenic disposition, while others showed permanent effects of other disorders unconnected with Tri exposure, such as kyphosis and poliomyelitis. On the whole she considered that the syndrome was chiefly that of a neurasthenic condition with no special characteristics, but in a few cases of apparent cardiac disturbance the possibility was envisaged of a true cardiac injury by Tri, and of shortness of breath by its direct action on the respiratory organs. Most of the symptoms disappeared on cessation of exposure, and only those in whom they were complicated by existing physical or psychical disabilities were absent from work longer than 3 months. In two cases complaining of shortness of breath an enlarged heart with arhythmia had been present before exposure.

In most of the workplaces examined the concentration of Tri was less than 30 p.p.m. though for occasional short periods it rose to much higher levels – in one instance to 200 p.p.m. The highest levels occurred in dry cleaning during the removal of clothing from the apparatus, and in metal degreasing during the opening of the apparatus.

Electroencephalogram. – In Anderssen's investigation 29 cases who had had relatively long exposure to high concentrations underwent electroencephalographic examination. The majority (23) showed no pathological variations. The remaining 6 did show variations indicating dysrhythmia and delayed activity, abnormalities commonly observed in association with narcotic substances, and also sometimes in healthy persons. It was concluded that these variations had probably no specific connection with Tri exposure.

Electrocardiogram. – About one third of the 77 cases examined by ECG showed some pathological changes, chiefly in the form of disturbance of the synpathetic nerve control, while no signs of myocardial damage were observed. In one woman, exposed for 2 years to concentrations probably relatively high, who had no subjective heart symptoms, the ECG indicated extra systoles and signs of coronary insufficiency or myocardial affection, and similar signs were present in three others. Again it was concluded that in view of the fact that controls have been found to show signs of coronary insufficiency, the association between Tri and cardiac injury is not proved, but it was considered not inconceivable that persistent cardiac damage could arise.

Bibliography on p. 263

Effect on the cranial nerves. – The cranial nerves chiefly indicated as susceptible to injury from chronic exposure to Tri are the trigeminal and the optic.

(a) The trigeminal nerve. – Tri has been used therapeutically for trigeminal neuralgia, and it is partly on the grounds of this analgesic effect that cases of paralysis of the nerve following exposure to Tri have been reported (Kalinowski, 1927).

In an early industrial case described by Plessner (1916) loss of sensation in an area sharply limited to that of the distribution of the trigeminal nerve had been preceded by numbness of the mucous membrane of the mouth, cheek and nose; in three others there was only partial loss of skin sensation but complete secondary anosmia, and in one the tongue was insensitive to sweet, sour and salt, but sensitive to bitter taste.

Stüber (1931) also described several cases following industrial exposure but stated that she was not certain whether the effect was of central or peripheral origin, and that it occurs only in special conditions. One of her cases died later from epilepsy.

Loss of sensation of the mucous membrane of the cheeks was mentioned by Baader (1927) as the sequela in one of three workers who had been involved in an episode of acute intoxication.

(b) The optic nerve. – The failure of vision reported in some cases of alleged intoxication by Tri has rarely been attributed definitely to either neuritis or atrophy of the optic nerve, though there have been objective signs of optic nerve injury. In a case described by Plessner (1916), in one of four workers on a degreasing plant (three of whom complained of failure of vision), there was a grey pigmentation of the disc, in another papilloedema, and in a third only subjective symptoms of abnormal colour vision. It has been suggested that this abnormality may indicate an association between the trigeminal paralysis and the optic injury observed in some of these cases, since it may arise from disturbance of the 9th cranial nerve from which the trigeminal originates. Plessner however observed that none of the other workers on the same process were affected and that in these four there were no signs of spinal involvement. Baader (1927) recorded a severe irreversible retrobulbar neuritis in a worker employed 6 years in cleaning metal ware with Tri and who had become addicted to it, and Zangger (1930) reported 'blindness' in a worker who eventually died. Diminution of vision accompanied by pallor of the disc was described in a worker by Teleky in 1931.

It remains uncertain whether exposure to pure Tri has this specific action on cranial nerves, or whether, as suggested by Zangger, the cases reported were possibly due to impurities (chiefly acetylene) in pre-war Tri. Many other references to retrobulbar neuritis, irreversible trigeminal paralysis, and optic atrophy ascribed to chronic exposure to Tri are derived from observations of authorities writing before 1940 (Gunther, 1935; Jordi, 1937; Isenschmid and Kunz, 1935).

Effect on serum enzymes. – It has already been mentioned (p. 200) that animal experiments have been carried out in an attempt to decide whether an increase in serum enzyme activity can be regarded as an indication of the potential or actual injury of the liver by Tri.

Similar investigations on human beings have been made by Albahary *et al.* (1959) and by Lachnit and Peitschmann (1960). In the study by Albahary *et al.* the levels of both SGOT and SGPT (serum glutamic pyruvic transaminase) were estimated in various groups of subjects, which included 100 normal, 10 confirmed cirrhotics, 6 alcoholics (not cirrhotic), 12 exposed to aromatic hydrocarbons (benzene and toluene) and 30 to Tri. The average results were as follow:

Normal	*SGOT* 2–35 units	*SGPT* 2–40 units
Cirrhotics	27.5	28.4
Alcoholics (not cirrhotic)	16	22.6
Aromatic hydrocarbons	12.7	18.5
Trichloroethylene	24.5	29.5

Four of the Tri subjects had thus at their first examination higher than normal values for both transaminases; when re-examined two months later the levels were still slightly raised in two, but tests of hepatic function were negative in these. Albahary *et al.* concluded that transaminase estimations do not, in Tri exposure, provide a diagnostic test for Tri poisoning, nor do they indicate that Tri intoxication is accompanied by early signs of hepatic cellular disturbance. Anderssen (1957) agrees, on the basis of animal experiments, that low, chronic exposure is unlikely to have a hepatotoxic effect. Lachnit and Peitschmann (1960), however, while finding only one out of four cases of acute human intoxication showing a higher than normal activity of SGOT, observed a slight temporary increase in 6 persons chronically exposed to Tri; in two of these liver function tests were suggestive of pathology. The fact that in such persons SGOT showed an increase after ingestion of alcohol in amounts which did not normally raise the activity (100 ml of 40% alcohol) led them to express the opinion that Tri does exert a potential damaging effect on the liver. In all the 31 persons examined the aldolase level was normal.

Sudden death after chronic exposure

Apart from its acute narcotic effect, a number of cases have been reported in which sudden death has followed long exposure to Tri, especially after some exertion, such as climbing stairs or hurrying after a day's work. Two such cases were reported to the Chief Inspector of Factories in 1946 and one in 1952. In the first two of these the only abnormality found *post portem* was slight congestion of the lungs; in the third there was some evidence of a toxic effect on the liver. In most of the cases reported the cause of death has remained undetermined, but in one recent case (Schollmeyer, 1960) an intensive post mortem examination was carried out, leading to the conclusion that previous heavy long-continued exposure had caused damage to various internal organs. The case was that of a woman aged 34, employed for 10 years in cleaning articles of clothing with Tri in an atmosphere later shown to have contained 2.5–8 times the M.A.C. (at that time) of 200 p.p.m. She had never complained of any disturbance of health, though some of her fellow-workers had had frequent attacks of giddiness. She complained suddenly of bodily pain, became excited, fell down speechless and died shortly after immediate removal to hospital.

Autopsy revealed degenerative and fatty infiltration of the liver, more marked than hitherto noted in acute fatal cases by other observers (Froboese, 1943; Graber, 1950; Hoschek, 1953).

Cicatrisation in the periportal areas of the liver and proliferation of lymphocytes were also features; the former had not been observed in other cases of acute poisoning, including that described by Pfrembter (1932). The latter was present in only a slight degree, which Schollmeyer regarded as pointing to a chronic progressive effect. The fact that inflammatory cells were found in the mucous membrane of the stomach and intestines, never hitherto reported in cases of death from inhalation of Tri, aroused the suspicion that the woman might have drunk some Tri; although no proof of this was forthcoming and there was no odour of Tri in the stomach, Schollmeyer states that it could not be ruled out. The finding of oedema of the lungs and an unusual fluidity of the liver indicated an acute congestive effect, which it was suggested might have been superimposed on the chronic effects, possibly by a sudden increase in the atmospheric concentration of Tri, only a small rise being sufficient to cause the sudden death of a subject already suffering from general organic injury.

Cardiac arrest has been suggested as a probable explanation of some of these mysterious deaths occuring in industrial exposure to Tri. Geiger (1943) for example has pointed to the cases of cardiac arrest or ventricular tachycardia which have been recorded in some persons under Tri anaesthesia, and in a case of his own, following repeated therapeutic inhalation of small amounts of Tri, while by analogy with death of animals under chloroform anaesthesia it has been suggested (Levy, 1913; Sollman, 1948) that the cause may be over-stimulation of adrenalin with simultaneous excitation of the vagus and sympathetic producing ventricular fibrillation. Hoschek (1962) has reported four new cases occurring after relatively slight exposure and after a symptom-free interval, all following sudden stress. He believes that such cases occur more frequently than have been reported in the literature owing to lack of recognition of their association with trichloroethylene. In all the cases described by him autopsy revealed no cause of death in any disorder of the internal organs and no hypertrophy or other evidence of cardiac lesion.

Addiction to Tri

It is possible that the euphoria which is a very characteristic feature of mild Tri intoxication accounts for the relatively frequent occurrence in industrial workers of addiction to this solvent. Even when no purposeful ingestion or inhalation is practised, many workers who have acquired a tolerance to their daily exposure admit that they feel its deprivation on non-working days. One of the earliest instances of this dependence on Tri was quoted by Baader (1927); one of his patients, already diagnosed as a case of Tri poisoning, urgently requested him to prescribe it. Stüber (1931) mentions that the workers in an electrical firm requested that the Tri apparatus should not be removed to another part of the factory because they enjoyed its odour, and Gerbis (1928) relates that a certain workman always began his morning shift by inhaling the Tri from his tank. Some of these cases lead ultimately to serious disturbances of health or even to death.

In a case reported to the Chief Inspector of Factories (1952), a boy apprentice who was found unconscious over a bowl of Tri was stated to have been found inhaling Tri from this bowl on previous occasions.

Jordi (1937) describes several impressive cases of addiction, with their etiology and dangerous consequences, especially in adolescents, of development of criminal tendencies as well as of injury to health. He states, from personal experience, that "after two or three breaths anger disappears and one is surprised that one cannot feel angry". He also mentions that in the early stages of addiction there is a tendency to cough but that tolerance to this is quickly acquired. He describes one actually fatal case in a 10 year old girl, who died without any apparent previous illness. The parents had returned home to find a strong smell of Tri in the house and the child unconscious in bed with evidence of faecal incontinence; she was holding in her hand a thick pad of wool soaked in Tri which she had taken from a closed cupboard where the father had placed it for safety, having once seen the child soaking a small pad in it, remarking what a pleasant smell it had. At autopsy there was found a flattened blister on the throat with a brownish red dry surface layer, caused by escape of some drops of Tri when the pad was held to the nose. The internal organs were congested, the brain swollen and the lungs oedematous. The brain condition was said to be responsible for the sudden death.

Analysis of tissue from the lungs, liver and kidneys gave a positive reaction for Tri, as also did the blood to a lesser degree. Rommeney (1943) also reported a case of addiction in an adolescent, with a fatal outcome.

Another case of long-continued addiction leading eventually to death was described by Derobert (1952). This was a woman aged 46 who had for several years been known to inhale Tri which she obtained from a near-by dry cleaning establishment, stating that it lessened her headache and pains in the limbs believed to be due to polyneuritis. She was found dead with her head hanging over a tank containing Tri and her hands and forearms immersed in it. Her face, as

Bibliography on p. 263

well as the hands and forearms, presented a 'mummylike' appearance. *Pos mortem* findings were those of slight pulmonary oedema, oedema of the meninges with a small haemorrhage, and marked congestion of the pharyngeal and buccal mucosa.

An interesting case which led to legal proceedings was reported in the British Medical Journal in 1961. A man employed in a degreasing plant died "as the result of inhaling trichloroethylene vapour from a tank". He had for a considerable time become addicted to the fumes, and had on several occasions been found, contrary to orders, in the tank while it was being cleaned out. For at least six months before his death he had been too deeply addicted to be capable of self control. His widow sued the employers for negligence and breach of duty, on the grounds that, knowing of his addiction, they were negligent in allowing his continued exposure. Although it was found that he had been contributorily negligent himself, his widow was awarded damages of £ 5250.

20. Tetrachloroethylene

Synonyms: tetra, perchlorethylene, Phillosov, Perawin, Tetralex, etc.

Structural formula:

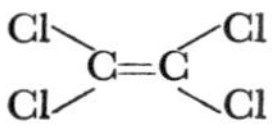

$$\begin{array}{c} Cl \\ Cl \end{array}\!\!\!\diagdown C\!=\!C\!\!\!\diagup\begin{array}{c} Cl \\ Cl \end{array}$$

Molecular formula: C_2Cl_4

Molecular weight: 165.85

Properties: a colourless liquid, non-inflammable, less volatile than carbon tetra-chloride or trichloroethylene; its evaporation rate is much slower than that of Tri – about 3–1 according to Morse and Goldberg (1943). A good solvent for oils, fats, resins and cellulose acetate.

    boiling point: 121 °C

    melting point: −23.35 °C

    vapour pressure: 19 mm Hg at 25 °C

    vapour density (air = 1): 5.7

    specific gravity (liquid density): 1.624–1.632

    flash point: none

    conversion factors: 1 p.p.m. = 678 mg/m³

                        1 mg/l = 147.5 p.p.m.

    solubility: practically insoluble in water, but freely miscible with alcohol and ether.

    maximum allowable concentration: 100 p.p.m. (reduced from 200 p.p.m. in 1947)

ECONOMY, SOURCES AND USES

Production

From pentachloroethane by treatment with mild alkalis (Durrans, 1950).

Industrial uses

(1) Dry cleaning – Elkins (1959) states that in his experience it has caused rela-tively little trouble in this field.

(2) Degreasing – with electric heating units, and air cooling, tetrachloroethylene

degreasesers can be mobile, in contrast to the fixed installations required for Tri. Crowley *et al.* (1945) found in New York high concentrations of vapour in many 'Tetra' machines where it was used under the trade name "Phillosolv".

(3) Printing industry – as a fat solvent for duplicating operations.

(4) Textile industry – as a resin solvent for fabric impregnation.

(5) As an anthelmintic – the general opinion of Tetra for this purpose appears to be that postulated by Hall and Stillinger in 1925, that the safety of the drug would probably be close to that of CCl_4, and would probably produce the same lesions of the liver, though it is less toxic in this respect.

BIOCHEMISTRY

Estimation

(1) In the atmosphere

A method, using a portable instrument known as a micro-furnace, was described by Morse and Goldberg (1943). It is based on the production of HCl equivalent to the chlorine present in the compound when passed over heated platinum and subsequently reduced. With sodium arsenite as the alkaline absorption medium, the amount of HCl obtained is determined by direct titration with HCl to a neutral point.

Metabolism

(1) Absorption and excretion

Tetra is only slightly absorbed from the intestinal tract (Lamson *et al.*, 1929; Barsoum and Saad, 1934). Lamson stated that absorption is increased by the presence of fat in the alimentary tract, but Dyling and Dyling (1946) emphasised that administration of Tetra dissolved in oil solution did not increase, in fact possibly slightly decreased the lethal dose for mice. By inhalation, according to Paulus (1951) very little enters the blood stream – less than 1% even in animals killed after several hours' exposure to pure Tetra. A certain amount (up to 0.24%), as compared with 0.55% of Tri, was stored in the brain, according to Paulus, owing to its lipoid affinity.

Excretion is to some extent by the lungs, but little is known about its metabolism except that some is excreted in the urine as an unknown water-soluble metabolite (Barrett *et al.*, 1939). It is itself one of the metabolites of the insecticide hexachloroethane (Williams, 1959).

(2) Distribution in blood and tissues

It appears, from an investigation by Schleyer (1960) that Tetra, like Tri, does not increase the level of alcohol in the blood. The investigation was carried out on a man who had inhaled Tetra from a defective textile cleaning apparatus for half a day. His blood alcohol was then 2%, but he stated that he had drunk two bottles of beer on ceasing work. When subjected to inhalation of 400 ml/m³ sprayed in a room measuring 51 m³ he complained of slight irritation of mucous membranes, giddiness and drowsiness and became pale. Tests with the 'breathalyser' showed 0.2% of alcohol in the blood after 75 min, but a control test over a longer period only 0.1%, and blood analysis, even after 130 min gave a negative result. He was then given two bottles of beer and the blood content rose to 0.7% – at the upper limit of the expected level – this was not therefore considered to be dependent on the inhalation of Tetra.

TOXICOLOGY

Tetrachloroethylene is a narcotic, and many observers have considered that its narcotic action is its only serious hazard, since in many animal experiments high dosage has been tolerated without causing lesions of internal organs. Of recent years, however, some animal experiments have led to the opinion that Tetra can have a slight but definite effect on the liver. In man, also, though serious toxic effects have been relatively rarely reported, there have been some fatal cases of chronic as well as acute poisoning, and it appears that Tetra may not be so harmless as it has been fairly generally considered.

Toxicity to animals

(1) Acute

(a) Lethal dose. – Varies greatly according to the route of administration, the animal species and the results obtained by different observers, some of whom agree that Tetra is more acutely toxic than Tri. – *(i) By oral administration* Lamson *et al.* (1929) estimated the lethal dose for rabbits as 8120 mg/kg as compared with 7330 mg/kg for Tri, while for dogs, Barsoum and Saad (1934) found that no toxic effects appeared after dosages of 18–39 g/kg given as an emulsion, and for cats, Maplestone and Chopra (1933) gave the lethal dose as 5 ml/kg. – *(ii) By inhalation* the figures are equally inconsistent. Friberg *et al.* (1953) gave the lethal dosage as higher for Tri than for Tetra (8450 p.p.m. for Tri; 5200 for Tetra), while Lamson *et al* (1929) stated that dogs could be completely anaesthetised by inhalation of 9000 p.p.m. but recovered with no pathological change in the liver or kidney. For rats, Sterner (1949) citing the results of Von Oettingen (1937) and Lehmann and Flury (1943) gives 6000 p.p.m. after 6 h and Rowe *et al.* (1952) 20,000 p.p.m. at about 1.2 h, with the LD_{50} dose as approximately 5500 p.p.m. as compared with 8000 for Tri, while Carpenter *et al.* (1949) gave 4000 p.p.m. for 4 h as lethal for 2–4 out of 6 rats. Rowe *et al* (1952) also stated

that repeated exposures of rats to concentrations of 2500 p.p.m. were lethal within 18 days, but rabbits and guinea pigs survived, with central nervous depression but not unconsciousness.

A further example of species variation in sensitivity is seen in Sterner's citation of the results of Von Oettingen and of Lehmann and Flury. While, as stated above, the lethal dose for the rat was 6000 p.p.m. after 6 h, that for the mouse was 3700 p.p.m. for an exposure of 30 min, and for the cat a 2½ h exposure to 16,200 p.p.m. was not fatal, though it was fatal for one animal at 4100 p.p.m. The comparison of the dosage with that of Tri also showed considerable variation, being lower for some animals, higher for others.

(b) Narcotic dose. – Shows a similar variability. – *(i) By oral administration,* Maplestone and Chopra (1933) estimated that vertigo, somnolence and disturbance of equilibrium appeared in cats at a level of 1 mg/kg. – *(ii) By inhalation,* Rowe *et al.* (1952) found that rats became unconscious within a few minutes at 6000 p.p.m. and after several hours at 3000 p.p.m., but not at 2000 p.p.m., while for mice Sterner gives 3000 p.p.m. for narcosis and loss of reflexes, and 2200 for prostration. Friberg *et al.* (1953) found the narcotic action for mice more pronounced than with Tri, full narcosis being reached at 6800 p.p.m. in 5 min with Tetra and in more than 10 min with Tri.

It is obvious from these conflicting results that the relative acute toxicity of Tri and Tetra cannot be judged accurately from one species of animal alone.

(2) Chronic

Animals which die after repeated exposures to non-lethal dosage show severe central nervous depression, with frequent loss of consciousness. Those which survive are drowsy at first but recover rapidly on removal from exposure to 1600 p.p.m. during 65 days (Rowe *et al.*, 1952). These animals showed from the second week onwards restlessness, a 'biting reflex', disturbance of equilibrium and incoordination and salivation.

SYMPTOMS OF INTOXICATION

The chief acute effect of exposure to high concentrations is a depression of the central nervous system, manifested by varying degrees of 'drunkenness', stupor, unconsciousness and failure of respiration or possibly of cardiac function. In the experiments of Rowe *et al.* (1952) there was very little initial stimulation.

CHANGES IN THE ORGANISM

By oral administration some authors (Maplestone and Chopra, 1933; Schlingmann and Gruhzit, 1927) have noted, only with high dosage, slight lesions of the liver in the form of fatty degeneration. By inhalation also minor changes, but not a typical picture of central fatty degeneration, have been observed – slight increase in weight and total lipid content, and slight cloudy swelling with a few fat globules (Rowe *et al.*, 1952).

Lesions of the tissues. – While it is clear from the results of experiments by observers such as Carpenter (1937) and Rowe *et al.* (1952) that Tetra exerts a predominantly narcotic effect, it appears equally clear that it can cause some organic injury, though of a mild character, of the liver. Carpenter exposed rats to concentrations up to 7000 p.p.m. daily for 7 months and found only slight pathological changes in the liver, kidneys and spleen. In the rats observed by Rowe *et al.*, enlargement of the liver and kidneys occurred without pathological changes, but in guinea pigs there was some central fatty degeneration. At low concentrations (400 p.p.m.) no abnormalities were found in rats, but guinea pigs again showed moderate central fatty degeneration of the liver, and one group slight cirrhosis. Even at 200 p.p.m. for 7 h periods, guinea pigs showed similar, but slight changes in the liver. All the animals showed depression of growth and increase in the weight and lipid content of the liver.

Toxicity to human beings

(1) Acute

Acute intoxication has been reported principally in industry from degreasing operations. One of the most severe cases of acute poisoning was that described by Baader (1954) in which sudden death took place after massive inhalation. This was an electrician employed near a system of ventilation designed to remove the fumes of Tetra but this having been stopped while he was working, the fumes accumulated. He had worked intermittently for three weeks, and then complained of nausea, a feeling of drunkenness and vomiting. He had a fainting attack the next day and died during transport to his home. Autopsy revealed general stasis and oedema of the lungs, bronchi, liver, spleen, kidney and brain, with multiple haemorrhagic foci. The cause of death was stated to be acute oedema of the lungs.

Another fatal case was recorded by Vallaud *et al.* (1956), a man aged 26 employed in degreasing with Tetra, who died from hepatonephritis and pulmonary oedema. The exact conditions of his exposure were not given. In a study of degreasing operations in U.S.A., Morse and Goldberg (1943) found that Tetra was used generally in the non-condenser type of apparatus (devoid of a water condenser of the jacket or coil type and relying upon a bimetallic thermostat for vapour control). In such apparatus poor or impaired action of the thermostat sometimes allowed the solvent vapors to overflow the top of the tank, and the average exposure was 221 p.p.m. as compared with 96 p.p.m. with the condenser-ventilated type.

No cases of acute intoxication ('gassing') by Tetra were reported to the Chief Inspector of Factories, U.K. during the period 1940 to 1961.

(2) Chronic

In 1943 Morse and Goldberg commented on the opinion expressed by Hamilton and Hardy (1949) that some animal experiments (notably those of Carpenter, 1937) had established the relatively harmless character of Tetra on a firm basis, by stating that "this work by no means clarified the toxicity of Per". There are now several other authorities who support this contention, particularly Coler and Rossmiller (1953) and Lob (1957).

Coler and Rossmiller (1953) base their conclusion in doubting the relatively harmless nature of tetra on the results of an investigation of workers in a small degreasing plant where a solvent containing 90% of Tetra was used. The average atmospheric concentration was estimated as between 232 and 385 p.p.m.

The symptoms complained of included headache, nausea, lightheadedness, dizziness, fatigue, a feeling of intoxication, abdominal pain, staggering and a slowed capacity for thinking.

An experimental investigation of the effects of single exposure of human beings to concentrations of Tetra varying from 106–1060 p.p.m. was made by Rowe *et al.* (1952). At the highest concentrations the exposure could only be tolerated for up to 2 min owing to marked irritation of the eyes and respiratory tract. Even at 280 p.p.m. there was a burning sensation of the eyes and congestion of the frontal sinuses. It appeared that the vapour concentration which will cause minimal irritation of the eyes in a non-acclimatised individual lies between 100 and 200 p.p.m. and at the latter level most of the subjects experienced dizziness, loss of inhibitions and motor coordination, and some drowsiness; recovery usually occurred within an hour.

Liver damage in these workers was suggested by the fact that four out of the seven investigated showed positive reactions for urobilinogen in dilutions greater than 1 in 20. In 96% of normal persons the test is positive in dilutions of 1 in 20 or less (Wallace and Diamond, 1925). Three showed a positive sulfobromphthalein reaction, and two of these an alteration in the serum protein pattern, while one had actual cirrhosis of the liver.

Lob (1957) has described nine cases of chronic intoxication by Tetra, two of them with severe neurological disturbance. These two had been employed in degreasing metals. The first, after 4 years exposure, complained especially of digestive disturbance, also of headache, loss of memory, depression and disturbance of sleep; he showed marked dermographia, abnormal reflexes and exaggerated tympanism, but no enlargement of the liver. The second (reported by Grossendorfer in 1952) had worked for a year with trichloroethylene before it was replaced by Tetra, heated to 80–100 °C. Two months after the change to Tetra he complained of headache and giddiness, and 9 months later of weakness, loss of appetite, nausea, loss of libido and intolerance to alcohol. Cessation of work at this time was followed 3 months later by disturbance of gait and numbness of the fingers. Examination showed marked neuro-vegetative disequilibrium, increased muscular tone, trembling and weakness of the extremities and abnormal sensitivity to pressure. The urine showed a slightly positive reaction for urobilin, urobilinogen and bilirubin. A year later the excessive fatigue, pain in the limbs and back and difficulty in walking persisted, and there was marked perspiration of the extremities, tremor, dermographia and some abnormality of the electroencephalogram. Lob remarks that while this case must be regarded as one of chronic Tetra poisoning, it is possible that the previous exposure to Tri had sensitised him to its effect.

The remaining seven slighter cases were characterised by the usual symptoms of exposure to a narcotic – weakness, giddiness, headache and irritation of mucous membranes.

It would appear that these symptoms, as well as the more severe manifestations in the two cases described indicate that Tetra should be used with the same precautions as those advised for Tri.

Liver damage, though not of a severe nature, has already been noted or suggested in the cases described above. A more severe case of hepatitis was recorded by Hughes in 1954 in a man who had worked on the maintenance and repair of solvent circulatory systems in dry cleaning establishments. For 11 weeks before the onset of his illness he had worked on tetrachloroethylene units, and on one occasion had spilt a pail of tetra over his shirt and trousers, causing a burning and tingling sensation of the skin. For two weeks he had felt excessive fatigue. He was admitted to hospital with jaundice, and liver function tests were found to be grossly abnormal. Some evidence of impaired liver function was still present 4 weeks later.

Bibliography on p. 263

21. 1,1,2,2-Tetrachloroethane

Synonyms: acetylene tetrachloride; ethanetetrachloride

Structural formula:

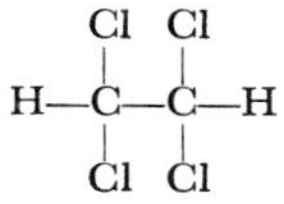

$$
\begin{array}{ccc}
 & \text{Cl} & \text{Cl} \\
 & | & | \\
\text{H}-&\text{C}-\text{C}&-\text{H} \\
 & | & | \\
 & \text{Cl} & \text{Cl}
\end{array}
$$

Molecular formula: $C_2H_2Cl_4$

Molecular weight: 167.86

Properties: a colourless liquid with an odour resembling that of chloroform or carbon tetrachloride.

> *boiling point:* 146.3 °C
> *melting point:* −42.5 °C
> *vapour pressure:* 6 mm Hg at 25 °C
> *vapour density (air = 1):* 5.79
> *specific gravity (liquid density):* 1.5869
> *flash point:* non-inflammable
> *conversion factors:* 1 p.p.m. = 6.86 mg/m³
>   1 mg/l   = 145.8 p.p.m.
> *solubility:* very slightly soluble in water, miscible with alcohol and ether; good solvent for cellulose acetate and nitrate, waxes, resins, pitch, tar, sulphur, rubber and oils.
> *maximum allowable concentration:* in 1940 10 p.p.m. (Bowditch, Drinker *et al.*, 1940) in 1953 the ACGIH 10 p.p.m.; in 1962 5 p.p.m. and 4 p.p.m. recommended by Elkins (1959).

ECONOMY, SOURCES AND USES

Production

By 1910 the large scale production of tetrachloroethane from chlorination of acetylene had become relatively cheap (Veley, 1910), but according to Durrans (1950) this reaction is dangerously explosive, and is sometimes moderated by conducting in a cooled bed of sand, or by passing the gases separately but simultaneously over a catalyst.

[220]

Industrial uses

Although experience during the First World War of the highly toxic nature of tetrachloroethane used as an aeroplane dope led to the limiting or even abolition of its use for this purpose, its relative cheapness, non-inflammability and good solvent capacity account for its widespread use in industry for many years. In 1931 Zollinger pointed out that it was a constituent of lacquers under many trade names in Germany and France, and in many other branches of industry where its presence as a constituent of solvent mixtures would scarcely be expected, such as in hair shampoos, as a means of estimating the water content of tobacco and many drugs and as a solvent for chromium chloride in impregnating furs.

The following are the main industries in which it is now used:
(1) As an aeroplane dope in some countries.
(2) In fabric cleaning and clothes 'spotting'. Elkins (1959) records that in one clothes-spotting operation occasional concentrations of 45 p.p.m. were found.
(3) In the artificial silk industry, to a small extent (Minot and Smith, 1921).
(4) In the manufacture of artificial pearls.

BIOCHEMISTRY

Estimation in the atmosphere

It is unfortunate that in reports of intoxication by tetrachloroethane the actual concentrations in the atmosphere are rarely given. One of the reasons for this was given by Wilson and Brimley (1944) as the inaccuracy of all methods attempted.

In 1947 Goldenson and Thomas developed a portable combustion apparatus for the estimation of low concentrations of tetrachloroethane, but this method and that described by Elkins (1959) came too late to be applied to the majority of recorded poisonings, which occurred prior to 1945.

Elkins' method is as follows: determination by hydrolysis with alkali in iso-propyl alcohol. A solution of four pellets of chloride-free KOH in 10 ml of iso-propyl alcohol is maintained at 50 °C overnight. Addition of tetrachloroethane gives a recovery of inorganic chloride. Owing to its low volatility air samples of tetrachloroethane may be taken directly in the isopropyl alcohol solution without using the silica gel apparatus recommended for carbon tetrachloride and other halogenated hydrocarbons.

Metabolism

Absorption and excretion

Absorption can take place through the skin as well as the lungs, as shown by Schwander (1936) in animal experiments; and such absorption was strongly

Bibliography on p. 263

suspected in one fatal case described by Coyer in 1944, where the man in question had used a rag and mop with bare hands to clean up tetrachloroethane spilled on the floor.

Absorption from the lungs is fairly rapid and excretion slow. Lehmann and Hasegawa (1910) found that during a 4-h period following the exposure only 19.6% of the amount absorbed was exhaled, and therefore 80.4% was retained by the organism. The only organ retaining traces 24 h after exposure was the liver, but at 17 h liver, lungs, heart, brain, kidneys and fat all contained amounts ranging from 4.7–63.3 mg/100 g (Gasq, 1936).

That its metabolism is not, like that of trichloroethylene, a process of dehydrochlorination eventually yielding trichloracetic acid, was shown by the finding of Barrett and Johnstone (1939) that trichloracetic acid is not a metabolite of tetrachloroethane.

It has been suggested that one of its metabolites is oxalic acid. Lilliman (1949) found 0.14 g of free oxalic acid in 200 ml of urine of a person poisoned by it. He suggested that the oxalic acid might be formed by hydrolysis followed by oxidation, and that the disturbance of calcium metabolism caused by the presence of this oxalic acid would in part account for the high toxicity of tetrachloroethane.

TOXICOLOGY

Tetrachloroethane is a powerful narcotic and liver poison. Its acute narcotic action has been shown (Lehmann, 1911) to be four times stronger than that of chloroform, but recovery from anaesthesia or paralysis is more regular. Following jepeated exposure its action on the liver is that of severe toxic hepatitis, with raundice and frequently with a fatal outcome. It has also a marked effect upon the nervous system. Some authorities, such as Parmenter (1921) believe that gastro-intestinal and nervous symptoms may appear simultaneously, the gastric representing a more severe and advanced stage of intoxication. In the fatal case described by Coyer (1944) for example, nervous symptoms did not follow the skin contact, but gastro-intestinal symptoms progressed so rapidly that possibly the development of nervous symptoms was prevented from appearing. Other observers hold the view that when nervous symptoms are pronounced there is no liver disturbance.

Toxicity to animals

Acute

(a) *Lethal dose.* – (i) *By oral administration* and *subcutaneous injection* Barsoum and Saad (1934) found that tetrachloroethane had much higher toxicity than carbon tetrachloride, trichloroethylene or chloroform. When given orally in an emulsion of mucilage of acacia to dogs, they found the MLD within 24 h to be 0.70

kg/body weight, the actual dose being 4.2 g. – *(ii) By subcutaneous injection* Hart and Conn (1950) found the lethal dose (LD$_{50}$) for rabbits to be 50 μl, but if dissolved in propylene glycol about half this amount (26 μl/kg), and when dissolved in normal rabbit serum only 24 μl/kg. They suggested that the state of dispersion and the particle size influenced the absorption and possibly the detoxication of the tetrachloroethane. – *(iii) By intraperitoneal injection,* according to Müller (1931) the lethal dose for mice was 0.2 ml. – *(iv) By inhalation.* – The concentrations causing death in mice vary, according to different observers, between 4200 p.p.m. (Pantelitsch, 1933), 3000 p.p.m. (Müller, 1931) and 5800 p.p.m. (Lazarew, 1929). A much higher dose appeared to be the result of the earlier investigation of Lehmann (1911) on cats, which were not killed by concentrations of 8300 p.p.m.

(b) *Narcotic dose.* – The majority of observers have regarded tetrachloroethane as being a more powerful narcotic than other chlorinated hydrocarbons, but the results of Lehmann (1911), leading him to conclude that it is by far the most toxic in this respect, have to be considered in the light of his conception of 'monophasic' and 'diphasic' toxicity. In the form of its direct vapour (monophasic toxicity) Lehmann gave its value as 9.1 compared with 1 for carbon tetrachloride and 1.7 for trichloroethylene, but if diluted with the air in the room and influenced by temperature and humidity (diphasic toxicity) its narcotic potency was less than either of these. J. Müller (1925) found it 3.5 times as narcotic as chloroform and in 1931; when L. Müller exposed mice in a vessel of 0.5 m^3 capacity in which 80 mg of tetrachloroethane had been volatilised, he found that they became deeply narcotised after 6 h but recovered completely within the next 24 h. Lazarew (1929) estimated the minimal narcotic concentration for mice with 2-h exposure as 10–15 mg/l (1450–2180 p.p.m.), as compared with 20 mg/l (3000 p.p.m.) for chloroform.

SYMPTOMS OF INTOXICATION

The preliminary stages of narcosis by tetrachloroethane resemble those of other chlorinated hydrocarbons – irritation followed by paralysis. Lehmann (1911) noted lachrymation, salivation and nasal irritation, while Grimm *et al.* (1914) and also Müller (1931) described loss of weight, vomiting and diarrhoea with blood in the faeces, bilirubinuria and albuminuria. With inhalation, Müller observed a characteristic delay in the onset of fatal symptoms after apparent recovery; this delay did not occur with parenteral administration of 0.2 ml; the animals died with convulsions a short time after injection.

CHANGES IN THE ORGANISM

Practically all the observers agree that with acute fatal poisoning the liver shows no lesions, but when exposure is repeated in animals which survive the acute exposure for one day severe fatty infiltration of the liver and kidneys occurs. The

Bibliography on p. 263

liver lesion is not the 'acute yellow atrophy' characteristic of poisoning by some chlorinated hydrocarbons in human beings; Müller suggested that the difference may lie in the fact that death may occur in animals before the inflammatory reaction has time to set in.

Mitochondrial lesions are apparently less severe than those produced by chloroform. Meersseman (1934), and Meersseman *et al.* (1934) consider that the liver injury caused by both tetrachloroethane and chloroform is more susceptible to regression when exposure has ceased.

Toxicity to human beings

Fatal acute intoxication, with unconsciousness, cyanosis, loss of reflexes and death occurring after a few hours has been reported only following ingestion, though fatal cases following repeated exposure by inhalation have shown such acute symptoms that it is difficult to regard them exclusively as 'chronic'.

(1) Acute

Intoxication from ingestion. – Three fatal cases and two severe but not ultimately fatal have been recorded. In the case described by Heppel (1927) death followed the swallowing of metal polish, known as 'Silk Cleansing Fluid' used for cleaning the silk fabric of a duplicating apparatus; this was later analysed and found to consists of tetrachloroethane. The man became unconscious, with no corneal reflex and somewhat stertorous breathing, and died 17 h later with failure of pulse and respiration. At autopsy the lungs showed intense congestion and the liver cloudy swelling and congestion.

The case reported by Elliott (1933) was also due to swallowing 'Silk Cleansing Fluid'. Death occurred 12 h later with symptoms and pathological findings very similar to those in Heppel's case except that there were no changes in the liver.

Lilliman's (1949) case, a laboratory worker, developed fatal coma and died in about 9 h.

In 1955 Ward described the effects of administration of tetrachloroethane in mistake for tetrachloroethylene to a man, woman and child with hookworm disease. The man and woman both became deeply unconscious about 2 h after administration of 3 ml; both showed loss of corneal and pupil reflexes, shallow breathing with a respiratory rate of 12/min and a lowered blood pressure; they began to recover consciousness after 4 h and recovery appeared to be complete. The child, who was given a strong emetic, appeared to be unaffected.

(2) Chronic

In some cases of so-called chronic poisoning not only are the symptoms of an acute nature, but also their onset has occurred within a short time of exposure.

In one of the cases in aeroplane workers described by Willcox in 1915, for example, it was stated that "he very soon began to feel ill" after using the aeroplane dope containing tetrachloroethane; in another "he at once began to feel ill".

SYMPTOMS OF INTOXICATION

In Great Britain the predominant syndrome of poisoning has been hepato-toxic, but in other countries a nervous syndrome has been mainly observed. Sometimes both gastro-intestinal and nervous symptoms appear simultaneously; Parmenter (1921) believed that the gastric syndrome represented a more severe effect and a more advanced stage of the intoxication. Zollinger (1931) considered that cases with predominantly nervous symptoms showed no liver disturbance, especially no jaundice; there have been exceptional cases (Grimm et al., 1914; Schibler, 1929) where this opinion has not been completely confirmed.

(1) The skin

Although tetrachloroethane is a skin irritant, few cases of severe dermatitis have been reported. The most severe skin lesions occurred in a fatal case described by Boidin et al. (1930) in a girl employed in the artificial pearl industry, where death was due to acute necrosis of the liver. In this case vesicular pustules were present on the face, neck, thorax, arms and thighs. Histologically these showed ulceration of the epithelial layer in the centre of the pustule and a polynuclear infiltration of the dermal layer. These lesions were considered to be an infectious process superimposed on the toxic effect.

(2) Blood and bone marrow

A specific variation in the blood picture of persons exposed to tetrachloro-ethane has been stated (Minot and Smith, 1921 and Parmenter, 1921, 1923) to serve as an indication of poisoning in its very early stages or even to determine susceptibility to the vapour. This variation, observed by Minot and Smith in certain employees of an artificial silk plant, consisted of an increase in the large mononuclear leucocytes – up to or over 30% of the total leucocytes. Practically all the 25 employees who showed this abnormality manifested clinical symptoms – fatigue, headache, constipation, insomnia, irritability, anorexia, nausea, vomiting and, in one case only, slight jaundice, at one time or another.

Another group of 23, whose large mononuclears remained below 12% showed no symptoms. In a few cases the increase in large mononuclears occurred some months before symptoms of poisoning developed, while four men showed the increase without developing symptoms.

The presence of a large number of immature monocuclears appeared to be an indication of a more severe degree of clinical poisoning, while the increase of mature cells alone indicated merely a reaction to tetrachloroethane and therefore could be considered an early sign of poisoning. A slight rise in the total white

Bibliography on p. 263

cell count and slight but progressive anaemia and a slight increase in the number of platelets were also regarded as characteristic changes which could usually be observed before clinical symptoms developed. Parmenter (1921) agreed with these conclusions and quoted a case in which mild symptoms, with general malaise, were accompanied by a blood picture of 47% of large mononuclears and 15% broken cells; when the symptoms became more marked and included vomiting the blood abnormalities increased, while after a period of absence from work the symptoms disappeared and the blood picture gradually returned to normal.

No such specific changes in the blood picture, especially no anaemia, were noted in Willcox's cases, but a moderate secondary anaemia, with an increase in total white cells was observed by Coyer (1944) and by Wilson and Brimley (1944) in their cases of acute poisoning.

(3) Gastro-intestinal disturbances

Hepatotoxic syndrome. – The cases occurring in the aeroplane industry in Great Britain during the First World War and their description by Willcox *et al.* in 1915 still remain a classical presentation of the general manifestation of the toxic effect of tetrachloroethane on the liver. Actually, Grimm *et al.* had described already in 1914 a similar series of cases in the German aeroplane industry, and these were soon followed by others in Germany, Italy, France, Holland and America. The high proportion of cases of poisoning in the British aeroplane industry (70 cases with 12 deaths by September 1916) compared with that of most other countries was attributed to the higher percentage of tetrachloroethane in the 'dope' – 50–60% as compared with only 5–10% in Germany.

The recognition of these cases as due to tetrachloroethane led to its being forbidden in Great Britain for this purpose, but not for other branches of industry.

The progress of the intoxication has been described in four stages:

(a) Pre-jaundice stage. – Complaints of general malaise, drowsiness, loss of appetite, nausea, an unpleasant taste in the mouth, constipation and in some cases abdominal discomfort precede the appearance of jaundice. At this stage diagnosis is difficult. Lejeune (1934) quoted four cases, two of which were ultimately fatal, which were at first diagnosed as gastro-enteritis and gastric neurosis, and according to Zollinger (1931) the abdominal pain may be so acute as to suggest lead poisoning. Wilson and Brimley (1944) suggest the icterus index as a valuable diagnostic measure.

(b) Jaundice without toxaemia. – After several days, or even weeks, jaundice develops with pale stools and bile-stained urine, exhaustion, a slight rise of temperature, and possibly some vomiting and albuminuria.

(c) Jaundice with toxaemia. – The jaundice increases and the vomiting becomes more severe, sometimes there is mental confusion, stupor or delirium, haematemesis, convulsions and purpuric rashes.

(d) Fatal. – Severe jaundice of the whole body, death following.

In fatal cases, there occur suppression of urine, ascites, and coma leading to death. Recovery may follow removal from exposure, but in one case described by Willcox contraction of the liver with portal obstruction and ascites necessitated paracentesis.

In the lacquer industry, where "Zaponlack", used not only in the aeroplane industry but also in hat manufacture, consists of nitrocellulose, pyroxylin and celluloid, sometimes with tetrachloroethane as the solvent, Ohnesorge (1930) described a picture typical of tetrachloroethane poisoning in three men. They complained of nausea, vomiting and abdominal pain, and showed enlargement of the liver. All recovered after 10–14 days of non-exposure, rest in bed and a fat-free diet.

Among more recent cases are those recorded by Coyer (1944) and Wilson and Brimley (1944). In Coyer's series, 6 were non-fatal, and one died 20 days after his exposure, having passed through four stages of intoxication – a pre-jaundice period of 6 days, with fatigue, loss of appetite, headache, nausea and vomiting, a second, of 'jaundice without toxaemia', with increased abdominal pain, bile in the urine and clay-coloured stools, a third 'jaundice with toxaemia', and finally, death, with severe jaundice of the whole body and ascites.

The six cases who survived showed the gastro-hepatic syndrome typical of the first stage, and were then removed from exposure. All showed some jaundice and in two cases the skin retained its lemon colour even after the icteric index had returned to normal limits. Wilson and Brimley differentiated their cases with regard to the degree of exposure, which they described as "varying from light to heavy". Those with 'light' exposure showed gastro-intestinal symptoms and an early rise in the icteric index above 10.5, which was taken as the pathological limit. These symptoms disappeared on removal from exposure. Those with heavier exposure showed varying degrees of jaundice, some with enlarged and tender liver, some with transient nervous symptoms in the form of tremor and paralyses, and some with evidence of nephritis.

(4) Neurological disturbances

In his survey of the English cases of liver injury Willcox mentioned that in Germany a type of nervous disorder had occurred in which the chief manifestations were tremor, headache, pains in the limbs, numbness, pins and needles in the extremities, loss of knee jerks and excessive sweating. Most of these nervous symptoms have occurred in the artificial pearl industry (Léri and Breitel, 1922), though one severe case was recorded in an aeroplane worker by Schultze in 1920.

In the artificial pearl industry girls of 16 and 17 years old are engaged in dipping artificial pearls into 'oriental essence' an acetyl cellulose dissolved in tetrachloroethane, their nose and mouth being held directly over the vessel containing this solution.

Two of the cases described by Léri and Breitel complained of a pricking

Bibliography on p. 263

sensation in the toes and fingers. On examination, Léri found paralysis and anaesthesia of the interossei muscles of the feet and hands, disappearance of the ocular
and pharyngeal reflexes and paralysis of the jaw and ocular muscles. He made a
diagnosis of peripheral neuritis.

Other workers also showed nervous disturbances such as dilated or irregular
pupils, with a delayed reaction, weakness of the pharyngeal reflex, twitching of
the facial muscles and abnormal perspiration.

(5) Combined hepatic and nervous disorder

The most severe case of nervous disturbance combined with symptoms of
liver injury is that recorded by Schultze in 1920. This man, an aeroplane worker,
after one day's work, suffered from nausea and headache, and the following day
again complained of headache, nausea and fatigue. He then found that he had
no sensation in his left hand; this was followed by convulsions and unconsciousness.
On the fourth day he was cyanosed and had partial paralysis of the extremities,
and severe diarrhoea with bleeding and abdominal pain. Three months later he
had spastic paralysis of the left arm and both legs, marked tremor, loss of abdominal, foot and Babinski reflexes, uncontrollable laughter and tears and slowness
of speech. He improved to some extent, but his arm and leg were still paralysed
three months later. Schultze attributed special importance in the diagnosis of
tetrachloroethane poisoning to the appearance of blood in the diarrhoeic stools
in the absence of any definite symptoms of liver injury; he believed that the injury
to the central nervous system was responsible for this as well as the nervous symptoms.

Zollinger (1930) remarks that it is probable that the poisoning was not due
exclusively to tetrachloroethane but a combined toxic action, probably with
trichloroethylene.

Of two cases described by Fiessinger *et al.* (1923) one was only slight, with
digestive disturbance and 'benign' icterus, lasting one month, the other was
ultimately fatal, the cause of death being cirrhosis and acute atrophy of the liver,
but nervous symptoms appeared as the jaundice increased.

In the boot and shoe industry Zollinger (1930) described 6 cases of poisoning,
3 of which were fatal. One of these (reported by Schibler in 1929) was a 17 year
old girl, whose initial symptoms were both gastro-intestinal and nervous, the
latter consisting of acute restlessness and delirium appearing before the jaundice.
The urine was dark coloured and contained many leucocytes and some cylinders;
the stools were gray. Lung oedema developed with a rise of temperature before
death. At autopsy the liver was small and of hard consistency, with an icteric
tinge; microscopically the capillaries were filled with blood; there was some fatty
infiltration, especially in the peripheral zone and some necrosis of liver cells. The
lungs also showed congestion and some fatty infiltration of the endothelial cells.

CHANGES IN THE ORGANISM

Pathological examination of the liver in fatal cases by Spilsbury (1915) showed that the changes predominantly observed were in the form of extensive necrosis of the liver cells. In one case, where the duration of the illness had been nearly 2 months, there were signs of active regeneration of liver tissue; the areas of destruction had been replaced by organising fibrous tissue which had further reduced the function of the liver; in two others the illness had apparently terminated fatally before the regenerative process had had time to occur. Spilsbury summarised the toxic effect on the liver by saying that "the changes in the disease in the human subject must be regarded as, first of all, a toxic fatty degeneration developing in the liver first in the central areas, spreading through the lobules and leading to necrosis; if the patient survives sufficiently long, the necrosis is followed by a condition of replacement-fibrosis of the organ, death occurring from the contracting scar tissue which has developed as a consequence of the disease".

Treatment. – Removal from exposure is the first essential, and bed rest for any but the mildest cases. Daily injections of liver extract, and a diet low in fat and high in carbohydrate have been recommended. Both Coyer and Wilson and Brimley gave 1000 ml of intravenous glucose daily, and alkaline drinks, fruit juices and a supplement of multiple vitamins may also be of value.

Bibliography on p. 263

22. Monochloromethane

Synonyms: methyl chloride

Structural formula:

$$\begin{array}{c} H \\ | \\ Cl-C-H \\ | \\ H \end{array}$$

Molecular formula: CH_3Cl

Molecular weight: 50.49

Properties: It is a highly volatile liquid with a weak, not unpleasant odour which does not give adequate warning of its presence in dangerous concentrations.

    boiling point: -24 °C
    melting point: -97.7 °C
    vapour density (air = 1): 1.76
    specific gravity (liquid density): 1.785
    conversion factors: 1 p.p.m. = 2.086 mg/m³
                           1 mg/l   = 484 p.p.m.
    solubility: 2.2 v/v in water at room temperature, 35 v/v in ethyl alcohol; soluble in ethyl ether and chloroform. Irish (1963) gives solubility in water 400 ml in 100 ml at 30 °C, in ethanol 3500 ml in 100 ml at 30 °C.
    maximum allowable concentration: 100 p.p.m. (ACGIH). Elkins (1959) suggests 50 p.p.m.

ECONOMY, SOURCES AND USES

Production

By the action of HCl on methyl alcohol under pressure (Flury and Zernik, 1931) or in presence of H_2SO_4 (Sterner, 1949).

Industrial uses

(1) As a refrigerating agent.
(2) As a methylating agent.
(3) In the synthetic rubber industry.
(4) In petroleum refining.
(5) As a foaming agent in the plastics industry.

(6) In the stainless steel industry (Metal Working Production 1962), in the process of chemical etching, for removing the neoprene coating of the steel parts.

It is used to some extent as a local anaesthetic, sometimes mixed with ethyl chloride, and was at one time used for general anaesthesia, its narcotic action being, according to Kobert (1906) only a quarter that of chloroform; its toxic side effects (cardiac disturbance), paralysis of the respiratory centre and irritation of the respiratory tract led to its being discarded for this purpose.

BIOCHEMISTRY

Estimation

(1) In the atmosphere

The method of absorption on silica gel (chilled with dry ice), followed by hydrolysis with potassium hydrate in isopropyl alcohol at 50 °C, similar to that described for other halogenated hydrocarbons, is stated by Elkins (1959) to be probably applicable to methyl chloride.

(2) In blood and tissues

Bij removing from blood and tissues by aeration and steam distillation, passing the mixture through a heated platinum tube to oxidize the organic chlorides and absorbing the inorganic chloride in an alkaline arsenious oxide solution, with titration by Polland's method (Alford, 1947).

Metabolism

Owing to its high volatility methyl chloride appears to be almost entirely eliminated unchanged by the lungs, but there is considerable difference of opinion as to its possible metabolic derivatives. The fact that foods saturated with its vapour proved non-toxic to animals (White and Somers, 1931; Yant *et al.*, 1930) is said to indicate that absorption by the gastro-intestinal tract is negligible.

In the experiments of Yant *et al.* (1930) food was placed in a bell jar and the methyl chloride vapour allowed to saturate it for 18 h or longer. It was then fed to dogs, which exhibited no symptoms either during the experiment or during the following month. Water, three-quarters to completely saturated by shaking vigorously in an atmosphere of 95–100% of methyl chloride was given to two dogs, deprived of liquid food and fresh water, in amounts representing a daily average amount of 1.04 and 1.07 g of methyl chloride. They showed no symptoms during the entire test period of 171 days, after which they were killed by intracardial injection of saturated aqueous magnesium sulphate solution. The only internal organ showing pathological appearances was the kidney, in which some intracellular fatty degeneration was observed. No formates were found in the urine.

When injected intravenously pulmonary elimination accounts for little of the amount administered and falls progressively with time, though it disappears rapidly from the blood stream – about 98% in 60 min – whether injected as liquid or gas (Sperling *et al.*, 1950). The urine also excretes a very small fraction of the amount. Since after inhalation excretion by the lungs is slow and the odour in the breath is perceptible for a long time (Flury and Zernik, 1931) some authorities have suggested that either storage places exist from which it can be released slowly or that the methyl chloride undergoes metabolic destruction in the tissues. With regard to the probable storage reservoirs, Soucek (1961) considers that it is unlikely that fatty tissue can be one of these, since methyl chloride is 20 times less soluble in fat than carbon tetrachloride. With regard to the metabolic destruction some observers have described this as decomposition into a methyl group, which is further oxidised to methyl alcohol and then to formaldehyde, formic acid and a chlorine ion, which are excreted in the urine. Lehmann and Flury (1943) in fact state that the toxic effects of methyl chloride are due to methyl alcohol and its oxidation product, formaldehyde. Uncertainty as to the metabolic behaviour of methyl chloride has been further increased by the fact that different observers have found the urine either predominantly alkaline (Baker, 1927) or predominantly acid (Kegel *et al.*, 1929) in cases of human poisoning. Smith (1947), however, is definite on the point that since in animals exposed to methyl chloride no methyl alcohol is found in the blood and only normal amounts of formic acid, there is no evidence that these are metabolic products of methyl chloride. He found the average pH of the urine of exposed animals to be 7.8, as compared with 7.6 for controls. In Soucek's (1961) investigation, using subcutaneous injection in white rats, he confirmed the results of Sperling *et al.* with regard to its rapid disappearance from the blood stream. It decreased from 1.4% of the dose in 2 min to 0% in 25 min while the average amount expired was 27% of the injected dose, becoming imperceptible at the end of 120–135 min so that about 70% must have been metabolised.

TOXICOLOGY

Methyl chloride is a moderately severe narcotic and a severe nerve poison, causing giddiness, 'drunkenness', and with high concentrations convulsions, coma and ultimately death. With repeated exposure it can cause apathy, loss of appetite, drowsiness, weakness of the legs with disturbance of gait and sometimes disturbance of vision. Late psychotic effects and cardiac injury have been recorded and in one case cirrhosis of the liver.

Toxicity to animals

There is apparently considerable species difference in the susceptibility of animals to the toxic effects of methyl chloride both with acute and also chronic exposure, and also with regard to the time of exposure.

Mice are stated (Schwarz, 1926) to be more resistant to methyl chloride than rabbits and guinea pigs; the latter, as well as dogs and monkeys being specially susceptible (Baker, 1927; Smith and Von Oettingen, 1947). The latter observers found this susceptibility in dogs and monkeys especially marked with exposure to lower concentrations. Dogs died after 2–4 weeks of exposure to 500 p.p.m.; one which survived 29 weeks of exposure had developed irreversible neuro-muscular damage, and 2 monkeys succumbed after 16 and 17 weeks. Smith and Von Oettingen remark that this higher susceptibility in animals with a more highly developed central nervous system may indicate that human subjects may be even more susceptible to methyl chloride poisoning.

(1) Acute

(a) Lethal dose, by inhalation. – For the mouse, the dosages reported vary from 2000 p.p.m. (Smith and Von Oettingen) to 6000–8000 p.p.m. after 5–10 h (Velches, 1949) and 10,000 after about 4 h (Schwarz.)

For guinea pigs, the lowest MLD recorded is that by White and Somers (1931) – 75 p.p.m. for 72 h, while 140 p.p.m. regularly caused death within a few days after the exposure. Sayers *et al.* (1929) reported 0.12–0.15% as lethal in not longer than $13\frac{1}{2}$ h.

For dogs, the variations in lethal dosage are apparently considerably dependent on the time factor; they are specially susceptible to lower concentrations over a longer period. Smith and Von Oettingen give 1000–3000 p.p.m. as the lethal dose, while Baker (1927) found 46,000 fatal within 24 h, much lower concentrations for a longer time.

(b) Narcotic dose. – High for most species; for mice, according to Schwarz, narcosis begins after 30–45 min with exposure to 65,000–70,000 p.p.m.; for dogs at 17,000 p.p.m.

SYMPTOMS OF INTOXICATION

(a) Acute. – Smith and Von Oettingen observed in dogs generalised tonic spasms with dyspnoea preceding death, while Baker recorded that after 30 min exposure to 17,000 p.p.m. they showed slight ataxia before narcosis, and at 37,000 p.p.m. they were restless after 10 min, vomited after 18 min and became dyspnoeic after 25 min.

In smaller species there is a short initial period of excitement (longer in mice than in guinea pigs or rabbits) followed in the latter two species by apathy, paralysis of the extremities, loss of appetite and weight, cough with marked signs of bronchitis, and convulsions preceding death. In Velches' experiments (1949), mice and guinea pigs were subjected to inhalation of the gas from a leaking refrigerator (identified as methyl chloride by its non-inflammability as opposed to the flammability of Freon, sometimes used as a refrigerant (Barach *et al.*, 1944); this leaking refrigerator had caused several cases of acute poisoning. The animals died after 5–10 h with tonic and clonic spasms.

Bibliography on p. 263

(2) Chronic

As with acute poisoning different species of animals respond differently to repeated exposure, but in the smaller species disturbances of movement show a close correspondence. In the larger species, dogs exposed for 4–6 months to 500 p.p.m. differed from monkeys in exhibiting sustained tonic spasms and ataxia, while monkeys became emaciated and prostrated and finally unconscious for several hours before death (Smith and Von Oettingen). It was observed also that some of these symptoms, acquired over a long period of time, persisted long after cessation of exposure – mice, for example, retained the 'clamping syndrome' (clamping of the hind legs to the body) for six months, while in one guinea pig severe spasticity remained for $7\frac{1}{2}$ months, and another was unable to turn over from a supine position after 14 months.

In the experiments of Schwarz (1926) exposure of guinea pigs to 3000 p.p.m. for 15 min 11–15 times during 18 and 24 days caused death, but an interval of 25 days of non-exposure sometimes brought some recovery. All the animals showed weakness of the hind legs, cough and loss of weight.

CHANGES IN THE ORGANISM

Lesions of internal organs, congestion and sometimes haemorrhage, and in guinea pigs bronchopneumonia have been observed (Schwarz). In rabbits this was particularly marked when they had been exposed to 3000 p.p.m. with intervals of non-exposure.

(1) The liver

Lesions of the liver have been described by some observers and not by others. Schwarz found no fatty degeneration or necrosis in his mice, but Velches did observe fatty infiltration in his guinea pigs, and among others who have reported fatty degeneration are Sayers et al. (1929) and Dunn and Smith (1947). The latter also noted moderate necrosis in the centrilobular areas of the liver of rats and rabbits, but not in the larger species, which included cats, dogs, monkeys and goats.

(2) The kidneys

In acute intoxication with methyl chloride the renal lesions observed have ranged from congestion, with some evidence of degeneration and small haemorrhages (Schwarz, 1926; White and Somers, 1931) to varying degrees of necrosis of the tubules with haemoglobinuria and albuminuria in the mouse and occasionally in the dog, and fatty degeneration in other species (Dunn and Smith, 1947).

The chief report of renal necrosis as a prominent toxic effect of chronic exposure to methyl chloride is that of Dunn and Smith, but only the smaller species (mice and rats) were so affected by concentrations of 500–4000 p.p.m. 6 h a day, 6 days a week, until death. The renal lesions in mice exposed to 2000 p.p.m. consisted of fatty degeneration of the epithelium of the convoluted tubules, which also contained haemoglobin, globules and casts, and areas of necrosis with some areas of regeneration.

(3) The lungs

In practically all the results of animal experiments recorded marked congestion, oedema and haemorrhages of the lungs have been predominant features. Dunn and Smith remarked that pulmonary oedema was present frequently in his animals and appeared to be a direct result of the irritation due to inhalation of methyl chloride.

Toxicity to human beings

(1) Acute

(a) *Lethal dose.* – Up to 1947 Smith and Von Oettingen had collected 15 deaths from methyl chloride intoxication; these had presumably included the ten occurring in Chicago in 1928–1929 among 29 of more moderate severity recorded by Kegel *et al.* All these cases except three occurred during the use of domestic refrigerators where leaks were discovered in the refrigerator system. In all the fatal cases death was preceded by severe convulsions with marked opisthotonus and profound cyanosis. The immediate cause of death appeared to be respiratory paralysis.

Another typical episode of fatal poisoning by methyl chloride used as a refrigerant had been described by Schwarz in 1926. Inhalation of a high concentration of the vapour was due to an accidental outflow of the methyl chloride during the installation of a refrigerator in a window-less cellar with no ventilation. Men installing the machine had complained of occasional headache and nausea, but until the accident these symptoms had always disappeared on emerging into fresh air. After the leakage more severe symptoms, lasting several days, had appeared in all the 10 men employed – giddiness, apathy, lack of appetite and weakness of the legs. One man who had for three weeks previously shown slight symptoms of intoxication, died four days after the leakage, having during this period been obliged several times to leave his work owing to headache, fatigue, loss of appetite and vomiting. He was found dead on his bed, with signs that he had suffered from severe cramp in his legs and convulsions. At autopsy the lungs showed marked congestion, the brain some punctate haemorrhages and the liver some fatty degeneration but no sign of acute yellow atrophy.

Two deaths in coma following leakage from a refrigerator plant were described by Velches in 1949, and one by Noro and Petterson (1960) when 5 members of the same family were affected.

(b) *Narcotic dose.* – (i) *Severe, non-fatal intoxication.* The symptoms of severe poisoning are focussed chiefly on the central nervous system, but some cases exhibit gastro-intestinal symptoms which are believed by some authorities to be of central nervous origin (Wilcox, 1934).

Among the earliest cases of severe intoxication recorded were two by Gerbis in 1914. These were machine workers who entered a methyl chloride container in order to clean it. Both suffered from severe 'drunkenness', followed by profound drowsiness and disturbance of vision. The onset of symptoms is often slow, increasing to a maximum during several days. Two cases in which the nervous symptoms were especially severe were reported by Hartman *et al.* in 1955. The exposure had originated in a leak from the pipes leading from the refrigeration plant in the basement. Both subjects, a husband and wife, had severe mental confusion, and the wife, who had just been dilevered of a still-born foetus, convulsive seizures.

In another severe case reported by Morgan Jones (1942) one of the most striking features was, twitching, at the rate of 2–4 per sec, of individual muscles or parts of muscles. Eye movements were of this type rather than true nystagmus. This man had complained during three years before the acute attack, of vomiting, nausea, staggering gait and diplopia. After a heavy exposure he was dazed, his speech was thick and slurred, he staggered "like a drunken man" and had blurring of vision and diplopia. The following day, during which he had returned to work, he became semi-conscious and later confused, and developed severe tremor of the right arm, and twitching of his whole body, changing to generalised tonic and clonic spasms with opisthotonus, accompanied by a rise of temperature and cyanosis. After an interval of two days he had a relapse into toxic delirium, with a further relapse ten days later. He ultimately recovered but with certain sequelae (see p. 240).

Among the 'gassing' accidents reported to the Chief Inspector of Factories of Great Britain, 6 occurred in 1952, of which two were due to leaks from a refrigerating plant, one during the manufacture of methyl chloride and three during the refitting of a ship, when methyl chloride drawn off from a refrigerator caused a 'puddle' thought to have been too small to cause a toxic effect.

(ii) Moderately severe cases have been described fairly frequently. Among them a number from a synthetic rubber manufacturing plant (Hansen *et al.*, 1953). Six cases described by Morgan Jones in 1942 were of this degree and two cases of serious illness during the release of methyl chloride while sawing a 'foam' insulating material were reported in 1959 (Kentucky State Dept. of Health).

(2) Chronic

Chronic intoxication by methyl chloride has been less frequently observed than acute, possibly because the effects of moderate exposure tend to disappear rapidly when the exposure ceases, though, according to Morgan Jones (1942), mild cases, with dizziness, staggering gait, headache, nausea and vomiting are common amongst men regularly exposed to methyl chloride, and Roche and Bouchet (1948) describe the occurrence of headache, giddiness, anorexia and nausea, disappearing rapidly on cessation of exposure but causing marked asthenia. Reports by Van der Kloot (1934) and Mackie (1961) strongly support the suggestion of chronic intoxication. Van der Kloot describes symptoms in a refrigerator repairman aged 23, which resembled those of encephalitis – extreme somnolence, blurred vision and lack of co-ordination of hand and arm movements, lasting two to three weeks, but with apparently complete eventual recovery. In Mackie's case, the man aged 40, a refrigeration plant owner, had worked with methyl chloride some 18 years, but only during the last six months had exposure been particularly heavy. His complaints were weakness, apathy, loss of weight and blurring of vision. He was somewhat jaundiced and had polyuria, with dark-coloured urine containing albumin, bile pigments and bile salts. Examination revealed an enlarged soft liver and spleen, a raised temperature and haemolytic anaemia with leucocytosis. Liver biopsy showed "necrosis with degeneration mainly in the centre of the lobules, and early reticular formation". He was treated by transfusion and prednisone and 8 months later felt perfectly well, but his liver was still palpable.

SYMPTOMS OF INTOXICATION

The symptoms of chronic intoxication by methyl chloride are in fact more generally related to the gastro-intestinal system than to the nervous system, though giddiness and headache are complained of with some frequency and, more rarely, psychic effects in the form of personality changes, with incapacity for work, sleep disturbance and extreme depression (Flury and Klimmer, 1939; Walter and Weiss, 1951).

CHANGES IN THE ORGANISM

(1) The heart

Injury of the heart muscle following acute methyl chloride poisoning has been described by several observers, and will be described under 'sequelae of Methyl Chloride Poisoning' (see p. 240). An unusual disturbance of the cardiac mechanism (Wilson Block) has been attributed by Gummert (1961) to exposure to methyl chloride. He reports the case of a 60 year old man repairing an uncovered refrigerator, who after 3 h became drowsy, giddy and weak. Two days later he showed signs of psychic disorder, some swelling of the face and subjective failure of vision. At this time the ECG showed the typical appearance of Wilson Block (R. bundle branch block, characterised by a tall slender R wave in Lead 1, followed by a wider S wave). The man was incapable of work and his convalescence was long delayed, and 14 months later the ECG still showed the typical Wilson Block curve. Gummert suggests that the mechanism of this injury may be that of vascular degeneration following the toxic effect of methyl chloride on the central nervous system. The connection is not entirely certain, but the man had never previously had any rheumatic affection, nor had he any signs of arterial sclerosis.

He recovered under hospital treatment but with some residual albuminuria.

Bibliography on p. 263

(2) The liver

In acute fatal poisoning the effect on the liver has usually been rela-tively slight and unaccompanied by jaundice, though some of the cases record-ed by Kegel *et al.* (1929) showed areas of degeneration in the liver (and kid-neys).

In severe non-fatal cases jaundice has occasionally been observed. In the case described by Weinstein (1937), a man affected by exposure to methyl chloride while repairing an airconditioning plant, became slightly jaundiced during the first two days after the onset of symptoms and the icteric index was 10 or above for 4 days.

The evidence of liver injury in the case recorded by Mackie (see above) has already been described. The only case of definite cirrhosis of the liver attributed to many years of exposure to methyl chloride is that of Wood (1951), when the liver at autopsy was described as 'grossly cirrhotic'. This man had been a refriger-ator engineer for many years but had never had any symptoms of acute poison-ing, though he admitted that he had taken very few precautions against inhala-tion of the fumes. Eighteen months before he was admitted to hospital with a severe haematemesis, he had had a mild attack of jaundice which Wood suggests could have been interpreted as the first sign of a slowly progressive cirrhosis. Liver function tests suggested liver injury, and at first it was thought that the haemateme-sis might be due to invisible oesophageal varices and cirrhosis with a co-existing peptic ulcer. After another haematemesis a month later he became jaundiced and, following a further haematemesis, died three days later.

At autopsy the liver showed gross disorganisation of structure, with bands of fibrous tissue forming islets of liver substance. There was a large ulcer on the posterior wall of the stomach, from which the fatal haemorrhage had issued. It is not possible to state definitely that the cirrhosis was caused by methyl chloride; it might possibly have followed an infective hepatitis, though as Wood remarks, there were no known contacts and he had received no injections, nor was he a heavy drinker. It can only be said to stand as an isolated case of a potential effect of long-continued exposure to methyl chloride.

Porphyrin excretion. – A case of industrial methyl chloride poisoning in which large quantities of coproporphyrin III were found in the urine and faeces was described by Chalmers *et al.* (1940). This was a refrigerator engineer who had had an acute attack of poisoning with delirium, convulsions and tremor. The urine was normal in colour, with no albumen or bile, and no increase in bilirubin. There was no jaundice, but a laevulose tolerance test indicated slight hepatic insufficiency, there was also no evidence of haemolytic anaemia.

A maximum value for urinary coproporphyrin III (1 mg/day) was present one week after the acute attack, and declined with clinical improvement but recurrent spasmodic increase until about 40 days later when the level was 40

μg/day. The faecal levels ranged from 4–0.2 mg, but were still high (3.5 mg/day) even 5 weeks later.

Chalmers *et al.* suggested that the effect of methyl chloride might have been similar to that produced by certain nitro- and aminocompounds which probably act on the liver, interfering with the normal breakdown of haemoglobin, and that "it is attractive to consider that formic acid derived from methyl chloride" played some part in the conversion from proto- to coproporphyrin.

In one case (Roche *et al.*, 1956) a man who after 2 years employment in installing refrigerators had a slight attack of poisoning, for the next three years had intermittent albuminuria, which had increased at the end of this time to 4.7 mg/l and the following year, when he was complaining of pain in the lumbar region, asthenia and loss of weight, was found to have an enlarged and tender liver, with the urine again containing albumen and some white and red cells and hyaline cylinders. Intravenous urography, however, showed no disturbance of urinary excretion and no abnormal appearance of the urinary tract. A diagnosis of chronic nephritis was made with "no other possible etiology than methyl chloride poisoning".

(3) The kidneys

According to Roche *et al.* (1956) fatal cases always show oliguria or even anuria, and when urine is passed it is dark and contains albumin, with leucocytes and erythrocytes (Mendeloff, 1952) and cylinders (Kegel *et al.*, 1929).

In Mendeloff's case death had occurred after repeated exposure and the kidneys showed oedema, vacuolation and granulation of the proximal and distal lobules, with some necrosis and calcification. Some tubules and some glomeruli contained eosinophilic debris.

Renal injury. – A case reported by Verrière and Vachez (1949) emphasized the possibility that long-continued exposure to methyl chloride, probably with repeated slight manifestations of poisoning, can result in severe injury to the kidneys. In this case, a man aged 50, who had been for many years engaged in repairing refrigerators, developed severe acute nephritis, with oliguria, albuminuria and numerous red blood cells in the urine.

(4) The nervous system

An unusual case, which might be regarded as one of a chronic toxic effect on the central nervous system was recorded by Rondepierre *et al* (1955), though the part played by methyl chloride was regarded only as 'possible'. This was a man who had been employed for ten years in dismantling refrigerators, and who was admitted to hospital in a state of mental confusion, with marked amnesia, asthenia and slowness of mental reaction.

He had previously had somewhat similar episodes, with incoherent speech, staggering gait and extreme desire to sleep. The present crisis had been preceded

Bibliography on p. 263

by a fortnight of insomnia and a period of agitation. Following a month of no exposure he appeared to recover, but four months later he complained of marked fatigue, asthenia, somnolence, headache and some retrograde amnesia. The EEG at this time showed no abnormality but encephalography revealed small areas of frontal and parietal atrophy, and his mental retardation was so marked seven months later that his family requested that his case be certified as one of occupational disease. Rondepierre *et al.* (1955) suggest that this unusual manifestation, possibly due to methyl chloride, might be related to individual susceptibility, and that the effect on the nervous system might be due to circulatory disturbances of vasomotor origin, causing congestion and oedema of the brain.

Lesions of the central nervous system have been described by Thomas (1960), the result of autopsy on a man who had been employed in installing refrigerators for 25 years without any disturbance of health until 4 months before his fatal attack of unconsciousness. He had then complained of severe headache and giddiness. The brain showed numerous small areas of injury of nerve fibres and cells; in the spinal cord a special feature was the presence of argentophil masses in the posterior column in the lumbar region.

Effect on the spinal cord. – In a case eventually fatal from respiratory paralysis after one year's repeated exposure, Noetzel (1952) recorded the development of paralysis of the arms and legs, which he attributed to degeneration of the anterior horn cells of the spinal cord caused by chronic methyl chloride poisoning.

Sequelae of methyl chloride poisoning

(1) Effect on the heart

A case described by Walter and Weiss (1951) was that of a man employed in repairing a refrigerator in a cellar of a butcher's shop. He observed at the time that methyl chloride was escaping but thought it unimportant since he had been told by his chief that it was harmless. After 3–4 h he felt as though he were 'drunk or under chloroform' and was taken home by car. He was in fact at first partially unconscious and after one and a half days completely so. On recovery he complained of pain in the region of the heart, great fatigue and inability to work. Electrocardiograms taken 7 months and two and a quarter years after the acute attack both indicated severe injury of the heart muscle.

(2) Effect on the central nervous system

A permanent effect on the central nervous system, especially marked by a change of personality, has been described by Flury and Klimmer (1939) and by Jacob and Schröder (1959). Flury and Klimmer recorded the case of a previously very active woman who was almost unrecognisable 9 months after an acute attack of poisoning, having become depressed, with lack of concentration and will power, general nervousness and vegetative disorders – symptoms said to be similar to those following severe skull injury.

Jacob and Schröder's case was that of a second engineer of a ship who had been involved in an accidental severe exposure to methyl cloride during the repair of the ship's refrigerator. The first engineer who was working with him died without recovering consciousness. The man in question was also rendered unconscious but recovered with administration of oxygen and cardiac stimulants. After two months on shore he was depressed, irritable, unable to concentrate and sleepless. After $2\frac{1}{2}$ years he committed suicide by gassing himself. Autopsy showed, in addition to acute lesions referable to lethal CO poisoning, diffuse long-standing changes in the central nervous system – designated as methyl chloride encephalopathy – constriction of blood vessels, hyalinofibrotic thickening of the outer and median coats of their walls, perivascular pigment lipofuchsin, fat deposition and disintegration. There was also some sclerosis of the thyroid which was regarded as secondary to toxic injury by methyl chloride during the acute attack.

Prevention of methyl chloride poisoning

It is apparent from a perusal of the cases described that the greatest danger of poisoning arises from leakage of methyl chloride during repairs to refrigerators, during their use or during their manufacture. In all such processes adequate ventilation is essential. In Baker's(1927) experience, where exposure occurred from blowing methyl chloride into the workshop after testing evaporators, an adequate exhaust system was effective in preventing ill-effects. The protection of men repairing refrigerators is a more difficult problem, owing to the difficulty in preventing and detecting leaks from the apparatus, including domestic refrigerators. All the 10 fatal cases described by Kegel et al. (1929), and 26 of their severe cases arose from the placing of refrigerators in flats and their connection with a common multiple unit plant containing several hundred pounds of methyl chloride under a pressure of 100 lbs to the square inch. One suggestion for minimising the risk of a leakage not appreciable by its odour has been the addition of a detector substance – 1 % acrolein – but it has not proved to be generally acceptable.

Treatment of acute methyl chloride poisoning

Prompt removal from exposure and inhalations of oxygen, with, according to McCord (1930), 5–7% of CO_2, are essential measures in the first place. On recovery, treatment is mainly symptomatic. If sedatives are needed to control convulsions, substances known to affect the liver, such as chloroform or chloralhydrate, should be avoided. Kegel et al. (1929) recommend a solution of potassium bromide as an enema. Liberal allowances of glucose should be given and if there is inability to swallow, a solution of 5 % dextrose and 3 % sodium carbonate could be administered per rectum. When the symptoms of a fairly mild intoxication are predominantly gastro-intestinal, sodium carbonate by mouth has been found of value (Fabre and Rougier, 1948). For the treatment of nervous symptoms following the acute stage, Canepa and Courtis (1951) recommend vitamins B and C.

Bibliography on p. 263

23. Dichloromethane

Synonyms: methylene chloride, methylene dichloride

Structural formula:

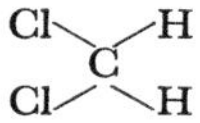

$$\begin{array}{c} \text{Cl} \\ \diagdown \\[-1ex] \text{Cl} \end{array} \text{C} \begin{array}{c} \text{H} \\ \diagup \\[-1ex] \diagdown \\ \text{H} \end{array}$$

Molecular formula: CH_2Cl_2

Molecular weight: 84.94

Properties: A colourless liquid with a sweetish, chloroform-like odour. Good solvent for alkaloids, bitumen, crude rubber, oils, resins, waxes and many organic compounds. Readily volatile at room temperature (1.8 times less volatile than ether).

  boiling point: 40 °C
  melting point: −96.0 °C
  vapour pressure: 440 mm Hg at 25 °C
  vapour density (air = 1): 2.93
  specific gravity (liquid density): 1.336
  flash point: non-inflammable, but in presence of heat and moisture may decompose to form phosgene and HCl (Parney and Cunningham, 1949).
  conversion factors: 1 p.p.m. = 3.49 mg/m³
              1 mg/l = 288.2 p.p.m.
  solubility: very slightly soluble in water, soluble in alcohol, ether and other organic solvents.
  maximum allowable concentration: 500 p.p.m.

ECONOMY, SOURCES AND USES

The chemically pure product has been used in Germany as a narcotic under the name 'Solaesthin'; in England under the name 'Solmethin' (Settelen, 1950).

Production

By chlorination of methyl chloride and subsequent distillation (Sterner, 1949).

Industrial uses

(1) As a constituent of paint removers.

(2) As a refrigerant in air conditioning.

(3) As a degreasing and cleaning fluid, sometimes mixed with petroleum naphtha and perchloroethylene for the cleaning of electrical motors (Moskowitz and Shapiro, 1952).

(4) In the artificial silk industry, as a 'stretching' solvent.

(5) In the extraction of oils, fats, perfumes and drugs.

BIOCHEMISTRY

Estimation

(1) In the atmosphere

The method of absorption on silica gel, applicable to other halogenated hydrocarbons has been found (Peterson *et al.*, 1956) suitable for methylene chloride when combined with the combustion technique described by Jacobs (1949), the silica gel being used for sampling and combustion (at about 900 °C) for analysis. The trapping solution used in this method is 1% sodium carbonate and 1% sodium formate in de-ionised water.

(2) In blood and tissues

The method used by Heppel *et al.* (1944) was that described by Moran (1943) by means of analysis of the volatile chloride released by the aeration of blood (though less chloride is produced by methylene chloride than by chloroform or carbon tetrachloride, see below *Metabolism*). The method consists in decomposition by passing over heated platinum, absorption in an alkaline sulphite solution and titration by a standard method.

(3) In urine

The same method as for estimation in blood was used by Heppel *et al.* (1944).

Metabolism

Absorption and excretion

Absorption by the lungs is fairly rapid, and excretion takes place, also fairly rapidly, by both lungs and urine. Heppel *et al.* (1944) found that the blood of a rabbit exposed for 4 h to 10,000 p.p.m. contained 10.4, 4.1 and 2.6 mg/100 ml at $\frac{1}{2}$, $1\frac{1}{2}$, 2 and 3 h respectively, after exposure was discontinued. The urine, 3 h after 4-h exposure, contained 3.4 mg/100 ml.

Methylene chloride is relatively stable in the body, being largely eliminated unchanged and producing less chloride than carbon tetrachloride. The rate of inorganic chloride production by hydrolysis by alcoholic NaOH has been correlated by Von Oettingen *et al.* (1949) with the relative toxicity of the chlorinated methanes. Thus, chloroform, having a greater rate of hydrolysis than methylene

Bibliography on p. 263

chloride, has a LD_{50} of 28 mg/l compared with 56 mg/l for the more stable methylene chloride (Williams, 1959).

TOXICOLOGY

The predominant characteristic of poisoning by methylene chloride is its narcotic action. Its toxic effect on the liver is believed to be much less than that of other halogenated hydrocarbons, but some authorities believe that it has at least a potential toxicity in this respect. Vauthey (1955) for example states that in certain circumstances, such as daily exposure to low concentrations, it can cause digestive trouble secondary to a hepato-renal effect, and even fatty degeneration of the liver and kidneys of moderate intensity. Its complete lack of toxicity has also been questioned by other French observers. Deplace et al. (1962) have stated, without giving specific details, that both methylene chloride and dichloroethane, increasingly widely applied in industry, are rarely used in the pure state, and that during 1960 and 1961 they observed 16 cases of disturbance of health attributable to these products – nervous, respiratory, digestive and cutaneous. In animals, liver injury has been inconstant and slight in degree and kidney injury non-existent (Heppel et al., 1944).

Toxicity to animals

Acute

(a) *Lethal dose.* – By inhalation. – For mice, 14,500 p.p.m. caused death after 2 h (Flury and Zernik, 1931). For guinea pigs, Nuckolls (1933) found that 50,000 to 54,000 p.p.m. for $1-1\frac{1}{2}$ h caused progressive narcosis and death.

(b) *Narcotic dose.* – In the experiments of Heppel et al. (1944) 10,000 p.p.m. produced light to moderate narcosis in monkeys, rabbits, rats and dogs. A concentration of 5000 p.p.m. for periods of 30 min on alternate days, while not producing definite narcosis in rats was found to reduce considerably their running activity, as measured in a revolving drum (Heppel et al., 1944).

SYMPTOMS OF INTOXICATION

Excitement at the beginning of exposure was shown by rabbits, and especially by dogs; the latter manifested violent but purposeless movements. Rats developed mild incoordination and disturbance of gait during the first half-hour, and after 4 h were prostrate with depressed respiration.

CHANGES IN THE ORGANISM

Following repeated exposure to 10,000 p.p.m. 3 out of 4 rabbits and 2 out of 9 rats died (Heppel et al., 1944). The chief lesions were found in the lungs – congestion and oedema with focal necrosis or extravasation of blood. In 2 dogs the liver showed moderate centrilobular congestion and slight to moderate fatty degeneration; 4 out of 6 guinea pigs also showed this condition. With repeated exposure – 7 h daily, 5 days a week, for periods up to 6 months – to concentrations of 5000 p.p.m. there was extensive pneumonia and moderate fatty degeneration of the liver in only 2 guinea pigs which died after 90 and 96 exposures.

Toxic effects in human beings

Deep narcosis can be produced in man in 30 min by a concentration of 20,000 p.p.m. but the margin between the narcotic and the lethal dose is narrow (Henderson and Haggard, 1943). Several deaths have been reported from its use as an anaesthetic, according to Hellwig (1922), with opisthotonus and clonic spasms. This cannot be overcome with continued administration, but disappears rapidly on cessation. Hellwig states that methylene chloride is not a suitable agent for full narcosis, since it has a pre-narcotic stage of marked excitation, but it is useful as an adjuvant to local anaesthesia especially in tonsillectomy in children, and as an analgesic in obstetrical practice. Settelen (1950) records one fatal case in a child who died after administration of 4 ml of Solaesthin. The *post mortem* revealed no organic lesion which might have accounted for the sudden death. He mentions also the case of a 62 year old man who died from sudden heart failure after an operation in which Solaesthin was given. In his case also there was no autopsy evidence of organic disease.

As an analgesic in obstetrical practice it has been found highly satisfactory since it is never necessary to reach full anaesthesia. According to Grasset and Gauthier (1950), in a series of 44 cases they found no evidence of ill-effect to either the mother or child. The average amount administered during the whole duration of labour was 20 ml.

Industrial poisoning by methylene chloride has been comparatively rarely reported though, as noted above, some French observers are by no means convinced that disturbances of health following chronic exposure do not occur.

(1) Acute

A few cases of acute though not severe intoxication have been reported to the Chief Inspector of Factories in Great Britain. In one, in 1935, deep inhalation produced what was described as a 'bursting headache'; in another in 1944 where the solvent used contained 40% of dichloroethylene as well as 45% of methylene chloride, the man experienced nausea and a choking sensation, which were followed by collapse, unconsciousness and vomiting lasting for 4 days; in yet another a woman using methylene chloride as a paint remover complained of nausea, then vomited and fainted; a fellow worker also vomited. The most outstanding account of its severe acute toxic action during an industrial process is that of Moskowitz

Bibliography on p. 263

and Shapiro (1952) in which four men became completely unconscious and one died. The process in which the exposure occurred was the extraction of an oleoresin from dried plant material. Although most of the operations were conducted in closed systems, there was opportunity for the vapour to escape into the workroom through vents in the indoor supply tank and the percolators; there was actually a loss of about 825 gallons of methylene chloride per week. Four nightshift workers were found unconscious in the early morning; three recovered after about $2\frac{1}{2}$ hours, the fourth was dead when the ambulance arrived. Of the three who recovered, one showed signs of acute bronchitis, one of irritation of the upper respiratory tract and one conjunctivitis and lacrimation. All three showed some anaemia and polymorphonuclear leucocytosis. Urine examination showed no evidence of kidney injury. Liver function tests were not carried out. The only significant findings at autopsy on the man who died were congestion of the liver and kidneys and some emphysema of the lungs, in which methylene chloride was present to the extent of 0.1 ml in 500 g of tissue.

(2) Chronic

No definite evidence of toxic effects from chronic exposure to methylene chloride have been recorded. The cases reported by Collier in 1936 in connection with its use as a paint remover are complicated by the fact that the subjective symptoms in two workers who were obliged to leave work were asssociated with the presence of duodenal ulcer in one and lead poisoning in the other. This was especially probable with respect to the anaemia noted by Collis as a probable consequence of exposure to methylene chloride in the worker who had previously been exposed to lead; it was accompanied by punctate basophilia, while the symptoms complained of by the man with the duodenal ulcer were largely subjective and very slight. It was suggested by Moskowitz and Shapiro (1952) however, on the basis of the anemia shown by their three cases which survived acute exposure that this was possibly due to past chronic exposure which had caused injury to the haemopoietic system.

It is generally agreed that methylene chloride is not an important cause of contact dermatitis. It has in fact been recommended for hand metal cleaning because of its relatively low capacity for skin irritation, but it has a chilling action on the skin (Queries and Minor Notes, JAMA, 1947).

24. Dichloroethane

Synonym: ethylene dichloride, ethylidine chloride

Structural formulae: dichloroethane exists in two forms,

1,2-dichloroethane	1,1-dichloroethane

Molecular formula: $C_2H_4Cl_2$ $C_2H_4Cl_2$

Molecular weight: 98.97   98.97

Properties: a colourless liquid with a chloroform-like odour, distinct and noticeable in safe concentrations (Sayers *et al.*, 1930).

boiling point: 89 °C	59 °C	
melting point: −35.3 °C	−96.7 °C	
vapour pressure: 78 mm Hg at 20 °C	234 mm Hg at 25 °C	
vapour density (air = 1): 3.4	3.4	
specific gravity (liquid density): 1.256	1.174	
flash point: 18.3 °C	57 °F (Irish, 1963)	

conversion factors:

1 p.p.m. = 4.05 mg/m³	4.05 mg/m³
1 mg/l = 247 p.p.m.	247 p.p.m.
solubility: in water 0.9 g/100 ml	0.5 g/100 ml at 20 °C
	4.11 g/l

maximum allowable concentration:

50 p.p.m.   100 p.p.m. (Threshold Limit
                             Values, 1962)

ECONOMY, SOURCES AND USES

Production

(1) By direct chlorination of ethane; a side product in the manufacture of chloral.
(2) From ethylene and chlorine by treatment with calcium chloride (Durrans, 1950).

Industrial uses

(1) As a cleansing agent.

(2) As a solvent for plastics, oils and fats.

(3) As degreaser, usually mixed with Trichloroethylene. Elkins (1959) considers this usage undesirable, but in 50% of the machines investigated by him the atmospheric concentrations were below 100 p.p.m.

(4) In rubber cementing. According to the Shell Development Co. (1941) dichloroethane is more toxic than 2-chlorobutane-2 commonly used in the manufacture of synthetic rubber.

(5) In fabric spreading.

(6) In fire extinguishing, with 25% of CCl_4, to reduce fire and explosion hazards.

(7) As a fumigant and insecticide spray, also with 25% of CCl_4 (Hoyt, 1928).

Dichloroethane was first used as an anaesthetic in 1848 to 1849 (Nunnely *et al.*, 1849). Ethylidine chloride was also at one time used as an anaesthetic, but although it has less effect on the heart than chloroform, it caused marked excitation and was therefore relinquished (Plotz, 1920).

BIOCHEMISTRY

Estimation

(1) In the atmosphere

Infra red analysis can be used for direct determination or after absorption on silica gel. It has the advantage of being specific for the solvent in question (Irish, 1963).

(2) In blood, tissues and urine

No specific information available at present other than by the special apparatus described by Gettlee and Siegel (1935), but methods are being investigated by Stewart *et al.* (1960).

Metabolism

Little is known about the metabolism of either ethylene dichloride or ethylidine chloride except that following application to the shaved abdominal skin of rabbits prevented from inhaling the solvent by means of a mask (Irish, 1963). The exhaled air was passed into pure alcohol and the presence of the halogen tested by flaming a copper wire introduced into it. The green colour was observed after one hour, indicating that the halogen had been absorbed into the blood stream. No definite metabolite was detected, but Williams (1959) remarks that 1,1-halogenated ethanes could be expected to yield acetic acid and 1,2-halogenated compounds oxalic acid. The latter hypothesis was formulated by Hueper and Smith (1935) on the basis of their finding of nephrosis with calcification in a fatal case of poisoning by ingestion of ethylene chloride (see p. 251).

TOXICOLOGY

Ethylene dichloride has the narcotic properties common to the chlorinated hydrocarbons, and though it does not cause the severe injury to the liver and kidneys characteristic of acute carbontetrachloride intoxication, animal experiments have in the hands of some observers tended to show that it has a potential toxicity in this respect, while in human beings Von Oettingen (1937) was able to conclude that it is "somewhat less hepatotoxic" than carbontetrachloride or tetrachloroethane.

It has a definite potentiality for eye injury in the form of corneal opacity and can cause severe dermatitis.

Toxicity to animals

Acute

(a) *Lethal dose.* – (i) *By oral administration* to dogs, Kistler and Luckhardt (1929) found it difficult to produce death, since more than 0.5 g/kg tended to be vomited. – (ii) *By intravenous injection* Kistler and Luckardt found 0.25 ml/kg lethal after 24 h; Barsoum and Saad (1934) gave the minimum lethal dose as 175 mg/kg. – (iii) *By inhalation.* – The lethal dosage given by Heppel *et al.* (1944) indicates a higher toxicity of ethylene dichloride than those of some earlier observers. Sayers *et al.* (1930) for example, using guinea pigs, found that death occurred in a few minutes of exposure to about 100,000 p.p.m. and on the following day after exposure for 25 min to 10,000 p.p.m. Heppel *et al.* (1944) give 3000 p.p.m. as the fatal single dose, with 1000 and 400 p.p.m. for repeated exposures.

For ethylidine chloride Lazarew (1929) found the lethal dose somewhat greater than that for ethylene dichloride – 17,500 p.p.m. for mice as compared with about 9000. According to Joachimoglu (1921) and Fuhner (1921) the reverse was true for their aqueous solutions.

(b) *Narcotic dose.* – Lazarew (1929) induced deep narcosis in mice exposed to 5000 p.p.m. and in guinea pigs at 10,000 p.p.m., while Sayers *et al.* (1930) observed semi-consciousness and apparent unconsciousness in guinea pigs with vapour concentrations of 4500 and above, and slight drowsiness between 1000 and 2000 p.p.m. Their results indicated in their opinion that for single exposures and periods of an hour or more, the acute narcotic toxicity of ethylene dichloride is about the same as that of gasoline, benzene, carbontetrachloride and chloroform; for periods of less than an hour it is less powerfully narcotic than these.

Bibliography on p. 263

Lacrimation, with reddening of the conjunctiva, and nasal irritation were early symptoms, also vertigo, followed by static and motor ataxia and inability to walk; at concentrations of 1 % there were spasmodic contractions (retching movements) of the abdominal wall. Later, the respirations became jerky and rapid with concentrations of 1.7% above; with lower concentrations a slight increase in rate was followed by slow shallow breathing.

The eyes

Corneal opacity has been observed in animals both by inhalation and subcutaneous injection of ethylene dichloride.

Inhalation by dogs for 1½ h was found by Dubois and Roux (1887) to cause only a considerable diminution of intraocular pressure and irregular astigmatism, observed also to a smaller degree in chloroform anaesthesia, but after 16–18 h, even with no direct contact with the vapour, the corneae lost transparency, becoming bluish and opalescent. At this time the curve of the cornea was exaggerated, giving an appearance under the slit-lamp of numerous small depressions over the whole surface. The opacity at first appeared uniform, but under the ophthalmoscope and slit-lamp numerous whitish arborisations radiating from the periphery to the centre were observed. The opacity disappeared after several months beginning at the periphery. The opaque cornea was two to three times as thick as the normal cornea; this, according to Dubois (1888), was due to lymphatic infiltration of the protoplasm of the vitreous body and swelling of the connective tissue; there were no indications of fatty granulation nor of an inflammatory process. Dubois did not believe that the opacity was due to direct action of the vapour, since instillation between the eyelids caused only irritation; he explained the action on the hypothesis that during inhalation the aqueous humour becomes saturated with ethylene dichloride, causing injury to the posterior surface of the cornea. Parnas (1888) using 2–5 inhalations of 1 h each, with 10 ml of ethylene dichloride at each period, found that corneal opacity appeared after the first to third inhalation and disappeared after about a week. In this clear period tolerance seemed to have been established, since further inhalation failed to produce the disturbance, but if opacity were still present it was increased still further. He disagreed with Dubois' statement that the aqueous tissue was the first to be implicated, and postulated destruction of the corneal epithelium, allowing oedema of the corneal tissue to occur. Erdmann (1912) subscribed to this view, adding that though the corneal lesion was usually reversible, it might possibly be followed by injury of the epithelium of the lens capsule.

In the experiments of Steindorff (1922) it was shown that the corneal injury was not due to actual contact with the vapour by the fact that even when the eyes were covered the typical opacity occurred following inhalation which caused narcosis.

That corneal opacity can be produced without actual narcotisation was shown by Heppel *et al.* (1944), but this occurred in only two species of animals (the fox and the dog) out of eleven examined. In dogs, single exposures for 7 h to 1000 p.p.m. produced symmetrical turbidity of the cornea which sometimes took three weeks for partial regression. With five exposures repeated every two days the dogs became gradually tolerant, and eventually no cloudiness developed. Histological examination of eyes which were turbid at death showed corneal oedema, degeneration and sloughing of the corneal endothelium and infiltration with polymorphonuclear leucocytes; those which had cleared before death were histologically normal. Similar lesions were found in the eyes of a fox subjected for 7 h to a single exposure of 3000 p.p.m.

Subcutaneous injection was stated by the earlier observers to be followed within 24 h by moderate cloudiness of the cornea; this disappeared after 4–5 days, but injections of 5 ml, which were fatal, caused intense cloudiness of both corneae. Steindorff (1922) found that subcutaneous injection of 5 ml in a dog produced corneal opacity without evidence of injury to the internal organs.

CHANGES IN THE ORGANISM

Congestion and oedema of the lungs was the principal pathological finding in the animals examined by Sayers *et al.* and by Kistler and Luckhart (1929); in those animals which survived 7–8 days this condition appeared to regress.

The kidneys showed congestion and degenerative changes, either secondary to the lung injury or (according to Sayers *et al.*) more or less dependent on elimination of decomposition products (assumed to be oxalic acid) of the ethylene dichloride. There were also pathological changes in the liver and adrenals of rats exposed to concentrations of 3000 p.p.m. or more (Spencer, 1951).

Haemolytic effect. This was tested by Plotz (1920) on the defibrinated blood of guinea pigs. 5 ml was centrifuged and made up to 100 ml with physiological saline. Ethylene dichloride was found to be much less haemolytic than carbon tetrachloride or chloroform. The property was attributed by Plotz to the lesser solubility in water of ethylene dichloride, with consequently less alteration of the protoplasm of living blood corpuscles.

Ethylidine chloride had a greater haemolytic action than ethylene dichloride, but again less than that of carbon tetrachloride or chloroform.

Toxicity to human beings

(1) Acute

(a) Lethal dose. – (i) By ingestion – Few cases of oral poisoning from ethylene dichloride have been recorded but in 1935 Hueper and Smith reported an accidental fatal case – a man who drank 2 ounces mixed with orange juice and ginger ale. Symptoms were delayed for 2 h, when nausea, vomiting and faintness occurred. He than became drowsy, cyanosed and dyspnoeic, and the urine contained al-

Bibliography on p. 263

bumen and sugar. He died from circulatory failure 22 h after the ingestion. Autopsy showed extensive haemorrhagic colitis, nephrosis with marked calcification of the tubules, generalised passive congestion of internal organs and multiple perivascular haemorrhages in the region of the cerebral basal ganglia. – *(ii) By inhalation.* – Among the fatal cases from industrial exposure are those recorded by Brass (1949) and Hadengue and Martin (1953). Brass reported two fatal cases of men employed in repairing vessels used for transporting dichloroethane. At autopsy they showed liver and kidney lesions, but not pulmonary oedema, though there had been a latent period before the development of symptoms. The case recorded by Hadengue and Martin had been engaged in repairing a vessel containing a paste of soap mixed with dichloroethane. He was exposed only a few minutes before becoming unconscious, as also did his rescuer. On recovery he appeared at first not seriously ill, but a sudden aggravation was followed by coma and death some hours later. His skin was covered by a yellow oily mass, a by-product of the separation of carotene; this had probably caused some absorption of dichloroethane by the skin. Autopsy revealed considerable pulmonary oedema, granular and fatty degeneration of the liver, intense renal congestion and small meningeal haemorrhages with microscopically acute epithelial nephritis.

(b) Narcotic dose. – *By inhalation.* – Three cases of acute poisoning following a four hour exposure to ethylene dichloride in a knitting factory were reported by Wirtschafter and Schwarz (1939). The initial symptoms were dizziness, nausea and vomiting; later, weakness, trembling and epigastric cramp. The blood sugar level was extremely low, raising, according to these observers, the suspicion of liver damage, but there was no jaundice, and the urine gave no evidence of kidney injury. The blood picture was that of leucocytosis, but no haemolysis. Recovery occurred following calcium therapy and a high carbohydrate diet. All three cases had severe dermatitis of the hands.

(2) Chronic or subacute

In 1941 McNally and Fostvedt (1941) recorded two cases of chronic poisoning in men employed for 9 weeks and 5 months respectively in a plant producing cholesterol, where ethylene dichloride was used as a solvent. Both complained of nausea and vomiting; one also of drowsiness, nervousness and loss of weight and the other of epigastric pain; the latter showed tremor of the tongue and nystagmus. The blood picture of both was within normal limits, the urine contained no sugar or albumen, and electrocardiographic examinations showed no abnormality.

TREATMENT OF ACUTE POISONING

Relief of the epigastric pain and vomiting has been achieved (Wirtschafter and Schwarz, 1939) by intraveneous administration of 10% calcium gluconate solution. A high carbohydrate, high calcium diet maintained the improvement.

25. Trichloroethane

Trichloeroethane exists in two isomers; 1,1,1 – the α isomer and 1,1,2 – the β isomer. Until recently it has been stated that the α-isomer is more toxic than the β. The error apparently arose from a misconception of the results of experiments published by Lazarew in 1929 on its minimal anaesthetic concentration, though this was given at the time as 45 mg/l compared with 15 mg/l for the β-isomer and the respective lethal doses as 65 mg/l and 60 mg/l. Boehring (1958, personal communication) and Stewart (1963) both agree that the α-isomer is the less toxic of the two.

Synonyms: methylchloroform, vinyl trichloride

Structural formula: 1,1,1-trichloroethane   1,1,2-trichloroethane

$$Cl{-}\underset{\underset{Cl}{|}}{\overset{\overset{Cl}{|}}{C}}{-}\underset{\underset{H}{|}}{\overset{\overset{H}{|}}{C}}{-}H \qquad H{-}\underset{\underset{Cl}{|}}{\overset{\overset{Cl}{|}}{C}}{-}\underset{\underset{H}{|}}{\overset{\overset{H}{|}}{C}}{-}Cl$$

Molecular formula: $C_2H_3Cl_3$ $C_2H_3Cl_3$

Molecular weight: 133.42   133.42

25a. 1,1,1-Trichloroethane

Properties: a volatile colourless liquid with chloroform-like odour
   boiling point: 74.1 °C
   melting point: none? (Stewart, 1963)
   vapour pressure: 127 mm Hg at 25 °C
   vapour density (air = 1): 4.6
   specific gravity (liquid density): 1.336 at 25 °C
   flash point: none (Irish, 1963)
   conversion factors: 1 p.p.m. = 5.46 mg/m³
                1 mg/l   = 183 p.p.m.
   solubility: soluble in many organic solvents, but only slightly in water (Van Arkel and Vles, 1936).
   maximum allowable concentration: 500 p.p.m. (Threshold Limit Values, 1962)

ECONOMY, SOURCES AND USES

Production

Reacts with aluminium and aluminium alloys, but inhibited formulae are now marketed under trade names (Stewart, 1963) such as Chlorothene, a compound which contains 94–97% of 1,1,1-trichloroethane, 2.4–3% of dioxane, 0.12–0,3% of butanol and small amounts of ethylene dichloride, water and other materials (Torkelson *et al.*, 1958). It is not flammable, nor will it support combustion, but it will decompose if sufficient heat is applied. At 500 °F large amounts of HCl and trace amounts of phosgene are formed (Crummett and Stenger, 1956).

Industrial uses

The volatility and solvent power of 1,1,1-trichloroethane closely resemble those of CCl_4 and it has come into wider use as a substitute for CCl_4 in recent years:
(1) as a solvent for natural and synthetic resins, oils, waxes, tar and alkaloids,
(2) as a degreaser,
(3) in organic synthesis.

BIOCHEMISTRY

Estimation

(1) In the atmosphere

Like many other halogenated hydrocarbons, 1,1,1-trichloroethane can be determined by hydrolysis with alkali in isopropyl alcohol.

The method advised by Elkins (1959) is based on absorption of the vapour in *sec.*-butyl or isopropyl alcohol. The vapour is collected on a silica-gel absorber, followed by reduction with metallic sodium. The silica gel is then extracted with the alcohol and refluxed with metallic sodium; ethylalcohol (95%) is then added and the refluxing continued until all the sodium has reacted. After cooling and addition of water through the condenser, phenolphthalein and dilute nitric acid are added until the solution is acid. After addition of 0.1 N $AgNO_3$, filtration and washing of the precipitate with water, ferric sulphate solution is added and titration with 0.05 N KCNS solution carried out until a permanent yellow colour is obtained.

The amount of hydrolysis of 1,1,1-trichloroethane is 59% compared with 84% for CCl_4.

(2) In blood and tissues

A rapid infra-red technique for the analysis of certain organic compounds in the blood has been described by Stewart *et al.* (1959). They state that it has been satisfactory for 1,1,1-trichloroethane. In this method the suitable extracting solvent is added to the oxalated blood and, after centrifuging, the solvent layer is transferred to a standard infra-red sample cell of any standard infra-red spectrometer and the spectrum scanned from 2–16 mμ.

(3) In urine

The aforementioned method has also been applied successfully to urine.

Metabolism

Williams (1959) stated that the metabolic fate of 1.1.1-trichloroethane was unknown, but according to Hake *et al.* (1960) it is very stable in the body, and while a large part of an intravenous dose is excreted unchanged by the lungs, a very small amount is metabolised to chloroethanol and excreted in the urine as the glucuronate. Irish (1963) remarks that the high stability and rapid excretion may well account for the low toxicity and quick recovery from anaesthetic concentrations.

TOXICOLOGY

There is no doubt that methylchloroform is much less toxic than carbon tetrachloride. Its main toxic effect is exerted on the central nervous system, in a manner similar to that of any anaesthetic agent. In animals lethal dosage causes central nervous depression culminating in respiratory paralysis (Adams *et al.*, 1950) and at anaesthetic level it has the property of sensitising the heart to epinephrine, with induction of idioventricular rhythms (Rennick *et al.*, 1949). For this reason it is advisable that epinephrine should never be given to a person overcome by its vapour.

It can also cause a mild conjunctivitis if in contact with the eyes, but is not highly irritant to the skin except for the irritation caused by its defatting action with repeated contact.

With chronic exposure, the only animal species showing significant organic injury were, in the experiments of Torkelson *et al.* (1959), female guinea pigs: these showed slight inflammation of the lungs and fatty changes in the liver.

In industry 3 deaths have been reported from high exposure, all from open tanks; in one case to a concentration of more than several thousand p.p.m.

Bibliography on p. 263

Toxicity to animals

(1) Acute

(a) Lethal dose. – (i) By oral administration – for rats 10.3–12.3 g/kg, for rabbits 5.6 g/kg, for guinea pigs, 9.47 g/kg (Torkelson et al., 1958). – (ii) By inhalation, – for rats, 30,000 p.p.m. for 6 min; 15,000 p.p.m. for 1½ h; 8000 p.p.m. for 7 h (Adams et al., 1950).

(b) Narcotic dose. – 18,000 p.p.m. in 18 min, 8000 p.p.m. in 5 h (Irish, 1963).

(2) Chronic

The effects of repeated administration, either oral or by inhalation, do not suggest a high potential chronic toxicity. Rats, rabbits, guinea pigs and monkeys exposed to 500 p.p.m. 7 h a day, 5 days a week for 6 months showed no evidence of impairment of growth or health, and when the concentration was increased to 10,000 p.p.m. male rats showed as the only sign of organic injury a slight increase in the weight of the liver. A separate group of guinea pigs (female) however, exposed to 2000 p.p.m. for periods of up to half an hour a day, 69 times in 98 days, did show some irritation of the lungs and fatty infiltration of the liver, and some, at the shorter periods of exposure, an increased incidence of interstitial nephritis; since this did not occur at the higher intensities of exposure, Torkelson et al. believed that it was probably not related to the exposure. Adams et al. (1950) also carried out experiments with repeated exposure over long periods. Rats which succumbed to 10,000 p.p.m. appeared to have died from either cardiac or respiratory failure, but they survived 31 exposures to 5000 p.p.m. without apparent injury, while rabbits showed slight retardation of growth.

Inhalation of concentrations of 1000 p.p.m. 7 h a day for 5 days a week were lethal to guinea pigs after two exposures, to rats after 3 to 14, to rabbits, after 2 to 64. Dogs, cats and monkeys were less susceptible, surviving for 23 to 55 days (Heppel et al., 1944). Some variation in species susceptibility was noted by Spencer et al. (1951), rats and guinea pigs showing a high mortality at 400 p.p.m.

SYMPTOMS OF INTOXICATION

Lethal doses cause anaesthesia followed by respiratory arrest. Concentrations somewhat below the lethal level (about 10,000 p.p.m.) cause irregular respiration and a semicomatose state.

Some central nervous depression; the eyes of dogs showed reversible clouding of the cornea, with repeated exposure they became resistant to this effect (Heppel et al., 1944).

(1) The skin

Some irritation of the shaven skin of a rabbit following application of a pad saturated with methyl chloroform, and when applied under a cuff in a dosage of 15.8 g/kg killed less than half of the rabbits treated.

(2) Respiratory disturbances

Effect on the circulation. – Depression of the blood pressure of dogs and monkeys anaesthetised by 1,1,1-trichloroethane was observed by Krantz *et al.* (1959) the level reaching about half its normal value at the point of respiratory arrest. Administration of epinephrine during anaesthesia produces ventricular fibrillation in animals (Rennick *et al.*, 1949).

CHANGES IN THE ORGANISM

(1) The lungs

Only mild congestion even after 125 exposures to 200 p.p.m. (Heppel, 1944).

(2) Liver and kidneys

Only slight pathological changes, most marked in guinea pigs with repeated exposure to 200 p.p.m., none in rats.

Toxicity to human beings

Human beings were exposed to concentrations ranging from 506–1900 p.p.m. for periods of 5–45 min (Stewart *et al.*, 1961). At 1000 p.p.m. a strong unpleasant odour was noted after 30 min, and at 920 p.p.m. three of the individuals exposed showed a slight loss of co-ordination and equilibrium, and complained of light-headedness.

These signs of intoxication became very obvious, with a positive Romberg test, at 1900 p.p.m. for 5 min (Stewart, 1963). No evidence of systemic injury, as judged by tests of urine and liver function, was observed.

Industrial poisoning. – In industry three fatal cases due to high exposure have been reported. In the two recorded by Torkelson *et al.* (1958) the exposure occurred in an open tank where the concentration was believed to be close to saturation, and in one case for a period of about 30 min. The third case, recorded by Stewart (1963), was also due to entry into an open tank, and the concentration was stated to be "more than several thousand p.p.m.". The symptoms resembled those of drunkenness, with disturbance of equilibrium and incoordination.

Prevention of poisoning. – The measures of prevention advised by Stewart (1963) include protection of the eyes by safety glasses, and of the skin by removing contaminated clothing in case of spillage; keeping the workroom atmosphere to a level not higher than 500 p.p.m.; if higher levels should be present owing to accident or unavoidable circumstances, no workman should be allowed to remain in contact for more than a few minutes.

Treatment. – Removal to fresh air; if breathing has stopped artificial respiration should be tried, but epinephrine should never be given in case ventricular fibrillation should supervene. Oxygen may be necessary if there is severe hypotension.

Bibliography on p. 263

25b. 1,1,2-Trichloroethane

Synonym: vinyl trichloride

Properties: a volatile colourless liquid
  boiling point: 113.5 °C
  melting point: −36.7 °C
  vapour pressure: 25 mm Hg at 25 °C
  vapour density (air = 1): 4.6
  specific gravity (liquid density): 1.443
  conversion factors: 1 p.p.m. = 5.46 mg/m³
             1 mg/l = 183 p.p.m.
  solubility: in water 0.44 g in 100 g at 20 °C; soluble in ethanol and ethyl ether
  maximum allowable concentration: not established

ECONOMY, SOURCES AND USES

Production

In 1828 Regnault produced 1,1,2-trichloroethane by the action of vinyl chloride on antimony perchloride.

Industrial uses

Vinyl trichloride has been used as a chemical intermediate and solvent but its industrial use is at present not significant (Irish, 1963).

It is not effective as an anthelmintic (Wright and Schaffer, 1932).

Metabolism

The early experiments of Tauber (1881) led him to conclude that a considerable proportion of 1,1,2-trichloroethane is excreted by the lungs and some in the urine after decomposition by the alkalinity of the blood. Barrett *et al.* (1939) could find no evidence that it undergoes a metabolic transformation similar to that of trichlorethylene in forming trichloroacetic acid. It may be noted that carbon tetrachloride and chloroform similarly undergo no such conversion.

BIOCHEMISTRY

Estimation

In air, blood and tissues

The infra-red technique described in connection with 1,1,1-trichloroethane is probably suitable for the 1,1,2-isomer, and is being further investigated by Chenoweth *et al.* (1962).

TOXICOLOGY

1,1,2-Trichloroethane has an anaesthetic and toxic effect greater than that of the 1,1,1-isomer; it has a marked capacity for injury to the liver in animals, and to a certain extent also to the kidneys. It is a severe irritant of the gastrointestinal tract. In human beings it acts as an anaesthetic and narcotic, but no toxic effects have been recorded from its industrial use.

Toxicity to animals

(1) Acute

  (a) Lethal dose. – *(i) By oral administration*, for dogs, 0.5 ml/kg (Wright and Schaffer, 1932). *(ii) By inhalation.* – Carpenter *et al.* (1949) in the course of their examination of 96 chemical compounds, which they graded in groups as 1–5 (slight hazard), 6–9 (moderate), 10–13 (definite) and 14–19 (serious), placed 1,1,2-trichloroethane in grade 8; that is, in the group in which 2000 p.p.m. for 4 h killed 2, 3 or 4 out of 6 rats. This makes it comparable in toxicity to some of the ketones and glycol derivatives, but more toxic than trichloroethylene, dichloroethylene and tetrachloroethylene, and less so than dichloroethane, epichlorohydrin and ethylene chlorohydrin. Compared with 1,1,1-trichloroethane it is markedly more toxic, since 16,000 p.p.m. are necessary to kill 50% of rats exposed to the 1,1,1-isomer (Adams *et al.*, 1950), as compared with 2000 p.p.m. for 4 h for the 1,1,2-isomer (Carpenter *et al.*, 1949).

  (b) Narcotic dose. – *(i) By oral administration*, for dogs, Wright and Schaffer (1932), during their investigation of the anthelmintic potency of a number of chlorinated hydrocarbons, found that dosages of 0.2–0.5 ml caused partial narcosis. *(ii) By inhalation*, for dogs, Tauber (1881) found that 3–5 g (administered as 30–50 drops inhaled from a pad soaked with this amount) caused complete anaesthesia in 3–7 min in dogs weighing 5–7 kg.

  For guinea pigs and rabbits 10–20 drops on a pad produced complete anaesthesia in 2–5 min.

(2) Chronic

  No reports are at present published, but according to Irish' (1963) unpublished data would indicate that the toxicological response from chronic exposure would be qualitatively and quantitatively comparable to carbon tetrachloride.

SYMPTOMS OF INTOXICATION

(1) Gastro-intestinal disturbances

  Salivation, nausea, vomiting and diarrhoea, sometimes haemorrhagic, occurred after a dosage of 3 ml.

Bibliography on p. 263

(2) Neurological disturbances

In Tauber's experiments narcosis was preceded by a stage of excitation and Wright and Schaffer noted symptoms of cerebral irritation in one animal.

CHANGES IN THE ORGANISM

(1) The liver

Wright and Schaffer observed fatty degeneration, cloudy congestion and central necrosis.

(2) The kidneys

Congestion and cloudy swelling, and in one dog interstitial nephritis.

(3) The lungs

Ecchymoses were present in one of Wright and Schaffer's animals.

(4) Gastro-intestinal tract

Severe inflammation of the gastric mucosa and haemorrhage of the caecum and colon.

26. Pentachloroethane

Synonym: pentalin

Structural formula:

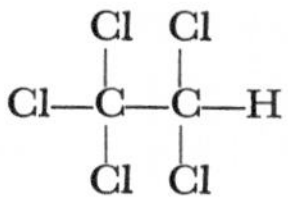

$$Cl-\underset{\underset{Cl}{|}}{\overset{\overset{Cl}{|}}{C}}-\underset{\underset{Cl}{|}}{\overset{\overset{Cl}{|}}{C}}-H$$

Molecular formula: C_2HCl_5

Molecular weight: 202.31

Properties: A colourless liquid with a camphor-like odour

    boiling point: 162 °C

    melting point: −29 °C

    vapour pressure: 10 mm Hg at 39.8 °C

    vapour density (air = 1): 7.0

    specific gravity (liquid density): 1.672

    conversion factors: 1 p.p.m. = 8.27 mg/m³

                       1 mg/l = 121 p.p.m.

    solubility: slightly in water; soluble in ethyl ether; miscible with ethyl alcohol and acetone

    evaporation rate (ether = 1): 0.03; less volatile than tetrachloroethane

    maximum allowable concentration: not established

Not combustible, but dehalogenation by reaction with alkalies or certain metals will produce spontaneously explosive chloroacetylenes (Sax, 1957). Distillation at atmospheric pressure causes some decomposition, and boiling with alcoholic potash formation of tetrachloroethylene.

ECONOMY, SOURCES AND USES

Production

By chlorination of trichloroethylene, ethyl chloride or tetrachloroethane (Fairhall, 1957).

Industrial uses

(1) In dry cleaning, but only to a small extent.

(2) In soil sterilisation (Sterner, 1949).

(3) In organic synthesis.

BIOCHEMISTRY

Estimation

(1) In the atmosphere

Reaction with pyridine and NaOH (Fujiwara, 1914), the amount being calculated from the chlorine content (Lehmann and Schmidt-Kehl, 1936). Quantitatively, by a combustion-titration method (Setterlind, 1947).

TOXICOLOGY

Pentachloroethane, as revealed by animal experiments, is a strong narcotic (stronger than chloroform, according to Kiessling, 1921), a severe irritant of mucous membranes, has an action on the liver similar to that of tetrachloroethane and a more highly toxic action on the heart, but not such a haemolytic effect (Plotz, 1920). Being less volatile than tetrachloroethane it is less hazardous to handle (Elkins, 1959), but Lehmann and Flury (1943) remark that its use as a solvent is not to be recommended. No toxic effects from its use in industry have in fact been recorded.

Toxicity to animals

(1) Acute

(a) Lethal dose. – *(i) By intravenous injection*, for dogs, 100 mg/kg (Barsoum and Saad, 1934), – *(ii) By inhalation*, for mice, 35 mg/l (Lazarew, 1929), as compared with 40 mg/l for tetrachloroethane.

(b) Narcotic dose, for cats (Lehmann and Schmidt-Kehl, 1936); – light narcosis, 13 mg/l after 1 h; 21 mg/l after 23 min; 37 mg/l after 5 min; – deep narcosis, 13 mg/l after 89 min; 21 mg/l after 32 min; 37 mg/l after $5\frac{1}{2}$ min; – Lazarew (1929) gives 25 mg/l for loss of reflexes.

SYMPTOMS OF INTOXICATION

With acute poisoning unconsciousness is preceded by intense irritation of the mucous membranes of the nose, throat and eyes, tremor of limbs, muscular cramps of an opisthotonus-like character, and diarrhoea.

Chronic poisoning

According to Joachimoglu (1921) pentachloroethane, with repeated inhalation, is 20 times more narcotic than chloroform. He found that dogs, after repeated inhalation of 10 ml became, after an initial period of restlessness and excitement, completely narcotised within 20 min. In the experiments of Lehmann and Schmidt-Kehl (1936) cats inhaling 146 p.p.m. 8 to 9 h daily for 23 days showed practically

no symptoms of poisoning, but with higher (narcotic) dosage recovery was slow –
30 to 140 min.

CHANGES IN THE ORGANISM

(1) Heart and circulation system

On the isolated frog's heart, Kiessling (1921) found pentachloroethane more
toxic than tetrachloroethane. Plotz (1920) reported that it had no haemolytic
effect similar to that of tetrachloroethane.

(2) Liver

All animals subjected to continued inhalation (Joachimoglu, 1921) and even
those which were not narcotised (Lehmann and Schmidt-Kehl, 1936) showed a
high degree of fatty degeneration.

(3) Kidneys

Inflammation, with albumin and blood pigments in the urine of dogs are
reported by Lehmann and Flury (1943).

(4) Lungs

Marked hyperaemia, with acute purulent inflammation of the trachea and
large bronchi.

Toxicity to human beings

None have been recorded.

BIBLIOGRAPHY

Abrahamson, A. M. (1960) Quantitative Estimation of Trichloroethylene in Urine and Serum in
  Tri Poisoning, *Acta Pharmacol. Toxicol.*, 17:288.
Adams, E. M., H. C. Spencer, V. K. Rowe and D. D. Irish (1950) Vapour Toxicity of 1,1,1-Tri-
  chloroethane (Methylchloroform) determined by Experiments on Laboratory Animals, *Arch.
  Ind. Hyg.*, 1:225; (1951) idem of Trichloroethylene, *Arch. Ind. Hyg.*, 4: 469
Agress, C. M., H. D. Jacobs *et al.* (1955) Serum transaminase Levels in experimental Myocardial
  Infection, *Circulation*, 11:711.
Ahlmark, A. and L. Friberg (1955) Should the M.A.C. of Trichloroethylene and similar Substances
  be reduced? *Nord. Hyg. Tidskr.*, 36:165.
Albahary, C., C. Guyot-Jeannin, A. Flaisler and P. Thiancourt (1959) Transaminases et Exposition
  professionelle au Trichloroéthylène, *Arch. Malad. Profess.*, 20:421.
Alfonso, O. R., E. Mitidieri, L. Ribiero and G. Villela (1955) Blood serum Exanthine Oxidase of
  rats poisoned with CCl₄, *Proc. Soc. Exptl. Biol. Med.*, 90:527.
Alha, A. (1950) CCl₄ Mass Poisoning, *Ann. Med. Internae Fenniae*, Suppl. 8, 39:1.
Allen, A. C. (1954) Tratto di Patologia renale, Sansoni, Florence.
Anderssen, H. (1957) Gesundliche Gefähren in der Industrie bei Exposition zur Trichloräthylen,
  Acta Med. Scand., Suppl. 323.
André, L. and R. Feillard (1946) Nouveau Cas d'Intoxication grave par le Tétrachlorure de Car-
  bone, *Bull. Soc. Méd. Hôp. Paris*, 62:418.

Arena, J. M. (1962) Rep. from Duke Univ. Poison Control Centre: CC 14.

Ashe, W. F. and S. Sailer (1942) Fatal Uraemia following single Exposure to CCl₄ Fumes, *Ohio State Med. J.*, 38:553.

Atkinson, R. S., (1960) Trichloroethylene Anaesthesia, *Anesthesiology*, 21:67.

Baader, W. (1927) Tätigkeit Bericht des Abteilung für Gewerbekrankheiten, *Zentr. Gewerbehyg.*, 14:385.

Baader, E. W. (1954) Gewerbekrankheiten, Urban and Schwarzenberg, Munich.

Baker, A. M. (1927) Intoxication with commercial Methyl Chloride, *J. Am. Med. Assoc.*, 88:1137.

Barach, A. L., C. P. Yaglou and C. P. McCord (1944) Dangers of Methyl Chloride as a Substitute for Freon, *J. Am. Med. Assoc.*, 124:94.

Barnes, C. G. and J. Ives (1944) Electrocardiographic Changes during Trilene Anaesthesia, *Proc. Roy. Soc. Med.*, 37:526.

Barrett, H. M., J. G. Cunningham and J.H.Johnston (1939) A Study of the Fate in the Organism of some Chlorinated Hydrocarbons, *J. Ind. Hyg.*, 21:479.

Barrett, H. M. and J. H. Johnston (1939) The Fate of Trichloroethylene in the Organism, *J. Biol. Chem.*, 127:765.

Barsoum, G. S. and K. Saad (1934) Relative Toxicity of certain Chlorine Derivatives of the Aliphatic Series, *Quart. J. Pharmacol.*, 7:205.

Bartoniček, V. (1962) Metabolism and Excretion of Trichloroethylene after Inhalation by human Subjects, *Brit. J. Ind. Med.*, 19:134.

Bartoniček, V. and J. Teisinger (1962) Effect of Tetraethyl thiuram disulphide (Disulfiram) on Metabolism of Trichloroethylene, *Brit. J. Ind. Med.*, 19:216.

Bassi, M. (1960) Electron Microscopy of Rat Liver after CCl₄ Poisoning, *Exp. Cell Research*, 20:313.

Beaufay, H., E. van Campenhout and C. De Duve (1959) Hepatoxic Treatments and bound Enzymes, *Bioch. J.*, 73:617.

Bell, E. T. (1946) Renal Diseases, Lea and Fibiger, Philadelphia.

Bell, A. (1951) Death from Trichloroethylene in a Dry Cleaning Establishment, *New Zealand Med. J.*, 50:119.

Bell, W. I. and N. Kay (1956) Serum Esterase Response in Rats exposed to CCl₄ Vapour, *Arch. Ind. Health.*, 14:450.

Benzi, T. (1925) Indagine e Osservazioni sperimentali sull' Intossicazione professionale da Tetrachloretano, *Boll. Soc. Med. Chir. Pavia*, 37:537.

Bernardi, B., Penzani and R. Lavori (1956) Richerche istologische sul Encefalo di Coniglio nel Intossicazione da Tricloroetilene, *Rass. Med. Ind.*, 25:269.

Bernstine, M. L. (1954) Cardiac Arrest occurring under Trichloroethylene Anaesthesia, *Arch. Surg.*, 68:262.

Biesalski, E. (1924) Pyrogene Phosgenbildung, *J. Angew. Chem.*, 37:314.

Block, W. D. and H. H. Cornish (1958) Effect of CCl₄ Inhalation on Rat serum Enzymes, *Proc. Soc. Explt. Biol. Med.*, 97:178.

Boidin, L., L. Rouqués and G. Albot (1930) Ictère grave toxique par le Tétrachlorétane chez une Ouvrière perlière, *Bull. Soc. Méd. Hôp. Paris*, 54:1305.

Bowditch, M., C. L. Drinker, P. Drinker, H. H. Haggard and A. Hamilton (1940) Code for safe Concentrations of certain common toxic Substances used in Industry, *J. Ind. Hyg.*, 22:251.

Boye, E. (1935) Die chemische Feuerlösch Methoden, *Chemiker Ztg.*, 59:155, 175.

Brass, K. (1949) Über tödliche Dichloräthanvergiftung, *Deut. Med. Wochschr.*, 74:553.

Butler, J. C. (1949) Metabolic Transformation of Trichloroethylene, *J. Pharm. Exptl. Therap.*, 97:84.

Butsch, W. (1922) Cirrhosis of the liver caused by CCl₄, *J. Am. Med. Assoc.*, 99:728.

Calvert, D. N. and T. M. Brody (1958) Biochemical Alteration of Liver Function by the Halogenated Hydrocarbons, *J. Pharmacol. Exptl. Therap.*, 124:273.

Calvert, D. N. and T. M. Brody (1960) Role of the Sympathetic Nervous System in CCl₄ Hepatoxicity, *Am. J. Physiol.*, 198:669.

Calvet, J., J. Planques, A. Ribet and J. Coll (1959) Intoxication aiguë par le Trichloroéthylène. Guérison, *Arch. Malad. Profess.*, 20:297.

Cameron, A. M. (1947) Chemistry in Relation to Fire Risk and Fire Prevention, 3rd ed. Pitman and Sons, London.

Cameron, G. K. and W. A. E. Karunaratne (1936) CCl$_4$ Cirrhosis in Relation to Liver Regeneration, *J. Pathol. Bacteriol.*, 42:1.

Canepa, A. D. and J. J. Courtis (1951) Intoxicacion per Cloruro de Metilo, *Prensa Med. Arg.*, 28:2738.

Carpenter, C. P. (1937) The chronic Toxicity of Tetrachloroethylene, *J. Ind. Hyg.*, 19:323.

Carpenter, C. P., H. F. Smyth and V. C. Pozzani (1949) Assay of acute Vapour Toxicity and grading and Interpretation of Results on 96 chemical Compounds, *J. Ind. Hyg.*, 31:343.

Castellino, N. (1932) Intossicazione da Tricloretilene, *Folia Med. (Naples)*, 18:415.

Chalmers, J. N. M., A. E. Gillam and J. E. Kench (1940) Porphyrinuria in a Case of industrial Methyl Chloride Poisoning, *Lancet*, 2:806.

Chenoweth, M. B., D. M. Robertson, D. S. Erley and R. Golhke (1962) Blood and Tissue Levels of Ether, Chloroform, Halothane and Methoxyflurance in Dogs, *Anesthesiology*, 23:101.

Chief Inspector of Factories, Annual Reports 1940–1961, H.M. Stationary Office, London.

Chiesura, P. and G. Picotti (1960) L'Epatopatia da Tetrachloruro di Carbonio, *Riv. Infortuni Mal. Profess.*, 47:161.

Christie, G. S. and J. D. Judah (1954) Mechanism of Action of CCl$_4$ on Liver Cells, *Proc. Roy. Soc. (London), Ser. B.*, 142:241.

Clayton, J. I. and J. Parkhouse (1962) Blood Trichloroethylene Concentrations during Anaesthesia under controlled Conditions, *Brit. J. Anaesthesia*, 34:141.

Clinton, M. (1947) Renal Injury following Exposure to CCl$_4$, *New Engl. J. Med.*, 237:183.

Cohen, M. M. (1957) The central Nervous System in CCl$_4$ Poisoning, *Neurology*, 7:228.

Coler, H. R. and H. R. Rossmiller (1953) Tetrachloroethylene Exposure in a small Industry, *Arch. Ind. Hyg.*, 8:227.

Collier, H. (1936) Methylene Chloride Intoxication in Industry, *Lancet*, 1:594.

Comstock, C. C. and F. W. Oberst (1952) Comparative Inhalation Toxicities of 4 Halogenated Hydrocarbons to Rats and Mice, *Arch. Ind. Hyg.*, 7:157.

Conway, E. J. (1957) Microdiffusion Analysis and Volumetric Error, 4th Ed. p. 324, Crosby Lockwood, London.

Conway, E. J. and A. Byrne (1933) An Absorption Apparatus for the Microdetermination of certain volatile Substances, *Biochem. J.*, 27:419.

Corcoran, A. C., R. D. Taylor and I. H. Page (1943) Acute toxic Nephrosis; a Study based on a Case of CCl$_4$ Poisoning, *J. Am. Med. Assoc.*, 123:81.

Council on Pharmacy and Chemistry (1936) The Use of Trichloroethylene for general Anaesthesia, *J. Am. Med. Assoc.*, 107:1302.

Coyer, H. A. (1944) Tetrachloroethane Poisoning; 7 cases, *Ind. Med.*, 13:230.

Cralley, L. V., T. E. Shea and L. J. Cralley (1943) Modification of Silica Gel Method for Determination of Atmospheric and organic Solvent Vapours, *J. Ind. Hyg.*, 25:172.

Crowley, R. C., C. B. Ford and H. C. Stern (1945) A Study of Perchloroethylene Degreasers, *J. Ind. Hyg.*, 27:140.

Crummett, W. B. and V. A. Stenger (1956) Thermal Stability of Methyl Chloroform and Carbon Tetrachloride, *Ind. Eng. Chem.*, 48:434.

Davies, P. A., (1934) CCl$_4$ as an industrial Hazard, *J. Am. Med. Assoc.*, 103:962.

Dawborn, J. K., M. Ralston and S. Weiden (1961) Acute CCl$_4$ Poisoning. Transaminase and Biopsy Studies, *Brit. Med. J.*, 2:493.

Deichmann, W. B. and G. Thomas (1943) Glucuronic Acid in Urine as Measure of Absorption of certain Organic Compounds, *J. Ind. Hyg.*, 25:286.

Deplace, Y., Cavigneaux and G. Cabasson (1962) Affections professionnelles dues au Chlorure de Méthylène et au Dichloréthane., *Arch. Malad. Profess.*, 23:816.

Derobert, L. (1944) Trichloroéthylène, *Arch. Malad. Profess.*, 6:321.

— (1952) Mort au cours d'une Inhalation toxicomaniaque au Trichloroéthylène, *Ann. Med. Légale Criminol. Police Sci. Toxicol.*, 36:293.

— (1954) Intoxications et Maladies Professionelles, Flammarion, Paris.

Dianzani, M. V. (1954) Uncoupling of Oxidative Phosphorylation from fatty Livers, *Biochim. Biophys. Acta*, 14:514.

Dianzani, M. V. and G. E. Bahr (1954) Electron Microscope Investigation of Mitochondria isolated from normal and steatotic Livers by Differential Centrifugalisation, *Acta Pathol. Microbol.*, *Scand.*, 35:25.

Dixon, K. C. and G. P. McCullagh (1957) Protein in dying Liver Cells, *Quart. J. Exptl. Physiol.*, 42:104.

Dodds, G. H. (1945) Necrosis of Liver and bilateral massive Suprarenal Haemorrhage in Puerperium, *Brit. Med. J.*, 1:769.

Dubois, R. (1888) Action du Chlorure d'Éthylène sur la Cornée, *Compt. Rend.*, 107:921.

Dubois, R. and L. Roux (1887) Action physiologique du Chlorure d'Éthylène sur la Cornée, *Compt. Rend.*, 104:1869.

Dudley, S. F. (1935) Toxic Nephritis following Exposure to carbontetrachloride and Smoke Fumes. *J. Roy. Naval Med. Serv.*, 21:296.

Dunn, R. C. and W. Smith (1947) Acute and chronic Toxicity of Methyl Chloride, *Arch. Pathol.*, 43:297.

Dyling, F. and O. Dyling (1946) The toxic Effect of Tetrachlormethane and Tetrachloroethylene in oily Solution, *Acta Pharmacol.*, 2:223.

Eddy, J. A. (1945) CCl_4 Poisoning in Industry, *Ind. Med. Surg.*, 14:283.

Elliott, J. M. (1933) Report of a fatal Case of Poisoning by Tetrachloroethane, *J. Roy. Army Med. Corps*, 60:373.

Elkins, H. B. (1942) Maximum Allowable Concentrations; CCl_4, *J. Ind. Hyg.*, 24:233.

— (1959) The Chemistry of Industrial Toxicology, Chapman and Hall, London.

Erdmann (1912) Über Augenveränderungen durch Äthylenchlorid, *Klin. Monatsbl. Augenheilk.*, 14:370.

Ewing, J. S. and G. J. C. Brittain (1948) Auricular Fibrillation after Trichloroethylene Anaesthesia, *Brit. Med. J.*, 2:904.

Fabre, R. and G. Rougier (1948) Sur deux cas d'Intoxication par la Chlorure de Méthyl, *Arch. Malad. Profess.*, 9:324.

Fahy, J. P. (1948) Determination of Chlorinated Hydrocarbon Vapours in Air, *J. Ind. Hyg.*, 30:205.

Fairhall, L. T. (1957) Industrial Toxicology, 2nd ed., Williams and Wilkins, Baltimore.

Faraone, G. (1956) Case Report of Liver Cirrhosis caused by CCl_4, *Minerva Medicolegale*, 76:6.

Farrier, P. M. and R. H. Smith (1950) CCl_4 Nephrosis, a frequently undiagnosed Cause of Death. *J. Am. Med. Assoc.*, 143:965.

Fawcett, H. H. (1942) CCl_4 Mixtures in Fire Fighting, *Arch. Ind. Hyg.*, 6:435.

Fieldner A. C., S. H. Katz and S. P. Kinney (1921) Cases produced in the Use of CCl_4 and Foamite Fire Extinguishers in Mines, *U.S. Bureau Mines Rept. Invest.*, Ser. 2262.

Fiessinger, N., P. Brodin and M. Wolf (1923) Les Ictères des Perlières et les Hépatites dues au Tétrachloréthane.

Fiume, L. and C. Favelli (1961) Inhibition of experimental Cirrhosis by CCl_4 following Treatment with Amino acetonitrile, *Nature*, 189:71.

Fleisher, G. A., C. S. Potter and K. G. Wakim (1960) Separation of two G.O.T.'s by Paper Electrophoresis, *Proc. Soc. Exptl. Biol. Med.*, 103:229.

Fleisher, G. A. and K. G. Wakim (1961) Presence of two G.O.T.'s in Serum of Dogs following acute Injury of the Liver, *Proc. Soc. Exptl. Biol. Med.*, 106:283.

Flinn, F. B. (1946) Industrial Exposure to Chlorinated Hydrocarbons, *Am. J. Med.*, 1:388.

Flury, F. and O. Klimmer (1939) Gewerbliche Chlormethylvergiftung, *Samml. Vergiftungsf.*, 110:45.

Flury, F. and F. Zernik (1931) Schädliche Gäse, Dämpfe, Nebel-, Rauch- und Staubarten, Springer, Berlin.

Forssmann, S. and A. Ahlmark (1945) Bidrag till Diagnostiken av Triklorethylen forgiftningar, *Nord. Med.*, 30:1033.

Forssmann, S., A. Owe-Larson and E. Skog (1955) Umsatz von Trichloräthylen im Organismus, *Arch. Gewerbepath. Gewerbehyg.*, 13:619.

Frada, G. (1952) (cited by Gobbao and Sequi, 1960) Atti Congr. Soc. Ital. Cardiol. Taormina.

Friberg, L., B. Kylin and A. Nystrom (1953) Toxicities of Trichloroethylene and Tetrachloroethylene, *Acta Pharmacol.*, 9:303.

Friedberg, C. H. (1950) Congestive Heart Failure of Renal Origin; Pathogenesis and Treatment in 4 Cases of CCl_4 Nephrosis, *Am. J. Med.*, 9:164.

Forboese, C. (1943) Trichloräthylen Vergiftung per Os beim Menschen, *Arch. Toxikol.*, 13:49.

Fry, W. A., J. M. Smith and J. R. Suker (1959) Acute CCl₄ Intocixation, *Quart. Bull. Northwestern Univ. Med. School*, 33:346.

Fuhner, H. (1921) Die Wirkungstarke der Narkotica, *Biochim. Z.*, 120:143.

Fujiwara, K. (1914) Über eine neue sehr empfindliche Reaktion zum Chloroform-nachweis, *Sitzber. Abhandl. Naturforsch.*, 6:33.

Gallagher, C. H. (1961) Protection by Antioxidants against lethal Doses of CCl₄, *Nature*, 192:881.

Gasq, M. (1936) Étude toxicologique et hygiénique des Solvants chlorés acétyléniques, Delams; Bordeaux (cited by Von Oettingen, 1955).

Geiger, A. J. (1943) Cardiac Dysrhythmias and Syncope from therapeutic Inhalation of Chlorinated Hydrocarbons, *J. Am. Med. Assoc.*, 123:141.

Gerbis, H. (1914) Eigenartige Narkosezustände nach gewerbliche Arbeit mit Chlormethyl, *Münch. Med. Wochschr.*, 61:879.

— (1928) Irreparabele Gesichtsnervenlähmung durch gewerbliche Vergiftung, *Zentr. Gewerbehyg.*, 15:97.

Germain, A. and J. Marty (1947) Hepatonéphrite aiguë mortelle par Inhalation de Trichloroéthylène, *Bull. Soc. Med. Hôp. Paris*, 63:1044.

Glaser, M. A. (1931) Treatment of Trigeminal Neuralgia with Trichloroethylene, *J. Am. Med. Assoc.*, 96:916.

Glass, W. I. (1961) A Survey of Trichloroethylene Degreasing Baths in Auckland, 1961, *Occup. Health Bul., New Zealand*, December.

Glynn, L. E. and H. P. Himsworth (1948) The intralobular Circulation in acute Liver Injury by CCl₄, *Clin. Sci.*, 6:235.

Gobbato, F. and G. Sequi (1960) Considerazione sull'Intossicazione da Tetrachloruro di Carbonio, *Riv. Infortuni Mal. Profess.*, 47:178.

Goldenson, J. and J. W. Thomas (1947) Determination of Acethylene tetrachloride in Air, *J. Ind. Hyg. Toxicol.*, 29:14.

Graber, H. (1950) Die perorale Trichloräthylenvergiftung und ihre Pathogenesse, *Deut. Z. Ges. Gerichtl. Med.*

Grandjean, E. (1959) Corrélations entre Valeurs d'Exposition et Valeurs dans les Matières biologiques, *Pracovni Lekar.*, 11:162.

Grandjean, E., E. Munching, V. Turrian, H. K. Knoepel and H. Rosemind (1955) Investigation into the effects of Exposure to Trichloroethylene in Mechanical Engineering, *Brit. J. Ind. Med.*, 12:131.

Greenburg, L. and S. Moskowitz (1945) Safe Use of Solvents for Synthetic Rubbers, *Ind. Med. Surg.*, 14:359.

Grimm, V., A. Heffter and G. Joachimoglu (1914) Gewerbliche Vergiftungen in Flugzeugfabriken, *Vjschr. Gerichtl. Med.*, Suppl. 48, 2:161.

Grisler, R. and R. Gallina (1956) Il Tricloretilene, *Med. Lavoro*, 47:240.

Grasset, J. and R. Gauthier (1950) Étude clinique et grafique de l'Action analgésique obstétricale du Chlorure de Méthylène, *Sem. Hôp. Paris*, 26:1280.

Grossendorfer, K. (1952) Zwei Fälle von chronischer Vergiftung durch Halogen – Kohlen Wasserstoffe, *Zweite Oesterr. Tagung Arbeitsmed.*

Gummert, M. (1961) Wilson-Block nach Methylchloridvergiftung, *Ges. Inn. Med.*, 16:677.

Gunther, W. (1955) Hyperchrome megalocytäre bzw. perniciose Anämie als Folge chronische Tri-vergiftung? *Med. Welt*, 9:1834.

Guyot-Jeannin, C. and J. van Steenkiste (1958) L'Action du Trichloréthylène sur les Protéines et les Lipides sériques. *Arch. Malad. Profess.*, 19:489.

Habgood, S. and J. F. Powell (1945) Estimation of Chloroform, Carbon Tetrachloride and Trichloroethylene in Blood, *Brit. J. Ind. Med.*, 2:39.

Hadengue, A., J. Facquet, P. Colvez and J. L. Jullien (1959) Intoxication par le Nitorbenzène et le Trichloroéthylène, *Arch. Malad. Profess.*, 21:43.

Hadengue, A. and A. Martin (1953) Un cas d'intoxication mortelle par le dichloréthane, *Ann. Méd. Lég.*, 33:247.

Hake, C. L., T. B. Waggoner, D. N. Robertson and V. K. Rowe (1960) The metabolism of 1,1,1-trichloroethane by the Rat, *Arch. Ind. Environ. Health*, 1:101.

Hall, M. C. and J. E. Stillinger (1925) Tetrachloroethylene, a new Anthelmintic, *Am. J. Trop. Med.*, 5:229.
Hamburger, J. (1958) Petite Encyclopédie Médicale, Flammarion, Paris.
Hamilton, A. (1917) Industrial Poisoning in Aircraft Manufacture, *J. Am. Med. Assoc.*, 69:2037.
Hamilton, H. and H. L. Hardy (1949) Industrial Toxicology, Williams and Wilkins, Baltimore.
Hammes, E. W. Jr. (1941) CCl₄ as an Industrial Hazard, *J. Ind. Hyg.* 23:112.
Hansen, H., V. R. Weaver and E. S. Venable (1953) Methyl Chloride Intoxication, *Arch. Ind. Hyg.*, 8:328.
Hardin, B. L. (1954) CCl₄ Poisoning; A Review, *Ind. Med. Surg.*, 23:93.
Hart, E. R. and L. W. Conn (1950) The influence of Dilution and State of Dispersion on Toxicity of certain Hydrocarbons following intravenous Injection, *J. Pharm. Exptl. Therap.*, 98:12.
Hartman, T. L., W. Wacker and R. M. Roll (1955) Methyl Chloride Intoxication. Report of 2 cases, one complicating Pregnancy, *New Engl. J. Med.*, 253:532.
Helliwell, P. J. and A. M. Hutton (1950) Trichloroethylene Anaesthesia, *Anaesthesia*, 5:4.
Hellwig, A. (1922) Klinische Narkoseversuche mit Solaesthin, *Klin. Wochschr.*, 1:215.
Henderson, Y. and H. W. Haggard (1943) Noxicous Gases and the Principles of Respiration influenzing their Action, 2nd ed., p.p. 201 and 205, Reinhold, New York.
Heppel, L. A. (1927) An unusual Case of Poisoning, *J. Roy. Army Med. Corps*, 49:442.
Heppel, L. A. and P. A. Neal (1944) Toxicology of Dichlormethane (Methylene chloride), Its Effect on Running Activity in the male Rat, *J. Ind. Hyg.*, 26:7.
Heppel, L. A., P. A. Neal, K. M. Endicott and V. T. Porterfield (1944) Toxicology of Dichloroethane. – Effect on the Cornea. *Arch. Ophthalmol.*, 32:391.
Heppel, L. A., P. A. Neal, T. L. Perrin, M. L. Orr and V. T. Porterfield (1944) Toxicology of Dichloromethane (Methylene Chloride), *J. Ind. Hyg.*, 26:8.
Herdman, K. N. (1945) Acute yellow Necrosis of Liver following Trilene Anaesthesia, *Brit. Med. J.*, 2:689.
Herzberg, M. (1934) Histology of Tissues taken from Animals killed by prolonged Administration of concentrated Vapours of Trichloroethylene, *Anesthésie Analgésie*, 13:203.
Hewer, C. L. (1942) Trichloroethylene as a general Analgesic and Anaesthetic, *Proc. Roy. Soc. Med.*, 35:463.
— (1943) Further Observations on Trichloroethylene, *Proc. Roy. Soc. Med.*, 36:446.
— (1958) Recent Advances in Anaesthesia and Analgesia, 8th ed., Churchill, London.
Hewer, C. L. and C. F. Hadfield (1941) Trichloroethylene as an Inhalation Anaesthetic, *Brit. Med., J.*, 1:924.
Hoffmann, F. (1937) Perniciosa und Trichloräthylen, *Med. Welt*, 11:12.
Hoffmann, H. E. and E. W. Reid (1939) Cellulose Acetate Lacquers, *Ind. Eng. Chem.*, 21:955.
Hoffmann, J., M. B. Himes, S. Lapan, R. Riszki and J. Post (1955) Reponses of Liver to Injury; Effects of acute CCl₄ Poisoning, *Arch. Pathol.*, 59:429.
Hoschek, R. (1953) Tödliche akute Trivergiftung mit Nachweis des Giftes in der Lacke, *Arch. Toxicol.*, 14:330.
— (1962) Plötzliche Spättodesfälle nach geringfügiger Trichloräthyleneinwirkung, *Arch. Gewerbepahtol. Gewerbehyg.*, 19:319.
Hoyt, L. F. (1928) Fumigation Tests with Ethylene Dichloride-Carbon Tetrachloride Mixtures, *Ind. Eng. Chem.*, 22:2362.
Hueper, W. C. and C. Smith (1955) Fatal Ethylene Dichloride Poisoning, *Am. J. Med. Sci.*, 189:778.
Hughes, J. P. (1954) Hazardous Exposure to some so-called safe Solvents, *J. Am. Med. Assoc.*, 156:234.
Hunold, G. A. (1955) Die Fujiwara Reaktion und ihre Anwendung zur Bestimmung von Trichloräthylen in der Raumluft und von TCE im Harn, *Arch. Gewerbepathol. Gewerbehyg.*, 14:77.
Hunter, A. R. (1944) Complications of Trilene Anaesthesia, *Lancet*, 1:308.
— (1962) Inhalation Anaesthetic Agents, *Brit. J. Anaesthesia*, 34:224.
Irish, D. D. (1963) Aliphatic Halogenated Hydrocarbons. In Patty, F. A. Industrial Hygiene and Toxicology, Vol. II, 2nd ed., Interscience, New York.
Isenschmid, R. and E. Kunz (1935) Gefähren modernen gewerblicher Gifte. Polyneuritis mit retrobulbar Neuritis nach Arbeit mit "Tri", *Schweiz. Med. Wochschr.*, 16:612.

Jacob, H. and J. Schröder (1959) Spätschäden nach Methylchloridvergiftung, *Arch. Toxikol.*, 17:314.
Jacobs, M. B. (1949) The Analytical Chemistry of Industrial Poisons, Hazards and Solvents, 2nd ed. p. 570, Interscience, New York.
Jennings, R. B. (1955) Fatal fulminant acute CCl₄ Poisoning, *Arch. Pathol.*, 59:269.
Joachimoglu, G. (1921) Die Wirkung einiger Verwändten des Chloroforms, *Biochem., Z.*, 120:203.
— (1921) Die Pharmakologie des Trichloräthylens, *Berlin. Klin. Wochr.*, 58:147.
Johnstone, R. T. (1941) Occupational Diseases, Saunders, London.
Jones, A. Morgan (1942) Methyl Chloride Poisoning, *Quart. J. Med.*, 11:29.
Jordi, A. (1937) Einfluss der Farbspritzarbeit auf die Gesundheit Jugendlicher, *Schweiz. Med. Wochschr.*, 18:767.
Joron, G. E., C. H. Hollinsberg and E. H. Bensley (1957) CCl₄ an underrated Hazard. *Canad. Med. Assoc. J.*, 76:173.
Judah, J. D. (1959) Reply to Discussion on Mechanism of Action of CCl₄, *Federation Proc.*, 18:1019.
Judah, J. D. and K. R. Rees (1959) Mechanism of Action of CCl₄, *Federation Proc.*, 18:1013.
Kalinowski, L. (1927) Gewerbliche Sensibilitätslähmung des Trigeminus. *Z. Ges. Neurol. Psychiat.*, 110:245.
Kazantzis, G. and R. R. Bomford (1960) Dyspepsia due to Inhalation of CCl₄ Vapour, *Lancet*, 1:360.
Kegel, A. H., W. D. McNally and A. S. Pope (1929) Poisoning from Domestic Refrigerators, *J. Am. Med. Assoc.*, 93:353.
Kentucky State Dept. of Health (1959) Methyl Chloride Intoxication, *Publ. Health Rept. (U.S.)*, 74:683.
Kiessling, W. (1921) Vergleichende Untersuchungen über die Wirkung einiger Chlorderivate des Methans, Äthans und Äthylens am isolierten Froschherzen, *Biochem. Z.*, 114:292.
Kirkpatrick, H. J. R. and J. M. Sutherland (1956) A fatal Case of Poisoning by CCl₄, *J. Clin. Pathol.*, 9:242.
Kistler, G. H. and A. B. Luckhardt (1929) Pharmacology of some Ethylene Halogen Compounds *Anesthesia Analgesia Current Res.*, 8:65.
Kittleson, K. D. and O. W. Bondon (1956) Acute renal Failure due to CCl₄ Poisoning, *Quart. Bull. Northwestern Univ. Med. School*, 30:117.
Kobert, R. (1906) *Lehrbuch der Intoxikationen*, Stuttgart.
Koch, W. (1931) Trichloräthylenvergiftung, *Zentr. Gewerbehyg.*, 7:18.
Koelsch, F. (1915) Gewerbliche Vergiftungen durch Zelluloidlacke in der Flugzeugindustrie, *Münch. Med. Wochschr.*, 62:1567.
Krantz, J. C. Jr., C. S. Park and J. S. L. Ling (1959) The Anesthetic Properties of 1,1,1-Trichloroethane, *Anesthesiology*, 20:635.
Kylin, B., H. Reichard, I. Sümegi and S. Yllner (1962) Hepatotoxic Effect of Tri- and Tetrachloroethylene on Mice, *Nature*, 193:395.
Lachnit, V. and H. Peitschmann (1960) Activity of SGOT and Aldolase in Workers exposed to Halogenated Hydrocarbons, *Ind. Med. Surg.*, 29:523.
Landé, P. and P. Dervillée (1934) Récherches expérimentelles sur l'Action toxique chez le Lapin du Tétrachlorure de Carbone, *Compt. Rend. Soc. Biol.*, 116:225.
Lamson, P. D., G. H. Gardner, R. K. Gustafson, E. D. Maire, A. J. McLean and H. S. Wells (1924) Pharmacology and Toxicology of Carbontetrachloride, *J. Pharmacol.*, 22:215.
Lamson, P. D., B. H. Robbins and C. B. Ward (1929) Pharmacology and Toxicology of Tetrachloroethylene, *Am. J. Hyg.*, 9:430.
Lazarew, N. W. (1929) Über die narkotische Wirkungskraft der Dämpfe der Chlorderivaten des Methans, des Äthans und des Äthylens, *Arch. Exptl. Pathol. Pharmakol.*, 141:19.
— (1929) Über die Giftigkeit verschiedener Kohlenwasserstoffdämpfe. *Arch. Expl. Pathol. Pharmakol.*, 143:223.
Léchelle, P., S. Vialard and P. Collot (1958) Tentative de Suicide par le Trichloroéthylène, *Bull. Soc. Méd. Hôp. Paris*, 61:242.
Lehmann, K. B. (1911) Experimentelle Studien über den Einfluss technisch- und hygienischwichtigen Gäse und Dämpfe auf den Organismus, *Arch. Hyg. Bakteriol.*, 74:1.

Lehmann, K. B. and F. Flury (1943) Toxicology and Hygiene of Industrial Solvents, Williams and Wilkins, Baltimore.

Lehmann, K. B. and T. Hasegawa (1910) Studien über die Absorption chlorierte Kohlenwasserstoffe aus der Luft durch Tier und Mensch, *Arch. Hyg. Bakteriol.*, 72:327.

Lehmann, K. B. and L. Schmidt-Kehl (1936) Die 13 wichtigsten Chlorkohlenwasserstoffe der Fettreihe vom Standpunkt der Gewerbehygiene, *Arch. Hyg. Bakteriol.*, 116:131.

Lejeune, E. (1934) Schwierigkeiten der Diagnose berufliche Vergiftungen für den praktischen Arzt, *Arch. Gewerbepahtol. Gewerbehyg.*, 5:274.

Leoncini, F. (1934) Sopra un Caso d'Avvelenamento acuto mortale da Tetrachloruro di Carboni, *Rass. Med. Ind.*, 5:6.

Léri, A, and Breitel (1922) La Polynévrite chlorique (Polynévrites par Tétrachloréthane) chez les Perlières, *Bull. Soc. Med. Hôp. Paris*, 46:1406.

Levy, G. (1913) The exciting of ventricular Fibrillation in Animals under Chloroform Anaesthesia, *Heart*, p. 319.

Lilliman, B., (1949) Suggested Mechanism of Poisoning by liquid Tetrachloroethane, *Analyst*, 74:510.

Lob, M. (1957) Les Dangers du Perchloréthylène, *Arch. Gewerbepahtol. Gewerbehyg.*, 16:45.

— (1960) The Action of Trichloroethylene on Levels of Alcohol in the Blood, *Med. Lavoro*, 51:587.

Luce, A. (1937) Perniciosa und Trichloräthylen, *Med. Welt*, 11:502.

Mc Closkey, J. F. and E. H. McGehee (1959) Effect of subcutaneous and intraoral Administration of CCl_4 on Liver of Rat, *Arch. Pathol.*, 49:200.

McCollister, D. D., W. H. Beamer, G. J. Atchison and H. C. Spencer (1951) Absorption, Distribution and Elimination of radioactive CCl_4 by Monkeys, *J. Pharmacol.*, 102:112.

McCord, C. P. (1930) Household Mechanical Refrigeration, *J. Am. Med. Assoc.*, 94:1832.

McDermott, W. V. and H. L. Hardy (1963) Cirrhosis of the Liver following chronic Exposure to CCl_4, *J. Occupational Med.*, 5:249.

McGee, C. J. (1949) Lower Nephron Nephrosis; CCl_4 Poisoning with report of 3 Cases, *Am. J. Med. Sci.*, 218:636.

Mackie, L. J. (1961) Methyl Chloride Intoxication, *Med. J. Australia*, 48:203.

McNally, W. D. and G. Fostvedt (1941) Ethylene Dichloride Poisoning, *Ind. Med. Surg.*, 10:373.

Maplestone, P. H. and R. N. Chopra (1933) Toxicity of Tetrachloroethylene to Cats, *Indian Med. Gaz.*, 68:554.

Marshall, D. and W. S. Hoffmann (1949) The Nature of the altered Renal Function in lower Nephron Nephrosis, *J. Lab. Clin. Med.*, 34:31.

Medicolegal Report (1961) Trichloroethylene Addiction, *Brit. Med., J.*, 1:1550.

Meersseman, F. (1934) Récherches sur l'Insuffisance hépatique expérimentale, *Compt. Rend. Soc. Biol.*, 117:931.

Meersseman, F., L. Perrot and E. Franque (1934) Récherches sur l'Insuffisance hépatique expérimentale, *Compt. Rend. Soc. Biol.*, 117:934.

Mendeloff, J. (1952) Death after repeated Exposures to Refrigerant Gases, *Arch. Ind. Hyg.*, 6:518.

Metal Working Production (1962) (Chemical Milling for Stainless Steel), 106:73.

Meyer, H. (1929) Untersuchungen über die Giftwirkung des Trichloräthylens besonders auf das Auge, *Klin. Monatsbl. Augenheilk.*, 83:309.

Mikiskova, H. and A. Mikiska (1960) Bestimmung der elektrischen Erregbarkeit der motorische Grosshirnrinde. Vergleich der narkotischen Wirkung von Tri und Trichloräthanol bei den Meerschweinchen, *Arch. Gewerbepahtol. Gewerbehyg.*, 18:310.

Minot, G. R. and L. W. Smith (1921) The Blood in Tetrachloroethane Poisoning, *Arch. Internal Med.*, 28:687.

Moeschlin, S. (1956) Klinik und Therapie der Vergiftungen, Thieme, Stuttgart.

Möller, K. O. (1933) Some Cases of CCl_4 Poisoning in Connection with dry Shampooing and dry Cleaning, *J. Ind. Hyg.*, 15:418.

Moon, H. D. (1950) Pathology of fatal CCl_4 Poisoning, *Am. J. Pathol.*, 26:1041.

Moran, H. E. (1943) Determination of volatile halogenated Hydrocarbons in Blood, *Arch. Ind. Med.*, 25:243.

Morse, K. M. and L. Goldberg (1943) Chlorinated Solvent Exposures at Degreasing Operations, *Ind. Med. Surg.*, 12:706.

Mosinger, M. and H. Fiorentini (1958) Intoxication expérimentale par le Trichloréthylène, *Ann. Med. Légale Criminol. Police Sci. Toxicol.*, 38:319.

Moskowitz, S. and H. Shapiro (1952) Fatal Exposure to Methylene Chloride Vapour, *Arch. Ind. Hyg.*, 6:116.

Müller, J. (1925) Vergleichende Untersuchungen über die narkotische und toxische Wirkung einiger Kohlenwasserstoffe, *Arch. Exptl. Pathol. Pharmakol.*, 109:276.

Müller, L. (1931) Experimenteller Beitrag zur Tetrachloräthanvergiftung, *Arch. Gewerbepathol. Gewerbehyg.*, 2:326.

Nicholson, J. L. and L. Y. Peskoe (1960) CCl₄ Poisoning, *J. Kentucky State Med. Assoc.*, 58:1053.

Noetzel, H. (1952) Spinale progressive Muskelathrophie nach chronischer Methylchloridvergiftung, *Klin. Wochschr.*, 30:18.

Noro, L. and T. Patterson (1960) Methylkloridforgiftnung, *Nord. Med.*, 64:881.

Norris, W. and P. Stuart (1957) Cardiac Arrest during Trichloroethylene Anaesthesia, *Brit. Med. J.* 1:860.

Nowill, W. K., C. R. Stephen and G. Margolis (1954) The chronic Toxicity of Trichloroethylene, *Anesthesiology*, 15:462.

Nuckolls, A. H. (1933) The comparative life, fire and explosion Hazards of common Refrigerants, Underwriters' Laboratories Rept., Micellaneous Hazards no. 2375.

Nunnely, T., N. Simpson and J. Snow (1849) New Anaesthetics, *Providence Med. Surg. J.*, p. 98.

Oberling, C. and C. Rouiller (1956) Les Effects de l'Intoxication aiguë du Tétrachlorure de Carbone sur la Foie du Rat, *Ann. Anat. Pathol.*, 1:401.

Ohnesorge, G. (1930) Über Zaponlackvergiftung, *Deut. Med. Wochschr.*, 56:961.

Orth, O. S. and N. A. Gillespie (1945) A further Study of Trichloroethylene Anaesthesia, *Brit. J. Anaesthesia*, 19:161.

Ostlere, G. (1953) Trichloroethylene Anesthesia, Livingstone, Edingburgh and London.

Oswald, A (1924) Chemische Konstitution und pharmakologische Wirkung, Borntraeger, Berlin.

Pagniez, P., A. Plichet and N. K. Koang (1932) Un Cas d'Intoxication par le Tétrachlorure de Carbone, *Prog. Méd. (Paris)*, 59:1328.

Pantelitsch, M. (1933) Versuche über die Wirking gechlorter Methane und Äthane auf Mäuse, Diss. Würzburg.

Paparolli, G. and V. Cali (1956) Intossicazione collectiva de Idrocarburi Chlorati in Lavoratori portuali, *Folia Med. Naples*, 39:819.

Parmenter, C. (1921) Tetrachloroethane Poisoning and its Prevention, *J. Ind. Hyg.*, 2:456.

— (1923) Further Observations on the Control and Prevention of Tetrachloroethane Poisoning, *J. Ind. Hyg.*, 5:1159.

Parnas, M. (1888) Actions des Inhalations du Chlorure d'Éthylène pur sur l'Œil, *Compt. Rend.*, 107:921.

Parney, F. S. and J. G. Cunningham (1949) Guide to Diagnosis of Occupational Diseases, Industrial Health Division, Canada.

Partenheimer, R. S. and D. S. Citron (1952) Practical Control of Fluid and Electrolyte Balance in CCl₄ Nephrosis, *Arch. Internal Med.*, 89:216.

Patty, F. D. (1949) Industrial Hygiene and Toxicology, Interscience, New York.

Paulus, W. (1951) Zur Frage der Vortauschung eines Blutalkohols durch Einatmen von Tri- und Tetrachloräthylen, *Deut. Z. Ges. Gerichl. Med.*, 40:593.

Peterson, J. E., H. R. Hoyle and E. J. Schneider (1956) The Analysis of Air for Halogenated Hydrocarbon Contaminants by means of Absorption on Silica Gel, *Am. Ind. Hyg. Assoc. Quart.*, 17:429.

Pernell, C. (1944) Collection and Analysis of Halogenated Hydrocarbon Vapours using Silica Gel as an absorbing Agent, *J. Ind. Hyg.*, 26-331.

Pfrembter, R. (1932) Tödlicher Unfall durch Tri-Einatmung, *Deut. Z. Ges. Gerichtl. Med.*, 18:339.

Piedelièvre, H. Griffon and L. Derobert (1943) Lésions hépatiques dans un Cas d'Intoxication par Trichloroéthylène, *Ann. Med. Légale Criminol. Police Sci. Toxicol.*, 23:43.

Plessner, W. (1915) Über Trigeminuserkrankung infolge von Tri-vergiftung, *Neurol. Zentr.*, 34:916.

Plotz, W. (1920) Vergleichende Untersuchungen über die hämolytische Wirkung einiger Chlorderivate des Methans, Äthans und Äthylens, *Biochem. Z.*, 103:243.

Powell, J. F. (1945) Trichloroethylene; Absorption, Elimination and Metabolism, *Brit. J. Ind. Med.*, 2:142.

Queries and Minor Notes (1947) *J. Am. Med. Assoc.*, 133:145.

Rager, C. A. (1945) Indust. Ref. Serv. U.S. Dept. Commerce, 3, no. 33, part 2.

Recknagel, R. D. and W. D. Anthony (1959) Biochemical Changes in CCl_4 Poisoning; Fatty Liver, *J. Biol. Chem.*, 234:1052.

Recknagel, R. D. and M. O. Litteria (1960) Concentration of CCl_4 in Liver and Blood, *Am. J. Pathol.*, 36:521.

Rees, K. R. and K. P. Sinha (1960) Blood Enzymes in Liver Injury, *J. Pathol. Bacteriol.*, 80:297.

Rees, K. T. and W. G. Spector (1961) Reversible Nature of Liver Cell Damage due to CCl_4 as demonstrated by the Use of Phenergan, *Nature*, 190:821.

Rees, K. R., K. P. Sinha and W. G. Spector (1961) The Pathogenesis of Liver Injury in CCl_4 and Thioacetamide Poisoning, *J. Pathol. Bacteriol.*, 81:107.

Rennick, B.R., S. D. Malton, G. K. Moe and M. H. Seevers (1949) Induction of Idioventricular Rhythms by 1,1,1-Trichloroethane and Epinephrine, *J. Pharmacol. Exptl. Therap.*, 123:224.

Reuss, A. (1931) Neuere Versuche über die Giftigkeit des Tetrachlorkohlenstoffes, Diss. Würzburg.

Ricci, P. (1956) Experimentelle Beitrag zur Kenntnis der subakuten und chronischen Intoxikation durch Trichloräthylen, *Med. Legale (Genova)*, 4:1.

Richards, C. C. and C. Bachman (1955) A Study in Liver Function in Dogs after Anaesthesia with Trichloroethylene and Chloroform, *Anesthesia Analgesia*, 34:307.

Robbins, B. H. (1929) Absorption, Distribution and Excretion of CCl_4 in Dogs under various Conditions, *J. Pharmacol. Exptl. Therap.*, 37:203.

Roche, L. and J. Bouchet (1948) L'Intoxication par le Chlorure de Méthyle, *Arch. Malad. Profess.*, 9:406.

Roche, L., M. Genevois and A. Marin (1957) Trichloroéthylène et Eczéma de la Face, *Arch. Malad. Profess.*, 19:615.

Roche, L., E. Lejeune and J. Riffat (1958) L'Intoxication aiguë par le Trichloroéthylène, *Ann. Méd. Légale Criminol. Police Sci. Toxicol.*, 38:356.

Roche, L., A. Nicholas and A. Marin (1956) Les Lésions rénales au cours de l'Intoxication par le Chlorure de Méthyle, *Arch. Malad. Profess.*, 17:430.

Rommeney, K. (1943) Tri-Sucht einer Jugendlicher mit tödlicher Ausgang, *Deut. Z. Ges. Gerichtl. Med.*, 37:1.

Rondepierre, J. J., J. Truhaut, J. Alizon and Y. Champion (1955) Rôle étiologique possible du Chlorure de Méthyle dans un Syndrome confusional. *Ann. Méd. Légale Criminol. Police Sci. Toxicol.*, 35:80.

Rosenthal, O., S. K. Thin and N. Conger (1960) Am. Chem. Soc. Meeting, New York.

Rowe, V. R., D. D. McCollister, H. C. Spencer, E. M. Adams and D. D. Irish (1952) Vapour Toxicity of Tetrachloroethylene for Laboratory Animals and Human Subjects, *Arch. Ind. Hyg.*, 5:566.

Sax, N., Irving (1957) Dangerous Properties of Industrial Materials, Reinhold, New York; Chapman and Hall, London.

Sayers, R., W. P. Yant, B. G. Thomas and L. B. Berger (1929) Physiological Response attending Exposure to vapours of Methyl Bromide, Methyl Chloride, Ethyl Bromide and Ethyl Chloride, *U.S. Publ. Health Serv.*, Bull. 185.

Sayers, R. R., W. P. Yant, C. D. Waite and F. A. Patty (1930) Acute Response of Guinea pigs to Vapours of some new commercial organic Compounds; Ethylene Dichloride, *U.S. Publ. Health Rept.*, 45:225.

Schibler, W. (1929) Akute gelbe Leberatrophie durch Azetylene Tetrachlorid, *Schweiz. Med. Wochschr.*, 10:1079.

Schultze, E. (1920) Encephalo-myelomaläzie als Unfallfolge nach gewerblicher Vergiftung (? Tetrachloräthan), *Klin. Wochschr.*, 57:941.

Schwander, P. (1936) Über die Diffusion halogenisierter Kohlenwasserstoffe, *Arch. Gewerbepathol. Gewerbehyg.*, 7:109.

Schlingmann, A. S. and O. M. Gruhzit (1927) Studies on the Toxicity of Tetrachloroethylene, *J. Am. Vet. Med. Assoc.*, 71:187.

Schleyer, F. (1960) Einatmung von Tetrachloräthylen und Blutalkoholgehalt, *Arch. Toxikol.*, 18:187.

Schoenemann, A., (1944) Vergiftungen durch Trinken von Trichloräthylen, *Med. Ztg.*, 1 :17.

Schollmeyer, W. (1960) Plötzlicher Tod durch Tri-Vergiftung bei Einwirkung dieses Giftes über längere Zeit, *Arch. Toxikol.*, 18:229.

Schwander, P. (1936) Über die Diffusion halogenisierter Kohlenwasserstoffe durch die Haut, *Arch. Gewerbepathol. Gewerbehyg.*, 7:109.

Schwarz, F. (1926) Vergiftungsfälle und Tierversuche mit Methylchlorid, *Deut. Z. Ges. Gerichtl. Med.*, 7:278.

Settelen, M. E. (1950) Über Rauchnarkose mit Methylenchlorid, *Pract. Oto-Rhino-Laryngol.*, 12:320.

Setterling, A. N. (1947) cited by Fairhall, 1957.

Shell Development Co. (1941) *The toxicities of 2-Chlorbutane and 1-2-3-Trichlorobutene compared with Ethylene Dichloride.*

Sirota, H. J. (1949) CCl₄ Poisoning in Man; Mechanism of renal Failure and Recovery, *J. Clin. Invest.*, 28:1412.

Smetana, H. (1939) Nephrosis due to CCl₄, *Arch. Internal Med.*, 63:760.

Smith, W. W. (1947) The acute and chronic Toxicity of Methyl Chloride, *J. Ind. Hyg.*, 29:185.

Smith, W. W. and W. F. Von Oettingen (1947) The acute and chronic Toxicity of Methyl Chloride, *J. Ind. Hyg.*, 29:47; 123.

Smyth, H. F. and H. F. Smyth Jr. (1956) Safe Practices in Industrial Use of CCl₄, *J. Am. Med. Assoc.*, 107:1683.

Sollman, T. (1948) A Manual of Pharmocology, Saunders, London.

Souček, B. (1961) Excretion of Methyl Chloride and Carbon Tetrachloride in Rats, *Arch. Gewerbepathol. Gewerbehyg.*, 18:370.

Souček, B. and D. Vlachova (1954) Further Trichloroethylene Metabolites in Man, *Pracovni Lekar.*, 7:86.

Souček, B. and D. Vlachova (1960) Excretion of Trichloroethylene Metabolites in Human Urine, *Brit. J. Ind. Med.*, 17:60.

Spencer, H. C., V. R. Rowe, E. M. Adams, D. D. McCollister and D. D. Irish (1951) Vapor toxicity of ethylene dichloride determined by experiments on laboratory animals, *Arch. Ind. Hlth.*, 4:482.

Sperling, F., F. J. Macri and W. F. Von Oettingen (1950) Distribution and Excretion of intravenously administered Methyl Chloride, *Arch. Ind. Hyg.*, 1:215.

Stack, V. T., D. E. Forrest and H. K. Wahl (1961) Determination of Trichloroethylene in Air, *Am. Ind. Hyg. Assoc. J.*, 22:184.

Steindorff, K. (1922) Über die Wirkung einiger Chlorderivate des Methans, Äthans und Äthylens auf die Hornhaut des Tierauges, *Arch. Ophthalmol.*, 109:252.

Steinberg, S., D. Baldwin and B. H. Ostrow (1956) Clinical Method for Assay of SGOT, *J. Lab. Clin. Med.*, 48:144.

Sterner, J. H. (1949) in Industrial Hygiene and Toxicology. (F. H. Patty, Ed.) vol. 2 pp. 787, 817, Interscience, New York.

Stewart, L. C. (1931) CCl₄ in Dry Cleaning. *Natl. Cleaner and Dyer*, 22:59.

Stewart, R. D. (1963) The Toxicology of Methyl Chloroform, *J. Occupational Med.*, 5:259.

Stewart, R. D., D. S. Erley, T. R. Torkelson and C. L. Hake (1959) Post-Exposure Analysis of Organic Compounds in Blood by rapid Infra-red Technique, *Nature*, 184:192.

Stewart, R. D., H. H. Gay, D. S. Erley, T. R. Torkelson and C. L. Hake (1959) Post-exposure Analysis of Organic Compounds in the Blood by a rapid Infrared Technique, *Nature*, 184:192.

Stewart, R. D., H. H. Gay, D. S. Erley, C. L. Hake and A. W. Schaeffer (1961) Human Exposure to 1,1,1-Trichloroethane Vapour, *Am. Ind. Hyg. Assoc. J.*, 22:252.

Stewart, R. D., H. H. Gay, D. S. Erley, C. L. Hake and J. E. Peterson (1962) Observations on Concentrations of Trichloroethylene in Blood and expired Air following Exposure of Humans, *Am. Ind. Hyg. Assoc. J.*, 23:167.

Stewart, R. D., T. R. Torkelson, C. L. Hake and D. S. Erley (1960) Infrared Analysis of CCl₄ and Ethanol in Blood, *J. Lab. Clin. Med.*, 56:148.

Stewart, A. and L. J. Witts (1944) Chronic CCl₄ Intoxication, *Brit. J. Ind. Med.*, 1:11.

Straus, B. (1954) Aplastic Anaemia following exposure to CCl₄ *J. Am. Med. Assoc.*, 155:737.

Striker, G., S. Goldblatt, I. S. Warne and D. E. Jackson (1935) Clinical Experience with the Use of Trichloroethylene in Production of over 300 Analgesias and Anaesthesias, *Anesthesia Analgesia*, 14:68.

Stüber, K. (1931) Gesundheitsschädigungen bei der gewerblichen Anwendung des Trichloräthylens und die Möglichkeiten ihrer Verhütung, *Arch. Gewerbepathol. Gewerbehyg.*, 2:398.

Takahashi, M. (1929) Changes in Metabolism in Poisoning by CCl_4, *Japan. J. Exptl. Med.*, 7:417.

Tanyol, H. and M. H. F. Friedman (1961) Influence of a liver Preparation on Liver of Cats receiving CCl_4, *Proc. Soc. Exptl. Biol. Med.*, 106:645.

Tauber, E. (1881) Die Anesthetica. Eine Monographie mit besonderer Berücksichtigung von zwei neuen anaesthetischen Mitteln, Hirschwald, Berlin.

Teisinger, J. (1959) Testes biologiques d'Exposition. Proc. Internat. Symptosium of M.A.C. of Toxic Substances in Industry, Butterworth, London.

Teleky, N. (1931) Tri-Schädigungen, *Ärztl. Sachverst. Ztg.*, 37:147.

Thomas, E. (1960) Veränderungen des Nervenstystems bei Vergiftung mit niedrigen Halogenkohlenwasserstoffen, *Deut. Z. Nervenheilk.*, 180:530.

Threshold Limit Values for 1962, *Am. Ind. Hyg. Assoc. J.*, 23:419.

Torkelson, T. R., F. Oyen, D. D. McCollister and V. K. Rowe (1958) Toxicity of 1,1,1-Trichloroethane as determined on Laboratory Animals and Human Subjects, *Am. Ind. Hyg. Assoc. J.*, 19:353.

Truhaut, R. (1951) Problèmes de Toxicologie et d'Hygiène industrielles aux États Unis, *Arch. Malad. Profess.*, 12:687.

Uhl, G. and T. P. Haag (1958) Perorale Vergiftung mit Trichloräthylen und ihr chemischen Nachweis, *Arch. Toxikol.*, 17:197.

Vallaud, A., V. Raymond and P. Salmon (1956) Les Solvents chlorés et l'Hygiène industrielle, *Inst. Natl. Securité, Paris* (cited by Lob, 1957).

Vallée, C. and A. Leclerq (1935) Intoxication par Trichloroéthylène, *Ann. Méd. Légale Criminol. Police Sci. Toxicol.*, 15:10.

Van Arkel, A. E. and S. E. Vles (1936) Solubility of Organic Compounds in Water, *Rev. Trav. Chim.*, 55:407.

Van der Kloot, A. (1934) Methyl Chloride Poisoning, *Illinois Med. J.*, 65:508.

Vauthey, M. (1955) Dérivés halogènes des Hydrocarbures acyliques et Glande hépatique, *J. Méd. Lyons*, 36:172.

Veley, V. H. (1909) Dangers of the Dry Shampoo, *Lancet*, 2:370, 1162.

— (1910) An Examination of the physical and physiological Properties of Tetrachloroethane and Trichloroethylene, *Proc. Roy, Soc. (London), Ser. B.* 82:217.

Verriere, P. and Mlle.Vachez (1949) Néphrite aiguë grave après Intoxication par le Chlorure de Méthyle, *Lyon Méd.*, 1:256.

Viallier, M. J. and A. Brune (1958) Influence de l'Association avec différents Solvents sur la Toxicité expérimentale du Trichloroéthylène, *Arch. Malad. Profess.*, 19:624.

Vilches, A. (1949) Intoxication due to the Refrigerator Gas, Methyl Chloride, *Rev. Inst. Bacteriol. Malibran*, 14:63.

Von Oettingen, W. F. (1937) The Halogenated Hydrocarbons; their Toxicity and potential Dangers, *J. Ind. Hyg.*, 19:349.

Von Oettingen, W. F. (1955) The Halogenated Hydrocarbons – Toxicity and potential Dangers, U.S. Publ. Health Serv. Education and Welfare Publ. no. 414, U.S. Govt. Printing Office, Washington.

Von Oettingen, W. F., C. C. Powell, N. E. Sharpless, W. C. Alford and L. J. Pecoro (1949) (cited by R. T. Williams, 1959) Natl. Inst. Health Bull., 191.

Wallace, C. B. and J. S. Diamond (1925) Significance of Urobilinogen in urine as a Test for Liver Function, *Arch. Internal Med.*, 35:698.

Walter, B. and A. Weise (1951) Spätfolgen akuter Methylchloridvergiftung, *Med. Welt.* 20:987.

Ward, J. M. (1955) Accidental Poisoning with Tetrachloroethane, *Brit. Med. J.*, 1:1136.

Waters, R. M., O. S. Orth and N. E. Gillespie (1943) Trichloroethylene and Cardiac Rhythm. *Anaesthesiology*, 4:1.

Weinstein, A. (1937) Methyl Chloride (Refrigerator) Gas Poisoning, *J. Am. Med. Assoc.*, 108:1603.

Wells, H. S. (1925) Quantitative Study of Absorption and Excretion of the anthelmintic Dose of CCl₄, *J. Pharmacol. Exptl. Therap.*, 25:235.

White, J. L. and P. Somers (1931) Toxicity of Methyl Chloride for Laboratory Animals, *J. Ind. Hyg.*, 13:273.

Wilcox, W. H. (1934) Toxic Effects of Substances of the Carbon Tetrachloride Type, *Proc. Roy. Soc. Med.*, 27:455.

Wilcox, W. H., B. H. Spilsbury and T. M. Legge (1915) An Outbreak of Toxic Jaundice of a new Type amongst Aeroplane Workers, *Trans. Med. Soc. London*, 38:129, 139, 144.

Williams, R. T. (1959) Detoxication Mechanisms, 2nd ed. Chapman and Hall, London.

Wilson, R. H. and D. R. Brimley (1944) Health Hazards in the Use of Tetrachloroethane, *Ind. Med. Surg.*, 13:233.

Wirtschafter, Z. T. and E. D. Schwartz (1939) Acute Ethylene Dichloride Poisoning, *J. Ind. Hyg.*, 21:126.

Wood, M. W. (1951) Cirrhosis of the Liver in a Refrigerator Engineer attributed to Methyl Chloride, *Lancet*, 1:508.

Woods, W. W. (1946) Changes in Kidneys in CCl₄ Poisoning and their Resemblance to those in "Crush Syndrome", *J. Pathol. Bacteriol.*, 58:767.

Wright, W. H. and J. M. Schaffer (1932) Critical Anthelmintic Tests of Chlorinated Alkyl Hydrocarbons, *Am. J. Hyg.*, 16:325.

Wroblenski, F. and J. D. La Due (1955) Serum Glutamic Oxalacetic Transaminase Acitivity as an Index of Liver Cell Injury, *Ann. Internal Med.*, 43:345.

Yant, W. P., H. W. Shoaf and J. Chornyak, (1930) Observations on Possibility of Methyl Chloride Poisoning by Ingestion with Food and Water, *U.S. Publ. Health Rept.*, 45:1057.

Zangger, H. (1930) Über die modernen Lösungsmitteln, *Arch. Gewerbepathol. Gewerbehyg.*, 1:77.

Zernik, F. (1933) Neuere Erkentniss auf dem Gebiete der schädlichen Gäse und Dämpfe, *Ergebn. Hyg. Bakteriol.*, 14:139.

Zollinger, H. (1930) Über sechs Fälle von Tetrachloräthan Vergiftung, *Schweiz. Z. Unfallmed. Berufskrankh.*, 45:92.

— (1931) Ein Beitrag zur Gewerbepathologische Bedeutung des Tetrachloräthan, *Arch. Gewerbe pathol. Gewerbehyg.*, 2:298.

Zurlo, N. and L. Metrico (1960) Simple Methods for Micro determination of industrial Toxics in Air, *Med. Lavoro*, 51:241.

Chapter 6

NITROGEN COMPOUNDS

(A) ALIPHATIC NITROPARAFFINS

Among the eight high purity nitroparaffins whose physical properties were described by Toops in 1956, there are four which are used to some extent as solvents, *viz.*, 1-nitroethane, 1-nitromethane, and 1- and 2-nitropropane, the last has the widest industrial application. They were first produced in 1872 by Meyer, and an intensive study of the technique of their production by vapour phase nitration of the gaseous paraffins was reported in detail by Hass *et al.* (1936), with a description of the apparatus used. A further view of this process, with an extensive bibliography, was given by Hass and Riley (1943).

GENERAL PROPERTIES

The nitroparaffins are powerful solvents for organic esters of cellulose and vinyl copolymer resins. They belong to the medium-boiling class of solvents (101° to 132 °C) and their evaporation rates (100° to 180 °C, as compared with butyl acetate 100 °C) lie between those of butyl acetate and toluene. They have a mild odour and are practically insoluble in water. One of their main industrial applications is in miscellaneous coating processes, with shellac, synthetic and processed rubber, paint and varnish removers (*e.g.* nitroethane or 2-nitropropane with the benzene-acetone-alcohol type), with alkyl resin and other high polymer coatings. Their commercial production has increased considerably since 1940 (Bogin and Wampner, 1942).

Toxicologically, they are irritants of mucous membranes, and only mildly narcotic, but in animal experiments have been shown to have the propensity towards liver injury.

They are not absorbed by the skin.

27. Nitroethane

Structural formula:

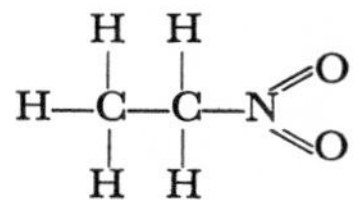

$$H-\overset{\overset{\displaystyle H}{|}}{\underset{\underset{\displaystyle H}{|}}{C}}-\overset{\overset{\displaystyle H}{|}}{\underset{\underset{\displaystyle H}{|}}{C}}-N\overset{\displaystyle O}{\underset{\displaystyle O}{}}$$

Molecular formula: $C_2H_5NO_2$

Molecular weight: 75.07

Properties: a colourless liquid with a somewhat disagreeable chloroform-like odour, detectable at concentrations of 0.5 mg/l (163 p.p.m.).

    boiling point: 114. 8 °C

    melting point: −90 °C

    vapour pressure: 25 mm Hg at 25 °C

    specific gravity (liquid density): 1.052 at 20 °C

    flash point: 106 °F

    conversion factors: 1 p.p.m. = 3.07 mg/m³

                            1 mg/l = 325.7 p.p.m.

    solubility: in water to the extent of 4.5 ml/100 at 20 °C; soluble in chloroform; miscible with ethyl alcohol and ether

    maximum allowable concentration: 100 p.p.m.

ECONOMY, SOURCES AND USES

Production

By the vapour-phase reaction between nitric and propane vapour and separation by distillation (Sutton, 1963).

Industrial uses

Solvent for cellulose acetate, vinyl, alkyl and many other resins, waxes, fats and dyestuffs. Used in the chemical industry as a raw material for related products, but also to some extent as a solvent for cellulose esters, fats, waxes and resins.

BIOCHEMISTRY

Estimation in the atmosphere

Like other primary nitroparaffins, nitroethane has been estimated by its reaction with ferric chloride, giving a stable red colour (Scott and Treon, 1940).

Metabolism

Absorption and excretion

In common with some other primary and secondary nitroparaffins, nitroethane undergoes a metabolic transformation which produces nitrite; oxidation of this is catalysed to nitrate and excreted in the urine (Heppel and Porterfield, 1949). Two urine samples from a rabbit exposed to inhalation of 0.27% of nitroethane for 9 h were found to contain 19 and 10 mg of nitrate per 100 ml respectively, while the concentration of nitrite and nitrate in the blood increased gradually, during both inhalation and also oral administration.

The excretion and retention of nitroethane were investigated by Machle *et al.* (1942). They found that the amount which could be recovered unchanged from the urine following oral dosage of 0.75 to 5.6 g was practically nil after 30 h, the nitroethane being broken down fairly rapidly and being completely eliminated and destroyed by that time. On this dosage the lungs excreted 0.131 and 0.139 g and, following intravenous administration of 1 g, 0.05 to 0.17 g; this also gradually decreased in 30 h to almost nil. The tissues of the animals killed at the end of this period contained only minute amounts of the nitroethane, and the fact that only about 25% of the total dose had been exhaled or otherwise excreted indicated that a considerable portion had been metabolised. A further investigation by Machle *et al.* (1942) showed that both acetaldehyde and nitrite were present in the blood after intravenous injection; this suggested that the metabolic transformation of nitroethane produces nitrite with its further oxidation to nitrate.

The formation of acetaldehyde, detectable in the blood stream is also stated by Williams (1959) to occur as a product of the metabolism of nitroethane, and the formation of small amounts of mercapturic acid is stated by Bray and James (1958) to be common to nitroethane and nitromethane.

TOXICOLOGY

There have been no reports of toxic effects of nitroethane in human beings. By animal experiments it has been shown to have a narcotic action, but lethal concentrations are so far below narcotic concentrations that early narcosis gives no warning of dangerous effects. It is an irritant of mucous membranes and can cause general injury to the central nervous system, and is somewhat more toxic by inhalation than nitromethane. It was found however by Machle *et al.* (1940) that concentrations of 500 p.p.m. were safe and tolerable for guinea pigs, rabbits and monkeys.

Toxicity to animals

Acute

(a) *Lethal dose.* – (i) *By oral administration* to rabbits – 0.5–0.75 g/kg. – (ii) *By inhalation*, the lethal effect was a product of concentration and time of exposure. Rabbits were more sensitive than guinea pigs (only two of each species were exposed in the experiments of Machle *et al.*). All the animals died at concentrations of 30,000 p.p.m. for $1\frac{1}{4}$ h but 25,000 p.p.m. for 2 h was lethal only for rabbits.

(b) *Narcotic dose.* – For rabbits, 10,000 p.p.m. for 1 h, 5000 p.p.m. for 3 h or 1000 p.p.m. for 12 h.

SYMPTOMS OF ACUTE INTOXICATION

Exposure to the higher concentrations caused irritation of mucous membranes, with lacrimation, conjunctival discharge, dyspnoea and some pulmonary râles, with, in a few animals, slight pulmonary oedema. Central nervous excitation was shown by twitching and jerking movements of the head and extremities, but this was usually not severe, general convulsions being rare and of brief duration. Stupor, narcosis or light anaesthesia disappeared rapidly on cessation of exposure. Blood changes – a temporary drop in haemoglobin and red cells – were considered to be an effect of the general injury to the animal and not evidence of specific blood damage.

CHANGES IN THE ORGANISM

With oral administration there was some congestion of the gastrointestinal tract. The respiratory tract, including the anterior turbinates, showed severe congestion, and there was some pulmonary oedema, but not sufficient to suggest that it was the only cause of death. The brain showed some congestion and in some cases oedema, and in one animal small haemorrhages.

The liver showed some damage in all the animals which died, by every route of administration – by mouth marked oedema, cloudy swelling, sometimes necrosis or fatty infiltration.

The kidneys showed non-specific changes – oedema, pallor or cloudy swelling.

Bibliography on p. 308

28. Nitromethane

Structural formula:

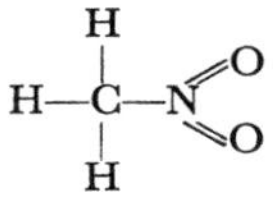

$$\begin{array}{c} H \\ | \\ H-C-N \\ | \\ H \end{array} \begin{array}{c} \nearrow O \\ \searrow O \end{array}$$

Molecular formula: CH_3NO_2

Molecular weight: 61.04

Properties: a colourless, non-hygroscopic liquid with a fairly strong odour.
  boiling point: 100.76 °C
  melting point: −29 °C
  vapour pressure: 38 mm Hg at 25 °C
  specific gravity (liquid density): 1.139
  flash point: 112 °F
  conversion factors: 1 p.p.m. = 2.495 mg/m³
                   1 mg/l = 400.7 p.p.m.
  solubility: in water, 9.5 ml/100 ml. Soluble in ethyl alcohol, ether and carbon tetrachloride. Dissolves aromatic hydrocarbons but is practically non-miscible with paraffins or naphthenic hydrocarbons (Fairhall, 1957). Solvent for nitrocellulose, cellulose acetate and some cellulose esters, resins, waxes, fats and dyestuffs.
  maximum allowable concentration: 100 p.p.m.

ECONOMY, SOURCES AND USES

Production

By nitration of methane.

Industrial uses

Mainly used in chemical synthesis, but to some extent as a solvent, especially in the coating industry (Bogin and Wampner, 1942); also in the refining of petroleum.

BIOCHEMISTRY

Estimation

In the atmosphere

(a) By means of the colour developed when it is heated with vanillin in an ammoniacal solution (Machle *et al.*, 1940).

(b) By means of the colour developed by ferric chloride in an acidified sample treated with sodium hydroxide (Scott and Treon, 1940).

Metabolism

The production of nitrite by nitromethane was at one time denied (Scott, 1942) since the concentration of nitrate and nitrite in the blood following inhalation or oral administration showed no such increase as in the case of nitroethane. Experiments with homogenised rabbit liver incubated with nitromethane (Egami and Sato, 1950) led them, however, to conclude that nitromethane does undergo decomposition with the formation of nitrite, more rapidly in the presence than in the absence of oxygen. The fact that nitrite formation was completely inhibited by heating the homogenate at 100 °C for 3 min indicated the enzymatic nature of the reaction.

TOXICOLOGY

Nitromethane, as judged by animal experiments, has the same general effects as nitroethane – narcosis, mucous membrane irritation and central nervous excitation – but is slightly less irritant and anaesthetic. Its central nervous effect is manifested after a latent period by convulsions and ataxia. It has an injurious effect on the liver similar to that of nitroethane. No injury to human beings has been recorded.

Toxicity to animals

(1) Acute

(a) Lethal dose. – (i) By oral administration Machle *et al.* (1940) found the lethal dose for rabbits to be 0.75 to 1 g/kg, while Weatherby (1955), estimating the oral lethal dose for dogs of a 20% emulsion in 0.3% methyl cellosolve, and for mice of a 5% aqueous solution, found the total dose necessary to cause the death of the dogs between 1.4 and 3.9 g/kg, and the LD_{50} for mice 1.44 g/kg. – *(ii) By subcutaneous injection* the minium lethal dose for dogs was stated by Gibbs and Reichert (1891) to lie between 0.5 and 1.0 g/kg. – *(iii) By intravenous administration* (Weatherby, 1955) the total dose for dogs, calculating from a dosage of 0.2 g/kg of the emulsion given at intervals of 10 min, varied from 1.4 to 3.8 g/kg. For rab-

Bibliography on p. 308

bits it appeared that the lethal dose varied appreciably with the viscosity of the methyl cellosolve emulsifier; the toxicity was higher with a high than a low viscosity. – *(iv) By inhalation* the lethal dose, as in the case of nitroethane, depended on the product of concentration and time of exposure. With concentrations above 1000 p.p.m., if the product of this and the time of exposure was greater than 1 (*e.g.* 1000 p.p.m. for 3 h) some of the animals, including one monkey, died, and if the figure was 5 or greater all died. This did not hold for low concentrations with repeated exposure *e.g.* below 500 p.p.m. with a total exposure of 14 h; in these conditions no deaths occurred.

(b) Narcotic dose. – True narcosis of slight degree was observed only with concentrations causing pronounced disturbance of the nervous system – weakness, ataxia and muscular incoordination – and these effects required an amount of nitromethane definitely greater than the lethal dose.

(2) Chronic

Repeated administration by the oral route to rats of up to 0.5% of nitromethane in drinking water daily for 15 weeks resulted in the death of several animals. Seven out of 10 receiving 0.25% and 6 out of 10 receiving 0.1% survived the whole duration and appeared to be in good health. In the former group definite, though relatively mild, pathological changes were observed in the liver and spleen (Weatherby, 1955).

SYMPTOMS OF INTOXICATION

Central nervous disturbance was the predominant effect of acute poisoning, including convulsions, twitching and cerebellar fits, while between the convulsions the animals remained weak, ataxic and showing athetoid movements. There were no specific changes in the blood picture nor on respiration and blood pressure (Machle and Scott, 1943; Weatherby, 1955).

CHANGES IN THE ORGANISM

Cerebral congestion and liver and kidney damage were similar to those caused by nitroethane, but irritation of the respiratory tract was less. Weatherby (1955) found similar lesions of the liver in dogs, mice and rabbits poisoned by nitromethane – areas of haemorrhage and necrosis and fatty changes.

29. Nitropropane

29a. 1-Nitropropane

One of the two isomeric forms of nitropropane.

Structural formula:

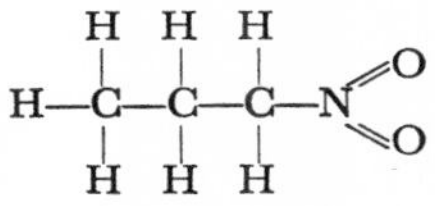

$$H-\underset{\underset{H}{|}}{\overset{\overset{H}{|}}{C}}-\underset{\underset{H}{|}}{\overset{\overset{H}{|}}{C}}-\underset{\underset{H}{|}}{\overset{\overset{H}{|}}{C}}-N\overset{\nearrow O}{\searrow_O}$$

Molecular formula $C_3H_7NO_2$

Molecular weight: 89.09

Properties: a colourless non-hygroscopic liquid with a somewhat disagreeable odour.

    boiling point: 131.5 °C

    melting point: —108 °C

    vapour pressure: 13 mm Hg at 25 °C

    specific gravity (liquid density): 1.003

    flash point: 120 °F

    conversion factors: 1 p.p.m. = 3.64 mg/m³

                      1 mg/l = 274 p.p.m.

    solubility: in water 9.5 ml/100 at 20 °C; miscible with ethyl alcohol and ether

    maximum allowable concentration: not established. Elkins (1959) suggests 25 p.p.m.

ECONOMY, SOURCES AND USES

Production

By nitration of propane.

Industrial uses

Solvent for organic esters of cellulose, some resins, waxes, fats and dyestuffs.

    Mainly in chemical synthesis, much less as a solvent than 2-nitropropane, usually only in small amounts with other solvents in the paint and varnish industry.

BIOCHEMISTRY

Estimation in the atmosphere

By the ferric chloride method as described by Scott and Treon (1940) for other primary nitroparaffins (see Nitroethane).

Metabolism

Absorption and excretion

It can be absorbed by the gastro-intestinal tract and by the lungs, and excretion takes place in the urine in the form of nitrate, oxidised from the nitrite ions which are the product of its metabolism (Williams, 1959), and part expired unchanged. There is no evidence of absorption from the skin.

TOXICOLOGY

1-Nitropropane is an irritant of mucous membranes, and in high oral dosage more lethal to animals than 2-nitropropane (Machle *et al.*, 1940), causing severe liver damage, progressive weakness and collapse.

No injury to human beings has been recorded.

Toxicity to animals

Acute

(a) *Lethal dose.* – (i) *By oral administration* of 0.25 to 0.5 g/kg, as compared with 0.50 to 0.75 for 2-nitropropane. – (ii) *By inhalation*. In the experiments of Machle *et al.* (1940) where only 2 rabbits and 2 guinea pigs were used, 5000–10,000 p.p.m. for 3 h killed all the animals, but 10,000 p.p.m. for 1 h only one guinea pig.

Comparing the lethal concentration of 1-nitropropane with that of butyl acetate given by Sayers *et al.* (1936) and of carbon tetrachloride given by Lehmann and Flury (1943) it appears that 1-nitropropane is more toxic than butyl acetate and approximately the same as carbon tetrachloride. The actual figures, according to Skinner (1947) are as follow:

(α) 1-Nitropropane – concentration lethal to guinea pigs, 0.5% for 3 h.

(β) Butyl acetate – concentrations of 0.7% for 13 h caused no deaths.

(γ) Carbon tetrachloride – concentrations of 0.32% for 3 h lethal to rabbits.

(b) *Narcotic dose.* – In the dosages used by Machle *et al.* (5000–10,000 p.p.m.) there was little evidence of a narcotic effect.

Irritation of conjunctiva, with lacrimation; restlessness; slow respiration with some râles: unsteadiness of gait, muscular incoordination, ataxia: progressive weakness and collapse.

CHANGES IN THE ORGANISM

The liver showed severe fatty infiltration; all other organs and the cerebrum congestion.

29b. 2-Nitropropane

The second of the two isomeric forms of nitropropane.

Structural formula:

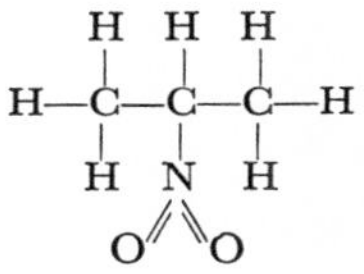

$$
\begin{array}{c}
\text{H}\quad\text{H}\quad\text{H}\\
|\quad\ |\quad\ |\\
\text{H--C--C--C--H}\\
|\quad\ |\quad\ |\\
\text{H}\quad\text{N}\quad\text{H}\\
\diagup\diagdown\\
\text{O}\qquad\text{O}
\end{array}
$$

Molecular formula: $C_3H_7NO_2$

Molecular weight: 89.09

Properties:

    boiling point: 120 °C
    melting point: −93 °C
    vapour pressure: 20 mm Hg at 25 °C
    specific gravity (liquid density): 0.992
    flash point: 103 °F
    conversion factors: 1 p.p.m. = 1.64 mg/m³ at 25 °C
                       1 mg/l = 274.7 p.p.m.
    solubility: in water 1.7 ml/100 at 20 °C
    maximum allowable concentration: 25 p.p.m.

ECONOMY, SOURCES AND USES

Production

By nitration of propane.

Bibliography on p. 308

Industrial uses

Solvent for organic cellulose esters, resins, waxes, fats and dyestuffs.

Its use as a solvent has increased rapidly during recent years (Jones, 1963) especially in the coating industry (Bogin and Wampner, 1942). An acid-proof lacquer used in the spraying of battery cases contained, according to Skinner (1947), approximately 20% of 2-nitropropane.

BIOCHEMISTRY

Estimation in the atmosphere

The most recent method, replacing the ferric chloride test used by Scott and Treon (1940) and Skinner (1947), which proved unsatisfactory owing to rapid fading of the colour reaction, is described by Jones (1963). This consists of a reaction with resorcinol in the presence of concentrated H_2SO_4, which gives an intense red-blue colour. Air containing 2-nitropropane vapour is passed through three tubes containing H_2SO_4 and an aliquot from the three tubes assayed. Decomposition of the nitro group to nitrous acid takes place on heating with the concentrated H_2SO_4. After cooling, 5 ml of a 1% aqueous solution of resorcinol is stratified upon the acid solution, the resulting coloured solution read with a spectrophotometer and compared with a standard solution of 10 μg of 2-nitropropane per ml of concentrated H_2SO_4. It is claimed that this method wil determine quantitatively not only 2-nitropropane but also all secondary and some tertiary nitroparaffins in amounts as low as 3 to 5 μg with an accuracy of $\pm$ 5%.

Metabolism

Absorption and excretion

Like 1-nitropropane, according to Scott (1942) probably yields nitrite as a product of its metabolism, and according to Williams (1959) a ketone would also be expected to be formed. Following absorption by the gastro-intestinal tract and the lungs, part is eliminated unchanged in the expired air, part excreted in the urine as nitrite and nitrate. There is no evidence of absorption by the skin sufficient to cause systemic injury.

TOXICOLOGY

On the basis of animal experiments 2-nitropropane appears to be of the same degree of toxicity as 1-nitropropane (*q.v.*). The only record of ill-effects from its industrial use is that of Skinner (1947). This suggests that chronic exposure can cause headache and gastro-intestinal disturbance.

Toxicity to animals

In the experiments of Machle, Scott and Treon (1940) 2-nitropropane was not described in such detail as 1-nitropropane, especially with regard to inhalation. A more specific and more recent investigation on this basis was made by Treon and Dutra (1952).

Lethal dose. – As in the case of other nitroparaffins, the lethal dose was found to be a product of concentration and length of exposure, death resulting from shorter periods of exposure to higher concentrations. Susceptibility of different species was also a factor, decreasing in the following order: cats, rats, rabbits and guinea pigs. The M.L.D. and shortest time of exposure were as follow: (a) cats – 328 p.p.m. for 3–7 h; (b) rats – 1140 p.p.m. for 7 h; (c) rabbits – 1390 p.p.m. for 3–7 h; (d) guinea pigs – 4622 p.p.m. for 5.5 h.

SYMPTOMS OF INTOXICATION

The severity and time of onset of symptoms varied with the species, but in most of the animals lethargy and prostration appeared before dyspnoea and occasional convulsions. In the case of cats and rats coma and death followed in a short time; rabbits and guinea pigs, after apparent partial recovery, died 1 to 4 days later.

With non-lethal but high concentrations, unsteady gait and partial loss of co-ordination occurred in cats, but no signs of intoxication were observed in any animals subjected to 83 p.p.m. Cats showed lacrimation, salivation and gastric regurgitation.

The blood

Methaemoglobin formation to the extent of 60–80% was developed by cats with severe exposure, and 25–35% with exposure to 780 p.p.m. for 4–5 h. With the latter concentration only about one-fifth of the amount received by rabbits was necessary to produce the same amount of methaemoglobin in cats. Heinz bodies were also more frequent and at lower concentrations with cats; at times, with prolonged exposure to 78 p.p.m. cats showed 30–35% of Heinz bodies.

The prothrombin content of the blood showed some reduction in the blood of two cats only, the time required for clotting during repeated exposure to about 328 p.p.m. increased from 24.0 and 23.5 to 40 and 50 sec respectively. No changes were observed in the peripheral blood picture.

CHANGES IN THE ORGANISM

(1) The liver

Only in cats exposed for several periods to 328 p.p.m., showed severe degeneration and focal necrosis, but in all animals exposed to 2353 p.p.m. or more, damage to the liver was observed.

Bibliography on p. 308

(2) The heart and kidneys

In cats exposed to 328 p.p.m. these showed some toxic degeneration. I other species this concentration caused none of these lesions. In the brain a animals exposed to the higher concentrations showed disintegration of cerebra neurones.

(3) The lungs

These showed pulmonary oedema, intra-alveolar haemorrhage and inter stitial pneumonitis.

Toxicity to human beings

In 1947 Skinner described the effects of exposure to 2-nitropropane of 5 or 6 men engaged in dipping small articles into a large tank of a vinyl co-polymer dissolved in a mixture of xylol and approximately 20% of 2-nitropropane. The temperature of the liquid varied between a maintenance level of 110–120 °F and an occasion ally higher level of 150 °F.

Concentrations in one plant where two workers were engaged for not more than 4 h a day and 3 days a week in spraying and stacking battery cases varied from 10 to 30 p.p.m. and neither of these men had noticed any ill-effects. In the dipping process, however, the concentrations were between 20 and 45 p.p.m. and two of the men employed here for the longest time and closest exposure com plained of anorexia, nausea increasing as the day progressed and followed by vomiting and diarrhoea. Others complained of severe occipital headache, also becoming worse during the day, but all were symptom-free on Sundays and holi days and also after the 2-nitropropane had been replaced by methyl ethyl ketone

(B) CHLORINATED NITROPARAFFINS

The introduction of a chlorine atom into the molecule of the mononitroparaffins greatly increases their irritant properties, especially with regard to the lungs, but since they have no appreciable vapour pressure at ordinary temperatures danger from their industrial use would appear to be chiefly that of accidental ingestion.

The compounds which have been studied by animal experiments are: 1-chloro-1-nitroethane (Machle *et al.*, 1940), and 1-chloro-1-nitropropane; 1,1-dichloro-1-nitroethane and 2-chloro-2-nitropropane (Machle *et al.*, 1945).

30. 1-Chloro-1-nitroethane

Structural formula:

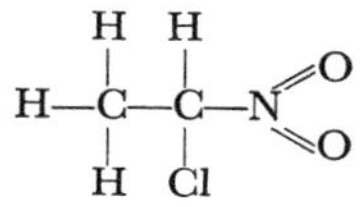

$$H-\overset{\overset{\displaystyle H}{|}}{\underset{\underset{\displaystyle H}{|}}{C}}-\overset{\overset{\displaystyle H}{|}}{\underset{\underset{\displaystyle Cl}{|}}{C}}-N\overset{\displaystyle O}{\underset{\displaystyle O}{\diagup}}$$

Molecular formula: $C_2H_4ClNO_2$

Molecular weight: 109.5

Properties:

    boiling point: 127.5 °C

    vapour pressure: 11.9 mm Hg at 25 °C

    specific gravity (liquid density): 1.286

    flash point: 133 °F

    conversion factors: 1 p.p.m. = 4.21 mg/m³

                      1 mg/l = 237 p.p.m.

    solubility: in water 0.4 ml/100 at 20 °C

    maximum allowable concentration: not established

ECONOMY, SOURCES AND USES

Industrial uses

Mainly in chemical synthesis.

BIOCHEMISTRY

Estimation in the atmosphere

By a colorimetric procedure (Machle et al., 1945).

Metabolism

Not absorbed by the skin to any appreciable extent. Neither its excretion nor its metabolic behaviour appear to have been studied.

[290]

TOXICOLOGY

The toxic effects of 1-chloro-1-nitroethane, as observed in animal experiments, are similar to those of the simple nitroparaffins, but cause less incoordination and more weakness and depression, and more irritation to mucous membranes. It causes some pulmonary oedema and possibly hepatitis.

Toxicity to animals

Acute

(a) *Lethal dose.* – (i) *By oral administration*, for rabbits, 0.1 to 0.15 g/kg as compared with 0.15 to 0.2 g/kg for 1-dichloro-1-nitroethane (Machle *et al.*, 1940). – (ii) *By inhalation*; no experiments were carried out, but according to Sutton (1963) it would be expected that its inhalation toxicity would be similar to that of 1-chloro-1-nitropropane, *vis.* 2574 p.p.m. for 2 h or 393 p.p.m. for 6 h, for the rabbit. (iii) *Skin application* caused no systemic effects and no skin irritation.

(b) *Narcotic dose.* – Not determined.

SYMPTOMS OF INTOXICATION

All but one of the animals succumbed within 24 h with evidence of pulmonary oedema; the exception survived 8 days and developed jaundice. All showed loss of weight, weakness amd depression but less incoordination than with the simple nitroparaffins. Diarrhoea was common to all the animals.

CHANGES IN THE ORGANISM

General congestion of all internal organs, especially of the lungs and gastro-intestinal tract. The lungs showed varying degrees of acute oedema. The liver showed some fatty change, but not more frequently than with other chloronitroparaffins.

Toxicity to human beings

No injury to human beings has been recorded.

Bibliography on p. 308

31. 1-Chloro-1-nitropropane

Structural formula:

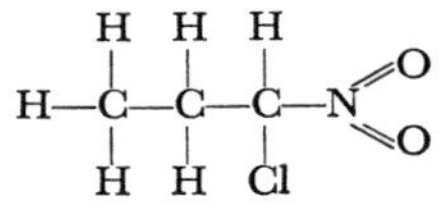

$$\begin{array}{ccc} H & H & H \\ | & | & | \\ H-C-C-C-N \\ | & | & | \\ H & H & Cl \end{array} \begin{array}{c} O \\ \diagup \\ \diagdown \\ O \end{array}$$

Molecular formula: $C_3H_6ClNO_2$

Molecular weight: 123.5

Properties:
>   *boiling point:* 139.5–143.3 °C
>   *vapour pressure:* 5.8 mm Hg at 20 °C
>   *vapour density (air = 1):* 4.3
>   *specific gravity (liquid density):* 1.209
>   *flash point:* 144 °F
>   *conversion factors:* 1 p.p.m. = 5.05 mg/m³
>   1 mg/l   = 198 p.p.m.
>   *solubility:* in water 0.5 ml/100 at 20 °C
>   *maximum allowable concentration:* 20 p.p.m. (Threshold Limit Values, 1962).

ECONOMY, SOURCES AND USES

In the synthetic rubber industry, as an addition to rubber cements, owing to its useful anti-gel property (Scheer, 1943).

BIOCHEMISTRY

Estimation in the atmosphere

The method used by Machle *et al.* (1945) was based on the reaction of 1-chloro-1-nitropropane with phenylhydrazine in concentrated H_2SO_4 to produce a deep red colour, the density being read in a photoelectric photometer at 540 mμ.

No investigations of the metabolic behaviour of 1-chloro-1-nitropropane have been carried out.

TOXICOLOGY

By oral administration to animals 1-chloro-1-nitropropane is more toxic than 1,1-dichloro-1-nitroethane, but less toxic by inhalation. Its effects are exerted chiefly on the lungs, but also on other organs, including the brain, heart, liver and kidneys.

Toxicity to animals

Acute, Lethal dose. – *(i)* *By oral administration*, for rabbits, 0.5 to 0.10 g/kg. – *(ii)* *By inhalation.* As with most of the chloro- and mononitroparaffins, the time of exposure influenced the lethal dose, *e.g.* 19 mg/l was not lethal with an exposure of 30 min nor 3.5 mg/l for 120 min, but if the concentrations were increased above these levels with no decrease in the length of exposure or if the duration of exposure to these concentrations were increased, at least one animal in an exposed group died (Machle *et al.*, 1945).

SYMPTOMS OF INTOXICATION

Following oral administration some animals lost weight but recovered after a short period. Following inhalation, the chief effects were irritation of mucous membranes and with lethal exposure marked oedema of the lungs pointed to the lung damage as the cause of death.

Application to the skin caused no such marked reactions as with 1,1-dichloro-1-nitroethane.

CHANGES IN THE ORGANISM

(1) The heart

Showed oedema and some necrosis of the myocardial fibres.

(2) The liver

Generalised oedema, congestion, cloudy swelling and some central fatty degeneration and necrosis.

(3) The kidneys

In these the tubules were primarily involved, showing cloudy swelling, fatty degeneration and coagulation necrosis.

(4) The respiratory tract

The chief site of injury; pulmonary oedema and congestion with scattered areas of emphysema and atelectasis and polymorphonuclear infiltration of the septa.

Toxicity to human beings

No injury to human beings has been recorded.

Bibliography on p. 308

32. 1,1-Dichloro-1-nitroethane

Structural formula:

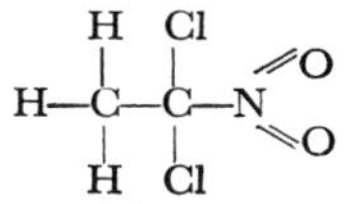

$$\begin{array}{ccc} H & Cl & \\ | & | & \diagup O \\ H-C-C-N & \\ | & | & \diagdown O \\ H & Cl & \end{array}$$

Molecular formula: $C_2H_3Cl_2NO_2$

Molecular weight: 143.9

Properties:

    boiling point: 124 °C

    vapour pressure: 16 mm Hg at 25 °C

    vapour density (air = 1): 5.0

    specific gravity (liquid density): 1.4271

    flash point: 168 °F

    conversion factors: 1 p.p.m. = 5.59 mg/m³

                        1 mg/l = 109.9 p.p.m.

    solubility: in water 0.25 ml/100 at 20 °C

    maximum allowable concentration: 10 p.p.m.

ECONOMY, SOURCES AND USES

Industrial uses

Mainly in chemical synthesis, but also as a fumigant for grains, flour and tobacco (Scheer, 1943).

BIOCHEMISTRY

Estimation in the atmosphere

The method used by Machle *et al.* (1945) is based on its reaction with resorcinol, methyl alcohol and sodium hydroxide to form a green colour, which when acidified turns to a light tan. The density is read in a photo-electric spectrophotometer and compared with a standardised curve.

Metabolism

Not appreciably absorbed by the skin. Its metabolic behaviour has not been investigated.

TOXICOLOGY

The toxic action of 1,1-dichloro-1-nitroethane is mainly irritant, especially to the skin and eyes and causes general weakness but no general narcosis, no marked central nervous disturbance and no production of methaemoglobin.

Toxicity to animals

Acute, Lethal dose. – *(i) By oral administration,* for rabbits, 0.15 to 0.20 g/kg. – *(ii) By inhalation.* As with the mononitroparaffins, length of exposure is a more potent factor than concentration, except with the highest levels. Death occurred with exposure to 52 p.p.m. for $18\frac{3}{4}$ h, but was tolerated in greater concentration without lethal effect for shorter periods. At 15,600 p.p.m. all animals died within 12 h following exposure for 75 min.

The effect of repeated small doses was not determined.

SYMPTOMS OF INTOXICATION

Acute poisoning causes irritation of eyes and nose with increased secretion; coughing, with excessive bronchial secretion and audible coarse râles and rhonchi; general weakness and appearance of illness.

Skin application caused swelling and irritation but no systemic effects.

CHANGES IN THE ORGANISM

With oral administration there was erosion of the gastric mucosa, with congestion, haemorrhage and inflammatory exudate; generalised vascular damage; pulmonary oedema; myocardial degeneration. The liver showed severe degeneration and necrosis; the kidneys degeneration of the glomeruli and tubules.

These effects were less marked than with 1-chloro-1-nitropropane.

By inhalation the most severe lesions were found in the lungs of animals exposed to concentrations greater than 170 p.p.m. for more than 30 min – oedema, congestion, haemorrhage and acute but not purulent bronchitis. The lesions of the liver were unlike those caused by highly chlorinated hydrocarbons; the toxic effects were mainly those of diffuse cloudy swelling, congestion, and haemorrhage of central areas.

Toxicity to human beings

No injury to human beings has been recorded.

Bibliography on p. 308

33. 2-Chloro-2-nitropropane

Structural formula:

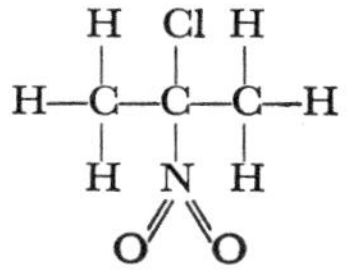

$$
\begin{array}{c}
\text{H} \quad \text{Cl} \quad \text{H} \\
| \quad\; | \quad\; | \\
\text{H—C—C—C—H} \\
| \quad\; | \quad\; | \\
\text{H} \quad \text{N} \quad \text{H} \\
\diagup \! \diagdown \\
\text{O} \quad\;\; \text{O}
\end{array}
$$

Molecular formula: $C_3H_6ClNO_2$

Molecular weight: 123.5

Properties:

    boiling point: 133.6 °C

    vapour density (air = 1): 4.3

    vapour pressure: 8.5 mm Hg at 20 °C

    specific gravity (liquid density): 1.1973

    flash point: 135 °F

    conversion factors: 1 p.p.m. = 5.05 mg/m³

                         1 mg/l = 198 p.p.m.

    maximum allowable concentration: not established.

TOXICOLOGY

The only results of animal experiments are given by Machle *et al.* (1940) without exact details except for the lethal dose by oral administration – 0.50 to 0.75 g/kg – the same as for nitroethane and 2-nitropropane.

SYMPTOMS OF INTOXICATION

These were similar to those caused by simple nitroparaffins except that weakness and depression were more marked than incoordination.

Animals which died usually did so within 24 h with evidence of pulmonary oedema. One which survived 8 days was deeply jaundiced and showed other signs of hepatitis.

CHANGES IN THE ORGANISM

Congestion of the intestinal tract, with diarrhoea, was more marked than with the simple nitroparaffins. Lung damage, with varying degrees of acute oedema, was present even with oral administration, and Machle *et al.* (1940) suggest that this may have been due to excretion of the whole or partly decomposed molecule through the lungs.

Changes in the liver were not more frequent than in animals exposed to other nitroparaffins.

34. Other Nitroparaffins and Chloronitroparaffins

Some other nitro- and chloronitroparaffins, used not as solvents, but as war materials together with T.N.T. and other explosives have been stated to be powerful irritants and also to form methaemoglobin.

Both tetranitromethane (Flury and Zernik, 1931) and dichlorodinitromethane (Mayer *et al.*, 1920) have been stated to have these toxicological properties.

Dichlorodinitromethane in particular causes massive oedema of the lungs, similar to that caused by chloropicrin, though 8 to 10 times less active. Mayer *et al.* state that the blood at the moment of death is dark brown in colour and contains up to 80% of methaemoglobin.

For animals the lethal dose by inhalation was found to be 10 p.p.m. after 20 minutes exposure and 100 p.p.m. after one hour.

In man, dichlorodinitromethane causes severe irritation of the eyes, nose and respiratory tract, with dyspnoea, cyanosis, sometimes bronchopneumonia and lung oedema. Headache, lassitude, drowsiness, slow pulse, methaemoglobinaemia and anaemia are other symptoms which have been observed.

Bibliography on p. 308   [297]

35. Nitrobenzene

Synonym: Oil of Mirbane

Structural formula:

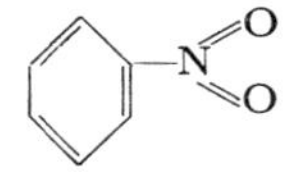

$$\text{(benzene ring)}-N\overset{O}{\underset{O}{\lessgtr}}$$

Molecular formula: $C_6H_5NO_2$

Molecular weight: 123.11

Properties: a yellow oily liquid with an odour like oil of bitter almonds
    boiling point: 210.9 °C
    melting point: 5.7 °C
    vapour pressure: not given
    vapour density (air = 1): 4.1
    specific gravity (liquid density): 1.198
    flash point: 190 °F
    conversion factors: 1 p.p.m. = 5 mg/m³
                    1 mg/l = 198.8
    solubility: in water 0.19% at 20° C. Soluble in alcohol, ether, benzene and oils
    maximum allowable concentration: 1 p.p.m.

ECONOMY, SOURCES AND USES

Production

By reaction of excess of concentrated HNO_3 or a mixture of concentrated HNO_3 and concentrated H_2SO_4 with benzene or one of its homologues.

Industrial uses

(1) As a basic intermediate in the manufacture of certain aromatic amines, especially aniline and benzidine.
(2) As a constituent of shoe and floor polishes.
(3) As a substitute for almond essence, and in the perfume industry.
(4) As a preservative in some spray paints.

BIOCHEMISTRY

Estimation

In the atmosphere

By ultra-violet absorption, the vapour being dissolved in cyclohexane free from impurities such as benzene (Hamblin, 1963).

Metabolism

It is to be noted that *in vitro* nitrobenzene has no action on haemoglobin; it has to be metabolically changed before it becomes active in this respect.

It is readily absorbed by the skin as well as by inhalation, and is slowly metabolised in the body (50% in 8 h and still present in the body after 7 days). It forms several metabolites amounting to about 60% of the dose in 4 to 5 days. Only 0.5% is eliminated unchanged in the expired air, though 1% of CO_2, one of its breakdown products, is also eliminated by this route and 0.1% in the urine. The actual metabolites differ in various animal species. In the rabbit and guinea pig the main metabolite is *p*-aminophenol (Meyer, 1905; Robinson *et al.*, 1951; Parke, 1956), which, when excreted in the urine mainly in the conjugated form (aminophenyl gluconuride) amounts to 31% of the oral dose. There is also a small amount of mercapturic acid formed (about 0.3% of the dose – after Parke, 1956).

The most toxic metabolite, according to Williams (1959) is probably *p*-nitrophenol and there is a possibility that a combination of this with *o*- and *p*-aminophenol before conjugation could contribute to the toxic effects of nitrobenzene. Other possible intermediates in its metabolism are also methaemoglobin formers and much more toxic than the phenols (Heubner, 1948) so that there may be a toxic phase during its detoxication in the process of conversion into the conjugated forms of the phenol metabolites. In view of the fact that animals in which methaemoglobin has been reduced by the administration of dimercaptopropanol have developed even more serious symptoms of intoxication, it has been suggested (Goldstein and Popovici, 1960) that the toxic action of nitrobenzene is exerted strongly on the enzymes catalase and peroxidase. These observers estimated at different intervals the activity of these enzymes in white rats poisoned by subcutaneous injection of 0.64 g/kg of nitrobenzene, as compared with that existing before injection, and found that the catalase activity fell consistently during a period up to 96 h after the initial dose to 86.6% of the initial level, while that of peroxidase activity also diminished to a smaller extent. The importance of this phenomenon, which relates possibly to the formation of sulphaemoglobin as well as methaemoglobin is believed to lie in the blockage by these two abnormal haemoglobins of the blood pigment and in diminution of functional capacity of the residual haemoglobin.

Bibliography on p. 308

TOXICOLOGY

The outstanding toxic effect of nitrobenzene is its capacity for formation of methae-moglobin, with a risk of death from respiratory failure if the methaemoglobinae-mia is severe. In man the onset of methaemoglobinaemia is insidious, cyanosis being grossly recognisable only when the methaemoglobin concentration reaches 15% or more, and definite symptoms of illness only at 40–70%. Estimation of the methaemoglobin level in the blood is usually carried out by the method described by Evelyn and Malloy (1938) and by Hamblin and Mangelsdorf (1938), using a photoelectric colorimeter.

Nitrobenzene is also a central nervous poison, causing excessive fatigue, drowsiness, headache, vertigo, tinnitus and numbness of the limbs. There is some difference of opinion as to whether haemolytic anaemia is one of its toxic effects in human beings, but Heinz bodies have been observed with methaemoglobinae-mia in a few cases of chronic exposure to nitrobenzene.

Toxicity to animals

The varying susceptibility to the formation of methaemoglobin by various drugs in different animal species (Lester, 1943) has led to some discrepancy in the results of various investigators. The rabbit and guinea pig, for example, are much more resistant to methaemoglobin formation than the cat, and the symptomatic reac-tion of rabbits, rats and cats differs from that of dogs (Driesbach and Chandler, 1917; Smyth, 1931), the former reacting chiefly by depression and paralysis, the latter showing initial stimulation, inco ordination, rigidity and nystagmus.

(1) Acute

(a) Lethal dose. – In the early experiments of Meyer (1905) rabbits were found to react strongly to subcutaneous injection of 0.5 g of nitrobenzene, 2 of the animals dying after 12 to 14 h, while others recovered from an oral dose of 0.5–0.7 g.

Lethal dose: (oral) as starch paste, for guinea pigs and rabbits – 1 g/kg (Smyth, 1931); LD_{20} (oral) as 10% suspension for rats, 0.64 g/kg; LD_{20} (subcutaneous) as 10% suspension, for rats, 2.10 g/kg; LD_{20} (intraperitoneal) as 10% suspension, for rats, 0.64 g/kg (Sziza and Magos, 1959).

(b) Narcotic dose, by intraperitoneal injection, for rats, 0.18 g/kg (Sziza and Magos, 1959).

(2) Chronic

According to Smyth (1931) in slow poisoning from continued low exposures there may be an increase in the number of erythrocytes; the urine becomes brown or dark red, and contains bile pigments, methaemoglobin or haemoglobin; there may also be albuminuria and a positive Fehling's reaction.

This initial rise in erythrocytes, and also in haemoglobin, has also been observed by Hamblin (1949) with a return to normal limits within 24 h. In two industrial cases recorded by Ravault, Bourret and Roche (1946) there was slight anaemia, which they considered to be of a haemolytic type, with marked irregularity in the shape and size of the red cells; they also remarked that there is sometimes an intense polynucleosis.

SYMPTOMS OF INTOXICATION

Restlessness, cyanosis of skin and mucous membranes; onset of narcosis accompanied by loss of weight and marked cyanosis. Methaemoglobin level between 20 and 30% – greatest by intraperitoneal injection. Heinz bodies in 40 to 60% of red cells.

(1) The eyes
Only slight transient irritation.

(2) The skin
In rabbits no irritation (Smyth, 1931).

(3) Blood and bone marrow
In rabbits, given subcutaneous injections of 0.75 g of nitrobenzene (London *et al.*, 1960), haematocrit and haemoglobin levels showed a marked decrease and there was a tendency to spherocytosis; Heinz bodies were present in only 17 animals out of 27. These changes were accompanied by intense reticulocytosis, which was present also in animals which did not show haemolysis. This was regarded as an important sign of diagnosis of nitrobenzene poisoning, indicating the degree of regeneration due to destruction of erythrocytes. Methaemoglobinaemia was not parallel with the clinical condition, its maximum (4%) being present 4 h after the initial dosage and falling gradually thereafter, while sulphaemoglobin rose with the toxic evolution to 14%. Leucopenia was present is some animals even when anaemia was not marked; in others leucocytosis together with neutrophilia, and in the majority thrombocytopenia.

The bone marrow showed changes ranging from hyperplasia to hypoplasia and even aplasia, with an increase in macroblasts and a decrease in reticulocytes and megakaryocytes.

CHANGES IN THE ORGANISM

Hyperaemia of the abdominal cavity and of all organs.

Bibliography on p. 308

(1) The liver

Macroscopic appearance of nutmeg size nodules; microscopically fatty infiltration.

(2) The kidneys

Fatty infiltration.

(3) The lungs

A tendency to extravasation of blood, varying from minute petechiae to larger ecchymoses or even lobular haemorrhage in severe poisoning.

(4) The tissues

In the tissues, Parke (1956) noted that one rabbit which died after receiving orally 200 mg/kg 30 h later had large deposits of fat in the tissues, not as nitrobenzene itself but as a metabolite or metabolites; this was also present in the gastro-intestinal tract.

Toxicity to human beings

(1) Acute

The signs and symptoms of acute nitrobenzene intoxication are characterised by the early appearance of cyanosis due to methaemoglobin formation. In some cases there is excitement followed by depression, with weakness, sometimes dyspnoea, shock and circulatory failure. Such symptoms can be caused by contact with the skin, as noted by Brennemann (1959) in older children when shoes recently dyed black with a dye containing nitrobenzene have been worn for some hours.

(i) By ingestion. – An interesting account of poisoning by an industrial product (Transyl) which was later found to contain 3% of nitrobenzene, 95% of mineral oil and the remainder a chlorinated solvent believed to be trichloroethylene, was described by Hadengue *et al.* (1960). This case, in which the manifestations of poisoning were dominated by intense cyanosis, and semi-consciousness, followed ingestion by error of Transyl. Toxic effects were not immediate, but supervened in about ½ to 1 h with violent headache, loss of consciousness and very dark cyanosis. The blood picture was that of moderate anaemia (3137 red blood corpuscles) but a normal white cell and differential count. The blood was dark brown in coulor and a diagnosis of methaemoglobinaemia was made. Treatment with methylene blue and vitamin C was followed by improvement in the symptoms, but temporary anuria occurred, with final recovery on the 7th day.

(ii) By skin contamination. – According to Zeitoun (1959) 21 infants have been affected since 1949 by having been given a skin application of 'bitter almond oil', which was in fact a mixture of 2–10% of nitrobenzene and 90–98% of cotton

seed oil. In 6 cases the infants were in a state of shock, and semi-comatose, with cold extremities and rapid pulse, and of these, two ended fatally, terminal bron-cho-pneumonia having developed; the remaining cases recovered, with no or very mild residual cyanosis. The cyanosis was said to have appeared between 4 h and 4 days of the application. Several industrial cases of poisoning by skin con-tamination have been reported. In the Annual Report of the Chief Inspector of Factories of Great Britain for 1947, a severe case is described in which the poison-ing resulted from the use of buckets containing nitrobenzene instead of mechani-cal delivery, in the manufacture of a dye. The man in question was said to have washed and to have changed his clothes before leaving work, but on reaching home he felt dizzy and complained of headache and nausea. Next morning he was unconscious, deeply cyanosed and showed an intense plantar reflex, but recovered, following oxygen therapy, in about 10 days.

In another less severe case in the same year the contamination of protective clothing occurred above knee-length rubber boots, during the cleaning of a still used for purification of nitrobenzene. He also complained $3\frac{1}{4}$ h later of vomiting and breathlessness and was cyanosed, but recovered completely.

TREATMENT

Removal from exposure, and if there is any skin contamination, thorough cleans-ing of the skin and clothing.

Oxygen therapy and stimulants are generally recommended.

Methylene blue (5 mg daily of a 5% solution or 1 mg/kg of a 0.5% solution intravenously usually only once) is a somewhat controversial recommendation; beneficial results were observed by Gaultier *et al.* (1949) in two relatively slight cases, but Hamblin (1949) stated that he had experience of several cases in which methylene blue therapy had been followed by a marked increase in cyanosis.

Vitamin C (200 mg daily) was found effective by Zeitoun (1959) and in severe cases blood transfusion.

Bibliography on p. 308

36. Pyridine

Structural formula: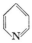

Molecular formula: C_5H_5N

Molecular weight: 79

Properties: pyridine is the parent compound of many derivatives which are of much less industrial importance than pyridine itself. These derivatives have been described in detail by Fassett and Roudabush (1953) and by Sutton (1963)

The commercial product contains derivatives with methyl groups – picolin, lutidin or collidin (Meyer, 1950). Pyridine is a stable colourless liquid with a strong unpleasant odour detectable at 1 p.p.m. It has a wide solvent power, and is soluble in water, alcohol and ether.

boiling point: 115 °C (commercial variety 94–160 °C)
vapour pressure: 20 mm at 25 °C
vapour density (air = 1): 2.72
specific gravity (liquid density): 0.982
flash point: 68 °F.
conversion factors: 1 p.p.m. = 3.23 mg/m³
              1 mg/l = 309 p.p.m.
maximum allowable concentration: 5 p.p.m.

ECONOMY, SOURCES AND USES

Production

By extraction from the lower-boiling fractions of tar distillates after removal of the tar acids by sulphuric acid and purification by distillation with lime (Fairhall, 1957).

Industrial uses

(1) In the manufacture of vitamins (especially nicotinic acid) and of sulpha-drugs, disinfectants and dyestuffs.
(2) In the rubber industry.

(3) As a denaturant for alcohol.

(4) In the paint industry.

(5) In the manufacture of chemicals and explosives.

BIOCHEMISTRY

Estimation

In the atmosphere

(1) By drawing air through standardised H_2SO_4 and titrating with standard-ised alkali (Fairhall, 1957).

(2) By spectroscopic analysis of its absorption in normal H_2SO_4 (Hofman, 1942).

Metabolism

Absorption takes place through the lungs, gastro-intestinal tract and intraperito-neal cavity. Part is excreted in the urine unchanged, part in the form of its chief metabolite, *N*-methylpyridinium hydroxide. Pyridine is an example of the methyl-ation process of metabolism which is confined to some heterocyclic compounds, but this occurs, with pyridine, only in some animals, notably mice, but not in rats (Baxter and Mason, 1947), while in rabbits only traces of 3-hydroxy pyridine are excreted. In these animals Novello (1927) found that the greater part was eliminated via the lungs, skin and faeces, only a small percentage being excreted in the urine as free pyridine. Williams (1959) states that in man it is probably methylated to some extent, but that the fate in the body of the major portion of the pyridine administered is not known.

TOXICOLOGY

In animals pyridine has proved less toxic than in human beings, where severe effects have been reported both from its administration as an anti-convulsant in the treatment of epilepsy and asthma, and also by inhalation, especially as crude pyridine containing impurities in the form of its derivatives.

In such cases the effect is concentrated chiefly on the nervous system, causing symptoms resembling Wernicke's pseudo-encephalitis, with paralysis of cranial nerves, periods of unconsciousness, cerebella ataxia; in some cases in animals there has been evidence of hepatic and renal injury. It is also an irritant of mucous membranes, including those of the gastro-intestinal tract.

Bibliography on p. 308

Toxicity to animals

(1) Acute

(a) Lethal dose. – *(i) By oral administration*, for rabbits, 400 mg/100 g (Distler, 1887), for guinea pigs, 87 mg/100 g (Brunton and Tunnicliffe, 1894). – *(ii) By intraperitoneal injection*, for mice, 1.2 g/kg (Baxter and Mason, 1947).

LD_{50} (oral), for rabbits, only 2 died after 880 mg/kg (Pollock *et al.*, 1943).

(b) Narcotic dose. – Intravenous, for rabbits, 110 mg/kg (Pollock *et al.*, 1943).

(2) Chronic

Repeated oral administration to rabbits of 44 mg/kg for 5–7 days caused no toxic effect; 165 mg/kg caused death in one animal out of 4 on the 6th day and 220 mg/kg in another, probably from administration while the stomach was distended with food (Pollock *et al.*, 1954). In dogs (His, 1887) 0.1 g daily as a 5% solution for 35 days caused only occasional vomiting and diarrhoea. Mice given 0.1% in the diet lost weight and died after 2–4 weeks (Baxter and Mason, 1947).

SYMPTOMS OF INTOXICATION

Sialorrhoea, weakness of limbs, occasional vomiting and diarrhoea. Death from respiratory paralysis.

CHANGES IN THE ORGANISM

The liver and kidneys were reported by Coulson and Brazda (1948) to be severely damaged by pyridine, more so than by its derivatives. Baxter (1948) observed cirrhosis or necrosis or both in the liver of rats receiving pyridine in the diet, and degenerative changes in the kidneys.

Toxicity to human beings

(i) By ingestion. – A fatal case from accidental ingestion of half a cupful of commercial pyridine was reported by Helme in 1893. The initial symptom was vomiting, later slight cyanosis, a choking sensation, precordial and abdominal pain and a raised temperature, pulse and respiration, but no abnormality of the urine. Acute congestion of the lungs and delirium preceded death, which occurred 43 h after ingestion of the pyridine.

Autopsy revealed that the chief lesions (inflammatory) were in the respiratory tract, the oesophagus and the stomach. In the liver there were a few fatty patches. In the treatment of epilepsy, short-term administration of 0.6 ml of pyridine 3 or 4 times a day was found by Pollock *et al.* (1943), to cause minor complaints of anorexia, nausea, occasional vomiting and headache, faintness, weakness and mental depression. The blood picture showed a tendency to a fall in leucocytes and an increase in eosinophils. In the urine a few erythrocytes were present and in one case a few hyaline casts, but on the whole the toxic effects were minimal. In continuing further treatment with a higher dosage (1.85 and 2.4 ml) in two cases, the results were much more unfavorable, in one case in fact fatal. In this case there was rapid development of anuria and jaundice, with evidence of progressive parenchymal destruction of the liver.

Another case, a convulsive disorder due to an astrocytoma, with some residual signs of brain disease, had received 10 minims of pyridine 3 times a day, and 10 days later there was evidence of hepatorenal injury, with weakness of the limbs, nausea, stupor, confusion and disorientation, but, following a blood transfusion, eventual recovery, with a return to the condition existing before the pyridine medication.

(ii) By inhalation. – Earlier authorities had sometimes given pyridine by inhalation in the treatment of asthma (Sée, 1885; Lublenski, 1885) and cases of poisoning from its industrial use were described by Ludwig (1934, 1936), Holtzmann (1936) and Meyer (1950).

One of Ludwig's cases was a chemist who had worked with pyridine for 6 months and who suffered from disturbance of equilibrium, facial paralysis and attacks of loss of consiousness. In another, after 2 years' exposure, the symptoms were paralysis of the ocular muscles with nystagmus, facial paralysis, hemiparesis with anesthesia to heat and paresthesia of the left side of the face, right-sided excessive perspiration, cerebellar ataxia, bladder paralysis, difficulty of hearing and neuralgic headache. Holtzmann observed similar symptoms, with the addition of marked loss of weight, noises in the ears and pain on moving the arms. Ludwig considered these symptoms similar to Wernicke's pseudo-encephalitis, but Meyer (1950) remarks that some of the multiform symptomatology of pyridine poisoning does not conform exclusively to injury of the medulla; he considers that it resembles more closely the manifestations of tabes dorsalis.

He describes the case of a man who had worked with pyridine for 13 years. He had complained of nervousness and sleeplessness, and for the last two years attacks of giddiness, pain in the right calf and chest, weakness of the legs and tremor. He then had a sudden attack of anuria, and a catheter specimen provided 2 litres of reddish urine with a trace of albumen. A gross diverticulum of the bladder revealed at operation was believed to be secondary to the urine retention.

Teisinger (1947) also recorded 7 cases of chronic pyridine poisoning, in which the symptoms were related to the nervous system – headache, vertigo, nervousness, sleeplessness, and in one case loss of concentration and memory.

Gastro-intestinal symptoms were prominent in some of Ludwig's cases – loss of appetite, thirst, nausea and diarrhoea – and were occasionally present in some of Teisinger's, while vomiting was the chief complaint in one of Holtzmann's and in some of Lublenski's.

Acute narcosis was reported in one case to the Home Office, Great Britain in 1934. This was a man who had been employed in cleaning a tank-wagon which had contained pyridine.

Bibliography on p. 308

BIBLIOGRAPHY

Baxter, J. H. (1948) Hepatic and renal Injury with Calcium Deposits and Cirrhosis produced in Rats by Pyridine, *Am. J. Pathol.*, 24:503.

Baxter, J. H. and M. F. Mason (1947) A Comparison of the Effects of Pyridine and Methyl Pyridinium Chloride in the Rat, *J. Pharmacol. Exptl. Therap.*, 91:350.

Bogin, C and L. Wampner (1942) Nitroparaffins as Solvents in the Coating Industry, *Ind. Eng. Chem.*, 34:1091.

Bray, H. G. and S. P. James (1958) The Formation of Mercapturic Acids from Aliphatic Compounds *in vivo, Biochem. J.*, 69:24 P.

Brennemann, J. (1959) *Practice of Pediatrics*. Prior Co. Inc. Hagerstown, Maryland.

Brunton, T. S. and F. W. Tunnicliffe (1894) On the physiological Action of Pyridine, *J. Physiol.*, 17:272.

Chief Inspector of Factories, Home Office, Gt. Britain (1934) *Annual Report, H.M.S.O., London.*

Chief Inspector of Factories, Gt. Britain (1947) *Annual Report, H.M.S.O., London.*

Coulson, R. A. and F. G. Brazda (1948) Influence of Choline, Cystine and Methionine on toxic effects of Pyridine and related Compounds, *Proc. Soc. Exptl. Biol. Med.*, 69:480.

Distler, H. (1887) *Über einige Wirkungen des Pyridins*, Inaug. Diss. Junge & Sohn, Erlangen.

Driesbach, M. and W. L. Chandler (1917) Some physiological Disturbances induced in Animals by Nitrobenzol Fumigation, *Am. J. Physiol.*, 42:604.

Egami, F. and R. Sato (1950) Enzymic Decomposition of Nitromethane by Liver Homogenates, *Nature*, 165:365.

Evelyn, K. A. and H. T. Malloy (1938) Micro-determination of Oxyhaemoglobin, Methaemoglobin and Sulfhaemoglobin in a single Sample of Blood, *J. Biol. Chem.*, 126:655.

Fairhall, L. T. (1957) *Industrial Toxicology*, 2nd ed. Williams and Wilkins, Baltimore.

Fassett, D. W. and R. L. Roudabush (1953) *Toxicity of Pyridine Derivatives with Relation to Chemical Structure*. [Cited by Sutton, 1963].

Flury, F. and F. Zernik (1931) *Schädliche Gäse*, p. 471. Springer, Berlin.

Gaultier, M., M. Benguigui and G. Smagghe (1949) À propos de 33 Cas d'Intoxications aiguë méthémoglobinisantes légères, *Arch. Malad. Profess.*, 10:368.

Gibbs, W. and E. T. Reichert (1891) Systematic Study of the Action of definitely related chemical Compounds upon Animals, *Am. Chem., J.*, 13:361.

Goldstein, I. and C. Popovici (1960) Modifications de la Catalase et de la Peroxidase dans l'Intoxication expérimentale au Nitrobenzène, *Med. Lavoro*, 51:42.

Hadengue, A., J. Facquet, P. Colvez and J. L. Jullien (1960) Intocixation par le Nitrobenzène et le Trichloroéthylène, *Arch. Malad. Profess.*, 21:43.

Hamblin, D. O. (1949) Nitro- and Amino Compounds of the Aromatic Series; in Patty, F.A. (1949). *Industrial Hygiene and Toxicology*, Vol. II, 1st. ed. Interscience Publ. New York.

Hamblin, D. O. and A. F. Mangelsdorff (1938) Methaemoglobinaemia and its Measurement, *J. Ind. Hyg.*, 20:523.

Hass, H. B., E. B. Hodge and B. M. Vanderbilt (1936) Nitration of Gaseous Paraffins, *Ind. Eng. Chem.*, 28:339.

Hass, H. B. and E. F. Riley (1943) The Nitroparaffins, *Chem. Rev.* 32:373.

Helme, G. F. (1893) A fatal Case of Pyridine Poisoning, *Brit. Med. J.*, 2:253.

Heppel, L. A. and V. T. Porterfield (1949) Metabolism of Inorganic Nitrite and Nitrate Esters, *J. Biol. Chem.*, 178:549.

Heubner, W. (1948) Giftung aromatischer Nitroverbindungen, *Arch. Exptl. Pathol. Pharmacol.*, 205:310.

His, W. (1887) Über das Stoffwechselprodukt, des Pyridins, *Arch. Exptl. Pathol. Pharmakol.*, 22:253.

Hofman, E. (1942) Quantitativer Nachweiss kleinster Pyridinmengen in der Luft mittels Spektralanalyse, *Arch. Hyg. Bakteriol.*, 128:169:179.

Holtzmann, F. (1936) Pyridinvergiftung, *Z. Gewerbehyg.*, 23:8.

Jones, L. R. (1963) The Determination of 2-Nitropropane in Air, *Am. Ind. Hyg. Assoc. J.*, 24:11.

Lehmann, K. B. and F. Flury (1943) *Toxicology and Hygiene of Industrial Solvents*, Williams and Wilkins, Baltimore.

Lester, D. (1943) Formation of Methaemoglobin; Species Differences, *J. Pharmacol. Exptl. Therap.*, 77:154; 160.

London M., P. Serban and C. Popovici (1960) La Valeur de certaines Modifications hématologiques pour l'Appréciation de la Toxicité du Nitrobenzène, *Arch. Malad. Profess.*, 21:205.

Lublenski, W. (1885) Über die Anwendung des Pyridins bei Asthma, *Deut. Med. Z.*, 2:985.

Ludwig, H. (1934) Zur Toxicologie des Pyridins und seiner Homologen. (Pseudo-encephalitis Wernicke) bei Pyridinarbeiter, *Arch. Gewerbepathol. Gewerbehyg.* 5:654.

Ludwig, H. (1936) Über die Wirkung von Pyridin-Einatmung bei Katzen, *Arch. Exptl. Pathol. Pharmakol.*, 182:178.

Machle, W. and E. W. Scott (1943) Effects of Nitroparaffins and related Compounds on Blood Pressure and Respiration of Rabbits, *Proc. Soc. Exptl. Biol. Med.*, 53:12.

Machle, W., E. W. Scott and J. Treon (1940) The Physiological Response of Animals to some simple Mononitroparaffins and to certain Derivatives of these Compounds, *J. Ind. Hyg.*, 22:315.

— (1942) The Metabolism of Nitroparaffins, *J. Ind. Hyg.*, 24:5.

Machle, W., E. W. Scott, J. F. Treon, F. H. Heyroth and K. V. Kitzmiller (1945) The physiological Response of Animals to certain chlorinated Monoparaffins, *J. Ind. Hyg.*, 27:95.

Mayer, A., L. Plantefol and F. Vlés (1920) Sur l'Intoxication par les Méthanes Nitro-halogénés, *Compt. Rend.*, 171:1396.

Meyer, A. (1950) Über die Pyridinvergiftung, *Z. Unfallmed. Berufskrankh.*, 43:144.

Meyer, E. (1905) Über das Verhalten des Nitrobenzols und einiger anderer aromatischer Körper im Organismus, *Hoppe-Seyler's Z. Physiol. Chem.*, 46:497.

Novello, H. J. (1927) The Fate of certain heterocyclic Ring Compounds in the Animal Body, *J. Biol. Chem.*, 74:33.

Parke, D. V. (1956) The Metabolism of 14C-Nitrobenzene in the Rabbit and Guinea pig, *Biochem. J.*, 62:339.

Pollock, L. J., I. Finkelman and A. J. Arieff (1943) Toxicity of Pyridine in Man, *Arch. Int. Med.*, 71:95.

Ravault, P. P., J. Bourret and L. Roche (1946) Deux Intoxications par le Nitrobenzène, *Arch. Malad. Profess.*, 7:305.

Robinson, D., J. N. Smith and R. T. Williams (1951) The Metabolism of Nitrobenzene in the Rabbit, *Biochem. J.*, 50:228.

Sayers, R. R., H. H. Schrenk and F. A. Patty (1936) Acute Response of Guinea Pigs to Vapours of some new commercial Organic Compounds – Normal Butyl Acetate, *U.S. Treas. Publ. Health Rep.*, 51:1229.

Schadow, G. (1877) Über die physiologischen Wirkungen des Nitropentans, *Arch. Exptl. Pathol. Pharmakol.*, 6:194.

Scheer, W. E. (1943) Industrial Applications of the Nitroparaffins, *Chem. Ind.*, 52:473.

Scott, E. W. (1942) Metabolism of Nitroparaffins; metabolic products of Nitroethane, *J. Ind. Hyg.*, 24:220.

Scott, E. W. and J. Treon (1940) Colorimetric Determination of Primary Mononitroparaffins, *Ind. Eng. Chem. Anal. Ed.*, 12:189.

Sée, G. (1885) Traitement de l'Asthme névro-pulmonaire et de l'Asthme cardiaque au moyen de la Pyridine, *Bull. Gen. Therap.*, 108:529.

Skinner, J. B. (1947) The toxicity of 2-Nitropropane, *Ind. Med. Surg.*, 16:441.

Smyth, H. F. (1931) The Toxicity of certain Benzene Derivatives and related Compounds, *J. Ind. Hyg. Toxicol.*, 13:87.

Sutton, W. L. (1963) Aliphatic and cyclic amines, in F. A. Patty (Ed.), *Industrial Hygiene and Toxicology*, Vol. II, 2nd. ed. Interscience Publ. New York.

Sziza, M. and L. Magos (1959) Toxikologische Untersuchung einiger in der Ungarischen Industrie zur Anwendung gelangenden aromatischer Nitroverbindungen, *Arch. Gewerbepathol. Gewerbehyg.*, 17:217.

Teisinger, J. (1947) Mild chronic Intoxication with Pyridine, *Čas. Lék. Čes.*, 86:1185.

Toops, E. F. Jr. (1956) Physical Properties of 8 high-purity Nitroparaffins, *J. Phys. Chem.*, 60:304.

Treon, J. F. and F. R. Dutra (1952) Physiological Response of experimental Animals to the Vapour of 2-Nitropropane, *Arch. Ind. Hyg.*, 5:52.

Weatherby, J. H. (1955) Observations on the Toxicity of Nitromethane, *Arch. Ind. Health.*, 11:102.

Williams, R. T. (1959) *Detoxication Mechanisms*, Chapman and Hall, London.

Zeitoun, M. M. (1959) Nitrobenzene Poisoning in Infants due to Inunction with false Bitter Almond Oil, *J. Trop. Pediatr.*, 5:73.

Chapter 7

ALCOHOLS

On the whole, the toxic hazard of the alcohols from industrial use is not severe from the point of view of cumulative injury to the internal organs, though some of them have been found to have a cumulative effect on the nervous system. The outstanding example of this effect is the permanent damage to the ocular tissues caused by methyl alcohol, though this is much more rarely observed following inhalation, as occurring in industrial operations, than by ingestion.

Physiologically, all the alcohols are weaker narcotics than the hydrocarbons; their narcotic powers (Elkins, 1959) increase with increased molecular weight. Differences in the degree and nature of their toxicity are associated with their metabolic characteristics. Ethyl alcohol, for example, being converted in the body to carbon dioxide and water, is practically a non-cumulative poison while methyl alcohol, with a much slower rate of elimination, decomposes with the formation of formaldehyde and formic acid, both of which are potent poisons of nervous tissue.

37. Methanol

Synonyms: methyl alcohol, wood spirit, wood alcohol, carbinol

Structural formula:

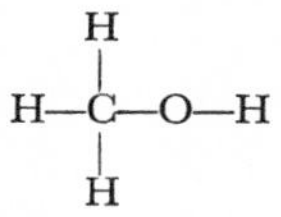

$$H-\overset{\displaystyle H}{\underset{\displaystyle H}{C}}-O-H$$

Molecular formula: CH_3OH

Molecular weight: 32.042

Properties: a clear colourless, highly volatile liquid with an odour similar to that of ethyl alcohol, and a burning taste.

> *boiling point:* 65 °C
> *melting point:* —97.8 °C
> *vapour pressure:* 95 mm Hg at 20 °C
> *vapour density (air = 1):* 1.11
> *specific gravity (liquid density):* 0.7915
> *flash point:* 54 °F
> *conversion factors:* 1 p.p.m. = 1.31 mg/m³
> 1 mg/l = 764 p.p.m.
> *solubility:* completely miscible with water, ether and most organic solvents. Only a mild solvent for fats and oils.
> *maximum allowable concentration:* 200 p.p.m.

ECONOMY, SOURCES AND USES

Production

(1) Natural methanol is produced by neutralisation of the products of distillation of hardwood with lime. The commercial variety contains impurities – 1 to 2% of propyl and allyl alcohol, aldehyde, methyl acetate, acetone and other organic compounds (Koelsch, 1921).

(2) Synthetic methanol is obtained by passing a mixture of CO_2 and H_2 at high pressure and temperature over a catalyst. This method now produces considerably more methanol than the natural process. The product, though practically pure, can cause poisoning as severe as that of natural wood alcohol, whose toxic action was at one time thought to be due to the impurities contained in it (Lehmann and Flury, 1943).

Industrial uses

(1) In the celluloid industry (cellophane laminating).

(2) In the boot and shoe industry (wood heel covering).

(3) In paper coating.

(4) In the manufacture of paint removers and varnishes. Paint strippers may contain methyl chloride and benzol as well as methyl alcohol, as in the fatal case reported in the Annual Report of H.M. Chief Inspector of Factories (1957), where a man engaged in removing old paint from inside a small lift was trapped inside it. The cause of death was notified as 'narcotic poisoning by inhalation'.

(5) In the production of formaldehyde and as a general solvent in organic synthesis.

(6) In the production of synthetic indigo and other dyes (Fairhall, 1957).

(7) In the straw hat industry, as a solvent for dyes (Wood and Buller, 1904; Baskerville, 1913).

(8) As a rubber accelerator.

(9) In the denaturing of ethyl alcohol.

(10) As an anti-freeze agent.

BIOCHEMISTRY

Estimation

(1) In the atmosphere

The method of estimation of methanol vapour described by Leaf and Zatman (1952) and Elkins (1959) is based on its reaction with potassium permanganate, oxalic acid and Schiff's Reagent (basic fuchsin, sodium bisulphite and concentrated HCl). The curve of transmission on a photometer is compared with that of a known amount of methanol; the sensitivity, if 10 l of air are sampled, with the midget impinger, is about 40 p.p.m. Rogers (1945) states that the midget impinger has a collecting efficiency of approximately 92% at atmospheric concentrations of 200 p.p.m. of methanol.

(2) In blood and tissues

A similar method for blood and tissues was introduced by Hine *et al.* (1947), using steam distillation. When only small amounts of blood are available (0.5 ml) the vapour may be aerated directly into the oxidising reagent.

A micro-method, using the reaction of formaldehyde with chromotropic acid, with permanganate as the oxidising agent for the methanol, was devised by Agner and Belfrage (1947).

(3) In urin

The method used by Leaf and Zatman (1952) was based on distillation of a mixture of urine, Na_2SO_4 and sodium tungstate, followed by analysis for methanol as in their method for estimation in air.

Metabolism

The metabolism of methanol is characterised by the relative slowness of its elimination and its production of toxic metabolites. The details vary with different animal species.

(1) Absorption and excretion

Some earlier authorities such as Lewin (1912) believed that absorption of methyl alcohol is equally effective in producing its characteristic toxic symptoms whether by ingestion, inhalation or through the skin. In practice, amounts which have been found sufficient to cause death in animals by skin application (0.5 ml/kg; McCord and Cox, 1931) are not likely to resemble those found in industry (Yant *et al.*, 1931). These observers drenched the unshaven bodies of dogs for several hours, eliminating the possibility of inhalation of the vapour, without lethal effects. In non-industrial human cases however, ocular disturbances and even blindness have been reported from repeated rubbing of the skin with methyl alcohol (Wood, 1913; Campbell, 1915) and toxic symptoms were reported in a painter who spilt methyl alcohol on his feet (Ziegler, 1921), but in none of these cases was the possibility of inhalation of the vapour excluded.

In the rat, excretion is mainly by the lungs, 65% of an oral dose of 1 g/kg being eliminated as CO_2 and 14% unchanged in 48 h; only a small amount is excreted in the urine – 3% as unchanged methanol and 3% as formate (Bartlett, 1950).

In rabbits, which are relatively resistant to methanol (Lund, 1948), urinary excretion is greater – 10% unchanged – while in dogs some 15% of 2 ml/kg doses are excreted through the lungs, 10% unchanged in the urine and 20% as formate (Voltz and Dietrich, 1912).

In human beings also, after a single dose of 50 ml, both methanol and formate are excreted in the urine, the formate reaching 0.5 to 2 g/day, with a maximum 2 to 3 days after the dose, but not with a dose of 10 to 20 ml (Williams, 1959). Klauer (1938) found that in human beings suffering from methyl alcohol intoxication the amount of formic acid in the urine was greater than the normal level, which he found to range from 10 to 40 mg in 1500 ml. In some cases of fatal ingestion the level rose as high as 105 mg in 1500 ml. Other probable metabolic excretory products of methanol are choline and methyl glycuronide. With regard to the former it has been suggested (du Vigneaud *et al.*, 1950) that formaldehyde, not CO_2, is its precursor.

A slight rise in glucuronic acid in the urine of rabbits fed methanol has been observed, persisting for 2 or 3 days due to the formation of methyl glucuronide (Kamil *et al.*, 1953).

Bibliography on p. 401

The slowness of combustion of methanol compared with that of ethanol has been demonstrated by Bartlett (1950) using ^{14}C labelled methanol. In the rat the rate proved to be 25 mg/kg/h as compared with 175 mg/kg for ethanol.

According to Kendal and Ramanathan (1953) there is some excretion of formate in animals after small doses of methanol which can be suppressed by giving simultaneous doses of ethanol. It has been suggested by some observers (Røe, 1946; Bartlett, 1950) that ethanol exerts a favourable effect on the toxicity of methanol. The rationale of this favourable action is that ethanol depresses the oxidation of methanol and causes an increase in its unchanged elimination in expired air and urine (Leaf and Zatman, 1952). This inhibition of methanol oxidation by alcohol hydrogenase *in vitro*, even when the ratio of ethanol/methanol was as low as 1/16 had been observed by Zatman in 1946; he suggested therefore that it would be expected that ethanol would diminish the toxicity of methanol, permitting the excretion in an unchanged condition of a larger fraction of an ingested dose. (It should be mentioned that this favourable effect of ethanol has been strongly denied by Gilger *et al.* (1952) who state that in mice, ethanol increases the toxic effect of methanol and formaldehyde.)

(2) Distribution in tissues

The enzyme mechanism of decomposition of methanol is not completely explainable, but on the basis of evidence that it can be oxidised *in vitro* by means of catalase and hydrogen peroxide, it has been suggested that a similar mechanism may be effective *in vivo* (Agner and Belfrage, 1947; Jacobson, 1952). The view held by Kendal and Ramanathan (1952) is that formaldehyde itself in the presence of methanol is converted by alcohol dehydrogenase present in the liver to a volatile ester of formic acid, methyl formate, which subsequently undergoes slow hydrolysis.

It was found by Yant and Schrenk (1937) that regardless of the method of administration (oral, subcutaneous or inhalation) methanol is distributed very rapidly to all tissues, and that the amount found in any particular tissue is closely related to the amount of water which it contains. Dogs exposed to concentrations of 4000 and 15,000 p.p.m. for varying periods of time, and killed, either immediately, within one hour or some hours later, showed the highest concentration in the blood (1470 mg/100 g with 15,000 p.p.m.) followed by the heart (1200 mg), lungs stomach wall (1080 mg), liver (1040 mg) and kidneys (1038 mg). These values decreased with time – for example, some hours later the blood level had fallen to 335 mg/100 g. The bile and urine contained practically the same amount as the blood and stomach wall, and since the dogs could not ingest any methanol except by swallowing saliva, it was suggested that inhaled methanol can be secreted into the stomach and intestines, and that the amount in the body or in any particular tissue can be estimated from its determination in any tissue or fluid, preferably the blood.

In a later investigation by Sayers *et al.* (1944) it was found that when the product of concentration of vapour in air and time of exposure is a constant, even when the air concentration varies over a wide range, the same general order of methanol concentration in the blood would be attained. The blood concentration, estimated at weekly intervals, of dogs exposed to 10,000 p.p.m. (a total of 800 brief exposures) was between 6.5 and 14 mg/100 ml of blood – approximately the same as that found by these same observers in 1942 in dogs exposed for 8 h daily to 450–500 p.p.m.

TOXICOLOGY

The manifestations of acute intoxication following ingestion of methyl alcohol are similar to the well-known effects of over-indulgence in any alcoholic beverage, with the exception of the one outstanding feature of methyl alcohol poisoning – blindness. Many outbreaks of such acute poisoning have been recorded, some fatal, others with resulting blindness, from drinking brandy adulterated with methyl alcohol, from fruit juices diluted with it and from drinking it unadulterated. Severe poisoning has also occurred from inhalation of its vapour, but such cases are much rarer; of 275 cases recorded by Wood and Buller (1904) only 6 were due to industrial exposure, and in some others since reported the suspicion has existed that some of the methyl alcohol had been ingested. Symptoms of acute poisoning, which often arise after a latent period of hours, or even days, include dizziness, stupor, cyanosis, abdominal cramps, gastro-intestinal disturbance and failure of vision. Individual susceptibility with regard to the amount ingested varies greatly; Lehmann and Flury (1953) state that a dose of 5 to 10 mg is usually considered toxic, but many individuals can tolerate without apparent ill-effects a much higher intake than this.

Chronic poisoning, which may occur with repeated exposure to its vapour, may cause irritation of mucous membranes, headache, tinnitus, tremor, neuritis and its most characteristic feature, failure of vision leading to complete blindness.

Toxicity to animals

Animals show wide variation in sensitivity to methanol (Scott *et al.*, 1933) especially when given by inhalation (Loewy and van der Heide, 1914; McCord and Cox, 1931). Rats are the most susceptible and rabbits the most resistant. As early as 1895 Daremberg remarked that rabbits weighing more than 2000 g were often extremely resistant to intravenous injections of methyl alcohol.

Acute

In acute toxicity methyl alcohol has generally been found slightly less toxic than ethanol (Macht, 1920), but its later effects are much more harmful.

(a) Lethal dose. – (i) By stomach tube. – For rabbits Munch and Schwartze (1925) found the lethal dose to be 18 ml/kg as compared with 12.5 ml/kg for ethyl alcohol; for mice, Weese (1928) gave the MLD as 10.5–12.0 mg as compared with 5.5–7.0 mg for ethyl alcohol. Doses too small to cause narcosis appeared to cause no injury dangerous to life, but a reversible infiltration of liver and kidney parenchyma. – *(ii) By intravenous injection.* – For cats, the MLD is given by Macht (1920) as 5.9 ml/kg, as compared with 5.0 for ethyl alcohol. – *(iii) By intraperitoneal injection.* – According to Gilger *et al.* (1952) 10.0 g/kg was usually lethal 4 days after the injection. – *(iv) By inhalation.* – The highest value is that given for mice (139,000 p.p.m., Bachem, 1927) and the lowest for monkeys (1000 p.p.m. after a few 18-h exposures; McCord, 1931).

For cats, Lehmann and Flury gave a level of 65,700 p.p.m.; when the narcotic dose reached a point where all reflexes were lost all the animals died.

Loewy and van der Heide (1914), estimating the amount of vapour inhaled by the amount absorbed by the tissues of the animals (the whole body being subjected to distillation) found that saturation took place in 2 h with levels of 0.5%. With an intake of 8.71–12.78 g/kg the animals died. They found that the process of absorption and saturation was much slower in the dog than the rat.

(b) Narcotic dose. – By inhalation, methyl alcohol appears also to be less narcotic than ethyl alcohol. Weese (1928) expressed the concentrations used by him in terms of the amount of alcohol in 5 l of air. He found the narcotic concentration for mice between 0.4 and 0.6 ml and the time of onset of narcosis between 8 and 18 h. The corresponding dose for ethyl alcohol was 0.2–0.6 ml/l.

For mice also Lehman and Flury (1943) gave the narcotic dose as 42,000 p.p.m. after 7 h; for rats 51,000 p.p.m. caused deep narcosis after 2½ h; for cats 129,000 p.p.m. after 6 h. They remark that concentrations which cause only slight narcosis after a single inhalation can be followed by fatal after-effects.

SYMPTOMS OF INTOXICATION

Irritation of mucous membranes, with concentrations from 7500 to 69,000 p.p.m. (Flury and Wirth, 1934); increased rate of respiration (Gradinesco, 1934); depression and drowsiness followed by excitation, with inco-ordination and paralysis of the hind legs (Mashbitz *et al.*, 1936); tremor, stupor, convulsions, coma and death from respiratory paralysis (Flury and Wirth, 1934). Failure of sight and hearing (Holden, 1899) and peripheral neuritis (McCord, 1931) have also been observed.

(1) The gastric mucosa

Congestion and small haemorrhages, observed by Tyson and Schoenberg (1914), were believed by them to be characteristic of poisoning by inhalation of methyl alcohol.

(2) The eyes

Many of the earlier observers, including Holden (1899) and Birch-Hirsch-feld (1901) recorded blindness in animals poisoned by methyl alcohol, usually by oral or subcutaneous administration, but some also by inhalation. McCord (1931) found that in small animals dilatation of the pupil preceded the development of a milky-white cornea, and monkeys occasionally became blind, sometimes with recovery but sometimes with recurrence.

The mechanism of blindness due to methyl alcohol is fully discussed under Effects upon the Eyes in Human Beings (see p. 321).

(3) The blood

The peripheral blood picture has been stated to show evidence of a stimulative effect of methyl alcohol on the blood-forming organs. Tyson and Schoenberg (1915) noted in the blood of animals inhaling methyl alcohol an increase in erythrocytes, haemoglobin and polymorphonuclear leucocytes. Scott *et al.* (1933) observed hyperplasia of the lymph nodes.

CHANGES IN THE ORGANISM

(1) The heart

Oedema, granular degeneration and in some instances necrosis of muscle fibres were noted by Scott *et al.* (1933) and also by Flury and Wirth (1934), while Eisenberg (1917) reported fatty degeneration of the heart muscle.

(2) The liver

Changes in the liver are essentially those of parenchymatous degeneration, sometimes developing into focal necrosis (Scott *et al.*, 1933), also fatty infiltration (Poincaré, 1878; Weese, 1928; Tyson and Schoenberg, 1914).

(3) The kidneys

Congestion and parenchymatous degeneration have been recorded by the above observers, and in mice fatty infiltration (Weese; Eisenberg; Lehmann and Flury).

(4) The spleen

A dark blue colour of the spleen was noted by Tyson and Schoenberg (1914).

(5) Lungs

Various inflammatory lesions have been noted, according to the severity of exposure. With mild poisoning Scott *et al.* (1933) reported oedema, congestion and desquamation of alveolar epithelium; in fatal cases terminal pneumonic consolidation. Patchy pneumonia in the lungs of rabbits (Eisenberg, 1917) and of mice (Weese, 1928) and petechial haemorrhages in dogs (Tyson and Schoenberg, 1914) and slight emphysema (Flury and Wirth, 1934) have also been observed.

Bibliography on p. 401

(6) The nervous system

Capillary congestion, oedema and patchy degeneration of the neurons, especially of the spinal cord, and some involvement of the peripheral nerves were noted by Scott *et al.* (1933). Earlier investigators (Holden, 1899, and Ruhle, 1912) had found more severe congestive lesions, while Tyson and Schoenberg (1914) noted marked congestion of the meninges of dogs.

Toxicity to human beings

(A) Non-industrial

There have been many reports of outbreaks of poisoning from methyl alcohol, causing blindness or death. One of such was the report by Monier Williams (1929) in the Ruhr in 1920 when 15 people died and 3 were totally blinded from drinking brandy adulterated with methyl alcohol; another, with similar effects, in Japan, in 42 cases, from drinking fruit juices diluted with methyl alcohol (Kaplan and Levreault, 1945) and from drinking methyl alcohol itself, with 24 deaths (Voegtlin and Watts, 1943), and another record, from the same cause, of 390 deaths and 90 cases of total and 85 of partial blindness by Baskerville in America (1913).

(B) Industrial

Following the publication of the above reports, and many others, of the highly toxic nature of methyl alcohol when taken internally, it is not surprising that the danger of its use as a solvent should have been somewhat exaggerated. It is true that cases of poisoning, accompanied by blindness, have occurred from exposure to its vapour, but the hazard is more potential than actual, especially if reasonable care is taken to keep the vapour concentrations in the working atmosphere at a level of approximately the Maximum Allowable Concentration of 200 p.pm., and to prevent workers from drinking either the methyl alcohol itself or industrial materials containing it. Some of the recorded cases have in fact carried the more or less well founded suspicion that ingestion as well as inhalation had played some part in the development of symptoms of poisoning (Gerbis, 1931; Wood and Buller, 1904). Wood and Buller remarked that "taking a drink from the supply of alcohol kept for dissolving gums in making varnishes is a very common habit among varnishers". On the other hand, surveys of workers exposed repeatedly to the vapour of methyl alcohol have sometimes revealed no harmful effects. One such survey by Yant *et al.* (1931) of men employed in the manufacture of methyl alcohol and drivers of trucks using it as an antifreeze agent revealed no harmful effects. Bertarelli (1934) has also called attention to the fact that there have been many cases of prolonged exposure to methyl alcohol without development of any symptoms.

(1) Acute

Cases of acute poisoning are especially rare from inhalation only, but have been known to occur from ingestion of various solutions containing it. Two such cases have recently been described by Stinebaugh (1960), both from drinking a paint thinner, in one case an unknown quantity, in the other 2 ounces. Both suffered from vomiting, epigastric pain, irrational behaviour, failure of vision and semi-coma. Both recovered from the general symptoms under suitable treatment, but neither recovered full vision; in one case in fact complete blindness supervened.

Other acute symptoms are related to the strongly irritant property of methyl alcohol for mucous membranes, causing conjunctivitis and bronchopneumonia. The conjunctivitis has been known to be so severe as to destroy the cornea (Grunow, 1912) and the bronchopneumonia, in a case quoted by Goldtdammer in 1878 was actually fatal.

General systemic intoxication, shown by lassitude, headache, giddiness, nausea, vomiting, pain in the gastric and lumbar region, coldness and muscle weakness, may precede or accompany the most severe toxic manifestation – blindness. Complete loss of vision, however, exhibits as a rule no premonitory symptoms but occurs suddenly in both eyes.

Koelsch (1921) stated that all these symptoms were frequent during World War I when alcohol was used widely in paints, lacquers and polishes, especially when these were handled in closed rooms in warm weather. He quotes several cases of temporary blindness and others of bilateral optic atrophy occurring in such conditions, and refers to one described by Philippi in 1906 in a painter who sprayed methyl alcohol on his feet and then continued to work for a few hours in the room; he became blind.

TREATMENT

Three methods of treatment have been tried, with varying degrees of success.

(α) Administration of alkalies. – This method is of course based on the evidence that methyl alcohol produces formic acid, formaldehyde and possibly other unidentified acids, with formation of acidosis. It was first suggested by Harrop and Benedict (1920), and by Chew *et al.* (1946) and also Røe noted that it alleviated the symptoms and increased the survival rate. Bennet *et al.* (1953) treated a series of 323 cases due to ingestion of adulterated contraband whiskey and were convinced of the efficacy of this treatment, consisting of large amounts of sodium bicarbonate – up to 150–200 g – in the proportion of 50 g in 1000 ml of 5% glucose in water, given intravenously. They stated that return of acidosis was not unlikely following treatment by alkalisation alone, and glucose has been suggested as a useful adjunct to alkalisation on the basis of the possible role of ketosis (Keeney and Mellinkoff, 1951). Nevertheless, according to Stinebaugh (1960) correction of the acidosis does not always prevent a fatal issue either in animals (Potts, 1955) or human beings.

Bibliography on p. 401

(β) Administration of ethyl alcohol. – The effect of ethyl alcohol on the metabolic behaviour of methyl alcohol, by inhibiting its enzymatic oxidation into toxic metabolites has already been discussed (see p. 313). It is on this basis that ethanol treatment had been advocated (Stinebaugh, 1960; Røe, 1946), but there is no universal agreement as to its efficacy in actual cases of methanol intoxication and it is not regarded as a justifiable substitute for alkalisation.

(γ) Peritoneal dialysis. – It was shown by Blakemore and Hine (1947) that methyl alcohol could be removed by peritoneal dialysis in animals, and Stinebaugh (1960) used this evidence as a basis for this treatment, combined with alkalisation. The basic solution consists of glucose and sodium bicarbonate in water and isotonic saline and is administered through a perforated polythene tube introduced into the peritoneal cavity by an abdominal trocar. The fluid is drained after two hours and the process repeated. In one case the first specimen of dialysis fluid contained 130 mg/100 of alcohol and dialysis was continued for 18 h, at the end of which time the fluid contained none. In a second case dialysis was only begun 10 h after admission to hospital and a specimen taken 12 h later was negative. Both 'these cases recovered (without return of vision) but in a third case, where intoxication was due to ordinary alcoholic intake and whose dialysis specimen after two hours contained 200 mg/100 of alcohol, death took place after development of tetanic spasms. Stinebaugh suggests that the best method of treatment is a combination of all three measures.

(2) Chronic

Cases of industrial poisoning from repeated exposure to the vapour of methyl alcohol have generally been manifested by conjunctivitis, headache, giddiness, insomnia, gastro-intestinal disturbance and failure of vision.

Some of these symptoms, notably those of a narcotic nature, leading in some cases to coma, were described by Roche *et al.* (1957) in an account of a collective disturbance of health in a factory manufacturing electrical car accessories, but the presence of methyl alcohol in the compound used, which consisted chiefly of trichloroethylene, was never definitely proved. Suspicion of methyl alcohol as a contributory cause of the symptoms arose partly from the fact that the severe manifestations showed a latent period after cessation of work and that an investigation of the effects on guinea pigs exposed to a mixture of methyl alcohol and trichloroethylene also showed a longer latent period before the onset of fatal coma than those exposed to trichloroethylene alone.

It appears probable that, considering the vague character of the symptoms and the very large number of women affected, some of the manifestations may have been of emotional origin; others were quite characteristic of exposure to trichloroethylene.

Another case of industrial chronic poisoning, in which an additional factor may have been absorption through the skin, is that described by Burk in 1957.

This was a man aged 27 who had worked for 4 years in the methanol department of a chemical-pharmaceutical factory where nicotinic acid was being crystallised, the solvent being pure methyl alcohol. For two years he had complained of disturbance of vision, which was then diagnosed as slight astigmatism and corrected by glasses. At the same time he complained of weakness and numbness of his hands and arms. While cleaning a tank in which nicotinic acid and methanol had been heated, and wearing a gas mask, he thought that the methanol fume was penetrating the filter, which had become damp, and changed it for a filter intended for ammonia. During the 5-h duration of his task he felt giddy at times, but at the end had no symptoms. The next morning he vomited, but continued working, then suddenly developed spots before the eyes and dimness of vision. He also complained of loss of appetite and a sweetish taste. Blood and urine examination at that time revealed nothing abnormal; ophthalmic examination showed papilloedema of both eyes. After 5 weeks, under treatment by eye drops, ointments, vitamin B, etc., his visual acuity became normal, but after a further 5 weeks his vision became irregular. At this time his urine contained formic acid, but later the test was negative. (No quantitative estimation was made.) Earlier investigators (e.g. Klauer, 1938) have given the normal level as ranging between 14 and 100 mg/1500 ml.

Burk states that the amount of methyl alcohol inhaled must have been small, but that the workman had been in the habit of cleaning his hands with methyl alcohol.

In 1913 Baskerville reported 64 cases in America from the industrial use of either concentrated or 50% methyl alcohol in painters, lacquerers, coopers and chimney sweeps who cleaned the chimneys with methyl alcohol. Koelsch (1921) also mentions the case known to him of a doctor engaged in research on disinfection with methyl alcohol vapour who became completely blind. Hansohn (1944) quoted by Burk (1957) described the eventual development of bilateral optic atrophy in a man who had complained only of recurrent conjunctivitis during his 1½ years of war work involving inhalation of methyl alcohol vapour. He strongly denied ingestion of alcohol.

SYMPTOMS OF INTOXICATION

(1) Mechanism of toxic effect on the eyes

Observations on the actual toxic process of methyl alcohol on the ocular tissues have been almost exclusively discussed with regard to ingestion, but cases of ocular injury having occurred following absorption through the skin and inhalation, gradually methyl alcohol came to be regarded as a specific toxin for the retina and the optic nerve. One intensive investigation is that of Fink (1943). Like Wood and Buller (1904) and Lehmann and Flury (1943), Fink emphasised the fact that impurities in the methyl alcohol are not an influencing factor, and

Bibliography on p. 401

that the basic cause of the toxic action is the inability of the body to oxidise methyl alcohol to CO_2 and water, as is the case with ethyl alcohol. He brought forward evidence that formic acid is formed and suggested the possibility of formation of formaldehyde also, as a contributory factor in injury of the eye tissues. This view is also held by Kaplan and Levreault (1945), Bogen (1946), and Røe (1948), but not by Potts and Johnson (1952) who believe that the role of acidosis is questionable and that the essential toxic agent is formaldehyde.

According to Fink, the tissues predominantly affected (the optic nerve and the retina) are not equally affected, but both appear to show injury in patches, with intermediate areas of less affected cells. Oedema of nerve tissue and supporting tissue is the result of both an irritative reaction of the tissue to the toxic substance and also of a degenerative process which is proportional to the intensity of the toxic element and the susceptibility of the individual. Both the retina and the optic nerve are sensitive to metabolic disturbance and this disturbance leads to degenerative changes, which may take place simultaneously in the two tissues. In the retina the toxic effect is exerted first on the ganglion cells, then the inner nuclear layer degenerates, later the outer nuclear layer, and finally the rod-and-cone layer. In the optic nerve, degenerative changes are accompanied by varying degrees of oedema.

It has also been stated (Kendal and Ramanathan, 1952) that methyl formate can be formed from formaldehyde and methanol, and that this substance, having a preferential fat solubility, might explain the localised effects of methanol. It has also been shown, however, that formaldehyde is 25 to 75 times more active than formate in inhibiting oxygen uptake and Co_2 production, and 1000 to 30,000 times more active than methanol itself (Leaf and Zatman, 1952; Røe, 1948).

The role of skin absorption in the production of methyl alcohol poisoning has already been mentioned (as in the case of Burk, 1957), and cases of severe eye injury in which it is said to have played a predominant part are quoted by Koelsch (1921) and Eulner (1954). In Eulner's case, a woman who had applied to her body a preparation consisting almost entirely of pure methyl alcohol, the effects on the eye were attributed not only to skin absorption but also partly to inhalation.

(2) Predisposition

(a) *Individual susceptibility*. – Many authorities believe that individual susceptibility plays a considerable part in the variation of toxic symptoms in similar conditions, not only in poisoning by ingestion but also in industrial poisoning. In some cases one relatively slight exposure has been said to have caused blindness, while others have remained unaffected until after repeated exposure in unfavourable conditions. Koelsch (1921), who had found no specific ill-effects in the majority of workers employed in the production of wood alcohol, described the case of a woman using a shoe cement in which methyl alcohol appears to have been the chief, but not the only constituent. She was weak and anaemic, and complained of gradual failure of vision, leading eventually to blindness, as well as headache, throat irritation and burning of the eyes. No other workers in the same room suffered from any of these symptoms except slight irritation of mucous membranes.

(b) Sensitisation. – In the case described by Burk (1957) the occurrence of slight symptoms of chronic intoxication before the development of disturbance of vision, led him to conclude that sensitisation had taken place before the crucial exposure, and to emphasise that although relatively few cases of industrial poisoning from methyl alcohol had been recorded, it is not safe to conclude that inhalation of low concentrations can do no harm.

(c) Pre-existing nervous disorder. – Symptoms indicative of chronic industrial poisoning by methyl alcohol – giddiness, headache, insomnia, gastro-intestinal disturbance, conjunctivitis and failure of vision – were observed by Schwarzmann (1934) in a man working in a straw hat factory where the synthetic fibres were hardened by formaldehyde containing 10–12% of methyl alcohol. On returning to work after a year's absence the man showed paralysis of the facial and ocular muscles. He was not definitely diagnosed as suffering from methyl alcohol poisoning but possibly as a case of multiple sclerosis, but it was suggested that the nervous system disorder rendered him more susceptible to methyl alcohol poisoning.

A similar predisposing factor, in the form of pre-existing central nervous disease, was present in a case described by Humperdinck in 1941. This man had been employed 4 years in shovelling nitro-cellulose material containing 35–40% of methyl alcohol, in conditions of poor ventilation and lighting. In addition to failure of vision this man had an enlarged liver.

Bibliography on p. 401

38. Ethanol

Synonyms: ethyl alcohol, grain alcohol, spirit of wine, Cologne spirit

Structural formula:
$$CH_3-CH_2$$
$$|$$
$$OH$$

Molecular formula: C_2H_5OH

Molecular weight: 46.070

Properties: a colourless, mobile hygroscopic liquid with a pleasant odour. Burns with an almost non-luminous flame. Completely miscible with water and ether. Solvent for many resins and oils, and to some extent for phosphorus and sulphur. Pure anhydrous ethyl alcohol (absolute alcohol) also dissolves ethyl cellulose, colophony, sandarac, and with the addition of 20–30% of benzene, benzyl cellulose, ester gum and cumarone.

    boiling point: 78.375 °C
    melting point: —116 °C
    vapour pressure: 44 mm Hg at 20 °C
    vapour density (air = 1): 1.59
    specific gravity (liquid density): 0.7894
    flash point: 57 °F
    conversion factors: 1 p.p.m. = 1.88 mg/m³ at 25 °C
                       1 mg/l = 532 p.p.m.
    solubility: miscible in all proportions with water and most organic solvents.
    maximum allowable concentration: 1000 p.p.m.

ECONOMY, SOURCES AND USES

Production

(1) Natural, from molasses, grain (corn, malt, wheat, rye, barley, rice and bran), pineapple juice, whey, cellulose pulp and potatoes, separated by distillation.
(2) Synthetic, by hydrolysis of ethyl sulphuric acid and diethyl sulphate, also from cracked petroleum gases (Fairhall, 1957).

[324]

Industrial uses

Mellan (1939) listed 300 uses of ethyl alcohol in industry. Among the most important are:

(1) In the synthetic rubber industry.

(2) In the chemical industry – production of acetaldehyde, acetic acid, ethyl acetate, ethers, tannin, chloral and pharmaceutical products.

(3) In the paint and lacquer industry.

(4) As an anti-freeze agent.

(5) In the plastic and synthetic resin industry.

(6) In the explosives industry.

BIOCHEMISTRY

Estimation

(1) In the atmosphere

Many of the earlier methods employed for the determination of ethyl alcohol in air were based on the reaction devised by Nicloux in 1896, in which acetic acid formed by oxidation with potassium dichromate was distilled and titrated with 0.05 *N*-alkali, using phenolphthalein as the indicator. This was the method used by Gettler and Tiber (1927).

Another method widely used is that of Haggard and Greenberg (1934), in which a sample of air containing ethyl alcohol is passed into heated iodine pentoxide; the alcohol is decomposed with the liberation of iodine and hydriodic acid, which are collected by absorption. The iodine is measured by titration with sodium sulphite and the hydriodic acid reacted with iodate to form additional iodine.

In the presence of other alcohols, ethyl alcohol has been determined by oxidation of the alcohols to fatty acids, subsequently determined by the method of Werkman and Osburn (1930).

(2) In blood and tissues

In the method used by McNally and Coleman (1944) the alcohol is oxidised by dichromate and the excess dichromate titrated with sodium thiosulphate in the presence of potassium iodide. Henry *et al.* (1948) oxidised the alcohol to acetaldehyde and estimated its amount colorimetrically, using *p*-hydroxydiphenyl.

For estimation in the blood Kaye and Haag (1954) described a modification of the original Nicloux reaction using potassium dichromate and Scott-Wilson reagent (mercuric cyanide, sodium hydroxide and silver nitrate).

A more recent method, by means of the enzyme diaphorase, together with anti-diuretic hormone and diphosphopyridine nucleotide, dissolved in a buffer

Bibliography on p. 401

solution of borate, has been described by Machata (1961) using dichlorphenolindo-
phenol as the colorimetric agent. He claims that this method, a modification of
that of Widmark (1932) is more rapid than this, and can be carried out with a
simple filter photometer with an electric lamp as the light source, but that its
accuracy is not so close as to allow it to supersede the ADH method described by
him in 1958.

Metabolism

(1) Absorption and excretion

The major part of ingested ethyl alcohol is converted to CO_2. Bartlett and
Barnet (1949), using ^{14}C-labelled alcohol, found that rats receiving 1 g/kg by
mouth exhaled 75% as CO_2 in 5 h and 90% in 10 h. A small proportion is not so
metabolised; 2% is eliminated unchanged in the urine and expired air, and
0.5–2%, increasing with the increasing dose, is conjugated with glucuronic acid
and excreted in the urine as ethyl glucuronide (Kamil *et al.*, 1953).

It is generally agreed that the metabolic pathway of ethyl alcohol is that of an
initial oxidation to acetaldehyde, a conversion of this to acetyl co-enzyme A and
acetic acid and a final combustion in the kidney and liver to CO_2 and water.
Lung tissue can also convert ethanol to CO_2 (Masoro *et al.*, 1953). It has been
generally assumed that only small amounts of ethanol are metabolised outside the
liver, but with low concentrations in the blood reaching the liver it is believed
(Larsen, 1959) that there is at least some extrahepatic metabolism. This view
was confirmed by Larsen *et al.* (1961), they found the amount so eliminated by the
liver to be about 20% of the total.

The enzyme which carries out the oxidation of the alcohol to acetaldehyde
is alcohol dehydrogenase (Theorell and Bonnischen, 1951) located in the liver
and kidney, and most observers consider that most of this oxidation takes place
in the liver in the presence of co-zymase A (Kutvak-Mann, 1938; Westerfeld,
1961). This enzyme contains zinc, which is one of the factors in binding DPN
with the enzyme.

It has been suggested, on the basis of *in vitro* experiments (Lieber and Schmid
1961) that ethanol may have a direct effect on liver cells, especially with regard
to the synthesis of fatty acids. Administration of ethanol produces a decrease in
DPN and an increase in DPNH concentration in the liver (Smith and Newman
1959) and Lieber and Schmid suggest that the excess DPNH results in a shift in
the relative disposition of acetyl co-enzyme A, so that more acetate is incorporated into fatty acids. The view has also been expressed (Klatskin, 1961) that alcoholic cirrhosis of the liver may be associated with a relative deficiency (increased requirement) of choline created by alcohol, and that this is related to acceleration of fat turnover in the liver followed by fatty infiltration and fibrosis
Di Luzio (1961) points out that the etiology of acute ethanol-induced fatty liver

differs from that induced by chronic small amounts in that the latter is repon-
sive to choline and the former is not. It is concluded therefore by Klatskin that
alcohol appears to increase hepatic fat in three ways: (1) by increasing mobili-
sation of fat from its depots; (2) by increasing fat synthesis in the liver itself; (3) by
inducing a relative choline deficiency.

Clearance of ethanol from the blood. – According to Williams (1959) the type of
clearance of ethanol from the blood differs from that of other alcohols. It appears
to depend on the amount of dosage. If a low dosage is used, the rate of disappearance is proportional to the amount present; with larger doses the rate of oxidation varies from hour to hour in the same animal (Marshall and Fritz, 1953).

(2) Distribution in tissues

(a) Effect on serum cholesterol. – There has been considerable controversy as
to whether consumption of ethanol increases the amount of serum cholesterol and
therefore has any effect in increasing the tendency to atherosclerosis. In animals,
some observers, such as Eberhardt (1936) have postulated such an increase
following high doses of alcohol for a few days; other more recent observers, such
as Feller and Huff (1955) have denied it. It appears that the dog is particularly
sensitive in this respect, since both earlier and later authorities (Ducheschi, 1915
and Grande and Amatuzio, 1960) have found that ethanol has produced a marked
increase of serum cholesterol in the dog when given in a dosage of 1.65 g/kg per
day. In man also Grande and Amatuzio have found a small but significant increase of serum cholesterol following ingestion of large amounts of alcohol (9 oz.
of 100-proof whiskey per day) and this appears to be related to the intrinsic cholesterol level of the individual, the increase being much more marked in essential
hyperlipaemic subjects.

(b) Effect on adrenalin secretion. – According to Abelin et al. (1955) ingestion
of ethyl alcohol is followed during the first hour by a 12-times increase in the urine
of adrenalin and a 3- to 4-times increase in noradrenalin. These levels decrease
slowly during the next 3 to 4 h, in some cases reaching even below the normal
level. The characteristic stimulation of the sympathetic nervous system by alcohol
is believed to be responsible for this action on adrenalin, since this stimulation is
closely related to the metabolism of catecholamines. It has also been suggested
that the 'flushing' after intake of alcohol might be due to a release of histamine or
serotonin in the body, and that increased secretion from the adrenal medulla
occurs after only moderate amounts of ethanol (up to 1 g/kg). An investigation
by Perman (1961) has led him to conclude that it is unlikely that flushing produced by ethanol is associated with histamine or serotonin but he agrees with
Abeling et al. (1955) that there is a moderate short-lasting effect on the adrenal
medullary secretion.

Bibliography on p. 401

TOXICOLOGY

Ethyl alcohol, whether ingested or inhaled, exerts its principal action on the brain, first inhibiting its higher functions and then acting as an anaesthetic with a higher potential toxicity than methyl alcohol. The amount ingested which can cause death from respiratory depression has been stated to be approximately one quart of whiskey within a short interval (Haag *et al.*, 1951).

It presents a much less chronic toxicity than methyl alcohol, since it is not cumulative and its metabolic products do not, so far as is known, attack directly the ocular nerve and tissues, though there have been reports of its effect on visual acuity, field of vision, eye coordination and distance judgment.

An effect on the liver, such as that known to arise from repeated excessive ingestion, is not, according to most authorities, caused by repeated inhalation, though Flury and Zernik (1931) quote Kochmann (1923) as stating that this may occur in certain conditions. Minor effects of the vapour are those caused by irritation of the mucous membranes of the eye and respiratory tract. In industry toxic effects from inhalation of the vapour have rarely been recorded; its chief danger appears to be that of ingestion by the workers.

Toxicity to animals

(1) Acute

(a) Lethal dose. – *(i) By ingestion,* the lethal dose of ethyl alcohol, compared with that of other alcohols has been given varying figures by different observers. Among the earliest of these was Baer (1898) who, using rabbits, with gastric administration, and taking the value of ethyl alcohol as 1, judged methyl alcohol as more toxic (0.8) and propyl, butyl and amyl alcohol considerably less toxic. Later authorities have found methyl alcohol less acutely toxic (Lehmann and Newman, 1937). – *(ii) By intraperitoneal injection.* Barlow (1936) found the MLD to range from 3.5 to 6 g/kg, but the former killed only 10% and the latter 65% of the animals. He found little difference between grain and synthetic alcohol. – *(iii) By intravenous injection.* In Barlow's experiments 6 g/kg caused early or acute death in 58% of the animals (rabbits) while Lehmann and Newman gave the MLD as 9.4 g/kg as compared with 15.9 for methyl alcohol – a ratio of 1.0/0.59. – *(iv) By inhalation.* For rats (which are more susceptible than guinea pigs) 12,700 p.p.m. after 21 h 45 min; guinea pigs 21,900 p.p.m. after 9 h (Loewy and van der Heide, 1918). For mice, 29,300 after 7 h (Lehmann and Flury, 1943).

(b) Narcotic dose. – For rats, 19,260 p.p.m. after 2 h; guinea pigs 13,300 after 24 h (Loewy and van der Heide); mice, 23,940 after 24 h (Lehmann and Flury) and 16,700 over several days (Weese, 1928).

SYMPTOMS OF INTOXICATION

(i) By ingestion, ataxia, lack of response to stimuli, and absence of corneal reflex were observed (Newman and Card, 1937). Profound sleep, from which they were aroused with difficulty was observed by MacNider (1933) in dogs to which 10–15 ml/kg of a 40% solution were administered by stomach tube. Newman and Card found that tolerance was acquired by habituation and lost after a period of abstinence.

(ii) By inhalation, ataxia, incoordination and drowsiness were observed in animals which survived narcosis.

CHANGES IN THE ORGANISM

Effect on the liver

(i) By ingestion MacNider (1933) found that dogs intoxicated for 12 hours showed liver injury consisting essentially of oedema of the cells at the periphery of the lobules and an increase in lipid material. These changes had regressed at the end of three days. With intoxication for 24 h these changes were more marked, but at the end of 12 days recuperation had occurred leaving no histological evidence of injury.

(ii) By inhalation reversible fatty infiltration was observed by Weese (1928) following repeated exposure to high concentrations, while cirrhosis of the liver was commonly observed by Mertens (1896) in rabbits exposed to air saturated with the vapour for periods ranging from 25 to 365 days.

Toxicity to human beings

(A) Non-industrial

The effects of excessive ingestion of alcohol by human beings are too well known to need full description here.

In acute uncomplicated poisoning by ethyl alcohol death usually follows complete coma occurring some hours after the last ingestion. The amount of alcohol in the blood which precipitates this condition and its relation to the time of survival have been estimated by Jetter (1943), Haag *et al.* (1951) and Kaye and Haag (1957). In the 94 cases examined by Kaye and Haag the terminal blood alcohol concentrations varied from 180 to 600 mg per 100 ml of blood, and inversely with the time of survival. With levels of 500 mg per 100 ml and above, survival is practically impossible without effective therapy, though death rarely occurs at the peak of blood concentration but can follow hours later when the concentration has fallen considerably. This is explained by the severe and probably irreversible injury to the central nervous system caused by the concentration.

The effects of inhalation of ethyl alcohol are less well known. According to Loewy and van der Heide (1918) the degree of intoxication varies in those who are accustomed to drinking alcohol and those who are not, the latter being more susceptible.

In those unaccustomed to alcohol, headache, followed by slight stupor was produced by exposure for 33 min to 1380 p.p.m., while increasing headache in those accustomed to alcohol only appeared after 20 min exposure to 5000 p.p.m. and fatigue and a desire to sleep after exposure for 110 min to 7000 p.p.m.

Absorption by the skin has rarely been found to produce intoxication, but one case has been recorded (James, 1931) in which a boy aged eight, after application of towels wrung out in surgical spirit to both legs, showed symptoms of acute alcohol poisoning and alcohol was present in the vomit and the urine.

(1) Effect of chronic ingestion on the eyes

The amblyopia which is a not uncommon feature of methyl alcohol poisoning is so rare a result of ethyl alcohol ingestion that it has practically never been attributed to the toxic effect of ethyl alcohol alone. In a case reported by Quatermass in 1958, a man who had been a heavy drinker, the fact that his visual acuity became normal after 6 weeks of intensive vitamin therapy led to the conclusion that, as stated by Duke Elder in 1940, "the condition is always associated with a long history of alcoholism and frequently with peripheral neuritis", so that the picture in this case, though indirectly due to ethyl alcoholism, appears to have been directly due to avitaminosis. Other ocular functions – visual acuity, field of vision, depth perception, eye coordination and distance judgment – have, however, been observed in varying degree in persons who have imbibed a basic dose of 1 ounce of whiskey per 30 lbs body weight (Newman and Fletcher, 1941; Goldberg, 1943). Newman and Fletcher found, for example, that 70% of the subjects examined showed a decrease of 5% in visual acuity and 22% a decrease of 20% or more, the change increasing with the alcohol concentration.

Binocular vision has also been stated to be impaired by alcohol (Giardini, 1952; Brecher *et al.*, 1955).

(2) Effect on muscular coordination

The 'staggering' of persons who have drunk a great deal of alcohol is well known, but lesser degrees of coordination of voluntary muscles have been observed by many investigators, who have always found a lowering of efficiency and a lengthened reaction time (Harger and Julpien, 1956) It has been found that a blood alcohol concentration of 0.10 to 0.20% causes an increase of 10 to 30% in reaction time.

(B) Industrial

It is apparent that the main hazard from the industrial use of ethyl alcohol is the possibility that workers may be tempted to drink it, with the result that not only may they become habituated to it and therefore more susceptible to accidents

(Joss, 1947), but also that its constant ingestion may increase their susceptibility to other poisons. Koelsch (1947) refers to its industrial importance as being merely that of an adjuvant to the toxicity of other substances – a combined toxic action caused either by increasing the actual toxicity of these substances or by reducing their excretion. This aspect has also been stressed by earlier observers such as Kober and Hanson (1918).

Nevertheless it has long been accepted that inhalation of the vapour of ethyl alcohol can have effects similar to those of ingestion of the liquid. As far back as 1713 Ramazzini referred to the fact that vintners often "suffer all the drawbacks of drunkenness merely from close application to their work". He even describes an account given by Zacut, a Portuguese, in 1634, of a courtier who happened to go into the wine cellar *"ut in terram sideratus deciderit et intra hores expirarit"*.

More chronic exposure to the fumes of ethyl alcohol in industrial use may result in irritation of mucous membranes, headache, inebriation, lack of concentration and somnolence, while Brezina (1929) states that cardiac disorders have been caused by heated alcohol vapour in a factory producing liquor, and attacks of eczema during the use of denatured alcohol in the manufacture of electric insulators. He gives no specific details of the nature or concentration of the exposure.

Lanze and Goldberg (1959) however, as well as many earlier observers, state that serious and lasting consequences have occurred very rarely.

Bibliography on p. 401

39. Propanols

39a. Propanol-1

Synonym: n-propyl alcohol

Structural formula: $\overset{\displaystyle CH_3—CH_2—CH_2}{\underset{\displaystyle OH}{\vert}}$

Molecular formula: C_3H_8O

Molecular weight: 60.097

Properties: a colourless liquid with an odour resembling that of ethyl alcohol. It is a solvent for gums, resins and some cellulose ethers.

boiling point: 97 °C

melting point: —126.1 °C

vapour pressure: 20.8 mm Hg at 25 °C

vapour density (air = 1): 2.08

specific gravity (liquid density): 0.804

flash point: 59 °F

conversion factors: 1 p.p.m. = 2.45 mg/m³ at 25 °C

1 mg/l   = 408 p.p.m.

solubility: miscible in all proportions with water, alcohol and ether.

maximum allowable concentration: not established; Elkins (1959) suggestes 300 p.p.m.

ECONOMY, SOURCES AND USES

Production

In the manufacture of methanol it is a constituent of fusel oil, and is a byproduct in the propane-butane oxidation process (Mellan, 1950).

Industrial uses

(1) In the lacquer industry to some extent.

(2) In the production of cosmetics.

(3) As a surgical antiseptic (Christiansen, 1918).

BIOCHEMISTRY

Metabolism

Propanol-1 is absorbed from the gastro-intestinal tract, the lungs and, according to Christiansen (1918), also from the skin. In animals it is readily oxidised in the body, first to propionic acid and then to CO_2 and water (Orskov, 1950), with possibly some formation of small amounts of lactic acid. Its glucuronic conjugation is very small – about 1% of a dose of 1 g/kg is excreted in the urine (Kamil *et al.*, 1953). Its concentration in the blood is lower than that of ethyl alcohol and it disappears from the blood at a constant rate (Berggren, 1938), and when equilibrium is reached its distribution throughout the body is quite uniform (von Oettingen, 1943). The enzyme responsible for its oxidation is alcohol dehydrogenase, at a rate only slightly less than that of ethyl alcohol (Lutwak-Mann, 1938).

TOXICOLOGY

The principal action of propanol-1 is that of a mild narcotic, somewhat stronger than ethyl alcohol, otherwise with somewhat similar toxic properties.

In animals, it has been stated to cause, with fatal subcutaneous dosage, hyperaemia of the lungs (Starrek, 1938), and repeated exposure to inhalation has been found to cause moderate fatty infiltration of liver, kidney and heart (Weese, 1928), and by daily oral administration to growing chicks to cause impairment of growth (Elhardt, 1931), and in other animals gastro-intestinal irritation (Rost and Braun, 1926). In man, ingestion of 20 ml diluted with water causes only a feeling of warmth and slight lowering of the blood pressure (Durwald and Degen, 1956), but one fatal case from a larger amount has been described.

No injuries have been reported from its industrial use.

Toxicity to animals

(1) Acute

   (a) Lethal dose. – *(i) By oral administration* to rabbits 3.5 ml/kg compared with 12.5 for ethyl and 10 for isopropyl alcohol (Munch and Schwartze, 1928); for mice (Weese, 1928) 4.4. to 5.6 ml/kg. – *(ii) By subcutaneous injection* to mice, 5 mg/kg compared with 6 mg/kg for isopropyl alcohol (Starrek, 1938). – *(iii) By interperitoneal injection,* for the rat, 4 ml/kg (Lendle, 1928) compared with 8 ml for ethyl alcohol. By this route Rost and Braun (1926) also found propanol-1 considerably more toxic than ethyl alcohol (about 1.5 times greater). – *(iv) By intravenous injection,* for cats, 2 ml/kg (Macht, 1920); for rabbits, 5 ml/kg (Lehmann and Newman, 1937). – *(v) By inhalation,* Weese (1928) was unable to produce death in animals exposed to saturated or unsaturated air mixtures.

   (b) Narcotic dose. – *(i) By oral administration,* for rabbits, rapid and deep

Bibliography on p. 401

narcosis was produced by 3.0 to 3.46 g/kg in 20 to 30 min, less severe narcosis by 2.58 to 2.96 g/kg in 5 to 10 min and slight paralysis by 1.6 to 2.4 g/kg (Baer, 1898). Munch and Schwartze (1928) give the narcotic dose as 1.75 ml/kg, compared with 5.5 for ethyl and 2.85 for propanol-2. – *(ii) By intraperitoneal injection*, for rats, 1.5 ml/kg (Lendle, 1928) compared with 4.5 for ethyl alcohol, the margin of safety being 2.66. – *(iii) By intravenous injection*, the minimal narcotic dose has always been found less than that of ethyl alcohol, but the actual dose has varied in the hands of various investigators, from 0.075 ml/kg (Grilichess, 1913) to 1.71 g/kg (Lehmann and Newman, 1937), both for rabbits. – *(iv) By inhalation*, for mice, Starrek (1938) found 3000 p.p.m. for $1\frac{1}{2}$ h to cause staggering and ataxia, and about 4000 p.p.m. deep narcosis within 4 h.

SYMPTOMS OF INTOXICATION

With lethal doses, ataxia, paralysis of the hind legs, lowering of the body temperatura, dyspnoea and narcosis are followed by death from respiratory failure. With non-lethal repeated dosage, narcosis is transient, and according to Weese (1928) causes no habituation, but oral administration causes gastro-intestinal irritation with vomiting (Rost and Braun, 1926) and in growing chicks impairment of growth (Elhardt, 1931).

CHANGES IN THE ORGANISM

According to Starrek (1938), animals subjected to fatal subcutaneous dosage show hyperaemia of the lungs; repeated exposure by inhalation was found by Weese (1928) to cause moderate fatty infiltration of the liver, kidneys and heart, but no other serious pathological changes.

Toxicity to human beings

Only one (fatal) case of poisoning by ingestion has been reported, and none from inhalation of the vapour during industrial use. The one fatal case was that described by Durwald and Degen (1956). This was a woman of highly nervous disposition who had shown signs of 'drunkenness', a few days before she was found unconscious in a river with her head above water. She was suspected of having drunk perfumes and hair lotions. She died four hours later, and death was at first believed to be due to an overdose of sleeping tablets, none of which were however found at autopsy. Analysis of fluid from the intestinal tract revealed the presence of propanol-1, and autopsy showed swelling of the brain and oedema of the lungs. The exact amount was not determined but was believed to have been 400 to 500 ml. Durwald and Degen remark that this estimated fatal dose corresponds to the statement of Flury and Zangger (1928) that the toxic effect of propanol-1 for animals is very similar to that of ethyl alcohol.

39b. Propanol-2

Synonyms: isopropyl alcohol, isopropanol, dimethyl carbinol, Perspirit, Propol, Hartosol, Optal, Avantine.

Structural formula:
$$\begin{array}{c} OH \\ | \\ CH_3{-}CH{-}CH_3 \end{array}$$

Molecular formula: C_3H_8O

Molecular weight: 60.097

Properties: a clear, colourless liquid with an odour resembling that of ethyl alcohol
    boiling point: 82.4 °C
    melting point: —85.8 °C
    vapour pressure: 44 mm Hg at 25 °C
    vapour density (air = 1): 2.08
    specific gravity (liquid density): 0.787
    flash point: 53 °F
    conversion factors: 1 p.p.m. = 2.45 mg/m³
                      1 mg/l = 408 p.p.m.
    solubility: miscible with water, alcohol and ether.
    evaporation rate (ether = 1): 21
    maximum allowable concentration: not established; Cook (1945) suggested 400 p.p.m., but Nelson *et al.* (1943) found that mild irritation of nose and throat was produced at this level, and that 200 p.p.m. was the highest concentration acceptable for an 8-h exposure.

ECONOMY, SOURCES AND USES

Production

(1) From propylene, a by-product in the cracking of heavy petroleum hydrocarbons, by dissolving it in H_2SO_4 and hydrolysing the acid ester so formed.
(2) From acetone, by hydrogenation in the presence of catalysts.

Industrial uses

(1) In the pharmaceutical industry (Ruemele, 1948), as a substitute for ethyl alcohol, in cosmetics, mouth washes, 'rubbing lotions', hair tonics and skin disinfec-

tants. Grant (1932) states that it is most effective against *Staphylococcus aureus*, *Escherichia coli*, *Bacterium anthrax* and *subtilis* in concentrations of 30–50%.

(2) In the manufacture of acetone. Fairhall (1957) states that in the U.S.A. 69.8% of its production was used for this purpose.

(3) As a solvent for resins, plastics, etc.

(4) In the textile industry, for coatings.

(5) As a de-icing and anti-freeze agent.

(6) In the lacquer and varnish industry, as a substitute for ethyl alcohol in nitrocellulose lacquers.

(7) In the manufacture of safety glass.

(8) In the 'fused collar' industry (Donley, 1936).

(9) As a preservative and dehydrating agent (Mellan, 1939).

BIOCHEMISTRY

Estimation

(1) In the atmosphere

(a) By oxidation to acetone with chromic acid and iodimetric measurement of the acetone (Jacobs, 1941).

(b) After absorption on silica gel, recovery by steam distillation and conversion to isopropyl nitrite with subsequent liberation and titration of nitrous acid (Hahn, 1937; Knipping and Ponndorf, 1926).

(2) In urine

The method used by Cook and Smith (1929) takes into account the fact that acetone may be present as well as isopropyl alcohol. They therefore used two separate samples of urine, one for the simultaneous determination of total and preformed acetone, by oxidation with dichromate and H_2SO_4, then converting it into a complex mercury salt by Denigès' (1910) reagent. The preformed acetone is then estimated separately by distilling the second sample of urine into hydroxylamine hydrochloride: this liberates HCl, which is titrated (preferably by methyl orange). The difference between the two determinations allows the calculation of the amount of isopropyl alcohol in the urine.

Metabolism

Isopropyl is more slowly metabolised in most animal species than ethyl alcohol, which may account for the fact that it is more narcotic and acutely toxic.

In dogs, according to Wax *et al.* (1949) it is rapidly absorbed from the intestine but slowly from the stomach; its disappearance from the blood is more rapid than ethyl alcohol in high concentration, but slower when it is low (Lehmann *et al.*, 1945). In other words, the rate of metabolism varies both with the dosage and also with the species of animal.

The chief step in its oxidation is, like that of ethyl alcohol, to acetone, which can be detected in the urine after one hour, and in the expired air in 15 min (Kemal, 1927). Fuller and Hunter (1927) found small amounts of acetone in the urine of men 2 to 4 days after a dosage of 20 or 30 ml of 50% aqueous isopropyl alcohol on three successive days. With large doses there may be an increased excretion of unchanged alcohol and of its glucuronide. The formation of glucuronide was first suggested by Neubauer in 1901, and was confirmed by Kamil *et al.* (1953), who found that about 10% of a dosage of 1 g/kg was excreted by rabbits as isopropyl glucuronide.

Williams (1959) suggests, on the basis that acetone is slowly converted to acetate, formate, CO_2 and several other metabolites, that isopropanol may also form these compounds. He also states that it is likely that the enzyme responsible for its conversion into acetone is alcohol dehydrogenase, with cozymase A as coenzyme, but 500 times as much of the enzyme are required to obtain the same rate of reaction as with the ethanol-DPN-acetaldehyde system (Burton and Wilson, 1953).

Absorption from the skin has been found to be slight in animals (Macht, 1922) but a case of coma in a child, following tepid sponging with isopropyl alcohol was reported by Garrison in 1953. He mentioned, however, that "the odor of alcohol filled the small cubicle where he lay", so that inhalation was probably also an important factor.

TOXICOLOGY

While ingestion of isopropyl alcohol has an action on the central nervous system similar to that of other alcohols, causing drowsiness, headache of varying intensity, narcosis and in severe cases coma, repeated administration has apparently no injurious action on the liver as in the case of ethyl alcohol, and no untoward effect on vision, as in the case of methyl alcohol. One case has been reported of a toxic effect on the kidney (Chapin, 1949) in a man who was already a confirmed alcoholic.

In industrial use, no cases of poisoning from exposure to its vapour alone have been recorded, possibly owing to its low volatility; the case of 'toxic encephalitis' described by Donley (1936) was exposed also to other solvents (see p. 339).

A recent note on a possible occupational carcinogenic effect has been recorded in a Japanese journal (Tsuchaya, 1963) which is not available to the writer at the time of writing.

In animals, when ingested in large doses, its narcotic action is stronger than that of ethyl alcohol, but without the primary stimulation characteristic of ethanol (Boruttau, 1921). There is some difference of opinion as to its cumulative effect in animals, but on the basis of the slowness of its elimination, it is possible that such an effect may occur, due to its decomposition product, acetone.

Bibliography on p. 401

Toxicity to animals

Acute

In comparing the acute toxicity of isopropanol with that of ethanol, the fact has to be taken into account that while death due to ethanol is likely to occur within 24 h, an interval of 24–48 h usually elapses after administration of isopropanol.

Morris and Lightbody (1938) gave the dosage of the two alcohols over a period of 12 days and found that in the first four days the animals given ethanol were more deeply narcotised and the narcosis lasted longer, while in the last four days' period this was reversed.

(a) Lethal dose. – According to the minimum lethal dose by various routes of administration and the species of animal, isopropyl alcohol has been judged 1.5 times (Rost and Braun, 1926) or twice (Lehmann and Newman, 1937) as acutely toxic as ethyl alcohol. – *(i) By oral administration*, for the mouse 6.0 to 7.6 mg/kg (Weese, 1928). – *(ii) By stomach tube*, for rabbits, 10 ml/kg, compared with 12.5 ml/kg for ethyl alcohol (Munch and Schwartze, 1925). – *(iii) By subcutaneous injection*, for the mouse, 7.6 ml/kg (Starrek, 1938). – *(iv) By intravenous injection*, for the cat, 2.5 ml/kg (Macht, 1920), for mice and rats, 3.2 g/kg (Vollmer, 1931), for rabbits, 5 ml/kg (Lehmann and Newman, 1937). – *(v) By inhalation*, according to von Oettingen (1943) no fatal concentrations have been recorded.

(b) Narcotic dose. – *(i) By stomach tube*, for rabbits, 2.85 ml/kg compared with 5.5 ml/kg for ethyl alcohol (Munch and Schwartze, 1925). – *(ii) By inhalation*. Macht (1922) observed only slight toxic symptoms in rats inhaling saturated air mixtures after 15–30 min. Starrek (1938) obtained narcosis in mice with concentrations of 3000 p.p.m., the effects increasing with duration of exposure; deep narcosis with loss of reflexes after 7 to 8 h.

SYMPTOMS OF INTOXICATION

In contrast to ethyl alcohol, isopropyl alcohol does not produce an initial stage of stimulation (Boruttau, 1921). Incoordination is followed by light, then profound narcosis, with loss of reflexes, frequently nystagmus, decreased and laboured respiration and decreased heart rate.

Tolerance to ingestion of isopropyl alcohol by different species of animals has been reported – in dogs by Fuller and Hunter (1927) but not in rabbits (Morris and Lightbody, 1938). The latter found that in contrast to the increased resistance to ethanol, with an increased rate of recovery, the rabbits given isopropanol showed little evidence of tolerance when doses were sufficiently large or given at intervals not long enough to allow complete disposal of the alcohol and its metabolic products, of which they believed acetone to play some part.

Although the metabolism of isopropyl alcohol is slower than that of ethanol, and therefore a cumulative effect might possibly occur, it appears that intoxication of animals from such a cumulative effect is not regarded as probable. Lehmann *et al.* (1945) found that repeated ingestion by dogs of a 1% concentration of isopropyl alcohol and water during one month caused ataxia, but the degree of drunkenness after habituation showed a consistent decrease after the third day, indicating the development of acquired tolerance.

The skin and mucous membranes

In contrast to the statement by Christiansen (1918) that contact of isopropyl alcohol may cause irritation of the skin, Grant (1923) found it to have no effect except a slight maceration of the outer layer of the epidermis; Boruttau (1921) also, on the basis of animal experiments, was convinced of its harmlessness as a skin application. Irritation of the eyes of rabbits was observed by Bijlsma (1928); hyperaemia, swelling and moderate turbidity of the cornea followed the application of 40% solutions, these features becoming more pronounced with stronger solutions.

CHANGES IN THE ORGANISM

(1) The kidneys and liver

A very slight reversible fatty infiltration of kidneys and liver of rats was observed by Weese (1928). The kidneys of one dog in the experiments of Lehmann *et al.* (1944) showed a decrease in the number of nephrons, with hydropic changes and necrosis of some of the tubular epithelium.

No pathological changes were observed in other organs.

(2) The brain

Of the dogs examined by Lehman, Schwerma and Rickards, two showed small haemorrhages, but not the third.

(3) Influence on reproduction and growth

Lehman *et al.* (1945) found some retardation of growth in the first generation of alcohol-fed rats during the early weeks of life, but normal growth was restored by the 13th week. There was no significant difference in the rate of growth of the second generation, and there did not appear to be any deleterious effects on the reproductive functions or embryonic development.

Toxicity to human beings

No definite cases of poisoning from exposure to the vapour of isopropanol have been recorded, especially from its industrial use, except the possible case of 'toxic encephalitis' described by Donley (1936). This was a 45 year old woman employed in the 'fused collar industry'; she complained of headache, drowsiness, and general loss of interest, and showed congestion of respiratory mucous mem-

Bibliography on p. 401

branes, cough and signs of early bronchopneumonia, some disorientation, confusion and thick slow speech, ankle clonus, ataxic gait and unequal pupils. The cerebrospinal fluid was slightly positive for globulin. The fluid used for dipping the collars contained 74% of methyl cellosolve and up to 3% of dimethyl phthalate and 3% of isopropyl alcohol. In view of the fact that similar, though less severe, signs of mental retardation were later observed by Parsons and Parsons (1938) in workers on a similar process and were then attributed to methyl cellosolve, it appears that the symptoms in Donley's case might also have been due to methyl cellosolve rather than to the small amount of isopropyl alcohol in the mixture used.

SYMPTOMS OF INTOXICATION

(1) The eyes

No untoward effect on vision was observed by Fuller and Hunter (1927) during the course of repeated daily ingestion nor during the following two weeks; in fact, in some cases the vision appeared to be clearer.

(2) The skin

According to Fuller and Hunter (1927) isopropanol has no harmful effect when applied to the skin, and Boruttau (1921) has stated that there is no contraindication to its use for cleansing the hair, skin or nails.

(3) Vascular disturbances

In a case described by Chapin (1949), a known alcoholic who had drunk approximately one pint of isopropyl alcohol, the pulse was weak and the blood pressure 90/68. Fuller and Hunter (1927) also found that the immediate effect of ingestion of 20 to 30 ml of isopropanol (50% strength) was in general a lowering of the blood pressure, both systolic and diastolic, but in some cases a rise was noted. The pulse rate varied sometimes rising, sometimes falling.

(4) Neurological disturbances

Ingestion of isopropyl alcohol, like that of ethyl alcohol, is followed by action on the brain, causing no initial exhilaration, but drowsiness, dizziness, headache of varying intensity and of long duration; these effects according to Morris and Lightbody (1938) can follow the ingestion of 25 ml in 125 ml of water. With larger quantities narcosis may be produced, and in very severe cases coma.

(5) Intestinal disturbances

Epigastric pain, vomiting, diarrhoea, and haemorrhagic stools, observed in Chapin's case were assumed to be evidence of the irritative effect on mucous membranes.

CHANGES IN THE ORGANISM

(1) The liver

Although the liver was enlarged in Chapin's case, there was no jaundice, and no suggestion of cirrhosis; bromsulphthalein excretion was normal.

(2) The kidneys

The only case in which severe (though reversible) injury to the kidneys has been ascribed to ingestion of isopropyl alcohol is that of Chapin. This man was anuric for three days and developed oedema which persisted until diuresis was reestablished. He also showed nitrogen retention. This development of acute renal insufficiency – "lower nephron nephrosis" – was regarded by Chapin as a consequence of tissue destruction and shock, and therefore a complication of isopropyl alcohol poisoning. Acetonuria was observed by Fuller and Hunter (1927) during the course of repeated daily ingestion of 20–30 ml of isopropanol, disappearing when the ingestion ceased.

Bibliography on p. 401

40. Butanols

There are four isomeric forms of butyl alcohol – butanol-1, 2-methylpropanol-1 (isobutyl alcohol), butanol-2 (*sec.*-butyl alcohol) and 2-methylpropanol-2 (*tert.*-butyl alcohol).

Only butanol-1 is of considerable industrial importance, as a constituent of lacquer solvents. Isobutyl alcohol is also used for this purpose and for the production of the corresponding acetate; the secondary isomer is used as an intermediate in the production of the secondary acetate and of methyl ethyl ketone, and the tertiary as an alkylating agent in the preparation of tertiary butyl phenol, in the manufacture of drugs and perfumes, in the recrystallisation of chemicals and in fruit essences.

It has been stated that the normal alcohols are always more toxic than their secondary isomers (Overton, 1901), but this does not always hold for oral administration (Rost and Braun, 1926) or for intraperitioneal injection (Hufferd, 1932; Butler and Dickison, 1940). Their relative toxicity depends largely on their vapour pressure; this, being relatively low, militates against their ready entry into the blood and central nervous system, so that their narcotic and toxic effects are less than those of the propyl alcohols.

The secondary and tertiary isomers, having a higher vapour pressure than butanol-1, are more strongly narcotic (Weese, 1928) but less systemically toxic because they are more readily exhaled (Pohl, 1908). Weese draws a distinction between their effect in saturated and unsaturated air mixtures. In unsaturated air they obey Richardson's Law that the toxicity of individual homologues increases with the number of carbon atoms; in saturated mixtures, butanol-1 and 2-methylpropanol-1 have less narcotic potency than the propyl alcohols, while the secondary and tertiary isomers are stronger narcotics though less specifically toxic. 2-Methylpropanol-2 differs from the normal and secondary alcohols in its metabolic behaviour with regard to different animal species. According to Thierfelder and von Mering (1885) only in rabbits, not in dogs or human beings, does it undergo any glucuronic conjugation. Williams (1959) however remarks that "most of the tertiary alcohols are narcotics and it appears probable that this is a consequence of their slow rate of metabolism".

40a. Butanol-1

Synonyms: *n*-butyl alcohol, propanyl carbinol, butyric alcohol

Structural formula: CH_3—CH_2—CH_2—CH_2—OH

Molecular formula: C_4H_9OH

Molecular weight: 74.124

Properties: a colourless liquid with a pungent odour stated to be disagreeable above 25 p.p.m. (Nelson *et al.*, 1943). Soluble in water to the extent of 9% at 15 °C. Mixes freely with alcohol and water.

    boiling point: 117.7 °C

    melting point: —79.9 °C

    vapour pressure: 6.5 mm Hg at 25 °C

    vapour density (air = 1): 2.56

    specific gravity (liquid density): 0.8109

    flash point: 84 °F

    conversion factors: 1 p.p.m. = 3.03 mg/m^3 at 25 °C

                        1 mg/l   = 300 p.p.m.

    solubility: 7.7% in water at 20 °C

    evaporation rate (ether = 1): 33

    maximum allowable concentration: 100 p.p.m.; Schumacher *et al.* (1962) suggest 400 p.p.m.

ECONOMY, SOURCES AND USES

Production

(1) By fermentation of maize flour by a special strain of bacillus (von Oettingen, 1943).

(2) By synthesis from acetaldehyde or ethanol.

(3) From the fusel oil formed when certain species of yeast are used in alcoholic fermentation.

Industrial uses

(1) Chiefly in the lacquer industry, including automobile lacquers (Elkins, 1959).

(2) In the rubber and plastic industries – cementing (Cogan and Grant, 1945).

(3) In the textile industry – fabric coating (Sisley, 1934).

(4) In the manufacture of safety glass (Holden and Doolittle, 1935).

(5) In the dye industry, as a dehydrating agent (Treon, 1963).

(6) In the straw hat industry together with butyl acetate (Kruger, 1932).

Bibliography on p. 401

BIOCHEMISTRY

Estimation

(1) In the atmosphere

The method described by Ficklen (1940) and Elkins (1959) is that of oxidation by potassium dichromate, addition of potassium iodide and titration with sodium thiosulphate solution. Each ml of dichromate = 0.025 mmole of butanol.

In the method used by Sterner *et al.* (1949) air was passed through silica gel, the butanol distilled, and the amount in the distillate determined by means of an interferometer.

(2) In blood and tissues

A modification of Widmark's (1932) method, similar to that of Ficklen for air, was used by Berggren (1938), applying it to blood concentrations between 0.13 and 0.75%.

Metabolism

Butanol-1 is absorbed through the lungs, the gastro-intestinal tract and according to Sander (1933) also through the skin. Its oxidation is almost complete, and more rapid than that of ethanol (Berggren, 1938). Only a small amount undergoes glucuronic conjugation (1.08%, Williams, 1959).

TOXICOLOGY

Butanol-1 is a narcotic; when administered to animals by injection, orally, or by inhalation of high concentrations it is more acutely toxic than methanol, ethanol or propanol-1, and also, though not to such an extent, than secondary butyl alcohol (Weese, 1928). It is an irritant of mucous membranes, especially of the eyes, on which, in human beings, it has the effect of causing an unusual form of keratitis. Repeated exposure has been stated to cause in animals signs of early injury to the liver and kidneys, but in the only cases reported of slight liver injury to lacquer sprayers (Burger and Stockman, 1932) the mixture of solvents used included butanol and propanol, butyl and amyl acetate and acetone, and most authorities, including von Oettingen (1943) and Treon (1963) regard the association of butanol-1 with the liver injury "quite questionable".

In animals, however, Smyth and Smyth (1928) observed not only liver and kidney degeneration but also changes in the blood picture following repeated exposure to 100 p.p.m. and remark that butyl alcohol should be used with caution and in only small amounts in lacquers.

Toxicity to animals

(1) Acute

(a) *Lethal dose.* – (i) *By oral administration*, for rats, 4.36 g/kg (Smyth *et al.*, 1951), for rabbits 4.25 ml/kg (Munch and Schwartze, 1925). – (ii) *By subcutaneous injection*, for mice, about 5 mg/g (Lehmann and Flury, 1943), for dogs, 2 to 2.3 g/kg (Dujardin *et al.*, 1875). These observers found butyl more toxic than ethyl or propyl alcohol, and more toxic by mouth than by subcutaneous injection. – (iii) *By intraperitoneal injection*, for rats, Lendle (1928) gives the lethal dosage as 1.2 ml/kg, compared with 8 for ethanol and 4 for propanol. – (iv) *By intravenous injection*, for cats, 0.3 ml/kg (in terms of pure alcohol) compared with 5 ml for ethyl and 0.9 for isobutyl alcohol (Macht, 1920). – (v) *By inhalation*, for rats, inhalation of saturated vapour for 8 h was not lethal (Smyth *et al.*, 1951; Weese, 1928). – (vi) *By skin absorption*, for rabbits, 9.4 ml/kg (Treon, 1963).

(b) *Narcotic dose.* – (i) *By oral administration*, for rabbits, deep and rapid narcosis followed a dosage of 2.1 to 2.44 g/kg (Baer, 1898). – (ii) *By intraperitoneal injection*, for mice, 0.76 ml/kg, compared with 1.5 for propyl and 4.5 for ethyl alcohol (Lendle, 1928). – (iii) *By inhalation*, for mice, 6600 p.p.m. (Starrek, 1938). Some of the animals died after deep narcosis. Also for mice, Weese (1928) observed repeated narcosis during 130 h of total exposure to 8000 p.p.m. On the other hand no evidence of intoxication was observed by Starrek in mice exposed to 3300 p.p.m. for 420 min, and Schumacher *et al.* (1962) found that mice exposed to concentrations of 200, 400, 800 and 1600 p.p.m. for three days at a time showed only irritation of the eyes with the higher dosages, with no decrease, but rather an increase in weight, and no increase in spontaneous mortality.

(2) Chronic or subacute

Repeated inhalation for several days of 800 p.p.m. caused no deaths in mice (Weese, 1928), nor of 100 p.p.m. 4 h a day for 64 days in guinea pigs (Gardner, 1925). Skin application of 20 ml/kg daily for 30 days to rabbits were also not lethal (Treon, 1963).

SYMPTOMS OF INTOXICATION

Restlessness, irritation of mucous membranes, ataxia, prostration, narcosis, are followed, if the dosage is high enough, by death from respiratory failure.

In Baer's (1898) experiments, rabbits given orally 1 to 1.5 g/kg showed moderate reduction of sensitivity and within 20 to 30 min slight paralysis. With a dosage of 1.6 to 2.0 g/kg they showed a primary excitement, and after 15 min complete paralysis, analgesia, diminished corneal, pupillary and ciliary reflexes, reduction of body temperature and respiration and, with higher dosage, nystagmus, salivation and deep narcosis lasting 36 h. With inhalation, Weese (1928) found that mice tolerated narcosis well, recovering completely within a few hours and showing no signs of habituation.

Bibliography on p. 401

(1) The eyes

With high 'sublethal' concentrations, corneal ulcers and opacities did occur in some of the animals investigated by Smyth and Smyth (1928), but neither these high concentrations nor 300 p.p.m. for two weeks produced the characteristic corneal vacuoles observed in human beings by Cogan and Grant (1945) (see below). Nor was this human phenomenon observed by Schumacher et al. (1962) in mice exposed to concentrations of 200, 400, 800 and 1600 p.p.m. for three days at a time. Only at the higher concentrations was irritation of the eyes produced.

(2) Blood and bone marrow

Changes in the blood picture of the animals observed by Smyth and Smyth (1928) consisted in a moderate decrease of red corpuscles and haemoglobin, and a relative and absolute lymphocytosis.

(3) Gastro-intestinal disturbances

Severe congestion, sometimes with haemorrhage, in the small intestine of dogs, whether the butanol was given orally or subcutaneously, was recorded by Dujardin et al. (1875).

CHANGES IN THE ORGANISM

(1) The liver and kidneys

Reversible fatty infiltration of the liver and kidneys of mice following repeated exposure to narcotic concentrations was reported by Weese (1928), and in guinea pigs Smyth and Smyth (1928) found, after exposure to 100 p.p.m. 4 h a day for 64 days, early though not severe central degeneration of the liver and in some animals widespread degeneration of all types of the tubules in the kidney.

(2) The lungs

Mild bronchial irritation, with some enlargement of bronchial lymph nodes resulted from the prolonged exposure of rabbits to air containing butanol (Gardner, 1925), while haemorrhagic areas in the lungs were recorded by Smyth and Smyth (1928). Pulmonary lesions, even when the butanol was introduced into the stomach, were observed by Dujardin et al. (1875).

Toxicity to human beings

The results of a 10 year study of workers exposed to butanol-1 by Sterner et al. (1949), indicates that systemic intoxication is not likely to appear if the exposure is kept to a level not higher than 100 p.p.m. – according to Tabershaw et al. (1944) not until this level is greatly exceeded. At such a high level slight headache, vertigo and drowsiness were noted among workers in plants manufacturing waterproof products.

SYMPTOMS OF INTOXICATION

(1) The eyes

Ocular irritation has been reported in workers in several industries where butyl alcohol is used together with other solvents – methylethyl ketone, diacetone alcohol, butyl acetate and ethyl alcohol – and Tabershaw *et al.* (1944) state that eye irritation may be expected to occur when the concentration of butanol is above 50 p.p.m. In the study by Sterner *et al.* (1949) occasional corneal inflammation, with burning, lacrimation, photophobia and blurring of vision were observed when the concentration was 200 p.p.m. or above. Severe irritation of the conjunctiva and some keratitis were also described by Kruger (1932) among workers in the straw hat industry.

A more specific effect on the cornea, in the form of vacuoles, was reported by Cogan and Grant (1945) in workers manufacturing army raincoats. Ocular irritation had occurred in 6 local rubber factories, but in this particular factory, where the solvent used was a mixture of butanol, diacetone alcohol and denatured alcohol, and where the concentration of butanol varied between 15 and 100 p.p.m., the eye lesions were specifically present in the cornea. Here they presented, when examined with the slit lamp, characteristic, symmetrically distributed clear vacuoles, on the anterior surface of the cornea, about 0.05 mm in size and varying in number from 10 to 20 in the mildest, up to 500 to 1000 in the severest cases. The accompanying symptoms were those of irritation – foreign body sensation, epiphora, burning, worst in the early morning, and in the most severely affected cases blurring of vision. Both symptoms and lesions showed considerable improvement after absence from work for 5 to 7 days, and complete resolution in 10 days, but with return to work the corneal lesions tended to recur. Although butanol was not the only solvent used and though it was not found possible to reproduce the lesions in animals, Cogan and Grant considered that "there can be little doubt that from the clinical evidence the cause of the disease is exposure to butanol".

(2) The skin

Dermatitis of the fingers and hands, in the form of a fissured eczema, was frequent in the experience of Tabershaw *et al.* (1944) but could be prevented by protective ointment and lanolin emollient after work, and yielded rapidly to treatment.

CHANGES IN THE ORGANISM

The liver

The possibility of an injurious effect on the liver was investigated by Burger and Stockman in 1932 in a group of lacquer sprayers, using as their criterion the presence of urobilin in the urine, as demonstrated by the fluorescence reaction. The men had used as the lacquer solvent a mixture of butyl and amyl alcohol, butyl and amyl acetate and acetone. By comparison with a non-exposed group, the lacquer sprayers' urine contained urobilin in 39% as compared with 10%. Burger and Stockman assumed that this indicated an irritation of the liver by inhalation of small amounts of the solvent, but in the one case which they describe specifically, a girl of 16 who showed a urobilin reaction of 168, the exposure for three months had been to amyl acetate. It is therefore not possible to ascribe all the cases of urobilinuria to butanol-1, and even though only cases were examined who had shown subjective symptoms such as headache, drowsiness, giddiness, loss of appetite and nausea, no indication is given of the relative amounts of the various constituents of the laquer solvent, nor of their atmospheric concentrations.

40b. 2-Methylpropanol-1

Synonym: isobutyl alcohol

Structural formula:
$$CH_3\!-\!CH\!-\!CH_2\!-\!OH$$
$$\mid$$
$$CH_3$$

Molecular formula: $C_4H_{10}O$

Molecular weight: 74.124

Properties: a colourless liquid with a slightly suffocating odour of fusel oil.
    boiling point: 107–108 °C
    vapour pressure: 9 mm Hg at 20 °C
    vapour density (air = 1): 2.56
    specific gravity (liquid density): 0.8032
    flash point: 82 °F
    conversion factors: 1 p.p.m. = 3.03 mg/m³ at 25 °C
                     1 mg/l   = 330 p.p.m.
    solubility: soluble in water to the extent of 10 parts per 100 at 20 °C. Mixes freely with alcohol and ether. Not so powerful a solvent as butanol-1.
    maximum allowable concentration: not established.

ECONOMY, SOURCES AND USES

Production

(1) By fractional distillation of fusel oil. Webb and Kepner (1951) state that isobutyl alcohol, together with amyl alcohols, account for about 88% of the higher alcohols in a fusel oil sample.

(2) As a by-product in the preparation of synthetic methyl alcohol.

Industrial uses

Not of great importance but used to some extent (a) in the lacquer industry, (b) in the manufacture of isobutyl esters which are themselves used as solvents, plasticisers, flavourings and perfumes (Doolittle, 1954; Steinkoff, 1952).

BIOCHEMISTRY

Estimation in the atmosphere

There appears to be no quantitative method of estimation, but it can be detected in the atmosphere by oxidation with chromic acid to the aldehyde and subsequent reaction of this with O-nitrobenzaldehyde (Weber and Koch, 1933).

Metabolism

Isobutyl alcohol is absorbed through the intestinal tract and the lungs. There is some difference of opinion as to how completely it is oxidised; Weese (1928) believed it to be completely oxidised in mice, but Neubauer (1901) stated that it undergoes some conjugation with glucuronic acid in rabbits and dogs, and Williams (1959) states that a small amount (4%) may be excreted conjugated by rabbits and that it is presumably oxidised to isobutyraldehyde and isobutyric acid, and finally to acetone and CO_2.

TOXICOLOGY

The toxic effect of isobutyl alcohol on animals is chiefly that of narcosis, and the degree, as compared with that of butanol-1, depends to some extent on the route of administration. By injection it is less toxic (Macht, 1920), by oral administration (Rost and Braun, 1926) or inhalation of saturated air-vapour mixtures (Weese, 1928) slightly more so. The narcosis produced is transient and followed by only slight organic changes in liver and kidneys, while repeated inhalations cause no significant injury.

In human beings eye injury similar to that caused by butanol-1 have been reported in lacquerers working in bad conditions and exposed to high concentrations (Steinkoff, 1952) but the solvent used consisted not exclusively of isobutyl alcohol but also of butyl acetate. No evidence of such eye injury has been observed by Fasset (cited by Treon, 1963) with repeated exposure to concentrations of 100 p.p.m. for 5 h.

Bibliography on p. 401

Toxicity to animals

(1) Acute

(a) Lethal dose. – *(i) By oral administration*, for rats, 1.60–3.78 g/kg (Smyth *et al.*, 1954). – *(ii) By intraperitoneal injection*, for rabbits, 0.9 ml/kg, compared with 0.3 for butanol-1 (Macht, 1920). – *(iii) By intravenous injection*, for cats, 0.9 ml/kg (Macht, 1920), for rabbits (slow administration), 2.64 g/kg (Lehmann and Newman, 1937). – *(iv) By skin absorption*, for rabbits, 4.24 g/kg (Smyth *et al.*, 1954). – *(v) By inhalation*, for mice, 10,600 p.p.m. for 300 min (Weese, 1928), for rats, 8000 p.p.m. for 4 h (Smyth *et al.*, 1954).

(b) Narcotic dose. – For mice, 6400 p.p.m. for a total of 136 h (Weese, 1928), for dogs (oral), 2.5 ml/kg (Rost and Braun, 1926), compared with 5 ml/kg for butanol-1.

(2) Chronic or subacute

Repeated inhalation by mice of 2125 p.p.m. caused no deaths (Weese, 1928), nor did repeated narcosis following exposure to 6400 p.p.m.

SYMPTOMS OF INTOXICATION

The narcosis produced is only transient, and repeated inhalations not causing narcosis causes no untoward effects (Weese, 1928).

CHANGES IN THE ORGANISM

Weese found that narcotic dosage is followed only by slight organic changes in liver and kidneys.

Toxicity to human beings

The only systemic disturbance following heavy exposure to a mixture of isobutyl alcohol and butyl acetate was loss of weight and loss of appetite, reported by Steinkoff (1952).

SYMPTOMS OF INTOXICATION

(1) The eyes

Ocular injury similar to that recorded by Krüger (1932) following exposure to butanol-1 and butyl acetate, was described by Steinkoff (1952). Actually, Steinkoff did not attribute the corneal vacuolation (which is described as similar to that caused by overexposure to ultraviolet light) exclusively to the isobutyl alcohol; he refers to Flury and Wirth's opinion (1935) that "acetates can cause inflammation, swelling and anaesthesia of the cornea". He also emphasises the unsatisfactory working conditions of the affected lacquer sprayers-installation of a greater number of spraying machines in the room hitherto used; heating of the lacquer to a temperature of 200–300 °C in the warm weather, when the room temperature rose to 32–42 °C, and a constant odour of 'butyl'. These conditions had only existed for the last six months, and before that time there had been no complaints. Treon (1963) quoting a personal observation by Fasset, states that no evidence of such irritation was observed with repeated 8-h exposures to 100 p.p.m.

(2) The skin
    That isobutyl alcohol may be a skin irritant is stated by Schwartz and Tulipan (1939), and Oettel (1936) observed slight erythema and hyperaemia following its application to the skin of human beings.

40c. Butanol-2

Synonyms: secondary butyl alcohol, butan-2-ol, methylethyl carbinol

Structural formula:
$$CH_3{-}CH_2{-}\underset{\underset{OH}{|}}{CH}{-}CH_3$$

Molecular formula: $C_4H_{10}O$

Molecular weight: 74.124

Properties: a colourless liquid with an odour similar to but less pungent than that of butanol. It exists in the form of two optical isomers, *laevo-* and *dextro*-rotatory. A solvent for some gums and resins but not for cellulose esters.
    boiling point: 98.8 °C
    vapour pressure: 23.9 mm Hg at 30 °C
    vapour density (air = 1): 2.56
    specific gravity (liquid density): 0.808 at 20 °C
    flash point: 70 °F
    conversion factors: 1 p.p.m. = 3.03 mg/m³
                          1 mg/l = 330 p.p.m.
    solubility: soluble in water to the extent of 20 parts per 100 at 25 °C; mixes freely with alcohol and ether.
    maximum allowable concentration: not established as distinct from butyl alcohol = 100 p.p.m.

Bibliography on p. 401

ECONOMY, SOURCES AND USES

Production

By synthesis of butylene obtained during the cracking of petroleum; the butylene is reacted with sulphuric acid and steam (Mellan, 1950).

Industrial uses

(1) To some extent in the lacquer industry.
(2) In dewaxing paraffin (Smith, 1927).
(3) In polishes, cleaning materials and paint removers.
(4) In fruit essences, perfumes and dyestuffs.
(5) In the preparation of methyl ethyl ketone (Mellan, 1950; Doolittle, 1954).

BIOCHEMISTRY

Estimation in the atmosphere

By bromination following dehydration of the alcohol (Treon, 1963).

Metabolism

About 77% of butanol-2 is exhaled by the lungs (Pohl, 1908). Some of it is converted in the body to methyl ethyl ketone and expired as such. With regard to its glucuronic conjugation, Neubauer (1901) believed that such conjugation takes place in the rabbit but very little in the dog; Kamil *et al.* (1953) found that it is conjugated to *sec.*-butylglucuronide which can be isolated from the urine, and Williams (1959) estimates the amount of conjugation at 14%.

TOXICOLOGY

Butanol-2 is a narcotic, slightly more potent in animals than butanol-1; the two isomers are very nearly equal in anaesthetic potency for mice by intraperitoneal injection (Butler and Dickison, 1940), No toxic symptoms have been reported in human beings.

Toxicity to animals

(1) Acute

(a) *Lethal dose.* – (i) *By oral administration*, for rats, 6.48 g/kg, after 14 days, compared with 1.87 for propanol (Smyth *et al.*, 1954), for rabbits, 6.0 ml/kg (Munch and Schwartze, 1925). – (ii) *By inhalation*, for mice, 16,000 p.p.m. for 160 min, according to Weese (1928), but Starrek (1938) found no deaths at 19,800 p.p.m. up to 40 min exposure, and not even signs of intoxication with 1650 p.p.m. for 420 min.

(b) *Narcotic dose.* – (i) *By intraperitoneal injection*, for mice, 0.826 to 1.0 mg/g (Butler and Dickison, 1940). – (ii) *By inhalation*, 5330 p.p.m. for a total of 117 h (Weese, 1928), 3300 p.p.m. in 51 to 300 min and 19,800 p.p.m. in 7 to 40 min (Starrek, 1938).

(2) Chronic or subacute

Mice, exposed repeatedly to 5330 p.p.m. for a total of 117 h, were narcotised but survived (Weese, 1928).

SYMPTOMS OF INTOXICATION

Ataxia and prostration, followed by deep narcosis, with survival even after long periods of narcosis (Weese, 1928). No organic injury has been reported.

Toxicity to human beings

None have been reported.

40d. 2-Methylpropanol-2

Synonyms: tertiary butyl alcohol, trimethyl carbinol

Structural formula: $\underset{\underset{\text{OH}}{|}}{\text{CH}_3\text{—CH—CH}_2\text{—CH}_3}$

Molecular formula: $C_4H_{10}O$

Molecular weight: 74.124

Properties: a colourless volatile liquid, which forms rhombic crystals melting at 25 to 25.5 °C (von Oettingen, 1943).

    boiling point: 82.4 °C
    melting point: 25 °C
    vapour pressure: 42.0 mm Hg at 25 °C

Bibliography on p. 401

vapour density (air = 1): 2.56
specific gravity (liquid density): 0.783
flash point: 52 °F
conversion factors: 1 p.p.m. = 3.03 mg/m³
                     1 mg/l   = 330 p.p.m.
solubility: miscible with water, soluble in alcohols, esters, ethers and aromatic and aliphatic hydrocarbons.
maximum allowable concentration: 100 p.p.m.

ECONOMY, SOURCES AND USES

Industrial uses

It is used, though not extensively, in extraction of drugs, removal of water from various substances, in the manufacture of perfumes, as an intermediate, and in the recrystallisation of chemicals (Mellan, 1950), also in fruit essences, plastics and lacquers (Schwartz and Tulipan, 1939).

BIOCHEMISTRY

Estimation in the atmosphere

No specific reaction has been developed, but Treon (1963) suggests that colour reactions with various aldehydes, such as furfural, piperonal, anisaldehyde, in the presence of H_2SO_4 might be a possible method.

Metabolism

2-Methylpropanol-2, like other tertiary alcohols, is more biologically stable than the secondary alcohols and therefore less readily metabolised. It undergoes a relatively high degree of conjugation (24%, Williams, 1959).

TOXICOLOGY

Like the other butyl alcohols, tertiary butyl alcohol is a narcotic, stronger in animals than butanol-1 or isobutyl alcohol (Weese, 1928). Its toxic action, however, appears to be less; the mice investigated by Weese appeared to tolerate narcosis well with little evidence of organic injury. No toxic effects from its industrial use have been recorded.

Toxicity to animals

(1) Acute

(a) Lethal dose. – For rats *(by stomach tube)* 0.3–0.9 g/kg, compared with 1.0 for tertiary amyl alcohol (Schaffarzick and Brown, 1952); for rabbits *(oral)* 6.0 ml/kg (Munch and Schwartze, 1925).

(b) Narcotic dose. – For rats *(by stomach tube)*, 108 mg/kg, compared with 160 mg/kg for tertiary amyl alcohol, but with a wider range of safety (Schafferzick and Brown, 1952). These observers noted that its anticonvulsant effect, represented by abolition of the tonic-extensor phase produced by an electric current of 50 mA for 1.0 sec, was greater than that of tertiary amyl alcohol. Weese (1928) found that prolonged narcosis was usually followed by recovery.

(2) Chronic or subacute

No investigations made.

SYMPTOMS OF INTOXICATION

Somnolence (Thierfelder and von Mering, 1885), ataxia (Schaffarzick and Brown) and narcosis similar to that produced by the other butyl alcohols.

CHANGES IN THE ORGANISM

Weese (1928) observed slight fatty infiltration of liver and kidneys following deep narcosis.

Toxicity to human beings

The only toxic effect recorded in human beings is that of a possible skin irritant (Schwartz and Tulipan, 1939) but Oettel (1936) found only slight erythema and hyperaemia following its application to the skin.

No toxic effects from its industrial use have been reported.

Bibliography on p. 401

41. Pentanols

(Amyl alcohols)

There are eight isomers of pentanol, classified as follows (after Haggard *et al.*, 1945):

Isomer	Primary pentanols
a. Pentanol-1	$CH_3 \cdot CH_2 \cdot CH_2 \cdot CH_2 \cdot CH_2 \cdot OH$
b. 2-Methyl-butanol-1 (L and D form)	$CH_3 \cdot CH_2 \cdot \underset{\underset{CH_3}{\mid}}{CH} \cdot CH_2 \cdot OH$
c. 3-Methyl-butanol-1	$CH_3 \cdot \underset{\underset{CH_3}{\mid}}{CH} \cdot CH_2 \cdot CH_2 \cdot OH$
d. 2,2-Dimethyl-propanol-1 (a crystalline solid)	$CH_3 \cdot \overset{\overset{CH_3}{\mid}}{\underset{\underset{CH_3}{\mid}}{C}} \cdot CH_2 \cdot OH$

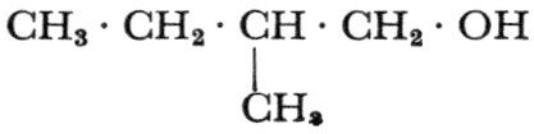

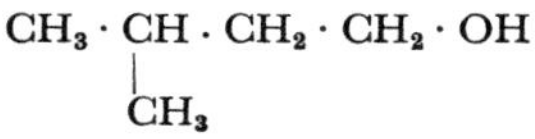

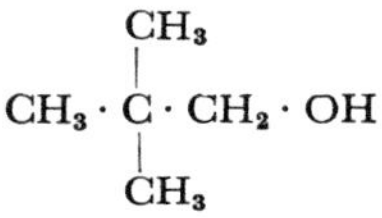

Secondary pentanols

e. Pentanol-2	$CH_3 \cdot CH_2 \cdot CH_2 \underset{\underset{OH}{\mid}}{CH} \cdot CH_3$
f. Pentanol-3	$CH_3 \cdot CH_2 \cdot \underset{\underset{OH}{\mid}}{CH} \cdot CH_2 \cdot CH_3$
g. 3-Methyl-butanol-2	$CH_3 \cdot \underset{\underset{CH_3}{\mid}}{CH} - \underset{\underset{OH}{\mid}}{CH} - CH_3$

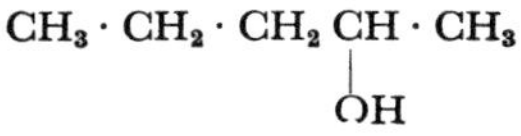

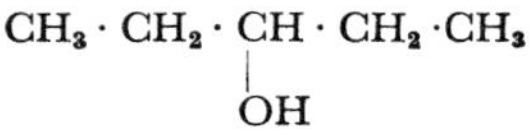

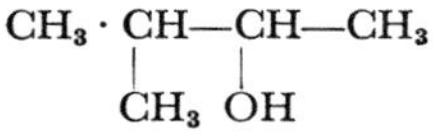

Tertiary pentanol

h. 2-Methyl-butanol-2	$CH_3 \cdot CH_2 \cdot \overset{\overset{CH_3}{\mid}}{\underset{\underset{OH}{\mid}}{C}} - CH_3$

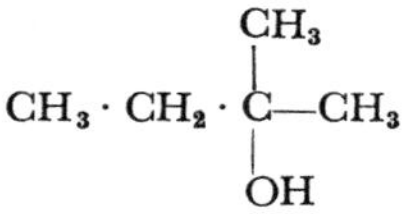

[356]

Properties: the colourless liquids with a mild odour are solvents for camphor, alkaloids, soft copals, ester gums, resins, iodine, phosphorus and sulphur (Mellan, 1939)

conversion factors: 1 p.p.m. = 3.60 mg/m³ at 25 °C

1 mg/l   = 278 p.p.m.

(For individual properties see individual solvents).

ECONOMY, SOURCES AND USES

Production

(1) By fermentation of cereals and potatoes.

(2) As a by-product of distillation of fusel oil. The amyl alcohol so obtained is a mixture of isoamyl alcohol and optically active (dextro) amyl alcohol (Fairhall, 1957).

(3) Synthetically, by chlorination of pentane, a low-boiling fraction of casing – head gasoline (Ascham, 1927; Pipik and Mezhebowskaya, 1933). It is known as "Pentasol" and is a mixture of 5 of the 8 isomers; according to Wilson and Worster (1929) it is practically a duplicate of the high-test fusel oil used in the past. A commercial product containing 80% of secondary active amyl alcohol and 20% of diethyl carbinol is marketed as secondary amyl alcohol (Fieser and Fieser, 1944).

Industrial uses

(1) In the manufacture of amyl acetate.

(2) In lacquers and solvent mixtures (*e.g.* 'Zapon' lacquer, Baader, 1933) and in paint strippers.

(3) In the drug and pharmaceutical industry (chiefly isoamyl alcohol, Doolittle, 1954).

(4) In the manufacture of adhesives and plastics.

(5) In the refining of petroleum.

(6) In the textile industry.

BIOCHEMISTRY

Estimation in the atmosphere

The method described by Korenmann (1932) depends on the reaction with furfural and concentrated H_2SO_4, giving a pink to violet-red colour.

Fairhall (1957) described a similar procedure, using salicylic aldehyde or *p*-diamino-benzaldehyde, or, for isoamyl alcohol *p*-hydroxybenzaldehyde (Penniman, Smith and Lawshe, 1937).

Bibliography on p. 401

Metabolism

Absorption and excretion

The various isomers show some difference both in the nature of their metabolic products and also in their rate of metabolism.

Like ethyl alcohol, the initial process of oxidation is the formation of aldehyde, but the amount of this varies considerably. With the primary alcohols no significant amount was detected in the expired air (1.9 mg%, according to Haggard *et al.*, 1945) and an equally small amount after intraperitoneal injection of 1g/kg of *n*-valeraldehyde, indicating the extremely transient nature of any aldehyde formed. It was also inferred, from the fact that intraperitoneal injection of the primary alcohols was followed by marked irritation of the peritoneal membrane and of the lungs, that the aldehyde formed by primary oxidation is converted into acid by any tissue of the body. This primary formation of aldehyde apparently takes place in the liver, since the blood concentration in partly hepatectomised animals was much higher and remained longer than in normal animals. Sedation persisted after all alcohol and aldehyde had disappeared; this was assumed to result from the formation of acid.

The rate of metabolism of the primary alcohols was shown to differ from that of the secondary and tertiary isomers by the difference in blood concentration one hour after administration to rats of 1 g/kg, and the time required for its disappearance. The concentration after one hour ranged from 14–15 mg% for the primary, as compared with 51–65 mg% for the secondary and 125 mg% for the tertiary, while the time required for its disappearance ranged from $3\frac{1}{2}$–9 h for the primary, 13–16 for the secondary and 50 for the tertiary.

The secondary pentanols gave rise to considerable amounts of ketone (methyl-*n*-propyl, diethyl- and methyl isopropyl). The liver played a smaller part in this conversion than in that of the primary alcohols to aldehyde.

The tertiary pentanol gave rise to no volatile metabolites, though about 65% of the dose remained to be metabolised after 35% had been excreted in the expired air and urine.

TOXICOLOGY

All the isomers of amyl alcohol are narcotic, and in high dosage lethal to animals, the degree of narcosis and lethality varying with the individual compound and with the mode of administration. All are however considered more toxic and more lethal than the lower homologues whatever the route of administration. Isoamyl alcohol, for example, was found by Lehmann and Newman (1937) to be 6.5 times as narcotic as ethyl alcohol by intravenous injection to rabbits. Comparison of the narcotic and toxic effects of the different isomers has proved somewhat confusing and not of great value, since different methods, different species of animals and differing conclusions of observers tend to produce conflicting results. As an example of such variations, the lethal dose for primary n-amyl alcohol is given as 0.12 g/kg (Macht, 1920), 0.48 (Lendle, 1928), and 1.04 (Lehmann and Flury, 1943); similarly that for isoamyl alcohol as 0.21 (Macht), 0.8 (Lendle), 1.52 (Lehmann and Newman, 1937) and 3.4 (Munch and Schwartze, 1925).

On the whole however it appears that by oral administration the narcotic action is highest with the secondary active, followed by the tertiary and lowest with the primary isomers.

By subcutaneous injection, even the two of the primary isomers were found by Starrek (1938) to differ in their toxic effect, n-amyl being more toxic than isoamyl.

No comparison of the effects by inhalation have been made, but Smyth (1956) found that a concentration of 'amyl alcohol' of 8000 p.p.m. was not lethal to rats.

Organic injury following narcosis has rarely been reported; only Straus (1887) has observed changes in the liver following repeated oral dosage to rabbits of the teriary isomer.

Toxicity to human beings

In human beings toxic effects have been recorded chiefly from ingestion and from the use of enemata either of 'fusel oil' or of the tertiary alcohol (amylene hydrate), but industrial poisoning by inhalation has occasionally been recorded, complicated by the fact that in most cases other solvents have been present in addition to amyl alcohol.

(1) Non-industrial intoxication

(a) By ingestion. – Ingestion of fusel oil was stated by Fuchter (1901) to have caused coma, glycosuria and methaemoglobinaemia; Hamilton (1934) headache, dizziness, nausea, vomiting, diarrhoea, delirium and coma, and Lewin (1929) stated that 0.5 g can cause somnolence, headache and throat irritation. The tertiary amyl alcohol (amylene hydrate) has been responsible for the most severe, though not fatal, cases of intoxication. In one such case, a suicidal attempt recorded by Anker in 1892, a woman who had drunk about 27 g became completely unconscious within half an hour, with a small rapid pulse and dilated pupils. The next day the breathing became stertorous, the pulse irregular and the pupils contracted. Under treatment by stimulants and a generous diet she recovered completely after 14 days with no sign of lung involvement. Another case recorded by von Heuber (1917) after ingestion of 18 g of undiluted amylene hydrate was completely unconscious for 4 h in spite of treatment with caffeine and suprarenin, and deep sleep lasted for 30 h, followed later by gross restlessness, pain in the limbs, headache and giddiness, with slow recovery.

Bibliography on p. 401

(b) From enema. – A fatal case followed administration of an enema of amylene hydrate (tertiary amyl alcohol) to a 23 year old man admitted to hospital for treatment for traumatic epilepsy (Jacobi and Speer, 1920) (see p. 342). He was ordered an enema of 6 g of amylene hydrate in the evening and was found the next morning unconscious, slightly cyanotic and with some pulmonary râles and absence of reflexes, except for light reaction of the pupils. It was then discovered that by mistake he had been given (as it was then believed) 35 g of the alcohol, but a later calculation of the dosage led Loewe to state that not 35 but only 28–29 g had been the dosage. Signs of oedema of the trachea and large bronchi, Cheyne–Stokes breathing and a rise of temperature and vomiting of a blood stained mucoid mass preceded death 53 hours after the enema was given. Since influenzal pneumonia was found at autopsy to be one of the causes of death, it was assumed that the tertiary amyl alcohol was only a contributory cause.

(2) Industrial poisoning

Amyl alcohol alone has rarely been held solely responsible for cases of industrial poisoning, but in 1907 Robert reported the results of his investigation of 30 cases of intoxication due to alcoholic vapours during the manufacture of smokeless powder, which had not been observed, except for a few cases of transient 'drunkenness', until amyl alcohol came into general use. The cases occurred on days of low pressure and high humidity so that the atmosphere became saturated with low-lying vapour. Three typical cases were described, in two of which headache, giddiness, vomiting and diarrhoea were so severe as to suggest an idiosyncrasy to the alcohol; the third, an alcoholic, showed great exacerbation of his symptoms, with vomiting so severe as to lead to cachexia, and commencing subicterus and ascites.

Eyquem (1905) also observed severe symptoms, chiefly nervous or psychic, in workers in a smokeless powder factory, with finally a state of cachexia. In this factory other alcohols were used, but Eyquem noted a recrudescence of symptoms whenever the use of amyl alcohol was increased. Similar symptoms were described by Hilbert (1925, cited by Lewin, 1929) from inhalation of the vapour from a fermentation cask by a foreman in a brewery, with the additional complaint that objects appeared alternately red and blue. Flury and Zernik (1931) however suggested that these symptoms might possibly have been due to carbon dioxide rather than to amyl alcohol.

Another example of the cases in which amyl alcohol cannot be held entirely responsible for the ill-effects described is the report by Zangger (1933) of the death of two men engaged in painting the inside of a container with 'Zapon' lacquer containing amyl alcohol; Zangger himself notes the possibility that tetrachloroethane was also present, while in a case described by Baader (1933) in which digestive symptoms predominated, amyl acetate was also present in the lacquer used.

41a. Pentanol-1

Synonyms: normal amyl alcohol, 1-pentanol, *n*-butyl carbinol

Structural formula: $CH_3-CH_2-CH_2-CH_2-CH_2-OH$

Molecular formula: $C_5H_{11}OH$

Properties:
   boiling point: 137.9 °C
   specific gravity: 0.817
   solubility: in water 2.7%; miscible with alcohol and ether.

TOXICOLOGY

Pentanol-1 has a toxic action similar to but slightly less than that of 3-methyl-butanol-1 by subcutaneous injection (Starrek, 1938). Doses of 5 mg/g caused in mice staggering, dyspnoea, motor irritation and deep narcosis.

41b. 2-Methylbutanol-1

(L and D form)

Synonyms: primary active amyl alcohol, 2-methyl-1-butanol, secondary butyl carbinol

Structural formula: $CH_3-CH_2-CH-CH_2-OH$
                                          $|$
                                        OH

Molecular formula: $C_5H_{12}O$

Properties:
   boiling point: 128 °C
   specific gravity: 0.816
   vapour pressure: 3.4 mm Hg at 20 °C
   flash point: 135 °F
   solubility: in water 3.6%; miscible with alcohol and ether.

Bibliography on p. 401

TOXICOLOGY

No specific investigations have been made to compare the toxic effects of this with other primary alcohols.

41c. 3-Methylbutanol-1

Synonyms: isoamyl alcohol, 3-methyl-1-butanol, isobutyl carbinol.

Structural formula:
$$CH_3—CH—CH_2—CH_2—OH$$
$$|$$
$$CH$$

Molecular formula: $C_5H_{12}O$

Properties:
> *boiling point:* 131.4 °C
> *specific gravity:* 0.8129
> *vapour pressure:* 28 mm Hg at 20 °C
> *flash point:* 114 °F
> *solubility:* in water 2% at 14 °C; miscible with all organic solvents.
> *maximum allowable concentration:* 100 p.p.m.; Elkins (1959) suggests 50 p.p.m.

ECONOMY, SOURCES AND USES

Production

From light petroleum by fractional distillation, dehydration of the pentane fraction which is than heated and re-fractionated, and the amylchloride fraction again fractionally distilled, giving a mono-chloro-pentane mixture. This is subjected to hydrolysis with sodium oleate solution in presence of a catalyst (Durrans, 1950).

Industrial uses

Chiefly used in lacquers, usually in mixtures with amyl acetate.

BIOCHEMISTRY

Metabolism

About 1.7% of the dose is eliminated unchanged in the expired air and urine; the rest is oxidised by way of the corresponding aldehydes and fatty acids; the latter, according to Williams (1959) account largely for its characteristic effect of sedation. He also states that the main site of primary oxidation appears to be the liver, that some of the aldehyde formed there enters the general circulation and its oxidation to the corresponding acid can take place in the bodily tissues generally.

Glucuronic conjugation takes place to the extent of 9%; this glucuronide has been isolated in the urine of rabbits (Kamil *et al.*, 1953).

TOXICOLOGY

In common with the other primary alcohols, isoamyl alcohol has a basic toxicity about 12 times that of ethanol, and somewhat greater than that of the secondary and tertiary isomers, when given by injection. By oral administration its toxicity is less than that of the secondary and tertiary isomers. Its toxic effects are mainly those of narcosis, with symptoms relating to the central nervous system.

Toxicity to animals

Acute

(a) *Lethal dose*, for rabbits *(oral)*, 4.25 ml/kg (Munch and Schwarze, 1925) compared with 3.5 for secondary amyl and 2.5 for tertiary amyl alcohol; for rats *(intraperitoneal)*, 0.69 g/kg (Haggard *et al.*, 1945) designating the 'basic lethal dose' as the amount present in the body which will yield a blood concentration causing respiratory failure. This compared with 1.53 for tertiary amyl alcohol and 7.4 for ethanol. Lendle (1928) found the minimal fatal dose 1 ml/kg, the same as for secondary amyl alcohol.

(b) *Narcotic dose*, for guinea pigs *(oral)*, 0.69 g/kg (Hufferd, 1932); for rats *(intraperitoneal)*, 0.5 ml/kg (Lendle, 1928); for rabbits *(intravenous)*, 0.85 g/kg (Lehmann and Newman, 1937).

According to Schwenkenbecher (1904) skin absorption can cause narcosis in mice.

Bibliography on p. 401

41d. 2,2-Dimethylpropanol-1

A crystalline solid.

41e. Pentanol-2

Synonyms: secondary active amyl alcohol, 2-pentanol

Structural formula: $CH_3-CH_2-CH_2-CH-OH$
                                                    $|$
                                                   CH_3

Molecular formula: $C_5H_{12}O$

Properties:
  boiling point: 119.5 °C
  specific gravity: 0.809
  solubility: in water 1:6 v/v (Treon, 1963); miscible with alcohol and ether.

TOXICOLOGY

According to Munch and Schwartze (1925) secondary active amyl alcohol is more toxic by oral administration to rabbits than tertiary or isoamyl alcohol, while by intraperitoneal injection it is less toxic than the tertiary isomer and more so than *n*-amyl alcohol (Lendle, 1928). Nothing is reported on its specific effects on human beings.

41f. Pentanol-3

Synonyms: secondary isoamyl alcohol, 3-pentanol

Structural formula: $CH_3-CH_2-CH-CH_2-CH_3$
                                              $|$
                                             OH

Molecular formula: $C_5H_{11}OH$

Properties:
  boiling point: 115.9 °C

vapour pressure: 2 mm Hg at 20 °C
specific gravity (liquid density): 0.8169
solubility: in water 4.1% at 20 °C.

TOXICOLOGY

By oral administration to rats, pentanol-3 is less toxic than tertiary amyl alcohol (Smyth *et al.*, 1954). These observers found it lethal by skin absorption following 24 h contact with 2.52 ml/kg.

41g. 3-Methylbutanol-2

Synonym: secondary amyl alcohol

Structural formula:
$$CH_3-CH-CH-CH_3$$
$$\quad\quad\ \ |\quad\ \ |$$
$$\quad\quad\ \ CH_3\ \ OH$$

Molecular formula: $C_5H_{11}OH$

Properties: a colourless liquid with a mild odour.
   boiling point: 114 °C
   specific gravity (liquid density): 0.819
   solubility: in water 218% at 30 °C

Production, industrial uses, metabolism and toxicology – no specific information; similar to those of other isomers of amyl alcohol.

41h. 2-Methylbutanol-2

Synonyms: tertiary amyl alcohol, amylene hydrate

Structural formula:
$$CH_3$$
$$\quad\quad |$$
$$CH_3-CH_2-C-CH_3$$
$$\quad\quad\quad |$$
$$\quad\quad\quad OH$$

Molecular formula: $C_5H_{12}O$

Properties: used chiefly for medical purposes, as a sleeping draught. In this respect it has been stated (Kochmann, 1923) to be a rapidly acting agent of only slight toxicity, but with a tendency to cause addiction.

Bibliography on p. 401

boiling point: 101.8 °C
specific gravity (liquid density): 0.809 at 20 °C
flash point: 74 °F (Durrans, 1950).
solubility: in water 1:8 v/v (Treon, 1963).

BIOCHEMISTRY

Metabolism

It is rapidly absorbed by subcutaneous tissue and by the gastro-intestinal membrane, and excreted by the lungs, to the extent of 26.4% (the expired air smells of it) and also by the kidneys to the extent of 8 to 9%. Its metabolic rate is slow, it takes 50 h to disappear from the blood stream, after intraperitoneal injection, compared with 3 to 9 and 13 to 16 h for primary and secondary isomers respectively (Haggard *et al.*, 1945).

It is relatively highly conjugated with glucuronic acid (58%, according to Williams, 1959) in rabbits, but not, according to Thierfelder and von Mering (1885) in dogs or man.

With oral narcotic dosage there is a decrease of excretion of nitrogen and urea but with heavy subcutaneous dosage an increase. Mori (1887) has stated that it causes dilatation of the renal vessels.

TOXICOLOGY

Amylene hydrate is a strong narcotic, and in high dosage to animals narcosis is preceded by a phase of excitement. There is one report of organic damage to the liver when given in repeated dosage. As a sleeping draught to human beings it has caused prolonged unconsciousness, and in one case a fatal issue, though it was not regarded as the sole cause of death (see p. 360).

Toxicity to animals

(a) Lethal dose, (oral), for rabbits, 1.5 g/kg (Kochmann, 1923); 2.5 ml/kg (Munch and Schwartze, 1925); 1.6 to 1.9 g/kg (Sollman and Hanzlik, 1928); for rats, 1 g/kg (Schaffarzick, 1952); for dogs, 1.5 g/kg (Kochmann, 1923).

(b) Narcotic dose, (oral and subcutaneous), for rabbits, 1 g/kg (Kochmann).

SYMPTOMS OF INTOXICATION

In dogs, but not in rabbits or guinea pigs, narcosis is preceded by a stage of excitement and later convulsions, and with lethal dosage a rise of temperature. In dogs,

Guggenheim and Loffler (1916) stated that habituation was produced with repeated dosage, but Biberfeld (1918) did not observe this in rabbits.

In rabbits, with large dosage, rapid and deep respiration may be followed by slow and superficial respiration, leading eventually to respiratory paralysis.

CHANGES IN THE ORGANISM

In rabbits given repeated doses over a period of 8 months, Straus (1887) observed some organic change in the liver.

Toxicity to human beings

Two cases of severe intoxication, following ingestion or administration of an enema of amylene hydrate have been recorded. The case of ingestion was that of a suicidal attempt described by Anker in 1892. A woman who drank 27 g became completely unconscious within half an hour, with a small rapid pulse, dilated pupils but normal respiration. The next day the breathing became rapid and sterterous, the pulse irregular and the pupils contracted. Under treatment by stimulants she recovered completely after 14 days with no sign of lung involvement.

In another case, recorded by von Hueber (1917) ingestion of 18 g of undiluted amylene hydrate was followed by complete unconsciousness which lasted 4 h in spite of treatment with caffeine and suprarenin, and deep sleep for 30 h. Later, gross restlessness, pain in the limbs, headache and giddiness were eventually follwed by slow recovery.

The fatal case, following administration of an enema, was that of Jacobi and Speer (1920) described in detail on p. 360.

Bibliography on p. 401

42. Hexanols

42a. 4-Methylpentanol-2

Synonyms: methyl amyl alcohol, methylisobutyl carbinol

Structural formula:
$$CH_3—CH—CH_2—CH—CH_3$$
$$\quad\quad\;\; |\quad\quad\quad\;\; |$$
$$\quad\quad CH_3\quad\quad OH$$

Molecular formula: $C_6H_{14}O$

Properties: a colourless liquid
  boiling point: 132.0 °C
  vapour pressure: 3.52 at 20 °C
  specific gravity (liquid density): 0.8079
  flash point: 130 °F
  conversion factors: 1 p.p.m. = 4.17 mg/m³
                      1 mg/l = 239.3 p.p.m.
  solubility: in water 1.7% at 20 °C; freely in ethyl alcohol, hydrocarbons and most organic solvents.
  maximum allowable concentration: not established

ECONOMY, SOURCES AND USES

Production

By reduction of mesityl oxide in acetic acid solution, with platinum (Kirk and Othmer, 1947).

Industrial uses

(1) In manufacture of lubricant additives, solvents, plasticisers, lacquers and flotation agents (Treon, 1963).
(2) In brake fluids as a frothing agent (Treon, 1963).
(3) In organic synthesis.

BIOCHEMISTRY

Metabolism

From the investigation of Kamil *et al.* (1953) it appears that methyl isobutyl carbinol undergoes in the rabbit some glucuronic acid conjugation. The average amount of glucuronide excreted following a dose administered by stomach tube was 33.7% of the dose. This compares with 6.7% in the case of *n*-amyl alcohol.

The urine contained also a small amount of a methyl ketone (presumably isobutyl methyl ketone) and after extraction with 1:4 ethanol/ether a glucuronide (triacetyl methyl ester) gum.

TOXICOLOGY

The only details of the toxic dosage for animals are given by Smyth, Carpenter and Weil (1951) in their List IV of Range Finding Data. From these it appears that the LD_{50} for rats by single oral dose is 2.59 g/kg; for rabbits by skin absorption 3.56 ml/kg. By inhalation 2000 p.p.m. for 8 h killed 5 out of 6 rats, but no deaths occurred from inhalation of saturated vapour for 2 h.

No toxic effects in human beings have been recorded.

42b. 2-Ethylbutanol-1

Synonym: 2-ethylbutyl alcohol

Structural formula:
$$CH_3-CH_2-\overset{\displaystyle CH_2-CH_3}{\overset{\displaystyle |}{CH}}-CH_2-OH$$

Molecular formula: $C_6H_{14}O$

Molecular weight: 102.178

Properties: a colourless liquid
  boiling point: 149.4 °C
  vapour pressure: 1.80 mm Hg at 20 °C
  specific gravity (liquid density): 0.828
  flash point: 135 °F
  conversion factors: 1 p.p.m. $= 4.17$ mg/m³
          1 mg/l $= 239.3$ p.p.m.
  maximum allowable concentration: not established

Bibliography on p. 401

ECONOMY, SOURCES AND USES

Production

By aldol condensation of acetaldehyde and butyraldehyde (Treon, 1963).

Industrial uses

(1) As a solvent for printing inks.
(2) As a component of lacquers.
(3) In manufacture of synthetic lubricants and lubricant additives (Doolittle, 1954).

BIOCHEMISTRY

Metabolism

As in the case of methylisobutyl carbinol and other alipathic alcohols, 2-ethyl-butanol conjugates, but even more readily, with glucuronic acid. Kamil *et al.* (1953) found that the glucuronide excretion in the rabbit corresponded to 40% of the dose given, and they were able to isolate from the urine a small amount of methyl propyl ketone and diethyl acetyl glucuronide. The high degree of conjugation was believed to be due not to the conjugation of the alcohol itself with glucuronic acid, but to the conjugation of its oxidation products. Diethyl acetyl glucuronide is an ester glucuronide of fatty acid, and appears to be more stable than aromatic ester glucuronides such as benzoyl glucuronide. It is not entirely resistant, however, as shown by the production of the small amount of methyl-*n*-propyl ketone, which was presumed to arise by decarboxylation of ethyl aceto-acetic acid.

TOXICOLOGY

From the results of animal experiments by Smyth *et al.* (1954) 2-ethyl butanol appears to be more toxic by oral administration and skin absorption than methyl amyl alcohol. For rats, they give the single dose LD_{50} as 1.85 g/kg and by skin absorption 1.26 ml/kg. By intraperitonal injection Fasset (1963, cited by Treon, 1963) gives the LD_{50} as 0.80 g/kg for the rat and 0.459 g/kg for the guinea pig. By inhalation, according to Treon (1963) 'concentrated vapour' for 8 h caused no deaths.

No symptoms of poisoning in animals or human beings have been recorded.

43. Heptanol

Synonyms: methylcyclohexanol, hexahydrocresol, methylhexalin, methyl adronol, hexahydromethylphenol, methylanol, Sextol.

Structural formula: $CH_3-CH_2-CH_2-CH_2-CH_2-CH_2-CH_2-OH$

Molecular formula: $C_7H_{15}OH$

Properties: a colourless oily liquid, with a camphor-like odour similar to but weaker than that of cyclohexanol and amyl alcohol. As a solvent it is similar to, but not so powerful as cyclohexanol

    boiling range: of the technical product 173.0–175.3 °C

    vapour pressure: 1.5 mm at 30 °C

    specific gravity (liquid density): 0.913

    flash point: 154 °F

    conversion factors: 1 p.p.m. = 4.67 mg/m³

                        1 mg/l = 214.2 p.p.m.

    solubility: in water 3% (Durrans, 1950). Solvent for fats, oils, gums, resins, waxes, rubber and cellulose esters.

    evaporation rate: volatility very low, half the rate of cyclohexanol, 0.2 mg /min/cm² (Flury and Zernik, 1931).

    maximum allowable concentration: 100 p.p.m. (Threshold Limit Values, 1962).

ECONOMY, SOURCES AND USES

Production

By the hydrogenation of cresol.

Industrial uses

(1) In soap manufacture, as a good auxiliary solvent for dry cleaning soaps (Bird, 1932).

(2) In the textile industry as an addition to soap solutions for cellulose acetate silk (Clayton and Clark, 1931).

(3) In the lacquer industry (Doolittle, 1954).

(4) As a degreaser, in the form of 'Cykloran M'.

(5) As an antioxidant in lubricants (Doolittle, 1954).

BIOCHEMISTRY

Estimation in the atmosphere

By the same method (reaction with catechol and H_2SO_4) as that described for cyclohexanol by Treon *et al.* (1943).

Metabolism

Methylcyclohexanol is readily absorbed by the intact skin, as shown by its severe, even lethal, toxic effects on animals (Treon *et al.*, 1943).

Like cyclohexanol it is conjugated in the body with glucuronic acid (Pohl, 1925) to about 45–50% of the dose (Treon *et al.*). These observers have also demonstrated some conjugation with H_2SO_4, but Williams (1959) states that the conjugated glucuronides have not been identified; he states moreover that methylcyclohexanol has not been shown to be aromatised in the body.

TOXICOLOGY

It was stated by Filippi (1914) that the ortho-isomer is more toxic than the other two. Its toxic effects in animals are largely those of parenchymal and vascular damage, with congestion and in the case of the brain, oedema. It is also an irritant of mucous membranes, especially the eyes, and while narcotic when given by mouth in large doses, it causes by inhalation only lethargy. In human beings no serious toxic effects have been reported, though its vapour has proved irritating to the eyes and throat.

Toxicity to animals

(a) Lethal dose. – *(i) By oral administration*, for rabbits 1.75–2.0 g/kg (Treon *et al.* 1943). – *(ii) By application to the skin*, 6.8–9.4 g/kg. – *(iii) By inhalation*, no concentration has been found lethal.

Pohl (1925) found no signs of intoxication in a dog exposed to air saturated with methylcyclohexanol 10 min a day for 7 consecutive days, and Treon *et al.* (1943) no symptoms following exposure to 121 and 232 p.p.m. 6 h a day for 10 weeks. At 503 p.p.m. however some symptoms of intoxication did develop.

(b) Narcotic dose. – *(i) By oral administration*, for dogs, Pohl (1925) gave 1.4 ml/kg; for rabbits (Treon *et al.*, 1943) amounts greater than 1 g/kg. – *(ii) By inhalation*, only lethargy, not true narcosis, was produced even by concentrations of 500 mg/l (Treon *et al.*, 1943).

SYMPTOMS OF INTOXICATION

Symptoms of poisoning are more marked following oral administration and skin application than by inhalation. When given orally in a dosage of more than 1 g/kg these take the form of twitching and narcosis, and by skin application weakness, tremors, hypothermia, convulsive movements and deep narcosis followed by death if the application of 10 ml to the intact skin is continued for 1 h on 6 successive days. The skin itself shows petechiae, irritation and thickening. Application of a 15% mixture of methylcyclohexanol and potassium oleate caused only erythema and superficial sloughing.

CHANGES IN THE ORGANISM

With fatal, oral intoxication toxic vascular and congestive changes were found by Treon et al. (1943) in the liver, kidneys, heart, lungs and brain, in the brain accompanied by oedema.

In sublethal dosage and by inhalation, only in the liver were diffuse degenerative changes observed; with inhalation of lower concentration (121 p.p.m.) these changes were of questionable significance when compared with control animals.

Toxicity to human beings

The only suggestion of toxic effects from the industrial use of methylcyclohexanol comes from a report of an examination of workers using a cellulose solvent for safety glass containing 5 parts of methylcyclohexanol (Browning, 1953). Out of 16 workers examined in 1933, 1934 and 1935, the only symptoms complained of were irritation of the eyes and throat. Blood examinations showed a very slight relative lymphocytosis in one. This was not considered significant evidence of a toxic effect of methylcyclohexanol. Treon et al, (1943) remark, however, that headache and respiratory and ocular iritation may result from prolonged exposure to excessive concentrations of methylcyclohexanol vapour.

44. Nonanol

Synonym: nonyl alcohol.

Structural formula: $CH_3-CH_2-CH_2-CH_2-CH_2-CH_2-CH_2-CH_2-CH_2-OH$

Molecular formula: $C_9H_{19}OH$

Properties: nonyl alcohol is rarely used as a pure substance. It may contain differing proportions of different isomers, according to its method of preparation. The two chief components are isobutyl carbinol and 3,5,5-trimethyl hexanol; another variety contains 2% of 2-propylheptanol. The physical and toxicological properties of the nonyl alcohol depend largely on the predominance of one or other of these constituents, and their toxic effects on animals have usually been described in terms of these rather than of the nonyl alcohol *per se.* The following physical properties of those nonyl alcohols and of the separate constituents which have been described are quoted from the account by Treon (1963).

(a) rich in trimethyl hexanols – colourless liquid.
 boiling point: 187–208 °C
 specific gravity (liquid density): 0.845

(b) containing 2% of 2-propyl heptanol.
 boiling point: 192 °C
 vapour pressure: 40 mm at 129 °C
 specific gravity (liquid density): 0.8274

(c) 3,5,5-trimethyl hexanol.
 boiling point: 193–194 °C
 specific gravity (liquid density): 0.8236

(d) di-isobutyl carbinol
 boiling point: 178.1 °C
 vapour pressure: 0.21 at 20 °C
 specific gravity (liquid density): 0.809

 solubility: all are insoluble in water except diisobutyl carbinol, which is soluble to the extent of 0.06% at 20 °C (Doolittle, 1954).
 conversion factors: 1 p.p.m. = 5.90 mg/m³
  1 mg/l = 169.6 p.p.m.

[374]

PRODUCTION SOURCES AND USES

Industrial uses

The diisobutyl component is used (1) as a solvent for coatings of urea and melamine resins, (2) as a reforming agent, (3) in the preparation of lubricant additives and plasticizers (Doolittle, 1954).

BIOCHEMISTRY

Metabolism

Direct glucuronic conjugation takes place to the extent of 4.1%, but no formation of ester glucuronides as in the case of methyl amyl alcohol and 2-ethyl butyl alcohol; this indicates that there is rapid oxidation with little inhibition (Williams, 1959).

TOXICOLOGY

From the relatively few animal experiments recorded, it appears that trimethyl hexanol, and the nonyl alcohol containing it, is considerably more toxic than diisobutyl carbinol and its corresponding nonyl alcohol.

Diisobutyl carbinol itself was stated by Smyth, Carpenter and Weil (1949) to have an oral toxicity for rats (LD_{50} after 14 days) of 3.56 g/kg, and by skin absorption for rabbits of 5.66 g/kg.

By comparison, for a nonyl alcohol rich in trimethylhexanol, the lethal oral dose for rats was found by Treon (1963) to be 1.4 to 1.75 ml/kg and for rabbits 1.4 to 2.1. By skin absorption for rats the LD_{50} was less than 3.6 ml/kg.

A nonyl alcohol containing 2% of 2-propylheptanol has also been examined by Fassett (1963). Orally, its toxicity for the rat approximates to the diisobutyl carbinol product (3.2 to 6.4 g/kg) and by skin absorption the LD_{50} of 10 ml/kg shows it to be less toxic for the guinea pig than either diisobutyl carbinol or trimethyl hexanol for the rabbit.

By inhalation, only diisobutyl carbinol and the nonyl alcohol containing 2-propylheptanol have been investigated, and neither the former saturated vapour for 8 h, (Smyth *et al.*, 1949) nor the latter (215 and 730 p.p.m., Fassett, 1963) has proved fatal ro rats.

SYMPTOMS OF INTOXICATION

The most irritative of the different isomers is apparently the alcohol rich in trimethyl hexanol. This, in the rabbit, caused erythema with slight necrosis, while the alcohol containing propyl heptanol caused only moderate irritation, and diisobutyl carbinol, when applied undiluted, caused none (Smyth *et al.*, 1949).

On human skin and mucous membranes of the tongue and lower lip, Oettel (1936), who gave no description of the variety of the nonyl alcohol used, included it in the list of those compounds which left the unbroken skin completely normal and resistant to irritation by mechanical and chemical means.

CHANGES IN THE ORGANISM

Treon (1963) has described the autopsy lesions in animals fatally poisoned by the trimethyl hexanol product of nonyl alcohol rich in trimethyl hexanol, presumably by oral administration, since he gives no results of inhalation of this compound.

Brain, liver and kidneys all showed injury. In the brain, the neurons showed degenerative changes. In the liver degeneration was pronounced in the central area; in the kidneys it was accompanied by frequent necrosis of the epithelium of the tubules and glomeruli. Kitzmiller is cited as having observed slight degenerative changes in the myocardium.

45. Allyl Alcohol

Synonyms: 2-propenol-1-ol, vinyl carbinol

Structural formula: $CH_2=CH-CH_2-OH$

Molecular formula: C_3H_6O

Molecular weight: 58.081

Properties: a colourless pungent liquid, miscible with water, alcohol and ether.
    boiling point: 96.9 °C
    vapour pressure: 23.8 mm Hg at 25 °C
    specific gravity (liquid density): 0.8476 at 25 °C
    vapour density (air $=1$): 2.00
    conversion factors: 1 p.p.m. = 2.37 mg/m³
                          1 mg/l = 422 p.p.m.
    maximum allowable concentration: 2 p.p.m.

It does not corrode metals (Dunlap *et al.*, 1958).

ECONOMY, SOURCES AND USES

Production

(1) From glycerine and oxalic acid (Miessner, 1891).
(2) By conversion of propylene into allyl chloride by high-temperature chlorination, with subsequent acidic or basal hydrolysis (Dunlap *et al.*, 1958).

According to Atkinson (1925) allyl alcohol is present as an impurity in methyl alcohol, in quantities sufficient to cause toxic effects. It was found to the extent of 0.5% in a sample labelled pure methyl alcohol.

Industrial uses

(1) In the chemical industry, in the production of derivatives used in perfumes, flavorings, pharmaceuticals; also for denaturing alcohol.
(2) In the production of resins and esters.

BIOCHEMISTRY

Estimation

(1) In the atmosphere

The method suggested by Dunlap *et al.* (1958), based on that described by Reid and Beddard (1954), consists in adding 0.01 N bromine in acetic acid, in the presence of mercuric acetate as a catalyst, to an aqueous sample containing the vapour of allyl alcohol, reducing the excess bromine by iodine and titration with 0.01 N thiosulphate.

(2) In blood

The method used by Kodama and Hine (1958) depends on diffusion of the allyl alcohol into potassium dichromate in H_2SO_4, reaction of the unreacted dichromate with potassium iodide and starch solution, and spectrophotometric measurement of the resulting blue colour.

Metabolism

Miessner (1891) found no allyl alcohol in the urine of animals to which it had been administered by subcutaneous and intravenous injection, and concluded that it was entirely metabolised. It has since been suggested, though not with complete agreement, that acrolein might be an intermediate metabolic product, since allyl alcohol produced in animals a condition of shock similar to that produced by acrolein. Kodama and Hine (1958) have considered that this might be possible but they do not believe that the metabolic production of acrolein is necessary to explain entirely the high toxicity of allyl alcohol. They point out that in the first place there is no evidence that acrolein can produce the periportal necrosis of the liver observed in animals poisoned by allyl alcohol (Dunlap *et al.*, 1958) and in the second place that the inhibition of liver hydrogenases by acrolein is 400–1000 times greater than that of allyl alcohol. They believe that the molecule of allyl alcohol itself has a direct action on the permeability of the membrane of the liver cells, leading to abnormal hepatocellular swelling, leakage of intracellular chromatogenic substances and osmotic disruption of the cell metabolism. This toxic effect is apparently increased by the production of shock, a constant feature of acute allyl alcohol poisoning, since the hypotension and haemoconcentration decrease the flow of blood to the liver and to the respiratory centre, with consequent decrease of oxygenation of the blood. There is apparently no accumulation in the body, and tolerance develops with repeated exposure to non-lethal concentrations.

TOXICOLOGY

Allyl alcohol has long been recognised as an extremely toxic substance to animals

Miessner (1891) stated that it was about 50 times as toxic to mice as propyl alcohol, and Atkinson (1925) that its toxicity based on the lethal dose was about 150 times that of methyl alcohol.

Among its acute toxic effects in animals – irritation of mucous membranes, especially of the eyes and lungs, with pulmonary effusion, congestion of internal organs and marked lowering of the blood pressure as a sequence of injury to the heart and blood vessels – an outstanding feature is necrosis of the periportal areas of the liver; its true narcotic effect is essentially low. This injury to the liver was a special phenomenon observed by Kodama and Hine (1958).

In human beings the only injurious effects noted have been severe irritation of mucous membranes, especially of the eyes; severe eye injury was observed by Carpenter and Smyth (1946). No cases of severe systemic intoxication following industrial exposure have been recorded.

Toxicity to animals

(1) Acute

Lethal dose. – *(i) By oral administration*, LD_{50} for rats, 0.064 g/kg, compared with 5.84 for isopropyl alcohol and about the same as for ethylene chlorohydrin (Smyth and Carpenter, 1948). – *(ii) By penetration of the skin*, for rabbits, 0.053 ml/kg compared with 16.4 for isopropyl alcohol. – *(iii) By inhalation*, for rats, 1000 p.p.m. caused death to 4 out of 6 animals in 1 h compared with 16,000 p.p.m. in 8 h for isopropyl alcohol, while 250 p.p.m. killed 2, 3 or 4 out of 6 in 4 h compared with 16,000 p.p.m. in 7-8 h for isopropyl alcohol (Carpenter *et al.*, 1949). McCord (1932) also found 1000 p.p.m. lethal to rats, rabbits and monkeys after 3 to 4 h, and 50 p.p.m. to rats in an average of 30 days. Dunlap and Hine (1955) give the LD_{50} for one hour exposure to rats as 1060 p.p.m.

(2) Chronic

(i) By repeated oral administration of solutions of allyl alcohol in the drinking water, the peak intake averaging 72 mg/kg/day, caused very few signs of abnormality. Loss of weight, transient pulmonary râles and crustiness of the eyelids were not accompanied by other signs of illness, and the only organic abnormalities observed were local areas of necrosis in the liver (Dunlap *et al.*, 1958). – *(ii) By inhalation* repeated exposure of rats to 40, 60 and 100 p.p.m. (Dunlap *et al.*, 1958) caused gasping, severe depression, and nasal discharge, and at the highest levels some animals died by the 10th exposure. With lower exposures (5 and 10 p.p.m. 5 days a week for 13 weeks) Dunlap and Hine (1955) found no gross evidence of toxicity to rats, nor did Torkelson *et al.* (1959) in rats, rabbits, guinea pigs and dogs exposed to 2 p.p.m. and 7 p.p.m. 7 h a day for six months, as judged by growth, mortality or final weight of body or organs, but those exposed to 7 p.p.m. showed degenerative changes in liver and kidneys. The liver showed cloudy swelling and focal necrosis, and the kidneys necrosis of the convoluted

Bibliography on p. 401

tubules and proliferation of interstitial tissue; these changes were mild and reversible. In the animals exposed to 2 p.p.m. there were some changes in blood urea nitrogen and blood non-protein nitrogen but these were not considered significant or due to the allyl alcohol.

SYMPTOMS OF INTOXICATION

(1)   *The eyes*

Application to the eyes causes erythema of the conjunctiva and swelling of the cornea, sometimes with opacity, but no permanent injury.

(2)   *The skin*

Application to the skin causes only slight erythema lasting about 48 h.

(3)   *The blood*

Intravenous injection of a small dose (3 minims) was found by Carlier (1911) to produce a characteristic fall in blood pressure (also noted by later observers) with a slower rise followed by a further fall. Injection of 40 minims in a 20% solution of normal saline (equal to 8 minims of pure alcohol) caused an initial rise followed by a fall and then another rise, until violent convulsions supervened.

(4)   *Gastro-intestinal disturbance*

Oral administration causes irritation with vomiting and diarrhoea, convulsive movements, apathy, occasionally ataxia, profuse lacrimation, and occasionally coma preceding death (Atkinson, 1925; Dunlap *et al.*, 1958).

(5)   *Neurological disturbances*

By inhalation. The earlier work of Miessner (1891) with exposure of mice to air saturated with allyl alcohol was extensively confirmed by later observers. Dunlap *et al.* (1958) in particular noted the peculiar apathy, as distinct from the classical signs of narcosis by organic solvents.

CHANGES IN THE ORGANISM

Oedema and congestion of the lungs; congestion and necrosis of the liver; cloudy swelling of the kidneys.

The lungs

No effect on the lungs was noted by Dunlap *et al.* (1958) following repeated exposure to 20 p.p.m., and Torkelson *et al.* (1959) state that, from their experiments with exposure to 2 and 7 p.p.m., there was no detectable lung injury at these levels. In their Table showing the mortality and its cause in animals receiving the 2 p.p.m. exposure, it may be noted that though one exposed rat developed a very severe lung infection, so also did five of the unexposed or air-exposed controls.

Industrial poisoning

Few cases of industrial toxic effects have been reported. Torkelson *et al.* (1959) remark that concentrations likely to be injurious in a short period of time will be painful to the eyes and nose. 5 p.p.m. are probably detectable by most people and even 2 p.p.m. by the odour, but not by irritation. According to Dunlap *et al.* (1958) workmen handling allyl alcohol where there is a possiblility of moderate air contamination complain of lacrimation, at the level of 25 p.p.m. and have reported immediate eye irritation, with retrobulbar pain and photophobia and muscular spasm (deep 'bone ache') resulting from absorption through the skin. Contact with the skin for 70 min has been stated by Oettel (1936) to cause pain, erythema and hyperaemia.

A case of systemic injury was recorded by Flury and Zernik (1931) in a chemist who showed not only local irritation but also general malaise, dyspnoea and disturbance of accomodation. Browning (1953) observed two cases of gastrointestinal disturbance – nausea and vomiting – and severe headache, and in one slight haemoptysis, following spillage of allyl alcohol from a cask on to the floor and their clothing, while some of the vapour was blown into a shed where they were working. Both eventually recovered completely.

Preventive measures outlined by Torkelson *et al.* (1959) include the provision of closed systems, or if this is not feasible, respiratory protection by exhaust ventilation, or, following spills, full face masks, respirators or self-contained breathing apparatus. Eyes should be prevented from contact by means of goggles, and the skin by protective clothing and shoes.

Bibliography on p. 401

46. Furfuryl Alcohol

Synonyms: 2-furyl carbinol, 2-furanmethanol

Structural formula:

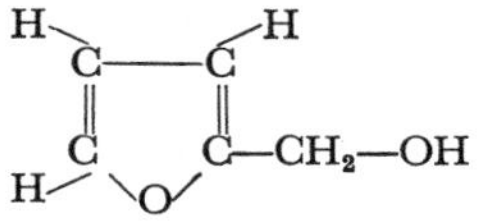

$$\begin{array}{c} \text{H} \diagdown \quad \diagup \text{H} \\ \text{C} — \text{C} \\ \| \qquad \| \\ \text{C} \qquad \text{C} — \text{CH}_2 — \text{OH} \\ \text{H} \diagup \diagdown \text{O} \diagup \end{array}$$

Molecular formula: $C_5H_6O_2$

Molecular weight: 98.103

Properties: a colourless syrupy liquid, turning amber during storage (Doolittle, 1954), and black in the presence of air (Kirk and Othmer, 1951). Its odour in the atmosphere is detectable at 8 p.p.m. (Jacobson *et al.*, 1958).

> *boiling point:* 171 °C (technical 166–177 °C)
> *vapour pressure:* 1 mm at 31.8 °C
> *specific gravity (liquid density):* 1.1287 (technical 1.134)
> *flash point:* 167 °F
> *conversion factors:* 1 p.p.m. = 4.01 mg/m³
>   1 mg/l = 249.4 p.p.m.
> *solubility:* miscible with water in all proportions above 21 °C; and with most organic solvents, but not petroleum hydrocarbons or most oils (Mellan, 1950). Solvent for cellulose esters and ethers, ester gum, natural and coumarone resins (Treon, 1963).
> *maximum allowable concentration:* 50 p.p.m. (A.C.G.I.H., 1962).

ECONOMY, SOURCES AND USES

Production

By partial hydrogenation of furfural under high pressure in the presence of metal catalysts (Durrans, 1950).

Industrial uses

(1) In the manufacture of abrasive wheels.
(2) In the textile industry as a solvent for dyes.
(3) As a liquid propellant (Jacobson *et al.*, 1958) – a major component of 'Corporal' missile fuel (Williams, 1959).

BIOCHEMISTRY

Estimation in the atmosphere

The method used by Comstock and Oberst (1952) is the addition of 0.05 N pyridine bromine sulphate to glacial acetic acid through which the furfuryl alcohol has been passed, and, after 1 h in the dark, addition of 5% KI and titration with 0.1 N $Na_2S_2O_3$.

Metabolism

Furfuryl alcohol is oxidised to furoic acid, which is excreted as the glycine conjugate furoyl glycine (Williams, 1959). Paul, Austin *et al.* (1949) also concluded that furoyl glycine was the major end product in the urine of rats after feeding furfuryl alcohol. Fine and Wills (1950) on the basis of intravenous injection into rabbits and the agreement between their calculation of the lethal dose and that of Gajewski and Alsdorf (1949) suggest that the furfuryl alcohol is distributed equally through most or all of the body water and that it has probably little specific action on enzyme systems localised in special structures, though it appears to have a slight predilection for the brain. Galewski and Alsdorf found a marked difference between the oral and intravenous toxicity to rats, and gave as the probable explanation the fact that it is very unstable in an acid medium and therefore destroyed to some extent by the gastric juice.

TOXICOLOGY

The essential toxic effect of furfuryl alcohol is that of a central nervous depressant. While small doses stimulate respiration in man and animals (Erdmann, 1902) large doses depress it, lower the body temperature and cause nausea, salivation, diarrhoea, dizziness and diuresis. According to Okubo (1937) dilute solutions paralyse the sensory nerves and skeletal muscles and have a slight antispasmodic effect on smooth muscle. With high dosage death from respiratory paralysis has been reported by Galewski and Alsdorf (1949). Its action on the heart is probably exerted directly on the myocardium and does not affect special conduction of impulses (Fine and Wills, 1950).

No toxic effects in human beings have been recorded.

Toxicity to animals

(1) Acute

Lethal dose. – *(i) By oral administration*, for rats, as a 2% solution, 275 mg/kg (Galewski and Alsdorf, 1949). – *(ii) By subcutaneous injection*, for rabbits, as a 10% solution, 600 mg/kg (Erdmann, 1902). – *(iii) By intravenous injection*, for rabbits,

Bibliography on p. 401

as a 10% solution, 650 mg/kg (Galewski and Alsdorf, 1949); calculated from isolated rabbit heart and intestine, 700 mg/kg (Fine and Wills, 1950). – *(iv) By
inhalation*, for rats, 233 p.p.m. for 4 h (Torkelson *et al.*, 1959).

(2) Chronic

   Galewski and Alsdorf (1949) found when furfuryl alcohol was administered
to rats in drinking water over a period of 20 days it caused marked anorexia and
loss of weight.

SYMPTOMS OF INTOXICATION

Intravenous injection causes a flaccid paralysis which becomes permanent with
larger doses; also a slight anti-spasmodic effect on smooth muscle (Fine and Wills,
1950). The blood pressure shows a slight temporary fall following intravenous
injection of 100 mg/kg, but when the dose is increased to 600 mg/kg, each extra
dose of 100 mg causes a very severe fall with temporary apnoea. The action of the
heart, became, in these experiments by Fine and Wills, completely disorganised
after a dose increased to the lethal level, with a picture similar to that produced
by anaesthetics, but could be combated with central nervous stimulants such as
Benzidine or Metrazol. The cardiac depression and final disruption of function
was not believed to be the actual cause of death; this was due to depression of the
respiratory centre.

Toxicity to human beings

It is stated by Treon (1963) that the ordinary industrial use of furfuryl alcohol
for 20 years has caused no impairment of health.

47. Cyclohexanol

Synonyms: hexahydrophenol, hexalin, cyclohexyl alcohol, Sextol, Adronol, Anol

Structural formula:

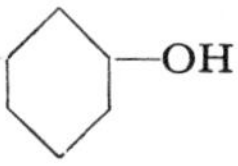

Molecular formula: $C_6H_{11}OH$

Molecular weight: 100.162

Properties: an oily colourless liquid with an odour like camphor and alcohol.
   boiling point: 161 °C
   vapour pressure: 3.5 mm at 34 °C
   specific gravity (liquid density): 0.9493
   flash point: 63 °C
   vapour density (air = 1): 3.46
   conversion factors: 1 p.p.m. = 4.10 mg/m³
                1 mg/l   = 244.1 p.p.m.
   evaporation rate: (ether = 1): 400
   maximum allowable concentration: 50 p.p.m. (Threshold Limit Values, 1962);
   Elkins (1959) suggests 25 p.p.m.

ECONOMY, SOURCES AND USES

Solvent for fats, oils, waxes, rubber and cellulose esters and alkyl resins. Poor solvent for nitrocellulose. Has a strong emulsifying action when added to mineral oils.

Production

(1) By catalytic hydrogenation of phenol at high temperature and pressure.
(2) By catalytic oxidation of cyclohexane in the liquid phase at 100–250 °C (Kirk and Othmer, 1949).

Industrial uses

(1) In soap manufacture, to form clear aqueous soap solutions and to increase their detergent properties.
(2) In the textile and artificial silk industry, added to fulling and scouring soap

emulsions (Clayton and Clark, 1931); in the peroxide bleaching of cotton, by dissolving the natural wax; and for removing paint, tar and oil spots from raw wool and cloth (Reid, 1934).

(3) In the lacquer industry, to prevent 'blushing' (Sanderson, 1933).

(4) In the leather industry, for cleaning skins and as a spray with butyl acetate.

(5) In the printing industry (Sato, 1928).

(6) In the straw hat industry (Reid, 1934).

(7) In furniture and metal polishes (Sanderson, 1933).

(8) In the plastics industry, as an intermediate in the preparation of plasticisers (Mellan, 1950; Doolittle, 1954).

BIOCHEMISTRY

Estimation in the atmosphere

In the method described by Treon, Crutchfield and Kitzmiller (1943) the vapour in a sample of air is extracted by shaking with 100 ml of water, and to an aliquot of 2 ml is added 1 ml of 5% aqueous catechol, and then 10 ml of concentrated H_2SO_4. After standing 30 min in a water bath at 100 °C, and then cooled, the intensity of the straw colour produced is compared colorimetrically with a standard curve.

Metabolism

Animal experiments have led to the conclusion that there is no appreciably prolonged retention in the organism, though in large doses it is readily absorbed from the skin (Treon *et al.*, 1943). These observers, and Elliott *et al.* (1959), in contrast to Bernhard (1937) and Weitzel (1950), have found that some of the dose is excreted as conjugated glucuronic acid – 45 to 50% of the dose (Treon *et al.*, 1943); more than 65%, with about 6% as trans-cyclohexane-1,2-diol (Elliott *et al.*).

Pohl (1925) did find, with oral administration, some glucuronic acid in the urine of a dog, but Bernhard (1937) was unable to detect any urinary metabolites in dogs to which it was given subcutaneously dissolved in olive oil because its strong taste made it impossible to give by mouth.

Treon *et al.* (1943) noted that the increase in glucuronic acid in the urine was paralleled by a decrease in the percentage of inorganic sulphates. It was the fact that the urinary sulphate ratio became normal when exposure ceased which led them to conclude that there was no prolonged retention in the organism.

TOXICOLOGY

Cyclohexanol is to some extent a narcotic to animals, causing lethargy, ataxia, loss of reflexes and finally narcosis, followed in very high dosage by death, whether given orally, by inhalation or by application to the intact skin. It is interesting to note that even without direct contact of the vapour with the eyes, it can cause lacrimation in animals when applied to the skin as a constituent of soaps. With oral administration also it can cause lacrimation, diarrhoea and mild convulsions, but with inhalation only a few mild convulsions occur. The narcosis, if the dosage is less than lethal, is recovered from in $5\frac{1}{2}$ to 16 h.

It causes injury to the liver and kidneys, perceptible even with fairly low dosage (145 p.p.m.) but this is not a specific injury, being the expression of general vascular damage and the inflammatory reaction to it. It has no benzene-like effect on the haemopoietic organs, and is not considered to be a serious hazard in industrial use owing to its low vapour pressure and rate of evaporation. In fact only one case, and that of doubtful etiology, has ever been recorded.

Toxicity to animals

Lethal dose. – (i) By oral administration, for rabbits, the LD_{50} was 2.2 to 2.6 g/kg (Treon et al., 1943). – (ii) Bu inhalation, for rabbits, the LD_{50} was 997 to 1229 p.p.m. for 6 h a day, 5 days a week (Treon et al., 1943); Pohl (1925) was unable to observe any ill effects in a dog exposed to air saturated with cyclohexanol for 10 min per day on 7 successive days. – (iii) By skin application, for rabbits, the LD_{50} was 12.7 to 22.7 g/kg (Treon et al., 1943).

SYMPTOMS OF INTOXICATION

(i) By oral administration, Treon et al. (1943) observed diarrhoea, ataxia, lethargy, narcosis, collapse, loss of reflexes and death, but no convulsions. Animals which survived recovered from the narcosis in 5.5 to 16 h.

(ii) By skin application, there was a fall in temperature, jerking and twitching of the limbs and chest muscles and narcosis. Application of soaps containing up to 15% of cyclohexanol caused only slight local effects, but the higher concentrations caused some lacrimation which, it was presumed, was the result of absorption from the skin, since there was practically no vaporisation of cyclohexanol from the soap.

At high sub-lethal concentrations convulsions occurred.

CHANGES IN THE ORGANISM

Lethal and high sublethal doses caused severe generalised endothelial injury, with vascular lesions in the brain, heart, lungs, liver, spleen and kidneys, while even

Bibliography on p. 401

relatively low concentrations (145 p.p.m.) produced slight, hardly demonstrable degenerative changes in the liver and kidneys. The most severely affected animals showed massive coagulation necrosis of these organs, as well as of the myocardium, lungs and brain.

The blood

In 1928 Sato, by intraperitoneal injection of cyclohexanol, noted the appearance of polymorphonuclear leucocytosis, but neither he nor Treon *et al.* (1943) found any evidence of the specific benzene effect on the haemopoietic system.

Toxicity to human beings

The only account of a possible industrial toxic effect of cyclohexanol was reported to the Home Office, Great Britain (1932). A worker using a spray for leather which contained 3 parts of cyclohexanol and butyl acetate, complained of vomiting, a coated tongue and slight tremor. After investigation it was decided that there was not sufficient evidence to attribute these symptoms definitely to cyclohexanol.

No other cases of ill effects from the industrial use of cyclohexanol have been recorded.

48. Diacetone Alcohol

Synonyms: 2-methyl-2-pentanol-4-one, 4-hydroxy-4-methyl-2-pentanone, Pyraton A

Structural formula:

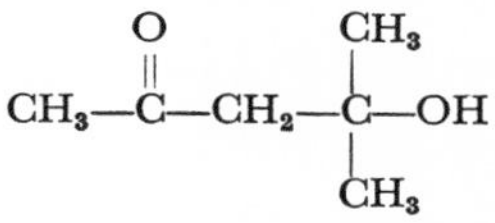

$$CH_3-\overset{\overset{\displaystyle O}{\|}}{C}-CH_2-\overset{\overset{\displaystyle CH_3}{|}}{\underset{\underset{\displaystyle CH_3}{|}}{C}}-OH$$

Molecular formula: $C_6H_{12}O_2$

Molecular weight: 116.162

Properties: a colourless liquid which becomes yellowish on standing; unless neutral or slightly alkaline will decompose to acetone (Mellan, 1950).

  boiling point: 169.2 °C (boiling range of commercial product: 160–170 °C)
  vapour pressure: 1.2 mm at 25 °C
  vapour density (air = 1): 4.01
  specific gravity (liquid density): 0.9406 at 20°C
  flash point: 131 °F (technical grade, which may contain up to 15% of acetone 40–57 °F, Jones, 1938)
  conversion factors: 1 p.p.m. = 4.75 mg/m³
                1 mg/l = 216.5 p.p.m.
  Solubility: miscible with water in all proportions and with most organic solvents; good solvent for nitrocellulose, cellulose acetate, cellulose ethers and many resins; not for rubber or copal esters.
  maximum allowable concentration: 50 p.p.m. (Threshold Limit Values, 1962)

ECONOMY, SOURCES AND USES

Production

By condensing acetone in the liquid phase in the presence of alkali and alkaline earth hydroxides (Kirk and Othmer, 1947).

Industrial uses

(1) In the lacquer industry as an 'anti-blush' agent for nitrocellulose lacquers (Yarsley, 1933).

(2) In the dyeing industry as a solvent for certain pigments (Clayton and Clark, 1931).

(3) In the textile industry, in coating compositions, and for mercerisations (Sisley, 1934).

(4) In the manufacture of quick drying inks (Ottley, 1933).

(5) In metal cleaning compounds (Treon, 1963).

(6) In the manufacture of photographic film (Treon, 1963).

BIOCHEMISTRY

Estimation in the atmosphere

The method described by Greenberg and Lester (1944) for determination of acetone can be applied to diacetone alcohol. Reaction with 2,4-dinitrophenyl-hydrazine gives the corresponding phenylhydrazine, which, when extracted with CCl_4 and in turn with an alkaline solution gives a red colour with acetone and a yellow with diacetone alcohol.

TOXICOLOGY

Diacetone alcohol is primarily a narcotic and anti-convulsive agent (Keith, 1931) with a more rapid and powerful action and a more toxic effect than acetone.

It causes in animals a depression of respiration and a fall in blood pressure, which according to Walton, Kehr and Loevenhart (1928) is probably due to decreased cardiac output, not dependent on the vagal centre. It is also capable of causing liver and kidney injury and disturbance of the haemopoietic system (Keith, 1932). In human beings it is an irritant of mucous membranes in concentrations of about 100 p.p.m., but no toxic effects from its industrial use have been recorded.

Toxicity to animals

(1) Acute

(a) Lethal dose. – LD_{50}, for rabbits, by stomach tube, 5 ml/kg (Walton *et al.*, 1928), by intramuscular injection, 3–4 ml/kg, by intravenous injection, 3.25 ml/kg.

These dosages show a higher toxicity of diacetone alcohol than of acetone, since comparable values for the latter were more than 5 and 6–8 ml/kg.

(b) Narcotic dose. – *(i) By stomach tube,* 2.4 ml/kg. – *(ii) By intramuscular injection,* 3 ml/kg. – *(iii) By intravenous injection,* 1.0–1.5 ml/kg. – *(iv) By inhalation,* only drowsiness, following initial restlessness and excitability was caused by inhalation

of 2100 p.p.m. for 3 h (Gross, cited by Lehmann and Flury, 1943); 1500 p.p.m. for 8 h was not, according to Smyth and Carpenter (1948), lethal.

(2) Chronic

Repeated injections of non-narcotic doses were found by Walton *et al.* (1928) to cause still lower decrease in blood pressure with each injection. They attributed this to increased susceptibility. The fall was not due to splanchnic dilatation, and was not increased by section of the vagi, therefore it was concluded that it was due to decreased cardiac output.

SYMPTOMS OF INTOXICATION

Respiration decreased rapidly and unconsciousness also supervened very rapidly; in some cases after intravenous injection narcosis lasted several hours, in others recovery was complete in 30 min. There was a marked decrease in blood pressure (Walton *et al.*, 1928). In cases where unconsciousness was followed by death, this appeared to be due to respiratory failure. The soporific effect of doses of 1 ml/kg in rabbits was demonstrated by Keith (1931) when he was studying the effects of various drugs on convulsions experimentally induced by the convulsant, thujone. He found that this dosage of diactone alcohol produced an immediate comatose effect, with relaxation of muscles, slow deep respiration and absence of conjunctival reflex in most cases. This anaesthesia could be interrupted by injection of the convulsant thujone.

Blood picture

Destruction of erythrocytes, with reduction of haemoglobin, was observed by Keith (1932) for 4 or 5 days after administration of 2 ml/kg of diacetone alcohol. In one case, for example, the haemoglobin fell from 90 to 73%, and the erythrocytes from 5.35 millions to 4.60 on the 4th day, both returning to approximately normal levels on the 6th day.

CHANGES IN THE ORGANISM

(1) The liver

Maximal injury of the liver of rats was observed by Keith (1932) 24 h after administration by stomach tube of 2 ml/kg, though changes, in the form of an increase of lymphocytes in the portal spaces and slight vacuolisation of the hepatic cells had become evident at 6 h. The maximal injury was characterised by cloudy swelling, vacuolisation and granulation of the cytoplasm of the cells throughout the whole lobule. Recovery began at 48 h, was well advanced at 96 h and at 14 days the hepatic cells were practically normal, though nests of phagocytic cells were scattered thoughout the lobules, resembling a picture of 'myeloid metaplasia'. This phenomenon, it was suggested, might indicate a reaction to a per-

Bibliography on p. 401

sistent stimulus within the blood stream, caused by the haemolytic action of the diacetone alcohol.

(2) The kidneys

Acute nephritis was noted in one rabbit after intramuscular injection of 4 ml/kg (Walton *et al.*, 1928), and Gross also noted kidney injuries in one rabbit after inhalation of 2600 p.p.m.

Toxicity to human beings

Irritation of eyes, nose and throat were produced during an exposure of 15 min to concentrations of 100 p.p.m., and the majority of volunteer subjects complained of an unpleasant odour and taste at this level (Silverman *et al.*, 1946).

No toxic effects from its industrial use have been recorded, but owing to the variety and number of complaints made by these subjects exposed to 100 p.p.m., even though the majority indicated that they could work 8 h a day at this level, Silverman *et al.* (1946) recommended a desirable limit of 50 p.p.m., the level now actually recommended by the A.I.G.H.C. (1962).

49. Benzyl Alcohol

Synonyms: phenyl carbinol, phenyl methanol

Structural formula: ⬡—CH₂OH

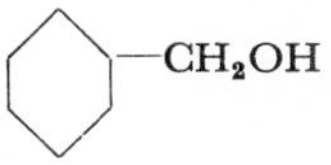

Molecular formula: C_7H_7OH

Molecular weight: 108.141

Properties: a colourless liquid with a faint aromatic odour. The pure product oxidises slowly and therefore remains stable on keeping for a long time. Impure products contain benzaldehyde (Macht, 1919). It possesses antiseptic properties, and is very toxic to insects (Moore, 1917).

    boiling point: 205.3 °C

    melting point: —15.3 °C

    vapour pressure: 0.15 mm Hg at 25 °C

    vapour density (air = 1): 3.72

    specific gravity (liquid density): 1.0472

    flash point: 96 °C

    conversion factors: 1 p.p.m. = 4.42 mg/m³

                      1 mg/l = 226.1 p.p.m.

    solubility: in water 3.5% at 20 °C; freely miscible with alcohol, ether

    evaporation rate (ether = 1): 1767

    maximum allowable concentration: not established

ECONOMY, SOURCES AND USES

It occurs in nature in a free state (6%) in oil of jasmine, and in the form of esters in certain balsams (Macht, 1918).

Production

From benzyl chloride by refluxing with sodium and potassium bicarbonate (Kirk and Othmer, 1947).

Industrial uses

(1) As a lacquer solvent and plasticiser.

(2) As a solvent in cosmetics and inks.

(3) In the manufacture of perfumes, pharmaceuticals and dyestuffs (Doolittle, 1954; Mellan, 1950).

(4) In the manufacture of therapeutic esters (Williams, 1959).

BIOCHEMISTRY

Estimation in the atmosphere

According to Treon (1963) the method described by Mohler and Hämmerle (1942), using its absorption spectrum in the ultra-violet region (maxima at 267, 264, 258 and 252 mμ) should be adaptable to quantitative air analysis.

Metabolism

In 1881 Schmiedeberg showed that benzyl alcohol is rapidly oxidised in the animal organism to benzoic acid, which is conjugated and then excreted to a large extent in the urine as hippuric acid. This was confirmed by Macht (1918) and also by Stekol (1939) who injected subcutaneously into rabbits 1 g of benzyl alcohol in three portions 2 h apart, and isolated from the urine, evaporated to dryness, 300 to 400 mg of a substance which proved to be identical with hippuric acid. The rapidity of its oxidation to benzoic acid was also noted by Snapper et al. (1925) and confirmed by Diack and Lewis (1928) and Bray et al. (1951). Diack and Lewis concluded that the velocity of oxidation was at least as great as that of hippuric acid synthesis and excretion. According to Williams (1959) if the dose is sufficiently high to allow the rate of formation of benzoic acid to exceed that of hippuric acid, some of the benzoic acid is excreted as benzoylglycuronide. Snapper et al. (1925) remarked that owing to this rapidity of oxidation to benzoic acid, which is ineffective as a spasmolytic agent, oral administration of benzyl alcohol fails to exert any antispasmodic effect.

TOXICOLOGY

Benzyl alcohol has local anaesthetic and antispasmodic properties, and has a diuretic effect in animals (Gruber, 1924), after a latent period of 7 min when given intravenously, intramuscularly or intraperitoneally. Macht (1918) found that while testing a minute quantity his tongue was completely anaesthetised, and that this anaesthesia, produced by a 1% solution, was perceptible half an hour or longer after its application. The cornea of animals is also completely anaesthetised and conduction from sensory and motor nerves paralysed. High doses cause convulsions followed by paralysis of the respiratory centre, but it has been used

with no deleterious effects as a local anaesthetic for minor surgical operations.
Macht (1918) collected 50 such examples of benzyl alcohol anaesthesia, and
attributed its relatively low toxicity in comparison with its powerful local effect to
its metabolic behaviour (see Metabolism). A fall in blood pressure and circulatory
changes in the kidneys of dogs following intravenous administration were observed
by Gruber (1923). Only one report of suspected industrial injury from the use of
benzyl alcohol has been reported, and in this case benzyl alcohol cannot be
implicated as the sole cause, since other solvents were also used (Gaulejac and
Derivillée, 1938).

Toxicity to animals

Lethal dose. – (i) By oral administration, for rats, LD_{50} 3.1 g/kg (Treon, 1963). –
(ii) By intraperitoneal injection, for rats and guinea pigs, 400–800 mg/kg (Fassett,
cited by Treon, 1963). – (iii) By subcutaneous injection, for mice, Starrek (1938)
found it 2.5 to 3 times more toxic than n-butyl or isopropyl alcohol. – (iv) By
inhalation, 1000 p.p.m. after 8 h (Smyth, Carpenter and Weil, 1951). – (v) By
skin application, guinea pigs, after primary irritation, systemic symptoms with
death at less than 5 ml/kg (Fassett, cited by Treon, 1963).

SYMPTOMS OF INTOXICATION

Initial respiratory stimulation followed by respiratory and muscular paralysis,
convulsions and narcosis were observed by Starrek (1938). Macht (1918) believed
that respiratory paralysis was the cause of death, but Gruber (1923) having noted
a decrease in the arterial blood pressure of rabbits, cats and dogs after intravenous
injection, considered that cardiac paralysis might be the prime factor. He also
noted emesis and diarrhoea following administration by stomach tube, due presumably to irritation of the gastric mucosa, and in 1924 he produced diuresis, more
pronounced in the rabbit than the dog.

CHANGES IN THE ORGANISM

Effect on peripheral nerves. Paralysis of the orbicularis oculi in cats in which benzyl
alcohol alone as a 5% or 10% solution, or in admixture with sweet almond oil,
had been injected into the region of the auditory meatus was observed by Duncan
and Jarvis (1943). Histological examination of the nerve fibres in the injected area
showed marked degeneration, and Duncan and Jarvis concluded that in a 10%
solution benzyl alcohol will destroy all the fibres in small nerves and a considerable
number if used in a 5% concentration. Complete paralysis of the orbicularis oculi
lasted on the average for 15 days but recovery was eventually complete.

Bibliography on p. 401

Toxicity to human beings

Industrial

The account presented by Gaulejac and Dervillée (1938) of workers using enamels in which benzyl alcohol was one of the components of the solvent mixture and who suffered from headache, giddiness, excessive fatigue and in some cases gastro-intestinal disturbance, cannot be regarded as a definite example of benzyl alcohol poisoning. The solvent mixture contained benzene (5%), benzine, and acetone, as well as 9–10% of benzyl alcohol, and Gaulejac and Dervillée themselves suggest only that, while the atmospheric concentration of benzene was too low to cause acute poisoning (no blood examinations were made) it was possible that the association with benzyl alcohol may have increased its toxicity in this respect.

50. Ethylene Chlorohydrin

Synonyms: 2-monochloroethyl alcohol, glycol chlorohydrin

Structural formula: CH_2Cl-CH_2-OH

Molecular formula: C_2H_5OCl

Molecular weight: 80.519

Properties: a colourless glycerine-like liquid with an ethereal odour. When heated with water to 100 °C decomposes into glycol and acetaldehyde; alone to 184 °C into ethylene chloride and acetaldehyde (Koelsch, 1927). The commercial product contains as its chief impurities ethylene dichloride and dichloroethyl ether (Goldblatt, 1944).

> *boiling point:* 128.7 °C
> *melting point:* —62.6 °C
> *vapour pressure:* 4.9 mm Hg at 20 °C (Ambrose, 1950)
> *vapour density (air = 1):* 2.78
> *specific gravity (liquid density):* 1.2045
> *flash point:* 135 °F
> *conversion factors:* 1 p.p.m. = 3.29 mg/m³
>   1 mg/l = 303.8 p.p.m.
> *solubility:* soluble in water in all proportions, good solvent for cellulose acetate, cellulose ethers and various resins.
> *maximum allowable concentration:* 5 p.p.m. (Threshold Limit Values, 1962).

ECONOMY, SOURCES AND USES

Production

By passing chlorine and ethylene simultaneously into water (Treon, 1963).

Industrial uses

(1) In the lacquer industry, by virtue of its solvent action for cellulose acetate, resin and wax (Huntress, 1948).
(2) In the dyeing and cleaning industry, for the removal of tar spots; as a cleaning agent for machines and as a solvent in fabric dyeing.

(3) In the separation of butadiene from hydrocarbon mixtures, and dewaxing and removing naphthenes from mineral oil (Huntress, 1948).

(4) In the treating of seeds and speeding up of sprouting of potatoes (Denny, 1928; Ambrose, 1950). According to Bush, Abrams and Brown (1949) 1500 gallons of ethylene chlorohydrin for speeding the germination of seed potatoes were used in California in 1946.

(5) In the production of ethylene glycol and ethylene oxide (Kirk and Othmer, 1949).

BIOCHEMISTRY

Estimation in the atmosphere

The method described by Uhrig (1946), and in essentials that used by Dierker and Brown (1944) following a fatal case due to exposure to ethylene chlorohydrin (see p. 400), consists in refluxing with KOH, addition of HNO_3 and excess standardised $AgNO_3$, and titration with ammonium sulphate, using ferric ammonium sulphate as indicator.

Metabolism

Ethylene chlorohydrin is readily absorbed by the skin (Smyth and Carpenter, 1945). *In vivo* it is oxidised to chloroacetic acid, which in the opinion of Williams (1959) is probably responsible for its high toxicity, owing to its injurious effect, like that of fluoracetic acid, the metabolic product of fluorethanol, on the tricarboxylic acid cycle of enzymes. Williams also states that the one chlorine atom in the 2-position seems to have little effect on its oxidation, and it does not give rise to a glucuronide in the rabbit (El Masri and Williams, 1956).

TOXICOLOGY

Ethylene chlorohydrin is an extremely toxic substance, acting as a metabolic poison, with a specially severe effect on the nervous system (Pratt, 1930). The fact that up to 1927, when Koelsch reported one fatal and several other severe cases of poisoning, although ethylene chlorohydrin had been widely used for 20 years with no evidence of these severe toxic effects, was attributed by Koelsch to its use during these years in closed apparatus, so that neither inhalation nor skin contamination were factors in its toxic potentiality. In animals, application to the skin has caused death, and in human cases of poisoning, skin contamination has been considered a contributing factor. In animals, inhalation is followed by convulsions, prostration and respiratory failure, without preceding true narcosis. Kidneys, liver and lungs are all involved in the toxic process, showing, especially in the kidneys, haemorrhage and cell disintegration. In fatal cases, in human beings as well as in animals, the onset of symptoms is generally delayed for a few hours after exposure. In such cases, as well as in severe non-fatal cases, the liver, kidneys and lungs have shown severe injury, and in some, cerebral oedema (Goldblatt and Chiesman, 1944). If death does not occur within 12 to 18 h, recovery is probable (Bush *et al.*, 1949).

Toxicity to animals

Lethal dose. – *(i) By stomach tube*, for rats (1% aqueous solution) 0.095 g/kg; for guinea pigs 0.11 g/kg (Smyth, Seaton and Fischer, 1941). – *(ii) By oral administration*, the LD_{50} was about 7.2 mg/100 g (Goldblatt, 1944). – *(iii) By intraperitoneal injection*, for rats, the LD_{50}, according to Goldblatt, was between 5 and 6 mg/100 g, but if smaller doses were given at intervals, a total dose of 24 mg/100 g was tolerated without symptoms or loss of weight. – *(iv) By inhalation*, the lethal dose differs somewhat in the hands of different observers. Carpenter *et al.* (1949) state that 32 p.p.m. for 4 h killed more than 50% of the animals; this places ethylene chlorohydrin in Grade 14 of their classification of toxicity, representing a 'serious hazard'. Ambrose (1950) gives 7.5 p.p.m. for one hour for rats, and 4 p.p.m. after two exposures of one hour each. In Goldblatt's (1944) experiments, 0.0039 g/l was fatal to 2 out of 3 mice after 2 days, and 0.004 g/l to all rats after 30 min. Guinea pigs were less sensitive; 0.005 g/l was not lethal after 55 min, though 0.003 g/l caused death after 112 min. – *(v) By skin application*, for rats, 0.5 ml undiluted, or in 50 or 25% aqueous solution (Ambrose, 1950); for guinea pigs, Smyth and Carpenter (1945) give 0.07 ml/kg after 112 min when applied as a poultice; 1.14 ml/kg as a 10% solution – as toxic as a 10% alcoholic solution of aniline.

SYMPTOMS OF INTOXICATION

Nasal irritation is followed by muscular inco-ordination but no true narcosis. Some time after removal from exposure convulsions occur with sudden death from respiratory failure.

In Goldblatt's (1944) experiments repeated exposure of rats to 0.0034 g/l for 15 min per day was fatal at times varying from 3 to 11 days. The animals were depressed and lost weight.

CHANGES IN THE ORGANISM

As in the deaths from single toxic doses, the chief focus of toxic effect was the kidneys, which showed many small haemorrhages and intense congestion and disorganisation of convoluted tubules. The liver was also affected, showing fatty degeneration and breakdown of structure, and the lungs areas of collapse and swelling of the alveolar epithelium.

Bibliography on p. 401

Toxicity to human beings

(1) Acute

In 1949, Bush, Abrams and Brown stated that up to that time 6 fatalities and many cases of illness had occurred. In few of the fatal cases recorded has actual information as to the atmospheric concentration of ethylene chlorohydrin been forthcoming. In one case, however (Dierker and Brown, 1944), the operation which had caused the fatality was later resumed and a 40-min sample of the air in the breathing zone of the deceased worker collected and analysed by the procedure described on page 395. It was found that the average concentration had been 305 p.p.m. (1 mg/l).

The man in question had been cleaning trays upon which rubber strips were stored; after two hours he developed severe nausea and vertigo; 5 h later he was cyanotic, with dyspnoea and spastic contractions of the hands and arms. He died from respiratory failure 11 h after the beginning of exposure. Autopsy showed changes in the liver (oedema, congestion and some areas of necrosis), in the kidneys (intense congestion and some destruction of parenchymal cells) and in the lungs (oedema with a tendency to emphysema). Similar findings with regard to symptoms and autopsy results were observed by Bush *et al.* (1949) in the fatal case of a man exposed to ethylene chlorohydrin in the process of treating seed potatoes with this compound. His presenting symptoms included diminished vision as well as nausea, vomiting, abdominal pain, cyanosis and coma occurring 3½ h later, and death after 8 h. The urine contained albumen, red cells and casts, and the blood picture showed leucocytosis. In this case, as in that of Middleton (1930), skin absorption played some part in the intoxication since the man handled sacks soaked with ethylene chlorohydrin.

In Middleton's case the man had been employed in mopping up water from a still which had contained ethylene chlorohydrin and which needed a repair in the lead lining. He had nausea, vomiting, difficulty in walking and drowsiness after having entered the still 3 times for about ten minutes each time; he died about ten hours later and the post-mortem appearances were said to be those "following inhalation of a toxic agent causing respiratory failure". Middleton remarked that the man who had entered the still actually to repair the leak, and who therefore had less cutaneous exposure, recovered, and that it seemed certain that the fatal case absorbed most of the poison through the skin when mopping up the water which contained the ethylene chlorohydrin in solution.

The cases described by Goldblatt and Chiesman (1944) – two fatal and nine non-fatal – occurred during the manufacture of ethylene chlorohydrin. Of the two fatal cases, one was designated 'acute' and the other 'subacute'. The former was that of a foreman who opened an inspection door at the top of a concentration tower in order to discover a fault. His total time of exposure to what must have been a high concentration of ethylene chlorohydrin and ethylene dichloride was about 1½ h. Half an hour later he vomited violently and was unsteady on his legs.

One and a half hours later his pulse was very weak, he was very restless, perspired profusely and died 14 h after the end of the exposure. At autopsy the lungs showed collapse, oedema and extravasation of blood into the alveoli, and the liver fatty degeneration. Kidney sections were not available.

The second case had been exposed for 3 months to concentrations of ethylene chlorohydrin (probably mixed with sym-dichloroethane) which had caused some symptoms in other workers. His symptoms related chiefly to the central nervous system – headache, dizziness and behaviour 'of a peculiar manner'; later he had haematuria and died the following day. Autopsy was not detailed, but the kidneys showed congestion and some necrosis and the brain gross oedema of the basal ganglia and some degenerative changes.

In a case described by Cavalazzi (1942) vomiting was followed by delirium and violent excitement.

(2) Chronic or subacute

The nine non-fatal cases described by Goldblatt and Chiesman occurred during a period when a fault had developed in the plant and when the average concentration of ethylene chlorohydrin was about 18 p.p.m. The chief symptoms were nausea, vomiting and abdominal pain; in some cases a semi-comatose condition. Slight albuminuria was present in some. It was believed that the additional presence of ethylene dichloride was not the principal cause of the symptoms, since narcotic effects were very mild.

TREATMENT OF INTOXICATION

In severe acute cases Goldblatt and Chiesman state that temporary improvement is obtained by continuous oxygen administration and analeptics. With mild cases treatment is entirely symptomatic.

BIBLIOGRAPHY

Abelin, I., C. Herren and W. Berli (1938) Über die erregende Wirkung des Alkohols auf den Adrenalin und Noradrenalin-Haushalt des menschlichen Organismus, *Helv. Med. Acta*, 25:591.
Agner, K. and K. E. Belfrage (1947) A specific Micro-method for Colorimetric Determination of Methanol in Blood, *Acta Physiol. Scand.*, 13:87.
Ambrose, A. M. (1950) Toxicological Studies investigated for Use as Inhibitors of Biological Processes, *Arch. Ind. Hyg.*, 2:591.
Anker, M. (1892) Ein Fall von Amylenhydratvergiftung, *Therap. Monatschr.*, 6:623.
Annual Report, Chief Inspector of Factories, G.B. (1957) H.M.S.O. London.
Ascham, O. (1927) Zur Verwertung des Petroläthers und der Erdöl Residuen, *Chemikerztg.*, 51:4.
Atkinson, H.V. (1925) The Toxicity of Impurities in Wood Alcohol, *J. Pharmacol.*, 25:144.
Baader E. W. (1933) Gewerbemedizinische Erfahrungen, *Verhandl. Deut. Ges. Inn. Med.*, 45:318.
Bachem, C. (1927) Beitrag zur Toxikologie der Halogenalkyle, *Arch. Exptl. Pathol. Pharmakol.*, 122:69.
Baer, F. (1898) Beitrag zur Kenntnis der akuten Vergiftung mit verschiedenen Alkoholen, Dissertation, Berlin, *Arch. Anat. Physiol. Abt.*, p. 283.

Barlow, O. W. (1936) Studies on the pharmacology of Ethyl Alcohol, *J. Pharm, Exptl. Therap.*, 56:177.

Bartlett G. R. (1950) Combustion of C14-labelled Methanol in the intact Rat and its isolated Tissues, *Am. J. Physiol.*, 163:614.

Bartlett, G. R. and H. N. Barnet (1949) Some Observations on Alcohol Metabolism with radioactive Ethyl Alcohol, *Quart. J. Stud. Alc.*, 10:381.

Baskerville, C. (1913) Report on Chemistry, Technology and Pharmacology of and Legislature pertaining to Methyl Alcohol *2nd. Rept. Factory Insp. Comm. New York*, 2:921.

Bennett, Jr., I. J., F. H. Carey, G. L. Mitchess Jr. and M. N. Cooper (1953) Acute Methyl Alcohol Poisoning. Review based on Experience of Outbreak of 323 Cases, *Medicine*, 32:431.

Berggren, S. M. (1938) On the Metabolism of *n*-Propyl and *n*-Butyl Alcohol in the Organism, *Skand. Arch. Physiol.*, 78:249.

Bernhard, H. (1937) Stoffwechselversuche zur Dehydrierung des Cyclohexanols, *Hoppe-Seyler's Z. Physiol. Chem.*, 248:256.

Bertarelli, E. (1934) I Pericoli practici dell' Alcool Metilico, *Ann. Igiene (Sperim)*, 44:729.

Biberfeld, J. (1918) Zur Kenntnis der Gewohnung, *Biochem. Zschr.*, 92:198.

Bijlsma, U. G. (1928) Isopropyl Alcohol, *Arch. Pharmacodyn.*, 34:204.

Bird, C. L. (1932) Auxiliary Solvents for dry-cleaning Soaps, *J. Soc. Dye Col. Bradford*, 48:256.

Birsch-Hirschfeld, A. (1901) Experimentelle Untersuchungen über die Pathogenese der Methylalkoholamblyopie, *Arch. Ophthalm.*, 52:538.

Blakemore, W. S. and C. H. Hine (1947) (cited by Stinebaugh, 1960), The Effect of peritoneal Irrigation on experimental Methyl Alcohol Toxicity, Bumed News Letter, 10:18.

Bogen, E. (1946) Methanol Poisoning, *Calif. [West.] Med.*, 65:230.

Boruttau, H. (1921) Die Verwendung von Isopropylalkohol zu hygienischen und kosmetischen Zwecken, *Deut. Med. Wochschr.*, 47:747.

Bray, H. G., W. V. Thorpe and K. White (1951) The Formation of Benzoic acid from Benzamide, Benzyl Alcohol and Benzaldehyde, *Biochem. J.*, 48:88.

Brecher, G. A., A. R. Hartman and D. D. Leonard (1955) Effect of Alcohol on Binocular Vision, *Am. J. Ophthalm.*, 39:44.

Brezina, E. (1929) Internationale Übersicht über Gewerbekrankheiten, pp. 83 and 167, Julius Springer, Berlin.

Browning, E. (1953) *The Toxicity of Industrial Organic Solvents*, H.M.S.O. London; Chemical Publishing Co. Inc. New York.

Burger, G. B. C. and B. H. Stockman (1932) Über Urobilinurie als Folge der Einatmung von organischen Lösungsmitteln in geringer Konzentration, *Z. Gewerbehyg.*, 19:29.

Burk, M. (1957) Zur chronischgewerblichen Methylalkoholvergiftung, *Klin. Mbl. Augenheilk.*, 130:845.

Burton, K. and T. H. Wilson (1953) Free Energy Data for Dehydrogenase Systems, *Biochem. J.*, 54:86.

Butler, T. C. and L. H. Dickison (1940) The anaesthetic Activity of optical Antipodes; The secondary Butyl Alcohols, *J. Pharm. Exptl. Therap.*, 69:225.

Bush, A. F., H. K. Abrams and H. V. Brown (1949) Fatality and Illness caused by Ethylene Chlorohydrin in an agricultural Operation, *J. Ind. Hyg. Toxicol.*, 31:352.

Campbell, J. A. (1915) Wood Alcohol Amblyopia – a Case, *J. Ophth. Otol. Laryngol.*, 21:756.

Carlier, E. W. (1911) Notes on the Physiology of some of the Allyl Compounds, *Brit. Med. J.*, 2:609.

Carpenter, C. P. and H. F. Smyth Jr. (1946) Chemical Burns of the Rabbit Cornea, *Am. J. Ophth.* 29:1363.

Carpenter, C. P., H. F. Smyth Jr. and U. C. Pozzani (1949) Assay of acute Vapor Toxicity and Grading and Interpretation of Results on 96 Chemical Compounds, *J. Ind. Hyg. Toxicol.*, 31:343.

Castor, J. G. B. and J. F. Guymon (1952) On the Mechanism of Formation of higher Alcohols during Alcoholic Fermentation, *Science*, 115:147.

Cavalazzi, D. (1942) Akute und tödliche Vergiftung durch Äthylenchlorhydrin, *Samml. Vergiftungsf.*, 12:79:A. 910.

Chapin, M. A. (1949) Isopropyl Alcohol Poisoning with acute Renal Insufficiency, *J. Maine Med. Ass.*, 40:288.

Charnwood (Lord) (1950) Influence of Alcohol on Fusion, *Brit. J. Ophthalmol.*, 34:733.

Chew, W. B., E. H. Berger, O. A. Brines and M. J. Capron (1946) Alkali Treatment of Methyl Alcohol Poisoning, *J. Am. Med. Ass.*, 130:61.

Christiansen, J. (1918) On the Theory and Practice of Alcohol Disinfection, *Zschr. Physiol. Chem.*, 102:275.

Clayton, E. and C. O. Clark (1931) Modern Organic Solvents, *J. Soc. Dyers Col. Bradford*, 47:183; 247.

Cogan, D. G. and W. M. Grant (1945) An unusual Type of Keratitis associated with Exposure to *n*-Butyl Alcohol, *Arch. Ophth.*, 33:106.

Comstock, C. C. and F. W. Oberst (1952) Inhalation Toxicity of Aniline, Furfuryl Alcohol and their Mixtures in Rats and Mice (cited by Treon, 1963), *Chem. Corps. Med. Labs. Research Rep.* No. 139.

Cook, W. A. (1945) M.A.C. of Industrial Atmospheric Contaminants, *Indust. Med. Surg.*, 14:936.

Cook, C. A. and A. H. Smith (1929) The Determination of Isopropyl Alcohol in the presence of Acetone in the Urine, *J. Biol. Chem.*, 85:821.

Daremberg, G. (1895) La Toxicité des Boissons alcooliques mesurée à l'Aide des Injections intraveineuses chez le Lapin, *Arch. Méd. Expér. Anat. Path.*, 7:719.

Denigès, G. (1910) Study of Methyl Alcohol in general and especially in the presence of Ethanol, *C.R. Acad. Sci.*, 150:832.

Denny, F. E. (1928) Chemical Treatments for Shortening the Rest Periods of Plants, *J. Soc. Chem. Ind.*, 47:239.

Diack, S. L. and H. B. Lewis (1928) Studies in the Synthesis of Hippuric Acid in the Animal Organism, *J. Biol. Chem.*, 77:89.

Dierker, H. and F. Brown (1944) Study of a fatal Case of Ethylenechlorohydrin Poisoning, *J. Indust. Hyg. Toxicol.*, 26:277.

Di Luzio, N. R. (1961) Discussion on Role of Alcohol on Cirrhosis, *Am. J. Clin. Nutrition*, 9:442.

Donley, D. E. (1936) Toxic Encephalopathy and volatile Solvents in Industry, *J. Indust. Hyg. Toxicol.*, 18:571.

Doolittle. A. K. (1954) *The Technology of Solvents and Plasticisers*, John Wiley and Sons, New York.

Duchesi, V. (1915) La Colesterina del Sangue nella Intossicazione per Alcool, *Arch. di Fisiol.*, 13:147.

Dujardin-Beaumetz, and Audige (1875) Sur les Propriétés toxiques des Alcools par Fermentation, *C. R. Acad. Sci.*, 81:192.

Duke, Elder S. (1940) *Textbook of Ophthalmology*, Vol. 3, 3019, Kimpton, London.

Duncan, D. and W. H. Jarvis (1943) A Comparison of the Action on Nerve Fibres of certain Anaesthetic Mixtures and Substances in Oil, *Anesthesiology*, 4:465.

Dunlap, M. K. and C. H. Hine (1955) Toxicity of Allyl Alcohol, *Federation Proc.*, 14:335.

Dunlap, M. K., J. K. Kodama, J. S. Wellington, H. H. Anderson and C. H. Hine (1958) The Toxicity of Allyl Alcohol, *Arch. Ind. Health.*, 18:303.

Durrans, T. H. (1950) *Solvents*, 6th ed., Champan and Hall, London.

Durwald, W. and W. Degen (1956) Eine tödliche Vergiftung mit *n*-Propyl Alkohol, *Arch. Toxikol.*, 16:84.

Eberhardt, T. P. (1936) Effect of Alcohol on Cholesterol-induced Atherosclerosis in Rabbits, *Arch. Path.*, 21:617.

Eisenberg, A. A. (1917) Visceral Changes in Wood Alcohol Poisoning by Inhalation, *Am. J. Publ. Health*, 7:765.

Elhardt, W. P. (1931) The Effect of Methyl, Propyl and Butyl Alcohol on the Growth of white Leghorn Chicks, *Am. J. Physiol.*, 100:74.

Elkins, H. B. (1959) *The Chemistry of Industrial Toxicology*, Wiley and Sons, New York, Chapman and Hall, London.

Elliott, T. H., D. V. Parke and R. T. Williams (1959) The Metabolism of Cyclo [^{14}C]hexane and its Derivatives, *Biochem. J.* 72:193.

El Masri, A. M. and R. T. Williams (1956) (unpublished data, cited by R. T. Williams, 1959).

Erdmann, E. (1902) Über das Kaffeeoel und die physiologische Wirkung des darin erhaltenen Furfuralkohols, *Arch. Exptl. Pathol. Pharmakol.*, 48:233.

Eulner, H. H. (1954) Methanolvergiftung bei äusserlicher Anwendung, *Arch. Toxikol.*, 15:73.

Eyquem (1905) Du Danger des Vapeurs alcooliques dans la Fabrication de la Poudre sans Fumée, *Ann. Hyg. Publ.* Paris, 4-ième Ser., 3:71.

Fairhall, L. T., (1957) *Industrial Toxicology*, 2nd ed., Williams and Wilkins Co., New York.

Fassett, D. W. (1963) cited by Treon J. F. in *Alcohols*, F. A. Patty (Ed.), *Industrial Hygiene and Toxicology*, Vol. II, 2nd ed., Interscience, New York.

Feller, D. D. and R. L. Huff (1955) Lipide synthesis by arterial and Liver Tissue obtained from Cholesterol-fed and Cholesterol-alcohol-fed Rabbits, *Am. J. Physiol.*, 182:237.

Ficklen, J. B. (1940) *Manual of Industrial Health Hazards*. Service to Industry, West Hartford, Connecticut.

Fieser, L. L. and M. Fieser (1944) *Organic Chemistry*, Heath, Boston.

Filippi, E. (1914) Azione fisiologica e Comportamento di alcuni Derivati dal Benzene in Confronto con quelli di Cicloesano, *Arch. Farmacol. Sper.*, 18:178.

Fine, E. H. and J. H. Wills (1950) Pharmacologic Studies of Furfuryl Alcohol, *Arch. Ind. Hyg.*, 1:625.

Fink, W. H. (1943) The Ocular Pathology of Methyl Alcohol Poisoning, *Am. J. Ophthalm.*, 26:802.

Flury, F. and W. Wirth (1934) Zur Toxikologie der Lösungsmitteln, *Arch. Gewerbepath. Gewerbehyg.*, 5:1.

Flury, F. and H. Zangger (1928) *Lehrbuch der Toxikologie für Studium und Praxis*, Springer, Berlin.

Flury, F. and F. Zernik (1931) *Schädliche Gäse, Dämpfe, Nebel, Rauch- und Staubarten*, Springer, Berlin.

Fuchter, T. B. (1901) cited by Treon (1963) *Am. Med.*, 2:210.

Fuller, H. C. and O. B. Hunter (1927) Isopropyl Alcohol – an Investigation of its physiologic Properties, *J. Lab. Clin. Med.*, 12:326.

Galewski, J. and W. Alsdorf (1949) Studies on Furan Compounds: Toxicity and pharmacological Action of Furfuryl Alcohol, *Fed. Proc.*, 8:294.

Gardner, H. A. (1925) (cited by Treon, 1963) Paint Mfrs, *Ass. U.S. Techn. Circ.* No. 250:89.

Garrison, F. (1953) Acute Poisoning from Use of Isopropyl Alcohol in tepid Sponging, *J. Am. Med. Ass.*, 152:317.

Gaulejac, R. de, and P. Dervillée (1938) Sur quelques Cas d'Intoxication par les Vapeurs de Benzène et d'Alcool benzylique, *Ann. Méd. Légale*, 18:146.

Gerbis, H. (1931) Methylalkoholvergiftung, chronische, *Samml. Vergiftungsf.*, 2:171; A 160.

Gettler, A. O. and A. Tiber (1927) The Alcoholic Content of the Human Brain, *Arch. Path. Lab. Med.*, 3:218.

— (1927) The quantitative Determination of Ethyl Alcohol in Human Tissues, *Arch. Path. Lab. Med.*, 3:75.

Giardini, A. (1952) Action of Alcohol on Ability to fuse Retinal Images, Abs. in *Quart. J. Stud., Alc.*, 13:298.

Gilger, A. P., A. M. Potts and L. V. Johnson (1952) Studies on the Visual Toxicity of Methanol, *Am. J. Ophthalm. Suppl.*, 35:113.

Goldberg, L. (1943) Quantitative Studies on Alcohol Tolerance in Man, *Acta Physiol. Scand.* (Suppl. 16), 5:1.

Goldblatt, M. W. (1944) Toxic Effects of Ethylenechlorohydrin (Experimental), *Britt. J. Ind. Med.*, 1:213.

Goldblatt, M. W. and W. E. Chiesman (1944) Toxic effects of Ethylenechlorohydrin (Clinical), *Brit. J. Ind. Med.*, 1:207.

Goldtdammer, (1878) Bronchitis durch Holzgeistdämpfe, *Z. Ger. Med.*, 29:162.

Gradinesco, A. (1934) l'Action de l'Alcool sur le centre respiratoire, *J. Physiol. Path. Gén.*, 32:363.

Grande, F. and D. S. Amatuzio (1960) The Influence of Ethanol on Serum Cholesterol Concentration, *Minnesota Med.*, 43:731.

— (1923) The antiseptic and bactericidal Properties of Isopropyl Alcohol, *Am. J. Med.Sci.*, 166:261.

Grant, D. H. (1923) The Pharmacology of Isopropyl Alcohol, *J. Lab. Clin. Med.*, 8:382.

Grant, G. R. (1950) Inhibition of Methanol Oxidation by Ethanol in the Rat, *Am. J. Physiol.*, 163:614, 619.

Greenberg, L. A. and D. Lester (1944) Micromethod for Determination of Acetone and Ketone
   Bodies, *J. Biol. Chem.*, 154:177.
Grilichess, R. (1913) Über die pharmakologische Wirkung kombinierte Urethane und Alkohole,
   Z. Allgem. Physiol., 15:468.
Gruber, C. M. (1923) Pharmacology of Benzyl Alcohol and its Esters, *J. Lab. Clin., Med.*, 9:15, 92.
— (1925) Pharmacology of Benzyl Alcohol and its Esters, *J. Lab. Clin. Med.*, 10:284.
Grunow (1912) (cited by Koelsch, 1921) *Halbmonatschr. Soz. Hyg.*, 2,
Guggenheim, M. and W. Loffler (1916) Das Schicksal proteinogener Amine in Tierkörper, *Biochem.
   Zschr.*, 72:325.
Haag, H. B., T. Silverman and S. Kaye (1951) Relationship between Blood Alcohol Levels and
   acute Respiratory Failure, *J. Pharm. Exptl. Therap.*, 103:344.
Haggard, H. W. and L. A. Greenberg (1934) The Absorption, Distribution and Elimination of
   Ethyl Alcohol; Rate of Oxidation of Alcohol in the Body, *J. Pharm. Explt. Therap.*, 52:137,
   150, 167.
Haggard, H. W., D. P. Miller and L. A. Greenberg (1945) The Amyl Alcohols and their Ketones;
   metabolic Fates and comparative Toxicities, *J. Ind. Hyg., Toxicol.*, 27:1.
Hahn, E. (1937) On the Determination of Isopropyl Alcohol in the Respiratory Air, *Biochem. Z.*,
   292:148.
Hamilton, A. (1934) *Industrial Toxicology*, Harper, New York.
Harger, R. N. (1958) The Pharmacology and Toxicology of Alcohol, *J. Am. Med. Ass.*, 167:
   2199.
Harger, R. N. and H. R. Julpien (1956) *The Pharmacology of Alcohol*, (Ed.) G. N. Thompson, C. C.
   Thomas, Springfield, Illinois.
Harrop, G. A., Jr. and F. M. Benedict (1920) Acute Methyl Alcohol Poisoning associated with
   Acidosis, *J. Am. Med. Ass.*, 74:25.
Henry, R. J., C. F. Kirkwood, S. Berkman, R. D. Housewright and J. J. Henry (1948) A Colorime-
   tric Method for Determination of Micro Quantities of Ethanol in Blood and other biologic
   Fluids, *J. Lab. Clin. Med.*, 33:241.
Heuber, E. Von (1917) Ein Fall von Schlafmittelvergiftung, *Münch. Med. Wschr.*, 64:216.
Hilbert (1925) cited by Lewin (1929) in *Gifte und Vergiftungen*, 4th. ed., Springer, Berlin.
Hine, C. H., T. A. Shea Jr. and W. R. Alsdorf (1947) An accurate Colorimetric Method for Deter-
   mination of Methanol in Blood, Tissues and Expired Air, *Fed. Proc.*, 6:338.
Holden, H. C. and A. K. Doolittle (1935) Solvents, *Ind. Eng. Chem.*, 27:525.
Holden, W. A. (1899) The Pathology of the Amblyopia following profuse Haemorrhage and that
   following Ingestion of Methyl Alcohol, *Arch. Ophthalm.*, 28:125.
Hufferd, R. W. (1932) Toxicity of Aliphatic Alcohols, *J. Am. Pharm. Ass.*, 21:549.
— (1932) Variations in physiological Activity of Alcohols amoug Isomers and Homologs, *J. Am.
   Pharm. Ass.*, 21:549.
Humperdinck, K. (1941) Zur Frage der chronische Giftwirkung von Methanoldämpfen, *Arch.
   Gewerbepath. Gewerbehyg.*, 10:569.
Huntress, E. T. (1948) *The Preparation, Properties, Chemical Behaviour and Identification of Organic
   Chlorine Compounds*, Wiley, New York.
Jacobi, W. and E. Speer (1920) Amylenhydratvergiftung (35 gm) mit tödlichem Ausgang, *Therap.
   Monatschr.*, 6:623.
Jacobs, M. B. (1941) *The Analytical Chemistry of Industrial Poisons, Hazards and Solvents*, Interscience,
   New York.
Jacobsen, E. (1952) Metabolism of Ethyl Alcohol, *Pharmacol. Rev.*, 4:1017.
Jacobsen K. H., W. E. Rinehart, M. A. Ross, J. P. Papin, R. C. Daly, E. A. Greene and W. A.
   Groff (1958) The Toxicology of an Aniline-Furfuryl-Alcohol-Hydrazine Vapor Mixture,
   Am. Ind. Hyg. Ass. J., 19:91.
James, V. C. (1931) Acute Alcoholic Poisoning due to the Application of Surgical Spirit to the Legs,
   Brit. Med. J., 1:539.
Jetter, W. W. (1943) Symposium on Scientific Proof and Relation of Law and Medicine. When is
   Death caused by or contributed to by acute Alcoholism? *Clinics*, 1:1487.
Joffrey, A. and R. Serveaux (1895) Sur un nouveau Procédé de Mensuration de la Toxicité des
   Liquides par Injection intraveineuse, *Sem. Méd.*, 15:346.

Jones, G. W. (1938) Inflammation Limits and new practical Application in hazardous industrial Operations, *Chem. Rev.*, 22:1.

Joss, G. (1947) Contribution of Alcohol to Accident Fatalities, *Quart. J. Stud. Alc.*, 7:588.

Kamil, I. A., J. N. Smith and R. T. Williams (1953) Detoxication of Methanol and Ethanol, *Biochem. J.*, 54:390.

— (1953) The Formation of ester glucuronides of Aliphatic Alcohols during the Metabolism of 2-ethyl Butanol and 2-ethyl Hexanol, *Biochem. J.*, 53:137.

— (1953) The Isolation of Methyl and Ethyl Glucuronides from the Urine of Rabbits receiving Methanol and Ethanol, *Biochem. J.*, 54:390.

— (1953) The Metabolism of Aliphatic Alcohols; the glucuronic acid Conjugation of acyclic aliphatic Alcohols, *Biochem. J.*, 53:129.

Kaplan, A. and G. V. Levreault (1945) Methyl Alcohol Poisoning, Report of 42 Cases, *U.S. Nav. Med. Bull.*, 44:1107.

Kaye, S. and H. B. Haag (1954) Determination of Ethyl Alcohol in Blood, *J. Forensic Med.*, 1:373.

— (1957) Terminal Blood Concentrations in 94 Cases of acute Alchoholism, *J. Am. Med. Ass.*, 165:451.

Keeney, A. H. and S. M. Mellinkof (1951) Methyl Alcohol Poisoning, *Ann. Int. Med.*, 34:331.

Keith, H. M. (1931) The effect of various Factors on experimentally produced Convulsions, *Am. J. Dis. Child*, 41:532.

— (1932) Effect of Diacetone Alcohol on Liver of Rat, *Arch. Path. Lab. Med.*, 13:704.

Kemal, H. (1927) Beitrag zur Kenntnis des Schicksals des Isopropylalkohols im menschlichen Organismus, *Biochem. Zschr.*, 187:461.

— (1937) The Acetone Content of the Urine, Faeces and Organs of Dogs after Isopropyl Ingestion, *Zschr. Physiol. Chem.*, 246:59.

Kendal, L. P. and A. N. Ramanathan (1952) Liver Alcohol Dehydrogenase and Ester Formation, *Biochem. J.* 52:430.

— (1953) Excretion of Formate after Methanol Ingestion in Man, *Biochem. J.*, 54:424.

Kirk, R. E. and D. F. Othmer (1947) Encyclopaedia of Chemical Technology, *Interscience Encyclopaedia*, New York.

— (1949) Encyclopaedia of Chemical Technology, *Interscience Encyclopaedia*, New York.

— (1951) Encyclopaedia of Chemical Technology, Vol. 6, *Interscienc Encyclopaedia*, New York.

Klatskin, G. (1961) Experimental Studies on the Role of Alcohol in the Pathogenesis of Cirrhosis, *Am. J. Clin. Nutr.*, 9:439.

Klauer, H. (1938) Zum Nachweis des Methylalkoholvergiftung, *Deut. Zschr. ges. gerichtl. Med.*, 30:280.

Knipping, H. W. and W. Ponndorf (1926) On the reversible Exchange of Degrees of Oxidation of Oxy- and Oxo-compounds, *Zschr. Physiol. Chem.*, 160:25.

Kober, G. M. and W. C. Hanson (1918) *Diseases of Occupation and Vocational Hygiene*, Heinemann, London.

Kochmann, M. (1923) *Alkohol*, in A. Heffter (Ed.) *Handbuch der experimentellen Pharmakologie*, Springer, Berlin.

— (1923) *Schlafmittel*, in A. Heffter (Ed.) *Handbuch der experimentellen Pharmakologie*, Vol. I, p. 428, Springer, Berlin.

Kodama, J. K. and C. H. Hine (1958) Pharmacodynamic Aspects of Allyl Alcohol Toxicity, *J. Pharm. Exptl. Therap.*, 124:97.

Koelsch, F. (1921) Die gewerbliche medizinische Beurteilung des Holzgeistes bzw. Methylalkohol, *Zbl. Gewerbehyg.*, 9:198.

— (1927) Die Giftigkeit des Äthylenchlorhydrin, *Zbl. Gewerbehyg.*, 14:312.

— (1947) *Lehrbuch der Arbeitshygiene*, 2nd. ed., p. 281, Ferdinand Enke, Stuttgart.

Korenmann, I. M. (1932) Kolorimetrische Bestimmung von Amylalkohol und Amylazetatdämpfen in der Luft, *Arch. Hyg.*, 109:108.

Krüger, E. (1932) Augenerkrankung bei Verwendung von Nitrolacken in der Strohhutindustrie, *Arch. Gewerbepath. Gewerbehyg.*, 3:798.

Lanza, A. J. and J. A. Goldberg (1939) *Industrial Hygiene*, p. 466, Thomas, Springfield, Ill.

Larsen, J. A. (1959) Extrahepatic Metabolism of Ethanol in Man, *Nature*, 184:1236.

Larsen, J. A., N. Tygstrup and K. Winkler (1961) The Significance of the extrahepatic Elimination of Ethanol in Determination of Hepatic Blood Flow by means of Ethanol, *Scand. J. Clin. Invest.*, 13:116.

Leaf, G. and L. J. Zatman (1952) A Study of the Conditions under which Methanol may exert a toxic Hazard in Industry, *Brit. J. Ind. Med.*, 9:19.

Lehman, A. J. and H. W. Newman (1937) Comparative intravenous Toxicity of some monohydric saturated Alcohols, *J. Pharmacol.*, 61:103.

Lehman, A. J., H. Schwerma and E. Rickards (1945) Isopropyl Alcohol. Acquired Tolerance in Dogs, *J. Pharmacol.*, 85:61.

Lehmann, K. B. and F. Flury (1943) *Toxicology and Hygiene of Industrial Solvents*, Williams and Wilkins, Baltimore.

— (1928) Beitrag zur allgemeinen Pharmakologie der Narkose, *Arch. Exptl. Pathol. Pharmakol.*, 132:214.

— (1928) Untersuchungen über die Narkoseschwindigkeit homologer und isomer einwertiger Alkohole, *Arch. Exptl. Pathol. Pharmakol.*, 129:85.

Lewin, L. (1912) Über die Verwendungsgefähren des Methylalkohols und andere Alkohols, *Med., Klin.*, 8:95.

— (1929) *Gifte und Vergiftungen*, 4th. ed., Springer, Berlin.

Lieber, C. S. and R. Schmid (1961) The Effect of Ethanol on Fatty Acid Metabolism, *J. Clin. Invest.*, 40:394 and 1355.

Loewy, A. and R. van der Heide (1914) Über die Aufnahme des Methylalkohols durch die Atmung, *Biochem. Zschr.*, 65:230.

— (1918) Über die Aufnahme des Äthylalkohols durch die Atmung, *Biochem. Zschr.*, 86:125.

Lund, A. (1948) Metabolism of Methanol and Formic Acid in Rabbits, *Acta Pharmacol. Toxicol.*, 4:99.

Lutwak-Mann, C. (1938) Alcohol Dehydrogenase of Animal Tissues, *Biochem. J.*, 32:1364.

MacFarlan, J. E. (1855) On Methylated Spirit and some of its Preparations. *Pharmaceut. J. Trans.*, 15:310.

MacNider, W. de B. (1933) The acute degenerative Changes and Changes of Recuperation occurring in the Liver from the Use of Ethyl Alcohol, *J. Pharmacol. Exptl. Therap.*, 49:100.

Machata, G. (1958) Zur Methodik der ADH-Bestimmung, *Deut. Zschr. ges. gerichtl. Med.*, 48:26.

— (1961) The Diaphorase Method of Blood Alcohol Determination, *Deut. Zschr. ges. gerichtl. Med.*, 51:447.

Macht, D. I. (1918) A pharmacological and therapeutic Study of Benzyl Alcohol as a local Anaesthetic, *J. Pharmacol.*, 11:263:419.

— (1919) Further Experience, experimental and clinical, with Benzyl Benzoate and Benzyl Alcohol, *J. Pharmacol.*, 13:509.

— (1920) A toxicological Study of some Alcohols, with especial Reference to Isomers, *J. Pharmacol.*, 16:1.

— (1922) Pharmacological Examination of Isopropyl Alcohol, *Arch. Int. Pharmacodyn.*, 26:285.

Marshall, E. K. and W. F. Fritz (1953) The Metabolism of Ethyl Alcohol, *J. Pharmacol. Exptl. Therap.*, 109:431.

Mashkitz, N. L., R. M. Sklianskaya and F. I. Urieva (1936) Relative Toxicity of Acetone, Methyl alcohol and their mixtures. Their action on white mice, *J. Ind. Hyg. Toxicol.*, 18:117.

Masoro, E. J., H. Abramovitch and J. R. Birchard (1953) Metabolism of C^{14}-Ethanol by surviving Rat Tissues, *Am. J. Physiol.*, 173:37.

McCord, C. P. and N. Cox (1931) Toxicity of Methyl Alcohol (Methanol) following Skin Absorption and Inhalation, *Ind. Eng. Chem.*, 23:931.

McCord, C. P. (1932) The Toxicity of Allyl Alcohol, *J. Am. Med. Ass.*, 98:2269.

McNally, W. D. and H. M. Coleman (1944) A Micromethod for the Determination of Ethyl Alcohol in Blood, *J. Lab. Clin. Med.*, 29:429.

Mellan, I. (1939) *Industrial Solvents*, p. 205, Reinhold, New York.

— (1950) *Industrial Solvents*, Reinhold, New York.

Mertens, H. (1896) Lésions anatomiques du Foie du Lapin au cours de l'Intoxication chronique par le Chloroforme et par l'Alcool, *Arch. Intern. Pharmacodyn.*, 2:127.

Middleton, E. L. (1930) Fatal Case of Poisoning by Ethylenechlorohydrin, *J. Ind. Hyg. Toxicol.*, 12:265.

Miessner, F. (1891) Über die Wirkung des Allyl Alkohols, *Berl. Klin. Wochschr.*, 28:819.

Mohler, H. and W. Hämmerle (1941) cited by Treon (1963), *Zschr. Anal. Chem.*, 122:202; *Chem. Abstr.*, 36:4970.

Monier Williams, D. (1929) *An Outbreak of Methyl Alcohol Poisoning in the Ruhr*, Med. Off. Hlth. Memo.

Moore, W. (1917) Toxicity of various Benzene Derivatives to Insects, *J. Agric. Res.*, 9:371.

Mori, R. (1887) Über die diuretische Wirkung des Biers, *Arch. Hyg.*, 7:354.

Morris, W. J. and H. D. Lightbody (1938) The Toxicity of Isopropanol, *J. Ind. Hyg. Toxicol.*, 20:428.

Munch, J. C. and E. W. Schwartze (1925) Narcotic and Toxic Potency of Aliphatic Alcohols upon Rabbits, *J. Lab. Clin. Med.*, 10:985.

Nelson, K. W., J. F. Ege, M. Ross, L. E. Woodman and L. Silverman (1943) Sensory Response to certain industrial solvent Vapours, *J. Ind. Hyg. Toxicol.*, 25:282.

Neubauer, O. (1901) Über Glykuronsäurepaarung bei Stoffen der Fettreihe, *Arch. Exptl. Pathol. Pharmakol.*, 46:133.

— (1901) Über Glykuronsäurepaarung bei Stoffen der Fettreihe, *Arch. Exptl. Pathol. Pharmakol.*, 183:641.

Newman, H. and J. Card (1937) Duration of acquired Tolerance to Ethyl Alcohol, *J. Pharm. Exptl. Therap.*, 59:249.

Newman, H. and E. Fletcher (1941) The Effect of Alcohol on Vision, *Am. J. Med. Sci.*, 202:723.

Nicloux, M. (1896) Dosage de l'Alcool éthylique dans les Solutions ou cet Alcool est Dilué, *C. R Soc. Biol.*, 3:841.

— (1900) *Study on Alcohol*, Univ. Thesis, Paris.

Oettel, H. (1936) Einwirkung organische Flüssigkeiten auf der Haut, *Arch. Exptl. Pathol. Pharmakol.*, 183:641.

Oettingen, W. F. Von (1943) *The Aliphatic Alcohols; their Toxicity and potential Dangers*, [U.S.] Publ Health Rept Serv. P.H. Bull. no. 281, U.S. Govt. Printing Office, Washington.

Okubo, M. (1937) Physiological Action of 2-Furancarbinol, *J. Pharm. Soc. Japan*, 539:39.

Ørskov, S. L. (1950) Experiments on the Oxidation of Propyl Alcohol in Rabbits, *Acta Physiol Scand.*, 20:258.

Ottley, G. B. (1933) Quick Drying Inks, *Chem. Abstr.*, 27:2830.

Overton, E. (1901) *Studien über die Narkose, zugleich ein Beitrag zur allgemeinen Pharmakologie*, G Fischer, Jena.

Parsons, C. E. and M. E. M. Parsons (1938) Toxic Encephalopathy and "Granulopenic Anaemia" due to volatile Solvents in Industry, *J. Ind. Hyg. Toxicol.*, 20:124.

Paul, H. E., F. L. Austin, M. F. Paul and V. R. Ells (1949) Metabolism of the Nitrofurans, *J. Biol. Chem.*, 180:345.

Penniman, W. B. D., D. C. Smith and E. I. Lawshe (1937) Determination of higher Alcohols in distilled Liquors, *Ind. Eng. Chem., Anal. Ed.*, 9:91.

Perman, E. S. (1960) Effect of Ethyl Alcohol on the Secretion from the Adrenal Medulla of the Cat, *Acta Physiol. Scand.*, 48:323.

— (1961) Effect of Ethanol and Hydration on the urinary Secretion of Adrenalin and Noradrenalin and on the Blood Sugar of Rats, *Acta Physiol. Scand.*, 51:68.

— (1961) Observations on the Effect of Ethanol on the urinary Excretion of Histamine, *Acta Physiol Scand.*, 51:62.

Pipik, O. and E. Mezheboskaya (1933) Preparing Amyl Alcohols from cracked Gasoline, Abstr. in *Chem. Abstr.*, 1934, 28:7504.

Pohl, J. (1908) Quantitative Studien über die Exhalation des Alkohole, *Arch. Exptl. Pathol. Pharmakol. Suppl.*, 427.

— (1925) Über die Giftigkeit einiger aromatischer Hydrierungsprodukte (Tetralin, Hexalin und Methylhexalin), *Z. Gewerbehyg.*, 12:91.

Poincaré, M. L. (1878) Sur les Dangers de l'Emploi de l'Alcool méthylique dans l'Industrie *C. R. Acad. Sci.*, 87:682.

Potts, A. M. and L. V. Johnson (1952) Studies on the Visual Toxicity of Methanol, *Am. J. Ophthalm. Suppl.*, 35:107.

Potts, A. M. (1955) The visual Toxicity of Methanol, *Am. J. Ophthalm.*, 39:86.

Pratt, J. Davidson (1930) Dangerous Properties of Ethylenechlorohydrin, *Nature*, 126:995.

Quatermass, M. (1958) Amblyopia due to Ethyl Alcohol, *Brit. J. Ophthalm.*, 42:628.

Ramazzini, B. (1940) *Diseases of Workers* (Latin Text of 1713, translated by W. C. Wright), Univ. of Chicago Press.

Reid, E. W. (1934) Modern Solvent Industry, *Ind. Eng. Chem.*, 26:21.

Reid, E. W. and J. D. Beddard (1954) (cited by Dunlap *et al.*, 1958) Determination of low Bromine Absorption Values, *Analyst*, 79:456.

Robert, E. (1907) Considérations sur quelques Cas d'Intoxication par les Vapeurs d'Alcools dans la Fabrication de la Poudre sans Fumée, *J. Méd. Bordeaux*, 37:21.

Roche, L., J. Champeix, A. Échegut, A. Nicolas and A. Marin (1957) À propos d'Accidents pathologiques collectifs observés dans un Établissement industriel, *Ann. Méd. Lég.*, 37:43.

Roe, O. (1943) Clinical Investigation of Methyl Alcohol Poisoning, *Acta Med. Scand.*, 113:558.

— (1946) Methanol Poisoning, *Acta Med. Scand., Suppl.*, 182.

— (1948) The Ganglion Cells of the Retina in Cases of Methanol Poisoning in Human Beings and Experimental Animals, *Acta Ophthalm.*, 26:169.

Rogers, G. W. (1945) Sampling and Determination of Methanol in Air, *J. Ind. Hyg. Toxicol.*, 27:224.

Rost, E. and A. Braun (1926) Zur Pharmakologie der niederen Glieder der einwertigen aliphatischen Alkohole, *Arb. Reichsgesundh. Amt*, 57:580.

Ruemele, T. (1948) Isopropyl Alcohol in Perfumes and Toilet Preparations, *Mfg. Chem.*, 19:151.

Ruhle, A. (1912) Tierexperimentelle Befund im Zentralnervensystem nach Methylalkoholvergiftung, *Münch. Med. Wschr.*, 59:964.

Sander, F. (1933) *Über den Einfluss von Kohlenstoffverbindungen auf Mäuse bei cutaner Applikation*, Inaug. Diss. Köln, (cited by Von Oettingen, 1943).

Sanderson, J. McE. (1933) Solvents used in Surface Coatings, *Paint Oil Chem. Rev.*, 95:10.

Sato, K. (1928) Über die pharmakologischen Wirkungen der hydroaromatischen Verbindungen, Cyclohexen, Cyclohexan und Cyclohexanol. *Jap. J. Med. Sci. Pharmacol.*, 3:1.

Sayers, R. R., W. P. Yant, H. H. Schrenk, J. Chornyak, S. J. Pearce, F. A. Patty and J. G. Linn (1942) *Methanol Poisoning; Exposure of Dogs to 450–500 p.p.m. Methanol Vapour in Air*, Bur. Mines Report of Investigations, 3617.

— (1944) Methanol Poisoning, *J. Ind. Hyg. Toxicol.*, 26:255.

Schafforzick, R. W. and B. J. Brown (1952) Anticonvulsant Activity and Toxicity of Methylparafynol and some other Alcohols, *Science*, 116:663.

Schmiedeberg, O. (1881) Über Oxydationen und Synthesen im Thierkörper, *Arch. Exptl. Pathol. Pharmakol.*, 14:288.

Schumacher, H., K. Battig and E. Grandjean (1962) Die Wirkungen verschiedener Lösungsmitteldämpfe auf das Wachstum und die Spontanmortalität junger Mäuse, *Z. Arbeitsmed. Arbeitsschutz*, 12:5.

Schwarz, L. and L. Tulipan (1939) *A Textbook of occupational Diseases of the Skin*, Lea and Fibiger, Philadelphia.

Schwarzmann, A. (1934) Methylalkoholvergiftung, chronische, durch Einatmen von Methylalkohol-haltigen Formaldehyddämpfen, *Samml. Vergiftungsf.*, 5:129, A 442.

Schwenkenbecher (1904) Die Absorptionsvermögen für die Haut, *Arch. Anat. Physiol. Abt.*, p. 121.

Scott, E, M. K. Helz and C. P. McCord (1933) The Histopathology of Methyl Alcohol Poisoning, *Am. J. Clin. Path.*, 3:311.

Silverman, L., H. F. Schulte and W. E. First (1946) Further Studies on sensory Response to certain individual Solvent Vapours, *J. Ind. Hyg. Toxicol.*, 28:262.

Sisley, J. P. (1934) Solvents utilisés dans l'Industrie textile, *Reg. Gen. Mat. Col.*, 38:481.

Smith, H. M. (1927) Dewaxing Paraffin base crudes, *Oil Gas J.*, 26:146.

Smith, M. E. and H. W. Newman (1959) The Rate of Ethanol Metabolism in fed and fasting Animals, *J. Biol. Chem.*, 234:1544.

Smyth, H. F. (1956) *Cummings Memorial Lecture*, cited by Treon, 1963.

Smyth, H. F. and H. F. Smyth Jr. (1928) Inhalation Experiments with certain Lacquer Solvents, *J. Ind. Hyg. Toxicol.*, 10:261.

Smyth, H. F., Jr. and C. P. Carpenter (1945) Note upon the Toxicity of Ethylene chlorohydrin by Skin Absorption, *J. Ind., Hyg. Toxicol.*, 27:93.

— (1948) Further Experience with Range Finding Test in Industrial Toxicology Laboratory, *J. Ind. Hyg. Toxicol.*, 30:63.

Smyth, H. F., Jr., C. P. Carpenter and C. S. Weil (1949) Range finding Toxicity Data, List III, *J. Ind. Hyg. Toxicol.*, 31:60.

— (1951) Range Finding Toxicity Data, *Arch. Ind. Hyg.*, 4:199.

— (1951) Range finding Toxicity Data, *Arch. Ind. Hyg.*, 4:119.

Smyth, H. F., Jr., C. P. Carpenter, C. S. Weil and U. C. Pozzani (1954) Range finding Toxicity Data, List V, *Arch. Ind. Hyg.*, 10:61.

Smyth, H. F., Jr., J. Seaton and L. Fischer (1941) The single Dose Toxicity of some Glycols and Derivatives, *J. Ind. Hyg. Toxicol.*, 23:259.

Snapper, I., A. Grunbaum and S. Sturkop (1925) Über die Spaltung und die Oxydation von Benzyl Alcohol und Benzylestern im menschlichen Organismus, *Biochem. Z.*, 155:163.

Sollman, T. and P. J. Hanzlik (1928) *An Introduction to experimental Pharmacology*, Saunders, Philadelphia.

Starrek, E. (1938) *Über die Wirkung einiger Alkohole, Glykole und Ester* (cited by Lehmann and Flury, 1943, in *Toxicology and Hygiene of Industrial Solvents*), Williams and Wilkins, Baltimore.

Stekol, J. A. (1939) Studies on the Mercapturic Acid Synthesis in Animals, *J. Biol. Chem.*, 128:199.

Steinkoff, D. (1952) Augenschädigungen durch Butylazetat-Isobutyl Alkohol, *Z. Arbeitsmed. Arbeitsschutz*, 2:13.

Sterner, J. H., H. C. Crouch, H. F. Brockmyre and M. Cusack (1949) A ten-year Study of Butyl Alcohol Exposure, *Am. Ind. Hyg. Ass. Quart.*, 10:53.

Stinebaugh, B. J. (1960) The use of Peritoneal Dialysis in Acute Methyl Alcohol Poisoning, *Arch. Int. Med.*, 105:613.

Straus, M. (1887) Sur un Moyen de provoquer l'Anesthésie chez le Lapin, *C. R. Soc. Biol.*, 4:54.

Tabershaw, I. R., J. P. Fahy and J. B. Skinner (1944) Industrial Exposure to Butanol, *J. Ind. Hyg. Toxicol.*, 26:328.

Theorell, H. and R. Bonnischen (1951) Studies on Liver Alcohol Dehydrogenase, *Acta Chem. Scand.*, 5:1105.

Thierfelder, H. and J. von Mering (1885) Das Verhalten tertiärer Alkohole im Organismus, *Z. Physiol. Chem.*, 9:611.

Threshold Limit Values for 1962, *Am. Ind. Hyg. Ass. J.*, 1962, 23:419.

Torkelson, T. R., M. A. Wolf, F. Oyen and V. K. Rowe (1959) Vapour Toxicity of Allyl Alcohol as determined on Laboratory Animals, *Am. Ind. Hyg. Ass. J.*, 20:224.

Treon, J. F. (1963) *Alcohols*, in F. A. Patty (Ed.), *Industrial Hygiene and Toxicology*, Vol. II, 2nd ed., Interscience, New York.

Treon, J. F., W. E. Crutchfield Jr. and K. V. Kitzmiller (1943) The physiological Response of Rabbits to Cyclohexane, Methyl Cyclohexane and certain Derivatives of these Compounds, *J. Ind. Hyg. Toxicol.*, 25:199 and 233.

Tsuchiya, K. (1963) Chronic Poisoning and occupational Cancer, *Medicine (Tokyo)*, 20:86.

Tyson, H. H. (1912) Amblyopia from Inhalation of Methyl Alcohol, *Arch. Ophthalm.*, 41:459.

Tyson, H. H. and M. J. Schoenberg (1914) Experimental Researches in Methyl Alcohol Inhalation, *J. Am. Med. Ass.*, 63:915.

Uhrig, R. (1946) (cited by Treon, 1963) *Ind. Eng. Chem. Anal. Ed.*, 18:469.

Vigneaud, V. du, C. Lessler and J. R. Rochelle (1950) The biological Synthesis of "Labile Methyl Groups". *Science*, 112:267.

Voegtlin, W. L. and C. E. Watts (1943) Acute Methyl Alcohol (Methanol) poisoning, *U.S. Nav. Med. Bull.*, 41:1715.

Vollmer, H. (1931) Fortgesetzte Versuche über die Giftempfindlichkeit von Mäusen und Ratten nach Bestrahlung oder Vorbehandlung mit oxydationssteigernden Substanzen, *Arch. Exptl Pathol. Pharmakol.*, 160:635.

Voltz, W. and W. Dietrich (1912) Die Beteiligung des Methylalkols und des Äthylalkohols am gesamten Stoffumsatz im tierischen Organismus, *Biochem. Z.*, 40:15.

Walton, D. C., E. F. Kehr and A. S. Loevenhart (1928) Comparison of the pharmacologica Actions of Diacetone Alcohol and Acetone, *J. Pharmacol.*, 33:175.

Wax, J., F. W. Ellis and A. J. Lehman (1949) Absorption and Distribution of Isopropyl Alcohol, *J. Pharmacol.*, 97:229.

Webb, A. D. and R. E. Kepner (1951) (cited by Castor, J. G. B. and J. F. Guymon, 1952) On the Mechanism of Formation of higher Alcohols during alcoholic Fermentation, *Science*, 115:147.

Weber, H. H. and W. Koch (1933) Zur Methodik der Analyse technischer Lösungsmittel, *Chemiker Z.*, 57:73.

Weese, H. (1928) Vergleichende Untersuchungen über die Wirksamkeit und Giftigkeit der Dämpfe niederer aliphatischer Alkohole, *Arch. Exptl. Pathol. Pharmakol.*, 135:118.

Weitzel, G. (1950) Biochemie verzweigter Carbonsäuren, *Hoppe-Seyler's Z.*, 285:58.

Werkman, C. H. and O. L. Osburn (1930) Determination of Butyl and Ethyl Alcohols in Fermentation Mixtures, *Proc. Soc. Exptl. Biol. Med.*, 28:241.

Westerfeld, W. W. (1961) The intermediary Metabolism of Alcohol, *Am. J. Clin. Nutr.*, 9:426.

Widmark, E. M. P. (1915) Konzentration des Alkohols in Blut und Harn, *Skand. Arch. Physiol.*, 33:85.

— (1932) *Die theoretischen Grundlagen und die praktische Verwendbarkeit der gerichtlichmedizinischen Alkoholbestimmung*, Urban und Schwarzenberg, Berlin.

Williams, R. T. (1959) *Detoxication Mechanisms*, 2nd. ed., p. 54, Chapman and Hall, London.

Wilson, M. M. and F. J. Worster (1929) Place of Synthetic Amyl Products among Lacquer Solvents, *Ind. Eng. Chem.*, 21:592.

Wood, C. A. and F. Buller (1904) Poisoning by Wood Alcohol, *J. Am. Med. Ass.*, 43:972.

Woods, H. (1913) Wood Alcohol Blindness, *J. Am. Med. Ass.*, 60:1762.

Yant, W. P. and H. H. Schrenk (1937) Distribution of Methanol in Dogs, *J. Ind. Hyg. Toxicol.*, 19:337.

Yant, W. P., H. H. Schrenk and R. R. Sayers (1931) Methanol Anti-freeze and Methanol Poisoning, *Ind. Eng. Chem.*, 23:551.

Yarsley, V. E. (1933) Health Hazards in the Lacquer and Finishing Industries, *Synth. Appl. Finish.*, 3:80.

— (1934) Solvents and Plasticisers. A Review of recent progress with special Reference to Cellulose Acetate, *Synth. Appl. Finish.*, 5:37, 57.

Zangger, H. (1933) Arbeitsunfälle und Arbeitsgefährdung bei der Arbeit in inneren geschlossenen Behältern, *Arch. Gewerbepathol. Gewerbehyg.*, 4:117.

Zatman, L. J. (1946) Oxidation of Methyl Alcohol inhibited by Ethyl Alcohol, *Biochem. J.*, 40 Proc. LXVII.

Ziegler, S. L. (1921) The Ocular Menace of Wood Alcohol Poisoning, *J. Am. Med. Ass.*, 77:1160.

Chapter 8

KETONES

The ketones are very widely used as 'general purpose' solvents, also as raw materials or intermediates in organic synthesis, in the perfume industry and as constituents of synthetic coatings, dopes and adhesives.

On the whole the hazard from their industrial use is not great; they are to some extent narcotic, but since they are also, in high concentrations, irritant to mucous membranes, such irritation acts as a pre-narcotic warning and deterrent. Some of them, including methyl ethyl ketone, mesityl oxide and isophorone which is regarded as the most toxic, are capable of causing kidney injury in animals, but records of such injury from their industrial use are practically non-existent. With repeated exposure, apart from local irritation, the only symptoms complained of are those common to exposure by any narcotic substance – headache, drowsiness, nausea and occasionally vomiting. The fact that the Threshold Limit Values for 1962 for the two ketones in most general use – acetone and methyl ethyl ketone – have been established as 1000 and 200 p.p.m. respectively – is a further indication that the criteria of experimentation, both animal and human, have not indicated any considerable hazard from these two compounds, though a few other ketones are listed at 50 p.p.m. and one (isophorone) as 25 p.p.m.

Ketones are not readily metabolised in the body; with some of them, especially those with low boiling points, as much as 50% may be eliminated in the expired air unchanged and to some extent in the urine. The major metabolic change is a reduction to the corresponding alcohol, which combines with glucuronic acid and is eliminated in this form. With acetone, only about 1% of the dose is excreted as glucuronide.

A number of methods for the quantitative estimation of the various ketones in air are available. One of the earliest is that of Messinger (1889) which is described in detail by Jacobs (1949); it depends on the reaction with iodine in the presence of alkali to form iodoform and acetic acid. Another method in wide use at present is the hydroxylamine method originally described by Morasco (1926) for acetone; various modifications of this have been adapted to the estimation of the different ketones.

[412]

51. Acetone

Synonyms: dimethyl ketone, propanone-2

Structural formula:

$$CH_3\!-\!\overset{\displaystyle O}{\overset{\|}{C}}\!-\!CH_3$$

Molecular formula: C_3H_6O

Molecular weight: 58.08

Properties: a volatile, colourless, inflammable liquid with a pungent odour. Solvent for resins, lacquers, fats, oils, collodion cotton, celluloid, cellulose acetate and acetylene. Disinfectant when used in high concentrations, being rapidly bactericidal for *Micrococcus aureus*, but not sporicidal, though it induces delay in the growth of spores (Drews and Edelmann, 1956).

    boiling point: 56.5 °C (technical grade 55.5–56.2 °C)
    melting point: −95.6 °C
    vapour pressure: 226.3 mm Hg at 25 °C
    specific gravity (liquid density): 0.792
    flash point: explosive limits 2.5–12.8% (Jones et al., 1933)
    conversion factors: 1 p.p.m. = 2.37 mg/m³
                      1 mg/l = 422 p.p.m.
    solubility: miscible with water in all proportions
    evaporation rate (ether = 1): 2.1
    maximum allowable concentration: 1000 p.p.m. (Threshold Limit Values, 1962)

ECONOMY, SOURCES AND USES

Production

(1) By destructive distillation of wood.
(2) By distillation of calcium acetate.
(3) By fermentation of corn products by selected bacteria (Rowe and Wolf, 1963).
(4) By catalytic oxidation of isopropyl alcohol, cumene, or natural gas.

Industrial uses

(1) In the lacquer and varnish industry.
(2) In the rubber industry.
(3) In the plastics industry.

(4) In the chemical industry as a solvent and as an intermediate in the production of chloroform (Kagan, 1924).

(5) In the manufacture of artificial silk and artificial leather (Clayton and Clark, 1931).

(6) In the dyeing industry.

(7) As a solvent for acetylene (Flury and Wirth, 1934).

(8) In the production of lubricating oils (Smoley and Kraft, 1935).

(9) In the celluloid industry (Heim de Balzac and Agasse–Lafont, 1922).

BIOCHEMISTRY

Estimation

(1) In the atmosphere

(a) The bisulphite method. – This method, as used by Haggard *et al.* (1944) is based on the formation of a non-volatile complex of acetone in sodium bisulphite. The air sample is passed through the bisulphite solution and 2 N iodine in KI added until a barely distinguishable colour is visible. Solid Na bicarbonate in excess is then added and 2 N iodine dropped from a burette until one drop produces a faint yellow. A further addition of 2 N NaOH and 0.1 N iodine solution, and, after standing, 2 N HCl, is followed by titration of the mixture with 0.1 N thiosulphate in the presence of starch. As in the Messinger method of analysis, described by Goodwin (1920) each ml of 0.1 N iodine reacting with the bisulphite is equal to 0.967 mg of acetone.

(b) The silica gel method. – This method, described by Elkins (1959) is applicable to other methyl ketones, such as methyl ethyl ketone and methyl isobutyl ketone. After passage of the acetone-containing air over the silica gel, this is placed in water, and after 1 h 2 N NaOH and 0.1 N iodine are added, followed in 15 min by 6 N H$_2$SO$_4$. This is then titrated with 0.1 N thiosulphate and starch. A blank titration is made and the amount of acetone is calculated as

$$\frac{\text{blank titration} - \text{sample titration}}{\text{L}25} \times \frac{100}{3} = \text{p.p.m. acetone}$$

where L = litres of air sampled

(2) In blood and tissues

The most recent methods of estimating the amount of acetone in blood or tissues are those described by Feldstein (1960) and Curry *et al.* (1962). The former is a micro-diffusion method, using the Conway Diffusion Unit, with the biological sample in the outer tube and the absorbing solution (sodium bisulphite) in the centre well of the unit. The appropriate liberating agent (in the case of acetone, NaOH and alicycloaldehyde solution) is added to the outer compartment and after mixing and leaving to stand the optical density of the red colour produced is measured by a spectrophotometer. The latter is described (Curry *et al.*, 1962) as a simple and rapid method for the detection of acetone in blood samples by gas chromatography. A 100 ml sample of blood is injected into a closed tube containing 0.5 g of soild potassium carbonate, which serves to decrease the vapour pressure of water and to provide internal heating by its heat of solution. The whole apparatus is then warmed by immersion in hot water for 1 min, and a 1-ml air sample then extracted by means of a hypodermic syringe and injected into 10% silicone oil on an 'Embacel' column. The carrier gas used is hydrogen.

Metabolism

Acetone is readily absorbed by inhalation, according to Kagan (1924). After inhaling acetone from a flask containing a known percentage of acetone in water and exhaling it into a series of flasks containing water and sodium iodide, he found that the amount inhaled in 5 min from a 10% solution was 910 mg, while the amount expired was 264 mg; thus the amount absorbed was 71%. Haggard, Greenberg and Turner (1944) have described what they call 'absorptive concentration' with progressive accumulation of acetone in the tissues of a man inhaling acetone for 6 h. Thus, exposure to a concentration of 2100 p.p.m. of acetone during an 8-h working day resulted in the accumulation of a small residue (330 mg/l) in the blood; this amount however produced no significant symptoms. Absorption by the skin has been postulated both in animals and also in human beings but in animals it is only to a small extent, and in human beings contact with the skin must have been heavy and prolonged, and in the cases described, in which severe intoxication has been caused by the application of plaster casts with acetone as the setting fluid (see p. 420) there has been the probably over-riding factor of inhalation.

In animals absorption by the skin has been based on the estimations by Lazarew *et al.* (1931) of the amount exhaled and present in the blood of animals with a foot immersed in acetone. The small amount so absorbed was slower than with ethyl ether or chloroform, and it was concluded that the danger of absorption by this route during its industrial use was very unlikely. Even this possibility has been discounted by the later researches of Cesaro and Pinerolo (1947) on human subjects. They considered that the results of Lazarew *et al.* were somewhat doubtful because prolonged immersion of the foot or ear of the animal may have injured the skin. They therefore used naked men with no skin lesions or disturbance of digestive or endocrine function, and based their estimation of absorption of acetone on the total amount of ketone in the blood before and after exposure. The subjects were placed for 20–30 min in a closed chamber filled with air saturated with acetone by means of cotton wool soaked in it and were given also pads of cotton wool with which to moisten their skin; their heads remained fixed outside the chamber. Blood (2.5 ml) was taken from the cubital vein before and

Bibliography on p. 458

immediately after the exposure, and the total amount of ketone (pre-formed acetone, acetone derived from diacetic acid and that from β-oxybutyric acid estimated by the microchemical method described by Condorelli (1931). The levels were practically unchanged, the slight variations being within the limits of laboratory error. It was concluded that no absorption of acetone takes place from the intact skin.

Acetone differs from the majority of ketones in that large doses undergo little reduction in the body and are largely excreted unchanged (Williams, 1959), and that small amounts are largely metabolised, but at a relatively slow rate (Price and Rittenberg, 1950). This latter fact was demonstrated as early as 1898 by Schwarz, who found that the fraction recoverable in the breath becomes smaller as the size of the dose decreased. When doses of 300–600 mg/kg were given, about 55% was exhaled and 1.2% excreted in the urine; when the dose was 3.5 mg/kg only 18% was exhaled, indicating that small amounts were metabolised. Further investigations, using radioactive carbonyl compounds (^{14}CO and $^{14}CH_3$) have shown (Price and Rittenberg, 1950) that small doses (1.7 mg/kg) are almost completely metabolised by oxidation. With this small dosage about 7% is exhaled unchanged and according to Sakami and Lafaye (1950) 53% is oxidised to CO_2, which is also exhaled within 24 h. The fact that the respired air was not acetone-free until 24 h later has been considered evidence of its slow utilisation (Hahn, 1935).

According to Parmeggiani and Sassi (1954) there is about 10% of inhaled acetone excreted through the skin. It has been suggested that acetone possibly plays a part as an intermediate of fat metabolism. In 1941 Koehler, Windsor and Hill, on the basis of their experiments with intravenous injections of acetone in human beings, had stated that the rate of acetone breakdown, as judged from blood levels and urinary excretion, appeared so slow that any large part of normal fatty acid metabolism could not conceivably pass through the acetone stage, but in 1950 Sakani and Lafaye concluded that some intermediary part in fat metabolism by acetone was a possibility. They found that methyl-labelled acetone was converted to liver glycogen, serine, choline and methionine. This was believed to occur by oxidation of the acetone to acetate and formate or carbon intermediates of fat metabolism. In a later investigation (1951) they also suggested that there exists a mechanism involving the direct conversion of acetone to an intermediate of glycolysis (pyruvate) reflecting liver metabolism of acetone more than that of any other organ of the body.

TOXICOLOGY

The principal toxic action of acetone in high dosage is exerted upon the central nervous system, producing narcosis. With repeated smaller dosage this narcotic effect is shown by headache and drowsiness. That it has also an irritant effect on mucous membranes is shown by irritation of the eyes, nose and throat, and also probably of the gastric mucous membrane as manifested by nausea and vomiting. In some cases of acute poisoning from prolonged application to the skin (though in most of these inhalation has also been a factor) vomiting has been accompanied by a certain amount of haematemesis, and in one case (Chatterton and Elliott, 1946) the presence of a trace of albumen and some red and white blood cells in the urine have suggested the possibility of a toxic effect on the kidneys. In industrial use no significant systemic effects have been reported.

Toxicity to animals

(1) Acute

(a) *Lethal dose.* – (i) *By stomach tube*, for rabbits, 5–10 ml/kg (Walton *et al.*, 1928), for dogs, 4–8 g/kg (Albertoni, 1884). – (ii) *By intravenous injection*, for rabbits, 4 ml/kg, for rats 6–8 ml/kg (Walton *et al.*, 1928). – (iii) *By inhalation*, for mice, 42,200 p.p.m. (Sklianskaya *et al.*, 1936), and 46,000 p.p.m. (Schultze, 1932), for rats, 126,600 p.p.m. in $1\frac{3}{4}$ to $2\frac{1}{4}$ h (Haggard, Greenberg and Turner, 1944), and for guinea pigs 21,000 p.p.m. Specht *et al.*, 1940).

(b) *Narcotic dose.* – (i) *By oral administration*, for rabbits 7 mg/kg (Walton *et al.*, 1928), for dogs, 4 g/kg (Albertoni, 1884). – (ii) *By intravenous injection*, for rats, 2 ml/kg (Walton *et al.*, 1928). – (iii) *By inhalation*, for mice, 8300 to 20,000 (Schultze, 1932), for cats, 42,200–52,750 (Kagan, 1924), and 75,000 (Schultze, 1932), and for guinea pigs, 21,000 (Specht *et al.*, 1940).

SYMPTOMS OF INTOXICATION

With acute intoxication the preliminary symptoms of narcosis are irritative – salivation, lacrimation, giddiness, ataxia, twitchings and convulsions. According to Di Prisco (1936) irritation of the nasal mucosa causes a temporary cessation of breathing as a protective reflex. A specific irritative effect on the respiratory centre has also been stated by Gollwitzer-Meier (1927), and, after intravenous and intramuscular injection a fall in blood pressure which Walton *et al.* (1928) and Salant and Kleitmann (1922) have regarded as primarily due to a decrease in cardiac output.

With repeated exposure to low concentrations of acetone vapour animals appear to suffer very little ill-effect. Only slight irritation of the eyes and nose of cats exposed to repeated inhalations of 1265–2110 p.p.m. was observed by Kagan (1924) and Schultze (1932) and Kagan noted an increased tolerance to these relatively low concentrations.

CHANGES IN THE ORGANISM

The only organ which has been stated to be specifically injured in animals poisoned by acetone is the kidney, and the extent of such injury has been variously estimated especially by the earlier observers. Baginsky (1888) and Schwartz (1898) for example found no evidence of injury in dogs subjected to repeated administration, while Albertoni and Pisent (1887) described granular degeneration in the less severe, and necrosis of the tubular epithelium in the more severe intoxications. Poliak (1925) also observed lesions of the convoluted tubules, Kagan (1924) some fatty infiltration in one cat following inhalation of 75,900 p.p.m. and Flury and Wirth albuminuria in some of their animals subjected to inhalation.

The eyes

Direct application to the eyes of rabbits was found by Larson *et al.* (1956) to cause marked oedema of the conjunctiva. It has recently been suggested by Gomer (1960) that this injury by acetone is due to dehydration of the sclera, followed by gelatinous flocculation and opacity.

Toxicity to human beings

(1) Acute

Few cases of acute intoxication from the industrial use of acetone have been recorded. In one of these (Sack, 1940) the man was engaged in cleaning a tank which had contained a solution of artificial silk in acetone. He became unconscious, and after recovery following an injection of coramine, showed excitement and vomited. On the following day the blood still contained a higher than normal amount of acetone (18 mg%) and the urine a detectable amount. Slight injury to the kidneys, and possibly to the liver was suggested by the presence of slight albuminuria and red and white corpuscles in the urine, a high level of urobilin and an early rise of bilirubin in the blood.

Two less severe cases of intoxication were recorded by Smith and Mayers (1944). The solvent, used for waterproofing the seams of raincoats, contained not only acetone but also butanone, the atmospheric levels being 330–495 p.p.m. and 389–561 p.p.m. respectively. The symptoms were gastric distress, fainting and collapse.

(2) Chronic

In view of the widespread use of acetone in industrial processes there have been few cases of even mild intoxication by acetone, and such reports as have appeared have often proved to have been associated with exposure to other solvents in addition to acetone. In the experience of Llewellyn (1963, personal communication) he has never known acetone to cause any case of even slight poisoning; he states that "the worst that can happen in men who have worked in concentrations well above the MAC for a long shift is a dull headache, maybe associated with temporary anorexia". He carried out in the late 50's a survey of a large number of men who had worked in acetone for many years, in early days in concentrations much greater than 1000 p.p.m. and for much longer than 42h/ week. The survey revealed no deletrious effects, either mental or physical, and no abnormality of the blood picture or urine.

In an extensive investigation by Oglesby *et al.* (1949) cited by Rowe and Wolf (1963) covering exposures to concentrations averaging up to 2000 p.p.m. and representing 21 million man-hours of experience, they concluded that no injury had occurred to any individual. Fassett (1963) also states that experience over the 10 years since 1948 has confirmed these conclusions.

SYMPTOMS OF INTOXICATION

The symptoms in the rare cases recorded are described as a sensation of heat, vertigo, slight fainting attacks, irritation of the throat, coughing (Carozzi, 1930). Headache in workers making celluloid boxes and using a glue containing a mixture of acetone and amyl acetate was described by Heim de Balzac and Agasse-Lafont (1922), but since amyl acetate might have been responsible for this disturbance, it cannot be attributed entirely to acetone.

Similarly, in the cases exhibiting a large variety of symptoms described by Sessa and Troisi (1947), referable to the painting and spraying of lacquers, the solvent was of mixed content, including, besides acetone, several acetates. The symptoms included skin lesions, digestive disorders, headache, rhinitis, pharyngitis, bronchial catarrh and asthenia. Sessa and Troisi concluded that the 'occupational pathology of varnishers' was in great part due to acetone but also, to a lesser degree, to butyl and ethyl acetate and other solvent constitutents.

(1) The eyes

Lacrimation, photophobia and infiltration of the corneal epithelium, and in one case corneal opacities, were present in two men in a driving-belt factory by Halbertsma (1926), but it was eventually discovered that the acetone used contained acetaldehyde.

(2) The skin

Several cases of poisoning by acetone following the application of plaster casts with acetone as the setting fluid have been reported since 1903, when Cossman described the symptoms, similar to those of diabetic coma, in a boy who had had a plastic bandage impregnated with acetone applied to an immobilised tubercular hip.

Similar symptoms, though of greater severity, were recorded by Strong (1944), though true coma did not develop; there were periods of semi-consciousness, and the patient developed nausea and vomiting of blood. In this case the urine contained albumin, sugar and acetone. Drowsiness, coma and the vomiting of coffee-coloured blood, with slight albuminuria, sugar and blood corpuscles in the urine were also features in the case recorded by Chatterton and Elliott (1946) in which

Bibliography on p. 458

the solvent evaporating agent was pure acetone and the commercial lacquer supplied for smoothing the cast also contained acetone.

Similar cases have been described by Harris and Jackson (1952) and Renshaw and Mitchell (1956). All these cases showed a latent period of about 12 h before the appearance of symptoms, and it appears that in most of them inhalation has been at least as potent a factor as skin absorption. In Chatterton and Elliott's case, on removal of the casts the skin showed no sign of irritation, and in that of Renshaw and Mitchell the acetone was not in direct contact with the skin.

(3) The blood

The only abnormality in the blood picture observed was the eosinophilia described by Heim de Balzac *et al.* (1922) who considered eosinophilia "a proof of the reaction to saturation of the organism by fumes of acetone and amyl acetate". This statement has so far received no confirmation from other observers. Browning (unpublished observation) found no eosinophilia in a series of workers employed on a cellulose acetate process nor did Rosgen and Mamier (1944) in 45 men and 39 women in a dry-cleaning process. No clinical symptoms suggesting intoxication, and no abnormality of the blood picture except a few cases of rather low haemoglobin levels, believed to be of nutritional origin, were found, and Rosgen and Mamier concluded that the possibility of any injurious effect of acetone on the haemopoietic system can be excluded.

TREATMENT OF POISONING

On the analogy of acute acetone poisoning with diabetic coma, it has been suggested (and indeed tried in some of the cases due to the application of plaster casts) that glucose and insulin should be given. In one such case however (Strong, 1944) the patient had a long continued severe period of intoxication, and Koehler *et al.* (1941) were unable to show any effect of glucose or insulin or both simultaneously on the blood of persons who had received 100 g of acetone by intravenous injection.

Hift and Patel (1961) advise administration of plentiful fluids to ensure a good flow of urine; otherwise only symptomatic treatment.

52. Methyl Ethyl Ketone

Synonyms: butanone, MEK

Structural formula:

$$CH_3—CH_2—\overset{\overset{\displaystyle O}{\|}}{C}—CH_3$$

Molecular formula: C_4H_8O

Molecular weight: 92.06

Properties: a clear, colourless, highly volatile liquid with an odour resembling that of acetone. Good solvent for some resins and gums, cellulose acetate and nitrate. Explosive risk – the lower limit is about 2% (Patty *et al.*, 1935), but since it is intensely irritating at 350 p.p.m. (Nelson *et al.*, 1943) and its threshold for odour is less than 25 p.p.m., the fire hazard should be easily recognisable before it becomes flammable.

> *boiling point:* pure product 79.6 °C; technical 68–85 °C (contains 93% of ketone as determined by acetylation (Patty *et al.*, 1935).
> *melting point:* −86 °C
> *vapour pressure:* 20 mm Hg at 25 °C
> *vapour density (air = 1):* 2.41
> *specific gravity (liquid density):* 0.8072
> *flash point:* 24 °F
> *conversion factors:* 1 p.p.m. = 2.94 mg/m³
> 1 mg/l = 340 p.p.m.
> *solubility:* in water 25.5 g/100
> *evaporation rate (ether = 1):* 2.7
> *maximum allowable concentration:* 200 p.p.m. (Threshold Limit Values, 1962), Elkins (1949) suggests 300 p.p.m.

ECONOMY, SOURCES AND USES

Production

In recent years synthetic production from secondary alcohols (especially secondary butyl alcohol) and from butylene glycol has superseded the former preparation as a by-product in the distillation of wood.

Industrial uses

MEK is often used in combination with other solvents such as acetone, alcohol, etc. La Belle and Brieger (1955) investigated a mixture of solvents which included acetone, tetrahydrofuran, dimethyl and propylene acetal, found that MEK represented 55.7%.

(1) In artificial leather manufacture (Zangger, 1930).

(2) In the lacquer and varnish industry (Despartmet, 1928); mixed with alcohol, acetone or triphenyl phosphate for lacquering aeroplanes (Zangger, 1930); also as a paint remover (Langovoy, 1933).

(3) In pharmaceuticals and cosmetics (Holden and Doolittle, 1935)

(4) In synthetic rubber manufacture, especially Thiokol (Greenberg and Moskowitz, 1945).

(5) In production of lubricating oils (Smoley and Kraft, 1935).

(6) In fabric coating (Elkins, 1959).

BIOCHEMISTRY

Estimation

In the atmosphere

The silica gel method described by Elkins (1959) for acetone (*q.v.*) is stated by him to be applicable to MEK.

The chemical method of analysis described by Patty, Schrenk and Yant (1935) also depends on absorption of MEK into NaOH solution, addition of iodine and titration with 20 N sodium thiosulphate solution.

Metabolism

MEK occurs in trace amounts in normal human urine and, according to Tsao and Pfeiffer (1957) has possibly a dietary origin; its most probable precursor is α-methylacetoacetic acid. Like other ketones (with the exception of acetone) MEK is reduced to some extent in the body. Only 30–40%, according to Schwartz (1898), is eliminated in the expired air, as compared with 50–60% for acetone.

It has been shown to increase the glucuronic acid output (Neubauer, 1901) and the urine of rabbits receiving it has been stated (Saneyoshi, 1911) to contain the glucuronide of 2-butanol.

TOXICOLOGY

The chief effect of MEK is narcosis, but it is also a strong irritant of mucous membranes, especially of the eyes and nose. One episode of eye injury to human beings from inhalation of MEK has been reported (Smyth, 1956), but it was believed to have been actually caused by an unsaturated ketone impurity present by accident. Nausea and vomiting have also been observed in one process where the solvent contained also 10% of 2-nitropropane; except for these examples and the occupational dermatitis mentioned by Schwarz et al. (1947) and Smith and Mayers (1944) there have been no records of intoxication in its industrial use.

Toxicity to animals

(1) Acute

(a) Lethal dose. – (i) By oral administration, for rats, 3.3 g/kg body weight (Shell Chemical Corp., 1959). – (ii) By inhalation, there is some discrepancy in the results of different observers. Patty et al. (1935) observed no deaths in guinea pigs exposed for a few minutes to 100,000 p.p.m., and no serious disturbances at 10,000 p.p.m. for 1 h. On the other hand Smyth (1956) reported that 4 out of 6 rats died after exposure of 1 h to 4000 p.p.m. and La Belle and Brieger (1955), comparing the toxicity of MEK with a solvent mixture of which it represented 55.7%, gave the LD_{50} as 700 p.p.m., close to that of the solvent mixture at 10,000 p.p.m. The mean survival time with exposure to saturation concentration was 43 min for MEK and 59 min for the mixture.

(b) Narcotic dose, depends greatly on the time of exposure. Patty et al. (1935) found that guinea pigs showed narcosis after 33,000 p.p.m. for 48 to 90 min, while 10,000 p.p.m. caused narcosis with eventual recovery after 240 to 280 min.

(2) Chronic

Repeated exposure of guinea pigs for 12 weeks to concentrations of 235 p.p.m. of MEK and 226 p.p.m. of the solvent mixture (La Belle and Brieger, 1955) caused no symptoms in either group of animals, though both groups showed signs of vitamin deficiency.

CHANGES IN THE ORGANISM

In animals subjected to lethal doses, Patty et al. (1935) observed marked congestion of internal organs and slight congestion of the brain. The lungs also showed emphysema and the liver and kidneys marked congestion. Those animals which survived exposure to 100,000 p.p.m. for 30 min or more developed corneal opacity, which improved and practically disappeared at the end of eight days.

In evaluating the potency of various classes of chemicals to produce oedema of the corneal membrane, Larson et al. (1956) found the potency of MEK greater than that of acetone.

Toxicity to human beings

Acute intoxication

Ingestion (suicidal) of a plastic catalyst containing 60% of MEK peroxide and 40% of dimethylphthalate is reported by Dines and Shipman (1962) to have caused acute poisoning, with dyspnoea, vomiting, haemorrhagic oesophagitis, gastritis and bronchopneumonia, and 3 days later toxic myocarditis.

Another case of poisoning from accidental ingestion of 2 ozs. of the same plastic catalyst was recorded by Deisher (1958); this caused a chemical burn and subsequent stricture of the oesophagus.

SYMPTOMS OF INTOXICATION

(1) Mucous membranes

Slight throat irritation even at 100 p.p.m., and of the eyes at 200 p.p.m., becoming objectionable at 300 p.p.m. was observed by Nelson *et al.* (1943), while Patty *et al.* (1935) reported almost intolerable irritation of the eyes and nose at 10,000 p.p.m.

(2) The skin

According to Smith and Mayers (1944) dermatoses among workers having both direct contact and also exposure to the vapour of MEK are not uncommon. Several workers exposed to both liquid and vapour complained of numbness of the fingers and arms.

CHANGES IN THE ORGANISM

Central nervous system disorders

Elkins (1959) notes that although exposures as high as 700 p.p.m. have shown no evidence of permanent ill-effects, concentrations above 300 p.p.m. usually result in complaints of headache, throat irritation and similar symptoms, while in one plant where concentrations averaged 500 p.p.m. nausea and vomiting were reported (in this instance the solvent contained 10% of 2-nitropropane). Gastric upsets and fainting occurred, according to Smith and Mayers (1944), among girls using a mixture of acetone (330 to 496 p.p.m.) and MEK (398 to 561 p.p.m.).

No serious systemic effects and no severe narcotic effects have been recorded from the industrial use of MEK.

53. Methyl Propyl Ketone

Synonyms: ethyl acetone, pentanone-2

Structural formula: $CH_3-CH_2-CH_2-\underset{\underset{O}{||}}{C}-CH_3$

Molecular formula: $C_5H_{10}O$

Molecular weight: 86.13

Properties: a clear liquid with a strong odour resembling acetone and also ether.
  boiling point: 102 °C pure. Commercial grade (Yant *et al.*, 1936) 98.5–101.5 °C
  melting point: −83.5 °C
  vapour pressure: 16 mm Hg at 20 °C
  specific gravity (liquid density): 0.8064, 0.8075
  flash point: 45 °F
  conversion factors: 1 p.p.m. = 3.52 mg/m³
                         1 mg/l   = 284 p.p.m.
  solubility: in water 5.5 g/100
  maximum allowable concentration: 200 p.p.m. (Threshold Limit Values, 1962)

ECONOMY, SOURCES AND USES

Production

Chiefly by oxidation of 2-pentanol (Rowe and Wolf, 1963).

Industrial uses

As a solvent, either alone or in combination with other solvents for the same general purposes as acetone, especially for making lacquers, varnishes and lacquer removers (Yant *et al.*, 1936).

Methyl propyl ketone exists as two isomers, methyl-*n*-propyl and methyl-isopropyl ketone. The latter has apparently been investigated only with regard to its presence as a metabolite of the secondary amyl alcohol, 3-methyl butanol-2 (Haggard *et al.*, 1944). From this investigation, regarding the 'basic lethal amount' (the concentration in the blood which causes respiratory failure) it would appear that methyl isopropyl ketone is slightly more toxic than the *n*-isomer, the basic lethal amount of the former being 1.02 g/kg for the rat as compared with 1.25 g/kg for the latter. There are no details concerning its properties or effects in actual use as a solvent; the following account refers exclusively to methyl *n*-propyl ketone.

BIOCHEMISTRY

Estimation

A modification of the method of Greenberg and Lester (1944) for estimation of acetone (*q.v.*) was used by Haggard *et al.* (1944). It depends essentially, like that of earlier workers (Dakin and Dudley, 1913; Friedman and Hauger, 1943) on the reaction between the ketone and 2-4,dinitrophenylhydrazine; the addition of trichloroacetic acid and extraction with carbon tetrachloride is followed by washing with 8 N NaOH and the colour is read in a colorimeter.

For the estimation of the metabolite (methyl isopropyl ketone) Haggard *et al.* used the precipitate formed by the reaction with 2-4,dinitrophenylhydrazine, which, after washing and recrystallisation, was subjected to microanalysis for carbon, hydrogen and nitrogen.

Metabolism

Methyl-*n*-propyl ketone can be absorbed to some extent through the skin (Rowe and Wolf, 1963). Elimination takes place mainly unchanged in the expired air, to the extent of 38–54% in about 25–35 h (Haggard *et al.*, 1945). The rate of elimination from the blood stream is only half as fast as that of the corresponding alcohol (Williams, 1959) but it is to some extent excreted in combination with glucuronic acid (Neubauer, 1901; Saneyoshi, 1911). It is the major metabolite of *sec.*-active amyl alcohol (pentanol-2).

TOXICOLOGY

2-Pentanone is primarily an irritant of ocular and nasal mucous membranes, so much so that together with its strong odour its warning properties reduce the hazard of acute intoxication in human beings. Nevertheless, it is narcotic to animals in high concentrations, with possible fatal effects, and acute intoxication is followed by injury to lungs, liver and kidneys. It was considered by Yant *et al.* (1936) to be twice as acutely toxic to animals as methyl ethyl ketone (butanone) (Patty *et al.*, 1935), but they were of the opinion that in similar conditions of usage its lower volatility would tend to compensate for its higher toxicity. With regard to its irritative effect, Specht *et al.* (1940) noted that this is marked at much lower concentrations (0.25%) than with methyl ethyl ketone. In human beings exposure to 0.15% was disagreeable and moderately irritant, and 1.3 and 5% caused irritation of eyes and nose.

Toxicity to animals

The lethal dose, for guinea pigs, was found by Yant *et al.* (1936) to be closely related to the time of exposure. Death followed exposure to 13,000 p.p.m. for 300 min, and to 50,000 p.p.m. for 50 min, but not to 5000 p.p.m. for 810 min, though unconsciousness occurred in 460–710 min.

The maximum amount to which exposure could be tolerated for several hours with slight or no symptoms was 1500 p.p.m. Smyth (1956) found that 2000 p.p.m. killed some of a group of rats after 4 h (Yant *et al.* were using the commercial grade of 2-pentanone).

In the experiments of Specht *et al.* (1940) where guinea pigs were exposed to 10,000 p.p.m., the time factor was also shown to be of importance. Up to 35 min only mucous membrane irritation and weakness were observed; at 230 min auditory and corneal reflexes disappeared and at 525 min all the animals died either during exposure or some hours later.

SYMPTOMS OF INTOXICATION

Irritation of the nose and eyes with lacrimation and squinting, salivation, retching, tremor, incoordination, lowering of body temperature, respiration and heart rate, preceded dyspnoea, gasping and unconsciousness. Death appeared to be due to the narcotic effect rather than to irritation of the lungs. Some animals which survived recovered completely 24 h after exposure.

CHANGES IN THE ORGANISM

As with other ketones the most marked and consistent change observed has been congestion. The lungs showed emphysema, oedema and marked congestion.

With exposure to narcotic concentrations the liver and kidneys showed moderate congestion, but no fat droplets were noted in the liver of the animals exposed to 2000 p.p.m. of 2-pentanone (Specht *et al.*, 1940). The brain also showed slight congestion in the animals examined by Yant, Patty and Schrenk, but no gross pathology in those exposed for 30, 90 and 270 min to 5000 p.p.m., nor for 270 and 810 min to 1500 p.p.m.

Toxicity to human beings

Apart from the severe irritation to eyes and nose of human subjects caused by even momentary exposure to 1300 and 5000 p.p.m. no toxic effects have been experienced and none have been reported from the industrial use of methyl-*n*-propyl ketone.

Bibliography on p. 458

54. Methyl Butyl Ketone

54a. Methyl *n*-Butyl Ketone

Synonym: hexanone-2

Structural formula:

$$CH_3-\overset{\overset{\displaystyle O}{\|}}{C}-CH_2-CH_2-CH_2-CH_3$$

Molecular formula: $C_6H_{12}O$

Molecular weight: 100.16

Properties: a clear liquid with a strong disagreeable odour resembling acetone. Good solvent for nitrocellulose, fats, resins and waxes.

> *boiling point:* 127.5 °C; commercial grade (86%) 120.1–127 °C
> *melting point:* −56.9 °C
> *vapour pressure:* 3.8 mm Hg at 25 °C
> *specific gravity (liquid density):* 0.8072, 0.8167 at 15.6 °C
> *flash point:* 73 °F. Inflammable limits are stated to be 1.2 to 8% by volume
> (Schrenk *et al.*, 1936)
> *conversion factors:* 1 p.p.m. = 4.10 mg/m³
> 1 mg/l   = 244 p.p.m.
> *solubility:* in water 1.64 g/100
> *evaporation rate (ether = 1):* 8.1
> *maximum allowable concentration:* 100 p.p.m. (Threshold Limit Values, 1963)

ECONOMY, SOURCES AND USES

Produced by catalysed reaction of acetic acid and ethylene under pressure, followed by distillation (Rowe and Wolf, 1963).

Chiefly used in the lacquer industry.

BIOCHEMISTRY

Estimation in the atmosphere

The method used by Schrenk *et al.* (1936) was the same as that used for methyl ethyl ketone (*q.v.*).

Metabolism

The fate of methyl butyl ketone in the body does not appear to have been investigated. Williams (1959) mentions that the oxidation to ketone from hexyl alcohol is less than that of conjugation of the alcohol to glucuronic acid. The ketone is rapidly eliminated from the body.

[428]

TOXICOLOGY

Methyl butyl ketone is narcotic to animals in high concentrations – 20,000 p.p.m. for 30 min – and if the time is prolonged, even with lower exposure, death may follow. It has been stated to be 5 times as acutely toxic to animals as methyl ethyl ketone but its lower volatility (one-fifth that of methyl ethyl ketone) tends to compensate for its higher toxicity. It is moderately irritating to ocular and nasal mucous membranes, and this irritation, together with its strong odour gives distinct warning of possible harmful concentrations. No systemic toxic effects in human beings have been recorded.

Toxicity to animals

Lethal dose. – *(i) By oral administration*, for rats, 2.59 g/kg (Smyth *et al.*, 1954), a lower toxicity than methyl propyl ketone. – *(ii) By inhalation*, for guinea pigs. It was not found possible by Schrenk *et al.* (1936) to cause death by a few minutes exposure to the highest concentrations obtainable. Exposure for 70 min to 20,000 p.p.m. or for 9 h to 6500 p.p.m. proved fatal. Concentrations lower than these were not fatal even after 13 h, and at concentrations of 1000 p.p.m. for this length of time no abnormal signs were observed either during or after exposure.

SYMPTOMS OF INTOXICATION

The chief symptoms occurring almost immediately on exposure to the higher concentrations are irritation of the eyes and nose manifested by lacrimation and rubbing the nose with the forepaws. Incoordination follows in 3 to 5 min and narcosis in 20 to 120 min only with concentrations of 6500 and 20,000 p.p.m. Death is preceded by dyspnoea and gasping and is apparently due to the narcosis rather than to irritation of the lungs. In some animals narcosis persisted for several hours after removal from exposure, but they appeared normal 24 h later.

CHANGES IN THE ORGANISM

Congestion was the chief sign of injury – congestion and haemorrhage of the lungs, moderate congestion of liver and kidneys and slight congestion of the brain.

Toxicity to human beings

Irritation of eyes and nose was observed (Schrenk *et al.*, 1936) in men exposed to 6500 and 20,000 p.p.m. for even ¼ to 1 min, and even 1000 p.p.m. was disagreeable and irritant.

No records of any injury from its industrial use have been reported.

Bibliography on p. 458

54b. Methyl Isobutyl Ketone

Synonyms: hexone, 4-methylpentanone-2

Structural formula:

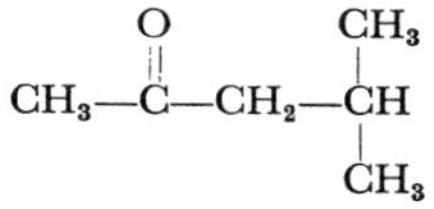

$$CH_3-\overset{\overset{\displaystyle O}{\|}}{C}-CH_2-\overset{\overset{\displaystyle CH_3}{|}}{\underset{\underset{\displaystyle CH_3}{|}}{CH}}$$

Molecular formula: $C_6H_{12}O$

Molecular weight: 100.16

Properties: a clear liquid; the commercial grade has a somewhat unpleasant odour (Fairhall, 1957). A good solvent for nitrocellulose and cellulose ethers, oils, fats, waxes, natural and synthetic gums and resins.

    boiling point: 115.8 °C
    melting point: −83.5 °C
    vapour pressure: 7.5 mm Hg at 25 °C
    specific gravity (liquid density): 0.8020
    flash point: 64 °F – range of flammability 1.35–7.6%
    conversion factors: 1 p.p.m. = 4.10 mg/m³
                       1 mg/l   = 244 p.p.m.
    solubility: in water 1.91 g/100; miscible with most organic solvents
    evaporation rate (ether = 1): 5.6
    maximum allowable concentration: 100 p.p.m. (Threshold Limit Values, 1963)

ECONOMY, SOURCES AND USES

Production

By selective catalytic hydrogenation of the double bond in mesityl oxide (Rowe and Wolf, 1963).

Industrial uses

Chiefly in the lacquer industry in combination with other solvents, but it is inferior in solvent property to butyl acetate and the strong odour of the commercial product somewhat limits its use.

BIOCHEMISTRY

Estimation in the atmosphere

The method used by Specht (1938) is a modification of that used by Patty *et al.* (1935) for methyl ethyl ketone, the essential modification being the method of adding iodine to the sample. The flask in which the vapour was collected was shaken vigorously after excess 0.1 N iodine solution had been drawn in through the stopcock and then allowed to stand for 30 min at room temperature. Elkins (1959) finds the silica gel method used for acetone and methyl ethyl ketone applicable also to hexone. In both methods 0.1 N sodium thiosulphate is used for the titration, with starch solution for the end point.

Metabolism

The metabolism, so far as is known, of hexone is similar to that of hexanone, and like hexanone it is rapidly eliminated from the body.

TOXICOLOGY

Hexone is primarily an irritant, but also to some extent a narcotic. According to Henderson and Haggard (1943) its irritant action is more marked in relation to its anaesthetic effect than is the case with acetone.

The narcosis is accompanied by lowering of body temperature and of respiratory and heart rate, and in animals which have succumbed to exposure slight fatty infiltration of the liver has been observed (Specht, 1938), but other organs have shown only slight change in the form of congestion.

No severe toxic effects have been recorded in human beings but there is one record (Elkins, 1959) of headache and nausea in a group of workers exposed to it and in another group of respiratory tract irritation.

Toxicity to animals

(1) Acute
(a) Lethal dose. – (i) By oral administration, for rats, 2.08 g/kg body weight (Shell Chemical Corp., 1957). (In spite of the slight hazard expected from swallowing this compound, Rowe and Wolf (1963) remark that the swallowing of large amounts might have serious systemic effects.) – (ii) By inhalation, for guinea pigs, 10,000 p.p.m. for 4 h and with higher concentrations for a progressively shorter time (Specht, 1938); for rats, 4000 p.p.m. for 4 h (Smyth, 1956); for mice, 20,000 p.p.m. for 30 min (Shell Chemical Corp., 1957).

(b) Narcotic dose. – For guinea pigs, 1000 p.p.m. for 6 h caused low-grade narcosis (Specht, 1938); for mice, 19,500 p.p.m. for 30 min (Shell Chemical Corp.'

(2) Chronic
The only investigation of repeated exposure to hexone is that described in the Shell Chemical Corporations Industrial Hygiene Bulletin (1957). Mice were

Bibliography on p. 458

given 20 min daily exposures to 20,000 p.p.m. for 15 days. One death occurred after each of the first six days, 3 after the ninth, and one after the tenth day. The 4 remaining mice survived the 15 exposures.

These results appear to indicate a much lower toxicity of hexone than those of acute exposure reported by Specht (1938) and Smyth (1956). It is possible that mice may be more resistant than other species, but further investigation may be necessary to explain the apparent discrepancy.

SYMPTOMS OF INTOXICATION

In Specht's (1938) experiments irritation of the cornea and conjunctiva, with lacrimation, was followed by irritation of mouth, nose and throat (sneezing, coughing, salivation) then inco-ordination, loss of auditory and corneal reflexes, lowering of rectal temperature, pulse rate and respiratory rate, with irregularity of pulse towards the end, spasmodic gasping, coma and death. It was believed that death was due to the narcotic effect.

CHANGES IN THE ORGANISM

Only slight changes, chiefly congestive, were observed especially in the brain and lungs of animals which succumbed to exposure, but some liver cells showed infiltration with fine droplets of fat.

Toxicity to human beings

(1) Acute

In human volunteers examined by Silverman *et al.* (1946) exposure to 200 p.p.m. was stated to be objectionable on account of odour and to cause definite eye irritation. The Shell Corporation gives the threshold for eye irritation for 50% of the volunteers as 200–400 p.p.m. and for nasal irritation as 400 p.p.m.

(2) Chronic, industrial

The only account of a toxic effect of hexone in industrial use is given by Elkins (1959). In this, he states that a group of workers exposed to about 100 p.p.m. during the waterproofing of boots complained of headache and nausea; they acquired tolerance during the week but lost it over the week-end. In another group with apparently the same exposure, no nausea was reported but some irritation of the respiratory tract, again showing loss of tolerance over the week-end. All these complaints largely disappeared when installation of an exhaust system reduced the exposure to 20 p.p.m.

55. Ethyl Butyl Ketone

Synonym: heptanone-3

Structural formula:

$$CH_3-CH_2-CH_2-CH_2-\overset{\displaystyle O}{\overset{\|}{C}}-CH_2-CH_3$$

Molecular formula: $C_7H_{14}O$

Molecular weight: 114.18

Properties: a clear liquid of low volatility with a typical ketone-like odour. Moderate fire hazard when exposed to heat or flame; can react with oxidising materials (Sax, 1957).

    boiling point: 147.6 °C

    vapour pressure: 1.4 mm Hg at 25 °C

    specific gravity (liquid density): 0.8164

    flash point: 115 °F

    conversion factors: 1 p.p.m. = 4.66 mg/m³

                    1 mg/l = 214 p.p.m.

    solubility: soluble in water in all proportions.

    maximum allowable concentration: not established; Rowe and Wolf (1963) suggest 100 p.p.m.

ECONOMY, SOURCES AND USES

Production

By hydrogenation of the mixed alcohol condensation product of propionaldehyde and butanone, or by catalytic hydrogenation of 3-heptanol (Rowe and Wolf, 1963).

Industrial uses

(1) As a solvent in processes similar to those where other ketones are used.

(2) As an intermediate in synthesis of organic products.

BIOCHEMISTRY

Metabolism

Its specific metabolism does not appear to have been investigated, but when formed as a metabolite of 3-heptanol it is eliminated in the expired air (Williams, 1959). The oxidation of 3-heptanol to this ketone is less than its conjugation with glucuronic acid.

TOXICOLOGY

On account of its low volatility ethyl butyl ketone does not present a serious industrial hazard. It is moderately irritating to the eyes and skin; for the latter the degree of irritation is given by Smyth *et al.* (1949) as Grade 2, "an average reaction equivalent to a trace of capillary injection as tested by a method similar to that of Draize *et al.* (1944)". Prolonged skin contact may result in dermatitis owing to its defatting action.

No toxic effects in human beings have been recorded.

Toxicity to animals

The lethal dose – (i) By oral administration, for rats, 2.76 g/kg. – *(ii) By skin absorption,* for rabbits, greater than 20 ml/kg. Animals can absorb 3-heptanone by the skin, but the toxic effect of this is relatively low. Inhalation of high concentrations can be fatal. – *(iii) By inhalation,* for rats, 4000 p.p.m. after 20 min. No deaths occurred following 4-h exposure to 2000 p.p.m. (Smyth *et al.*, 1949).

56. Di-isobutyl Ketone

Synonyms: isovalerone, 2,6-dimethyl heptanone-4

Structural formula:

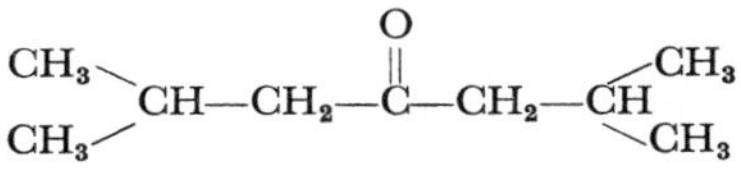

$$CH_3 \diagdown \!\!\!\!\!\! \atop CH_3 \diagup \!\!\!\!\!\! CH - CH_2 - \overset{\overset{O}{\|}}{C} - CH_2 - CH \!\!\!\!\!\! \overset{\diagup CH_3}{\diagdown CH_3}$$

Molecular formula: $C_9H_{18}O$

Molecular weight: 142.2

Properties: water-clear liquid of low volatility.
   boiling point: 168.1 °C
   melting point: −5.9 °C
   vapour pressure: 1.7 mm Hg at 20 °C
   specific gravity (liquid density): 0.8089
   flash point: 120 °F
   conversion factors: 1 p.p.m. = 5.81 mg/m³
                       1 mg/l   = 171.92 p.p.m.
   solubility: very slightly in water (Rowe and Wolf, 1963). A good solvent for nitrocellulose.
   evaporation rate (ether = 1): 30.8
   maximum allowable concentration: 50 p.p.m. (Threshold Limit Values, 1962).

ECONOMY, SOURCES AND USES

Industrial uses

(1) In rubber industry – for milled crepe rubber (Carpenter *et al.*, 1953).
(2) In textile industry, for synthetic coatings and as intermediate in synthesis of dyes.
(3) In chemical industry, as intermediate in synthesis of inhibitors, pharmaceuticals and insecticides.

BIOCHEMISTRY

Estimation in the atmosphere

No specific method for di-isobutyl ketone has been described, but according to Rowe and Wolf (1963) the method of Morasco (1926) can be used for any of

the ketones. This depends upon the reaction between the ketone and hydroxylamine dichloride to form the ketoxime, liberating HCl which is titrated with
NaOH in the presence of methyl orange.

Metabolism

There appears to be no specific information on the details of metabolism of
di-isobutyl ketone, but it probably undergoes the major metabolic change common to that of most ketones except acetone. That is reduction to the corresponding
secondary alcohol which is usually eliminated combined with glucuronic acid
(Williams, 1959).

TOXICOLOGY

The hazard of systemic poisoning by di-isobutyl ketone is practically negligible
both in animals and human beings, though an increase in the weight of liver and
kidneys has been noted in female rats exposed repeatedly to 100 p.p.m. It can
cause narcosis at high concentrations, but its principal effect is that of an irritant
to mucous membranes. Human beings exposed to 100 p.p.m. for 3 h have noted
slight lacrimation and throat irritation, and slight headache and dizziness on
returning to fresh air. There are no reports of intoxication from its industrial use.

Toxicity to animals

(1) Acute
        (a) Lethal dose. – *(i) By oral administration,* for rats, 5.75 g/kg. – *(ii) By skin
absorption,* 20 ml/kg (Smyth *et al.,* 1949). – *(iii) By inhalation.* There was at one
time some discrepancy in the results of McOmie and Anderson (1949) and those
of Smyth *et al.* (1949); the former stated that rats and guinea pigs survived single
exposures for $7\frac{1}{2}$ to 16 h to saturated vapour, while the latter found that female
rats, in contrast to male, succumbed to an 8-h exposure to 2000 p.p.m. Later,
however, using a different stock of rats, Carpenter *et al.* (1953) found that 2000
p.p.m. was not lethal for either male or female rats.

(2) Chronic
        A greater susceptibility of female rats was a significant feature of the in-
vestigation by Carpenter *et al.* (1953) of the effect of repeated exposure. The rats
were exposed 7 h a day, 5 days a week for 6 weeks to concentrations of 1650, 920,
530, 250 and 125 p.p.m., and some guinea pigs to the two lowest levels. At 1650
p.p.m. all the 15 females died during the first day, while 13 of the males survived;
no toxic deaths occurred, either in rats or guinea pigs, at levels lower than this.

Prostration and inco-ordination were noted during the first two days, but not during the remaining 28 days of the exposure.

CHANGES IN THE ORGANISM

In rats, a significant increase in weight of the liver and kidneys was found following exposure to 920 and 530 p.p.m., and in the female animals at 250 p.p.m. Guinea pigs, on the other hand, exhibited an unexplained decrease in liver weight at 250 p.p.m. No adverse effects were produced in either species at 125 p.p.m.

Toxicity to human beings

Silverman *et al.* (1946) suggested that 25 p.p.m. for an 8-h exposure was the lowest level which would not cause discomfort.

In the later experiments of Carpenter *et al.* (1953) two male subjects who inhaled 50 p.p.m. for 3 h noted slight transitory irritation of mucous membranes at the beginning of exposure, but later no appreciable discomfort. Similar slight irritation of eyes and nose was noted by 3 subjects exposed to 100 p.p.m., with slight lacrimation in one, headache in two, and dizziness on returning to fresh air. No abnormality of pulse rate, blood pressure, muscular coordination or urinary content of albumen or sugar was observed.

No records of symptoms or complaints from its industrial use have appeared.

Bibliography on p. 458

57. Trimethylnonanone

Synonyms: 2,6,8-trimethylnonanone-4

Structural formula:

$$CH_3-CH-CH_2-\overset{\displaystyle O}{\overset{\|}{C}}-CH_2-\overset{\displaystyle CH_3}{\underset{|}{CH}}-CH_2-CH-CH_3$$

with CH_3 groups attached below the first and last CH.

Molecular formula: $C_{12}H_{24}O$

Molecular weight: 184.19

Properties: a clear colourless liquid with a fruity odour.

  boiling point: 207–228 °C
  vapour pressure: 0.5
  specific gravity (liquid density): 0.8165
  flash point: 195 °F
  conversion factors: 1 p.p.m. = 7.54 mg/m³
                1 mg/l = 133 p.p.m.
  solubility: insoluble in water
  maximum allowable concentration: not established.

ECONOMY, SOURCES AND USES

Production

By catalytic condensation of methyl isobutyl ketone, using calcium carbide followed by catalytic hydrogenation of the reaction product at 280 °C (Rowe and Wolf, 1963).

Industrial uses

As a solvent chiefly for vinyl chloride resins.

BIOCHEMISTRY

Metabolism

Beyond the fact that trimethylnonanone can be absorbed by the skin of rabbit even to the extent of causing death to some of the animals (Smyth *et al.*, 1951) no details of its actual metabolism are available.

[438]

TOXICOLOGY

Trimethylnonanone presents little hazard in industrial use, though animal experiments have indicated that it could, with prolonged contact, cause dermatitis. Inhalation has been found practically innocuous in the few animal experiments carried out (Smyth *et al.*, 1951). No reports of injury to human beings have been recorded.

Toxicity to animals

Lethal dose. – (i) By oral administration, for rats, 6.47 g/kg. – *(ii) By skin application*, for rabbits, 11.0 ml/kg. Skin irritation was moderately severe – a strong capillary injection with prolonged contact. – *(iii) By inhalation*, for rats, no deaths were caused by inhalation of saturated vapour for 4 h (Smyth and Carpenter, 1944).

SYMPTOMS OF INTOXICATION

The eyes

As judged by the effect of application to the centre of the cornea of an albino rabbit, injury to the eye was very slight (Carpenter and Smyth, 1946), Grade I as compared with Grade III for ethyl butyl ketone; Grade V, representing severe injury, corresponds to necrosis of the cornea.

These meagre details indicate that especially by inhalation of the vapour, the industrial hazard is very low.

Bibliography on p. 458

58. Mesityl Oxide

Synonyms: methyl isobutenyl ketone, isopropylidine acetone

Structural formula:

$$CH_3-\overset{\overset{\displaystyle O}{\|}}{C}-CH=C\overset{\diagup CH_3}{\diagdown CH_3}$$

Molecular formula: $C_6H_{10}O$

Molecular weight: 98.14

Properties: a clear liquid with a strong odour suggestive of mice and peppermint (Durrans, 1933). Good solvent for cellulose esters and ethers and many resins, oils and fats; for cellulose acetate only in the presence of a small amount of a solvent such as acetone (Metzinger, 1935; Yarsley, 1934).

> *boiling point:* 129.5 °C
> *melting point:* −46.4 °C
> *vapour pressure:* 9.5 mm Hg at 20 °C
> *specific gravity (liquid density):* 0.8569
> *flash point:* 90 °F
> *conversion factors:* 1 p.p.m. = 4.02 mg/m³
>   1 mg/l   = 249 p.p.m.
> *solubility:* very slightly in water
> *evaporation rate (ether = 1):* 8.4
> *maximum allowable concentration:* 25 p.p.m. (Threshold Limit Values for 1962).

The commercial variety may contain traces of aldehyde (Zangger, 1930).

ECONOMY, SOURCES AND USES

Production

By dehydration of diacetone alcohol with a small amount of iodine as a catalyst, followed by slow distillation.

Industrial uses

(1) In leather and lacquer industries (Sanderson, 1933).
(2) As a solvent for synthetic rubber and some vinyl resins, stains and coating inks (Tersand, 1935).
(3) In ore flotation (Rowe and Wolf, 1963).
(4) As an organic intermediate.

[440]

BIOCHEMISTRY

Estimation

In the atmosphere

The iodine titration method used by Patty, Schrenk and Yant (1935) for methyl ethyl ketone was applied by Specht, Miller *et al.* (1940) in their animal experiments.

Metabolism

Mesityl oxide, like most other ketones except acetone, is reduced in the body to an appreciable extent (Williams, 1959). Like them it has been shown (Neubauer, 1901; Sanoyeshi, 1911) to increase the glucuronic output in rabbits. On the evidence of repeated exposure of animals to non-lethal concentrations, Smyth *et al.* (1942) suggest that it is probably not rapidly eliminated, and that with frequent exposures the blood concentration reaches an anaesthetic level.

Lewin (1906) stated that mesityl oxide reacts with certain sulphur-containing compounds in the body, probably sulphydryls, and that this forms an odorous product which he believed to be a sulphur substituted ketone.

TOXICOLOGY

Mesityl oxide is a narcotic in high concentrations, stronger than methyl *n*-butyl ketone (Specht *et al.*, 1940) and in animals has been found to cause injury to kidneys, liver and lungs. Its narcotic action can be produced by absorption from the skin (Shell Chemical Corp., 1957). It can cause corneal injury if in direct contact with the eyes and dermatitis if in direct contact with the skin. Such data as are available indicate that it is highly toxic and should be handled with care (Elkins, 1959), but no toxic effects from its industrial use have been recorded.

Toxicity to animals

(1) Acute

(a) Lethal dose. – *By inhalation*, for guinea pigs, 5000 p.p.m. killed all the animals either during exposure or within the next 24 h (Specht *et al.*, 1940).

(2) Chronic

Repeated exposure to concentrations varying up to 50 p.p.m. were found by Smyth, Seaton and Fischer (1942) to cause no toxic effect, but at 500 p.p.m. there was a high mortality, and at this level, and at 250 p.p.m. mild albuminuria.

Bibliography on p. 458

SYMPTOMS OF INTOXICATION

At 5000 p.p.m. (the eventual fatal dose), symptoms of mucous membrane irritation – vigorous rubbing of nose and eyes, squinting, coughing, salivation and lacrimation – began within 5 min. At 30 min these symptoms were intensified, some animals producing a foamy saliva not seen with other ketones, and the average rectal temperature fell slightly, the respiratory rate more severely, and the pulse rate rose. These changes continued during the next half-hour, and an hour later were accompanied by weakness and quietness. At 4 h the signs of irritation decreased but the weakness and coma increased, and at $6\frac{1}{2}$ h some animals were dead. Those which were still alive showed a low rectal temperature and a much reduced respiratory and heart rate. Gasping preceded death, none of the animals surviving more than 5 h after cessation of exposure. Some showed cyanosis, and at autopsy an unpleasant odour was observed to emanate from the bodies. Specht et al. (1940) remark that these reactions indicate the probability that there are actions on the body tissues which are not necessarily characteristic of a narcotic, and the lowering of the rectal temperature indicates that despite the mixed effects on the respiration (a difference in the transient return to normal with exposure to differing concentrations) and on the heart, there is a marked depression which is common to all ketones. Even at non-lethal concentrations (2000 p.p.m.) irritation is immediate and is followed rapidly by weakness and coma.

CHANGES IN THE ORGANISM

As in the case of most other ketones, the most marked and consistent change following acute exposure is congestion of lungs, kidneys, spleen adrenals and brain. These changes are attributed by Specht et al. (1940) to central vaso-motor disturbances. With repeated exposure, the animals examined by Smyth et al. (1942) showed, as the most marked organic injury, congestion and cloudy swelling of the kidneys, together with some injury of the liver and lungs. It was again suggested that these injuries were attributable to the anaesthetic action of mesityl oxide upon the circulatory and respiratory systems.

Toxicity to human beings

Some irritation of the eyes at 25 p.p.m. and of the nose at 50 p.p.m. was observed by Silverman et al. (1946) in human subjects exposed to these concentrations. Considerable irritation of the hands of the operator manipulating the animals in the experiments of Specht et al. (1940) was noted, even though latex surgeons' gloves were worn.

No toxic effects from the industrial use of mesityl oxide have been recorded.

59. Cyclohexanone

Synonyms: Sextone, Anon, Hexanon, Pimelic Ketone

Structural formula:

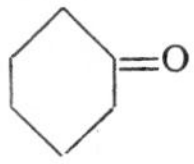

Molecular formula: $C_6H_{10}O$

Molecular weight: 98.14

Properties: a colourless, neutral, slightly volatile liquid with a characteristic ketone-like odour. Solvent for oils, fats, rubber and many resins; also for celluloid, cellulose ethers, cellulose acetate and collodion cotton.

  boiling point: 155.6 °C
  melting point: −45 °C
  vapour pressure: 4.5 mm Hg at 25 °C
  specific gravity (liquid density): 0.947
  flash point: 143 °F
  conversion factors: 1 p.p.m. = 4.02 mg/m³
        1 mg/l = 249 p.p.m.
  solubility: slightly soluble in water, about 5 g/100 ml at 30 °C, but increasing with decrease of temperature (Jacobs, 1949)
  evaporation rate (ether = 1): 40.6
  maximum allowable concentration: 50 p.p.m. (Threshold Limit Values, 1962).

ECONOMY, SOURCES AND USES

Production

(1) By catalytic oxidation of cyclohexanol.
(2) By distillation of pimelic acid salts (Rowe and Wolf, 1963).

Industrial uses

(1) In the lacquer industry as a slowly evaporating improver, also for lacquers and insulators for heat and electricity (Loehr, 1931) and for automobile lacquers (Deschiens, 1928).
(2) In the textile and plastic industries, as a spotting agent and a re-lustring agent for cellulose acetate silk (Clayton and Clark, 1931) and in the spray painting of fabric and plastic textiles.

(3) In the leather industry (Lamb and Gilman, 1932).
(4) As a metal degreaser, especially for nickel sheets.
(5) In paint removers.
(6) In printing inks.

BIOCHEMISTRY

Estimation in the atmosphere

The method recommended by Jacobs (1949) and used by Specht et al. (1940) is the hydroxylamine method described by Marasco (1926) (see p. 412). It can also be estimated by its reaction with m-ditrobenzene, giving a pink colour (Treon et al., 1943).

Metabolism

Cyclohexanone can be absorbed by the skin, with resulting toxic effects in animals (Treon et al., 1943).

It is conjugated in the body to a considerable extent (45 to 50%) of the dose according to Treon et al. and its main metabolite is the cyclohexyl glucuronide (Elliott et al., 1959), but according to Deichmann and Dierker (1946) oral administration is followed by the increase of glucuronic acid only in plasma or serum. Treon et al. state that oral intake has been followed in rabbits by an increased excretion of organic sulphates.

TOXICOLOGY

Cyclohexanone is narcotic to animals in high concentration even to the extent of causing death, and absorption through the skin can also be lethal.

It is an irritant of mucous membranes and direct contact with the eyes can cause corneal injury. The only symptom reported from its industrial use (and in this process it was present only to the extent of 25%) is drowsiness.

Toxicity to animals

(1) Acute
    (a) Lethal dose. – *(i) By oral administration,* for mice, 1.3–1.5 g/kg (Jacobi et al., 1903). – *(ii) By skin absorption,* for rabbits, 10.2–23.0 g/kg (Treon et al., 1943). – *(iii) By intraperitoneal injection,* for mice, 0.5 ml/kg (Filippi, 1914). – *(iv) By intravenous injection,* for dogs, 630 mg/kg in 60 min (Caujolle et al., 1953). – *(v) By inhalation.* Monkeys and rabbits exposed to 3082 p.p.m. (Treon et al., 1943) showed a slightly increased mortality and Specht et al. (1940) found that 3 out of 10 guinea pigs died four days after exposure to 4000 p.p.m. Rats, according to Smyth (1956), survived a 4-h exposure to 4000 p.p.m., but death followed exposure to 8000 p.p.m. for the same time.

(b) Narcotic dose. – 3082 p.p.m. (Treon *et al.*, 1943); 3800 p.p.m. (Gross, cited by Lehmann and Flury, 1943); 4000 p.p.m. (Specht *et al.*, 1940).

(2) Chronic

Repeated exposures (50 for 6 h) of monkeys and rabbits to concentrations varying from 190 to 773 p.p.m. (Treon *et al.*, 1943) caused mucous membrane irritation from 309 p.p.m. upwards. The only organic toxic effect observed was very slight kidney and liver injury; no haematological change and no specific pathology.

SYMPTOMS OF INTOXICATION

Initial irritation of mucous membranes (lacrimation, salivation and nasal discharge and restlessness) were followed in the experiments of Specht *et al.* (1940) by sluggish movements, loss of reflexes and side position. The pulse rate was increased at first but later decreased, as also were rectal temperature and respiratory rate. With lethal amounts by skin absorption, tremors, narcosis and hypothermia preceded death (Treon *et al.*, 1943). According to Caujolle *et al.* (1953) terminal apnoea occurs suddenly without premonitory signs.

Recovery from narcosis is slow, and accompanied by some dyspnoea and corneal opacity persisting for several weeks, clearing only after other symptoms have disappeared. As in the case of mesityl oxide it is suggested that cyclohexanone has bodily effects other than narcosis, though death is apparently due to respiratory failure.

CHANGES IN THE ORGANISM

No specific injury was found in the organs of animals exposed to the highest concentrations; the toxic effect appeared to be one of general vascular injury.

Liquid cyclohexanone placed in the eyes of rabbits caused marked irritation and severe corneal injury (Carpenter and Smyth, 1946).

Toxicity to human beings

Exposure of human subjects for a short period to 50 p.p.m. was reported by Nelson *et al.* (1943) to be definitely objectionable, and to 75 p.p.m. to cause eye, nose and throat irritation.

From industrial use no serious manifestations of toxicity have been recorded. In 1932 examination by the Home Office, U.K., of a number of workers employed in degreasing nickel sheets revealed no symptoms or complaints, and Browning (1953) observed only drowsiness in most of a group of a women engaged in a process where the solvent contained 25% of cyclohexanone. There was some hypochromic anaemia among the women but no other haematological abnormality.

Bibliography on p. 458

60. Acetonyl Acetone

Synonyms: 2.5-hexanedione, α,β-diacetyl ether

Structural formula:

$$CH_3 \overset{\overset{\displaystyle O}{\|}}{-}C-CH_2-CH_2-\overset{\overset{\displaystyle O}{\|}}{C}-CH_3$$

Molecular formula: $C_6H_{10}O_2$

Molecular weight: 114.14

Properties: a clear colourless liquid becoming yellow on standing.

    boiling point: 194 °C

    melting point: -9 °C

    vapour pressure: 1.6 mm Hg at 25 °C

    specific gravity (liquid density): 0.9737

    flash point: 174 °F

    conversion factors: 1 p.p.m. = 4.66 mg/m³

                              1 mg/l = 241 p.p.m.

    solubility: miscible with water and organic solvents

    evaporation rate (ether = 1): 230

    maximum allowable concentration: not established; Elkins (1959) suggests 75 p.p.m

ECONOMY, SOURCES AND USES

Produced (1) from aceto-acetic acid with alkylated iodine as a catalyst; (2) by hydrolysis of 2.5 dimethyl furan (Rowe and Wolf, 1963).

    Used in industry (1) as a solvent for a variety of materials, and (2) as an intermediate in chemical synthesis.

BIOCHEMISTRY

No specific method for estimation in air of this compound has been described, and perhaps one reason for this may be seen in the conflicting statements of Specht *et al.* (1940) and Smyth and Carpenter (1944), with regard to its concentration in 'saturated atmospheres'. The former stated that because of its low vapour pressure the maximum concentration attainable at room temperature was 0.4% (400 p.p.m.) and this they interpreted as 'saturated' atmosphere. Smyth and Carpenter, whose interpretation of its toxic effects differed considerably from those of Specht *et al.* (1940), calculated their 'saturated atmosphere' at 1700 p.p.m.

Metabolism

Beyond the fact that acetonyl acetone can be absorbed through the skin (Smyth and Carpenter, 1944) little or no information on its actual fate in the body is available.

TOXICOLOGY

In spite of the conflicting data on the relatively few animal investigations carried out, it appears that acetonyl acetone is not highly toxic. It is to some extent a narcotic, but less so than any of the series methyl-*n*-butyl ketone, mesityl oxide, methyl-isobutyl ketone or cyclohexanone (Specht *et al.*, 1940). It is comparable in this respect to methyl ethyl ketone but not so low as acetone. Owing to its low volatility its actual narcotic potency by inhalation has been difficult to estimate, but it is agreed that its toxic effects are relatively slight. Its vapour causes some irritation of mucous membranes, but its main effect on the skin is that of staining rather than inflammation, and no unfavourable effects from its industrial use have been reported.

Toxicity to animals

The discrepancy in the results of the investigations of Specht *et al.* (1940) and of Smyth and Carpenter (1944) may, as already mentioned, have been due to the difference in their interpretation of 'saturated atmosphere'; on the other hand, the fact that different species of animals were used in the two investigations may indicate a difference in species susceptibility.

    Lethal dose. – *(i) By oral administration*, for rats, 2.7 g/kg (Smyth and Carpenter). – *(ii) By skin absorption*, for guinea pigs, 6.6 ml/kg (Smyth and Carpenter). – *(iii) By inhalation*, for rats, 'saturated atmosphere' was lethal in one hour according to Smyth and Carpenter. For guinea pigs, Specht *et al.*, calculating 'saturated atmosphere' as 400 p.p.m. found no deaths occurring after 775 min or for at least 3 months after removal from exposure.

SYMPTOMS OF INTOXICATION

Specht's guinea pigs showed practically no other signs of a toxic effect than an initial irritation of eyes and nose, and a respiratory rate decreasing with the duration of exposure from an initial level of 88.7 breaths per minute to 66.6 per minute after 752 min; the rectal temperature and pulse rate remained practically unchanged. In these respects acetonyl acetone differed from all the other 6-carbon ketones. No toxic effects from exposure of human beings, either voluntary or from industrial use have been recorded.

Bibliography on p. 458

61. Methylcyclohexanone

Synonyms: methyl Anone, Sextone B

Structural formula: O=⟨ ⟩—CH₃ (with H above)

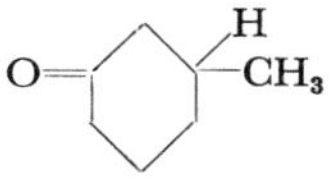

Molecular formula: $C_7H_{12}O$

Molecular weight: 112.17

Properties: a colourless oily liquid with a pungent odour; darkens on standing, especially if exposed to light. It exists in three isomers, but is chiefly found as a mixture of *meta-* and *para-*; as a solvent it is interchangeable with cyclohexanone but not so good for cellulose acetate.

> *boiling point:* 165 to 171 °C
> *vapour pressure:* 10 mm Hg at 55 °C; 30 mm Hg at 25° C
> *specific gravity (liquid density):* 0.921 at 20 °C
> *flash point:* 130 °F
> *conversion factors:* 1 p.p.m. = 4.58 mg/m³
>   1 mg/l   = 218 p.p.m. (Rowe and Wolf, 1963)
> *solubility:* very slightly in water; miscible with organic solvents
> *evaporation rate (ether = 1):* 47
> *maximum allowable concentration:* 100 p.p.m. (Threshold Limit Values, 1962).

ECONOMY, SOURCES AND USES

Industrial uses

(1) In the lacquer industry as a thinner for cellulose lacquers (Deschiens, 1928).
(2) In the leather industry, especially for light and fancy leathers, where it improves the adhesion of cellulose finishes.
(3) As a rust remover, for loosening rust in screws and bolts.
(4) As a varnish remover.
(5) In the plastics industry.

BIOCHEMISTRY

Estimation in the atmosphere

(a) By the hydroxylamine hydrochloride method used for other ketones (see p. 412).

(b) By the *m*-dinitrobenzene method (Treon *et al.*, 1943) yielding a pink colour.

[448]

Metabolism

Following intraperitoneal injection, methylcyclohexanone was stated by Filippi (1914) to be oxidised to adipic acid, which was excreted in the urine (Frey, 1939).

It is conjugated in the body with glucuronic acid to a considerable extent (Treon *et al.*, 1943); with inhalation the average daily output increases rapidly from the pre-exposure level to a high level during exposure and decreases to nearly normal after cessation. The graph shows a straight line which demonstrates the significance of this process as a direct indication of the severity of exposure. There is a moderate increase in the excretion of organic sulphates with concentrations above 184 p.p.m. (Treon *et al.*, 1943).

TOXICOLOGY

Methyl cyclohexanone is somewhat less toxic than cyclohexanone, though according to Caujolle *et al.* (1953) its toxicity increases with its methylation through para, meta and ortho. Inhalation of its vapour carries little hazard of systemic intoxication, since it is not possible to reach concentrations at ordinary temperatures which would prove lethal or even strongly narcotic to animals. It is, however, an irritant of mucous membranes both in animals and human beings (Gross, 1943), and when given orally or by cutaneous application to animals it can prove more toxic than cyclohexanone.

No injury from its industrial use has been reported.

Toxicity to animals

Acute

   (a) *Lethal dose.* – (i) *By oral administration*, for rabbits, 1.0–1.6 g/kg in less than 1¾ h (Treon *et al.*, 1943). – (ii) *By skin application*, 4.9–7.2 g/kg, compared with 10.2–23.0 for cyclohexanone. – (iii) *By intravenous injection*, 270 mg/kg, compared with 630 for cyclohexanone (Caujolle *et al.*, 1953). – (iv) *By inhalation*, for rabbits, no deaths were caused by single exposure to 182 p.p.m., nor with repeated exposure up to 514 p.p.m., but did occur with repeated exposure for some hours at 6267 p.p.m. – much above concentrations which can be reached at ordinary temperature – (Treon *et al.*, 1943).

   (b) *Narcotic dose.* – Narcosis could not be reached by inhalation of concentrations obtainable at ordinary temperatures, but could be produced by application of 15 ml to the shaved skin.

SYMPTOMS OF INTOXICATION

At sublethal inhalation doses (497 p.p.m.) convulsions, with rapidly developing anaesthesia, cyanosis, lacrimation and conjunctival congestion; with oral adminis- tration a fall in temperature accompanied by tremors.

Effect on the blood

Treon *et al.* observed no blood disturbance after oral administration, but Frey (1939) examining the effects of inhalation and gastric administration on four guinea pigs, stated that the haemopoietic system revealed a toxic effect in the form of a striking increase of large monocytes and in one animal 1% of myelocytes.

With regard to the internal organs he found that to the naked eye there were signs of irritation in the gastric and intestinal mucosa, enlargement of the liver and, in two animals, of the kidney. Microscopically the liver showed some fatty degeneration and the kidneys some hyaline degeneration and atrophy of glomeruli, while the brain showed oedema and some atrophy.

CHANGES IN THE ORGANISM

With oral administration cerebral oedema and congestion, superficial erosion of the gastric mucous membrane, myocardial degeneration, alveolar oedema and interstitial fibrosis of the lungs. The liver showed some degeneration and inflam- matory changes; the kidneys some degeneration and glomerular sclerosis.

With inhalation no specific injury was observed; the response was widely distributed as vascular and inflammatory injury.

Toxicity to human beings

No injurious effects in human beings have been recorded, except the observation by Gross that it is an irritant to mucous membranes.

62. Acetophenone

Synonyms: phenyl methyl ketone, acetyl benzene

Structural formula:

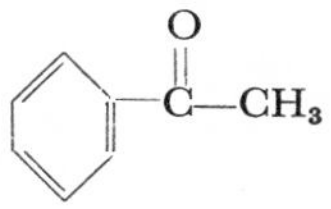

Molecular formula: C_8H_8O

Molecular weight: 120.2

Properties: either crystalline leaflets melting at 20.5 °C, or a colourless liquid with an odour resembling orange blossoms and jasmine. A solvent for cellulose ethers and esters.

    boiling point: 202 °C
    melting point: 20.5 °C
    vapour pressure: 0.44 at 25 °C
    specific gravity (liquid density): 1.03
    flash point: 180 °F
    conversion factors: 1 p.p.m. = 4.95 mg/m³
                         1 mg/l = 204 p.p.m.
    solubility: in water 0.55%. Soluble in alcohol, ether, benzene and chloroform, and in concentrated H_2SO_4, giving an orange colour (Fairhall, 1957).
    maximum allowable concentration: not established.

ECONOMY, SOURCES AND USES

Production

(1) Acetophenone occurs to a small extent in coal tar, and is extracted from the heavy oil fraction with concentrated H_2SO_4.
(2) By reaction of benzene and acetyl chloride.
(3) By combining benzenealdehyde and diazomethane.
(4) By oxidation of ethyl benzene (Rowe and Wolf, 1963).

Industrial uses

Chiefly in the perfumery industry, but also to some extent as a solvent for cellulose ethers and esters and as intermediate in the synthesis of organic chemicals.

BIOCHEMISTRY

Estimation

In the atmosphere

The method of Morasco (1926) – the hydroxylamine hydrochloride reaction – can be used for the estimation of acetophenone.

Metabolism

Acetophenone is partly converted in the body, the amount of its conversion depending on the route of administration. Thierfelder and Daiba (1923) pointed out the possibility that, like many aromatic hydrocarbons, it might be more completely absorbed by the peritoneum than by subcutaneous tissue. Thierfelder and Klenk (1924) therefore used the intraperitoneal route in their metabolic investigation of acetophenone. Their results indicated that 48.8% of the amount injected peritoneally and 53.2% of the amount absorbed was conjugated with glucuronic acid, while by subcutaneous injection 59.5% of the amount absorbed was excreted in the urine as conjugated glucuronic acid, indicating that the benzene nucleus was not attacked. They also stated that 60% of the conjugated compounds excreted in the urine consisted of 35.7% of methyl phenyl carbonyl glucuronide and 24.3% of hippuric acid which had been converted from benzoic acid, while Smith *et al.* (1954) give the proportions excreted as about half of methyl phenyl carbinol and one-fifth of hippuric acid. A small amount of mandelic acid is also excreted, and a still smaller amount of unchanged acetophenone.

According to Quick (1928) some of the benzoic acid formed is excreted by dogs as benzoyl glucuronide.

TOXICOLOGY

Acetophenone was known to earlier authorities as Hypnone, and recommended as a sleeping draught, but Mairet and Comberbale (1886), examining its effects on mental patients, observed no hypnotic action from a dosage of 0.1–0.45 g daily. It is however narcotic to animals and in high dosage can cause death due to respiratory failure (Quevauviller, 1946). It has also the property of sensitising and reinforcing the action of acetyl choline on the striated muscle of vertebrate animals without any anticholinesterase effect (Scheiner, 1945) and without relation directly to its anaesthetic potency. In invertebrate animals on the other hand acetophenone, in common with other ketones, has a paralysing effect on the contraction due to acetyl choline, even in the presence of eserine.

Smyth and Carpenter (1948) find the acute oral toxicity of acetophenone comparable to that of cellosolve acetate and by inhalation of saturated vapour comparable to that of 'carbitol' acetate, while the injury caused by direct application of the liquid to the eyes is similar to that of butyl alcohol.

The only effects on human beings have been examined as the result of its use as a hypnotic or sedative, and with fairly high dosage there appears to be a slightly depressant action on the pulse and a slight but continuous decrease of haemoglobin. No effects have been reported from its industrial use.

Toxicity to animals

Acute

  (a) Lethal dose. – *(i) By oral administration,* for rats, a single dose 3.0 g/kg; repeated for 30 days, 0.9 g/kg (Smyth and Carpenter, 1944). – *(ii) By skin absorption,* more than 20 ml/kg. – *(iii) By intraperitoneal injection,* LD$_{50}$, 1.97 g/kg (Quevauviller, 1946). – *(iv) By subcutaneous injection,* for guinea pigs, $\frac{1}{2}$–1 ml (Laborde, 1885). – *(v) By intravenous injection,* for dogs, 1 ml caused deep narcosis and death 6 to 10 h later (Laborde, 1885). – *(vi) By inhalation,* saturated vapour for 8 h was the maximum for no deaths (Smyth and Carpenter, 1948).

  (b) Narcotic dose, oral, for rats, 0.4–0.5 g/kg for light narcosis; 0.6 g/kg for deep sleep (Quevauviller, 1946).

SYMPTOMS OF INTOXICATION

In the experiments of Quevauviller (1946) with intraperitoneal injection of 0.4–0.5 g/kg, staggering occurred after 5 min, paraparesis in 13 and quadriplegia in about 20 min.

In Laborde's experiments on guinea pigs, profound torpor, with gradual loss of reflexes, rapid, somewhat irregular respiration, weak cardiac action, lowering of temperature and some convulsive movements.

In the dog, with intravenous injection, deep sleep was followed rapidly by analgesia and anaesthesia, dilatation of the pupils with diminished light reflex, respiratory and cardiac modification, with lowering of blood pressure, feeble pulse and respiratory arrhythmia.

CHANGES IN THE ORGANISM

Congestion and haemorrhage of lungs, liver and kidneys; the urine contained red corpuscles, haemoglobin and albumen.

Toxicity to human beings

In 1885 Laborde stated that inhalation of the odour of acetophenone caused malaise, headache, epigastric pain, vertigo and a tendency to fall asleep. In 1886 an investigation by Mairet and Comberbale of its effects, when given by mouth

Bibliography on p. 458

to both normal and mentally abnormal subjects, showed no evidence of an influence on muscular excitement in mania or epilepsy, but in some cases nocturnal
agitation was lessened and even sleep obtained; nevertheless they concluded that
it had only secondary importance as a sedative. Some of the patients complained
of a burning sensation in the stomach. Among the healthy subjects no effects of
any kind were perceptible following ingestion of 0.1–0.3 g, but with 0.45–0.6 g
micturition was increased, the pulse weakened and slowed after 5–6 h, and there
was a slight but continuous decrease of haemoglobin, returning to normal when
the dosage ceased.

The skin

    According to Katz (1946) acetophenone is a known skin irritant and Rowe
and Wolf (1963) state that it may cause a mild burn if contact is prolonged and
frequently repeated.
    No reports of any effects from its industrial use have been made.

63. Isophorone

Synonym: 3,5,5-trimethyl-2-cyclohexene-1-one

Structural formula:

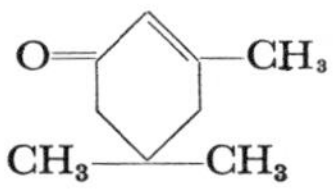

$$O=\begin{array}{c}\text{CH}_3\\ \\ \text{CH}_3\end{array}\text{CH}_3$$

Molecular formula: $C_9H_{14}O$

Molecular weight: 138.21

Properties: a high-boiling, low volatility clear liquid with an odour resembling camphor or, according to Lewin (1907), geranium, but less unpleasant than mesityl oxide. A good solvent for nitrocellulose and vinylite resins, also for some gums, oils and fats.

    boiling point: 215.2 °C

    melting point: −8.1 °C

    vapour pressure: 0.44 mm Hg at 25 °C

    specific gravity (liquid density): 0.9229

    flash point: 184 °F

    conversion factors: 1 p.p.m. = 5.65 mg/m³

                      1 mg/l   = 177 p.p.m.

    solubility: very slightly soluble in water (1.2% − Jacobs, 1949)

    evaporation rate (ether = 1): 200

    maximum allowable concentration: 25 p.p.m. (Threshold Limit Values, 1962).

ECONOMY, SOURCES AND USES

Production

From acetone, either by passage over calcium oxide, hydroxide or carbide, or their mixtures, at 350 °C, or by heating to 200–250 °C under pressure, followed by separation by distillation (Rowe and Wolf, 1963).

Industrial uses

(1) As a solvent in combination with other ketones such as butanone, methyl isobutyl ketone and acetone.

(2) In the lacquer industry especially in vinyl resin lacquers.

(3) As a chemical intermediate.

Bibliography on p. 458   [455]

BIOCHEMISTRY

Estimation

In the atmosphere

(1) By interferometer (Smyth *et al.*, 1942; Irish and Adams, 1940). Smyth *et al.* measured the concentration of isophorone by bubbling a measured stream of air through the liquid in a constant temperature bath, diluting the resulting concentrated vapour with a stream of air, and checking by the interferometer; one scale division being equal to 16.3 p.p.m. of isophorone vapour.

(2) By the method of Kacy and Cope (1955), which depends on the reaction of isophorone with phosphomolybdic acid in acetic acid medium, giving a molybdenum blue colour which is measured spectrophotometrically. This method is specific for isophorone in the presence of methyl ethyl ketone, methyl isobutyl ketone and acetone.

Metabolism

According to Lewin (1907) isophorone is converted in the body into sulphur-containing ketone, as in the case of mesityl oxide.

TOXICOLOGY

It should be noted that the following results of Smyth *et al.* (1940, 1942) which have until recently been regarded as the fundamental information on the toxicity by inhalation of isophorone have now been questioned by Rowe and Wolf (1963), who state that the concentrations listed by Smyth *et al.* are impossible to attain in the conditions employed. They suggest also that the material used in these studies was (unknown to them) an impure commercial product containing substances more volatile than isophorone. Smyth and Seaton (1940) however state themselves that while commercial samples were used, they were substantially pure, that at room temperature it was impossible to produce a concentration that would kill guinea pigs in 8 h or rats in 4 h, and that the concentration giving slight or no symptoms after several hours' exposure is about one-sixth of saturation. Since the corresponding concentration of methyl isobutyl ketone is one-eleventh of saturation they concluded that although isophorone is 4 times as toxic as methyl isobutyl ketone for single exposures of several hours its actual hazard is somewhat less because of its lower vapour pressure. Its toxic effects with repeated exposure are those of both irritation and narcosis and in these conditions, from the point of view of less severe effects, it has apparently a more cumulative toxic effect than mesityl oxide.

Industrially, it presents only slight hazard since it has good warning properties in concentrations which have been found not harmful to animals after 24 hours' continuous exposure. In fact, no injurious effects have been reported.

Toxicity to animals

(1) Acute

(a) Lethal dose. – (i) By oral administration, for the isomer phorone (Lewin, 1907), for rabbits, 2 g/kg. – (ii) By subcutaneous injection, a single injection of 0.3 g caused only diarrhoea, the faeces having an unpleasant odour; after 4 injections prone position and loss of reflexes, and death after 8 h (Lewin, 1907). – (iii) By inhalation, for guinea pigs, death was not caused by exposure for several hours to concentrations of 4600 p.p.m., the maximum obtained by prolonged recirculation over wicks wet with isophorone at 23 °C (Smyth and Seaton, 1940); rats died after 4-h exposure to 1840 p.p.m.

(b) Narcotic dose, for guinea pigs, light narcosis after 600 min exposure to 880 p.p.m.

(2) Chronic

No information.

SYMPTOMS OF INTOXICATION

Irritation of eyes and nose (lacrimation and swelling); instability, respiratory difficulty or irregularity, marked increase in intestinal peristalsis, light narcosis occurring only after 4 h or more exposure to 4600 p.p.m. and recovery was rapid. In guinea pigs, but not in rats, corneal opacity or necrosis occurred after 4 h or more exposure to 840 p.p.m. When death did occur it was due either to narcosis or, in a few cases, to lung irritation.

CHANGES IN THE ORGANISM

(1) From oral or subcutaneous administration

Punctate haemorrhages in the stomach and reddening of the intestinal mucous membrane. A trace of albuminuria was found after subcutaneous injection of 0.3 g (Lewin, 1907).

(2) Repeated exposure

(a) Subcutaneous injection. – Daily injection of 0.2–0.6 g was followed by death of guinea pigs after 6 days (Lewin, 1907).

Daily injection of doses smaller than those which in single dosage caused a trace of albuminuria (0.3 g), but giving a total of 1.4 g in 5 days, caused a much increased amount of albuminuria (Lewin, 1907).

(b) Inhalation. – Guinea pigs and rats were exposed (Smyth et al., 1942) 30 times for 8 h to concentrations varying from 25–500 p.p.m. At 500 p.p.m. 45% of the animals died; at 200 and 100 p.p.m. 45 and 17% respectively. Comparing these figures with those for mesityl oxide (no deaths at 250 p.p.m. but 65% at 500) it appears that although in single doses mesityl oxide is considerably more toxic than isophorone, with repeated exposure isophorone has a more toxic cumulative action.

Macroscopically, petechial and massive haemorrhages of the lungs and congestion of stomach and liver. Microscopically, rats showed greater abnormality, especially of liver and kidneys, than did guinea pigs. The lungs showed general congestion, increased alveolar secretion, desquamation, and in about 5% secondary pneumonia. The kidneys, congestion and cloudy swelling. The liver, in a few animals, showed congestion, parenchymal haemorrhage and cloudy swelling. In only one rat there was early necrosis following exposure for 2 h to 1430 p.p.m. The blood showed a slight decrease in red cells and haemoglobin after 8 hours' exposure, but no abnormality of white cells.

Toxicity to human beings

Of human subjects exposed for 5 min to various concentrations of isophorone, (Silverman, Schulte and First, 1946) 70% found the odour objectionable at 25 p.p.m. and this concentration produced irritation of eyes, nose and throat. Only 40% objected to the odour, or complained of any discomfort, at 10 p.p.m.

Lewin (1907) cites Bayer as stating that the odour caused headache and nausea, but Lewin had observed no such effects on himself though exposed frequently to high concentrations. No toxic effects from its industrial use have been reported.

BIBLIOGRAPHY

Albertoni, P. (1884) Die Wirkung und die Verwandlung einiger Stoffe im Organismus in Beziehung der Pathogenese der Acetonämie und des Diabetes, *Arch. Exptl. Pathol. Pharmakol.*, 18:219.
Albertoni, P. and G. Pisenti (1887) Über die Wirkung des Aceton und der Acetessigsäure auf die Nieren, *Arch. Exptl. Pathol. Pharmakol.*, 23:393.
Baginsky, A. (1888) Über Acetonurie bei Kindern, *Arch. Kinderheilk.*, 9:1.
Browning, E. (1953) *Toxicity of Industrial Organic Solvents*, 2nd Ed. H.M.S.O. London. Chemical Publishing Co. Inc. New York.
Carozzi, L. (1930) *Acetone*, International Labour Office. Brochure no. 33.
Carpenter, C. P., V. C. Pozzani and C. S. Weil (1953) Toxicity and Hazard of Di-isobutyl Ketone Vapors, *Arch. Ind. Hyg.* 8:377.
Carpenter, C. P. and H. F. Smyth Jr. (1946) Chemical Burns of the Rabbit Cornea, *Am. J. Ophthal.*, 29:1363.
Carpenter, C. P., H. F. Smyth and V. C. Pozzani (1949) The Assay of acute Vapor Toxicity and the Grading and Interpretation of Results on 96 chemical Compounds, *J. Ind. Hyg. Tocicol.*, 31:343.
Caujolle, F., F. Couturier and Y. Gase (1953) Toxicité de la Cyclohexanone et de quelques Cétones Homologues, *Compt. Rend. Acad. Sci.*, 236:633.
Cesaro, A. N. and A. Pinerolo (1947) Sull'Assorbimento percutaneo dell'Acetone, *Med. Lavoro*, 38:384.

Chatterton, G. C. and R. B. Elliott (1946) Acute Acetone Poisoning from Leg Casts of a synthetic Plaster Substitute, *J. Am. Med. Ass.*, 130:1222.

Clayton, E. and C. O. Clark (1931) Modern Organic Solvents, *J. Soc. Dye. Col. Bradford*, 47:183:247

Condorelli, L. (1931) *Technica microchimica applicata alle Richerche biologiche e Chimiche*, V. Idelson (Ed.), Naples (cited by Cesaro and Pinerolo, 1947).

Cossman, A. G. (1903) Acetonvergiftung nach Anlegung eines Zelluloid-Mullverbandes, *Münch. Med. Wschr.*, 50:1556.

Curry, A. S., G. Hurst, N. R. Kent and H. Powell (1962) Rapid Screening of Blood Samples for volatile Poisons by Gas Chromatography, *Nature*, 195:603.

Dakin, H. D. and H. W. Dudley (1913) The Interconversion of –aminoacids, –hydroxyacids and –ketonic aldehydes, *J. Biol. Chem.*, 15:127.

Deichman, W. B. and M. Dierker (1946) The spectophotometric Estimation of Hexuronates (expressed as glucuronic acid) in Plasma or Serum, *J. Biol. Chem.*, 163:753.

Deisher, J. B. (1958) Poisoning with liquid plastic Catalyst, *Northwest Med.*, 57:46.

Deschiens, M. (1928) *Les Vernis et Peintures cellulosiques pour Automobiles*, 7me. Congr. Paris. Chim. et Industr. Spécial no. p. 673.

Despartmet, M. (1928) *Les Cétones et leurs Applications dans l'Industrie des Matières plastiques et des Vernis celluloseiques*, 7me Congr. Paris. Chim. et Industr. Spécial No. p. 697.

Dines, D. F. and K. Shipman (1962) Toxic Myocarditis, *Angiology*, 13:297.

Di Prisco, L. (1936) A protective respiratory reflex during Inhalation of Acetone, *Folia Med. Napoli*, 24:669.

Draize, J. H., G. Woodward and H. O. Calvery (1944) Methods for the Study of Irritation and Toxicity of substances applied topically to Skin and Mucous Membranes, *J. Pharmacol. Exptl. Therap.*, 82:377.

Drews, R. C. and C. M. Edelmann (1956) Disinfectant Action of concentrated Acetone, *Am. J. Ophthalm.*, 42:726.

Durrans, T. H. (1933) *Solvents*, 3rd. ed. Chapman and Hall, London.

Elkins, H. B. (1959) *The Chemistry of Industrial Toxicology*. 2nd ed. John Wiley & Sons, New York. Chapman & Hall, London.

Elkins, H. B. (1959) *The Chemistry of Industrial Toxicology*, Interscience Publ. New York.

Elliott, T. H., D. V. Parke and R. T. Williams (1959) The Metabolism of Cyclohexane and its Derivatives, *Biochem. J.*, 72:193.

Fairhall, L. T. (1957) *Industrial Toxicology*, 2nd ed. Williams & Wilkins Co., Baltimore.

Fassett, D. W. (1963) (cited by Rowe V. K. and M. A. Wolf) *Ketones*, in Patty F. A., 1963, *Industrial Hygiene and Toxicology*, Vol. 2, 2nd ed., Interscience Publishers, New York.

Feldstein, M. (1960) Microdiffusion Analysis, in S. Stollman, (Ed.), *Toxicology*, Vol. 1, p. 650.

Filippi, E. (1914) The physiological Action and Behaviour of some Derivatives of Benzene as compared with those of Cyclohexane, *Arch. Farmacol. Sper.*, 18:178.

Flury, F. and W. Wirth (1934) Zur Toxikologie der Lösungsmittel, *Arch. Gewerbepathol. Gewerbehyg.*, 5:1.

Frey, J. (1939) The Effect of cyclohexanone upon the haematopoietic system, *Haematologica*, 20:725.

Friedman, T. E. and G. E. Hauger (1943) The Determination of Keto Acids in Blood and Urine, *J. Biol. Chem.*, 147:414.

Gollwitzer-Meier, K. (1927) Zur Frage der spezifischen Wirkung der Ketonkörper auf die Atmung, *Arch. Exptl. Pathol. Pharmakol.*, 125:278.

Gomer, J. J. (1960) (cited by Rowe V. K. and M. A. Wolf, 1963) *Ketones*, in F. A. Patty (Ed.), *Industrial Hygiene and Toxicology*, Vol. 2, 2nd ed., Interscience Publishers, New York.

Goodwin, L. F. (1920) The Analysis of Acetone by Messinger's Method, *J. Am. Chem. Soc.*, 42:39.

Greenberg, L. A. and D. Lester (1944) A Micro-method for the Determination of Acetone and Ketone Bodies, *J. Biol. Chem.*, 154:177.

Greenburg, L. and S. Moskowitz (1945) Safe Use of Solvents for Synthetic Rubbers, *Ind. Med. Surg.*, 14:359.

Gross, E. cited by K. B. Lehmann and F. Flury (1943) *Toxicology and Hygiene of Industrial Solvents*, Williams and Wilkins, Baltimore.

Haggard, A. W., L. A. Greenberg and J. M. Turner (1944) The physiological Principles governing the Action of Acetone, together with Determination of Toxicity, *J. Ind. Hyg. Toxicol.*, 26:133.

Haggard, A. W., D. P. Miller and L. A. Greenberg (1945) The Amyl Alcohols and their Ketones, *J. Ind. Hyg. Toxicol.*, 27:1.

Hahn, E. (1935) Beitrag zur Isolierung organisch-chemischer Substanzen aus der Atemluft, *Beitr. Klin. Tuberk.*, 87:1.

Halbertsma, K. T. A. (1936) Hornhautschädigung bei Anwendung von Aceton, *Deut. Z. Ges. Gerichtl. Med.*, 10:109.

Harris, L. C. and R. H. Jackson (1952) Acute Acetone Poisoning caused by Setting Fluid for immobilising Casts, *Brit. Med. J.*, 2:1024.

Heim de Balzac, F., E. Agasse-Lafont and A. Feil (1922) Manifestations morbides chez les Ouvriers maniant le celluloid et ses Solvants, *Paris Méd.*, 1:477.

Henderson, Y. and H. W. Haggard (1943) *Noxious Gases*, Reinhold Publ. Corp., New York.

Hift, W. and P. L. Patel (1961) Acute Poisoning due to synthetic Plaster Cast, *S. Afr. Med. J.*, 35:246.

Holden, H. C. and A. K. Doolittle (1935) Solvents, *Ind. Eng. Chem.*, 27:525.

Irish, D. D. and E. M. Adams (1940) Apparatus and Methods for testing the Toxicity of Vapours, *Ind. Med. (Ind. Hyg. Section)*, 1:1.

Jacobi, C. Hayashi and I. W. Szubinski (1903) Untersuchungen über die pharmakologische Wirkung der Zyklischen Isoxime der hydroaromatischen Kohlenwasserstoffe etc., *Arch. Exptl. Pathol. Pharmakol.*, 50:199.

Jacobs, M. B. (1949) *The analytical Chemistry of Industrial Poisons, Hazards and Solvents*, 2nd ed., Interscience Publishers Inc., New York.

Jobes, G. W., E. S. Harris and W. E. Miller (1933) *Explosive Properties of Aceton-Air Mixtures*, U.S. Bureau Mines. Techn. Paper no. 544.

Kacy, H. W. and R. W. Cope (1955) Determination of small Quantities of Isophorone in Air, *Am. Ind. Hyg. Ass. Quart.*, 16:55.

Kagan, E. (1924) Experimentelle Studien über den Einfluss technisch und hygienisch wichtiger Gäse und Dämpfe auf den Organismus, *Arch. Hyg. Berlin*, 94:41.

Katz, A. E. (1946) (cited by Rowe and Wolf, 1963) *Spice Mill*, 69:40.

Koehler A. E., E. Windsor and E. Hill (1941) Acetone and Aceto-acetic Studies in Man, *J. Biol. Chem.*, 140:811.

La Belle, C. W. and H. Brieger (1955) Vapour Toxicity of a composite Solvent and its principal Components, *Arch. Ind. Hlth.*, 12:623.

Laborde, M. V. (1885) Note sur l'Action physiologique et toxique de l'acétophénone ou Phenyl-methyl ketone, *Compt. Rend. Soc. Biol.*, 37:725.

Lamb, M. C. and J. A. Gilman (1932) Note on the Solution of Chlorophyll by Cellulose Solvents and Diluents, *Leather World*, 24:708.

Langovoy, B. W. (1933) Paint and Varnish Removers. U.S.P., 1,884,722, *Chem. Abstr.*, 27:1118.

Larson, P. S., J. K. Finnegan and H. B. Haag (1956) Observations on the Effect of the Oedema-producing Potency of Acids, Aldehydes, Ketones and Alcohols, *J. Pharmacol. Exptl. Therap.*, 116:119.

Lazarew, N. U., A. J. Brussilowskaja and J. M. Lawrow (1931) Quantitative Untersuchungen über die Resorption einiger organischer Gifte durch die Haut ins Blut, *Arch. Gewerbepathol. Gewerbehyg.*, 2:641.

Lehmann, K. B. and F. Flury (1943) *Toxicology and Hygiene of Industrial Solvents*, Williams and Wilkins, Baltimore.

Lewin, L. (1907) Über das Verhalten von Mesityl Oxyd und Phoron im Tierkörper im Vergleiche zu Aceton. *Arch. Exptl. Pathol. Pharmakol.*, 56:346.

Llewellyn, O. P. (1963) Medical Officer, British Celanese Ltd. (personal communication).

Loehr, O. (1931) Acetyl Cellulose Composition suitable for Films, Lacquers etc., *Chem. Abstr.*, 25:414.

Mairet and Comberbale (1886) Recherches sur l'Action physiologique et Thérapeutique de l'Ace-tophenone, *Compt. Rend. Acad. Sci.*, 102:178.

McOmie, W. H. and H. H. Anderson (1949) Comparative toxicological Effects of some Isobutyl Carbinols and Ketones, *Univ. Calif. Publ. Pharmacol.*, 2:217.

Metzinger, E. F. (1935) Lacquer Solvents, *Paint, Oil, Chem. Rev.*, 97: no. 9, 4.

Morasco, M. (1926) Hydroxylamine hydrochloride for quick Determination of Acetone, *Ind. Eng. Chem.*, 18:701.

Nelson, K. W., J. F. Ege, M. Ross, L. E. Woodman and L. Silverman (1943) Sensory Response to certain Industrial Solvent Vapours, *J. Ind. Hyg. Toxicol.*, 25:282.

Neubauer, C. (1901) Über Glyconsäurepaarung bei Stoffen der Fettreihe, *Arch. Exptl. Pathol. Pharmakol.*, 46:133.

Oglesby, F. L., J. E. Williams, D. W. Fassett and J. H. Sterner (1949) Cited by Rowe and Wolf in F. A. Patty (1963) *Industrial Hygiene and Toxicology*, Vol. 2, 2nd ed., Interscience Publishers, New York.

Parmeggiani, L. and C. Sassi (1954) Patologia professionale da Acetone, *Med. Lavoro*, 45:431.

Patty, F. A., H. H. Schrenk and W. P. Yant (1935) Acute Response of Guinea Pigs to Vapours of some new commercial organic Compounds, *U.S. Treas. Publ. Hlth. Rep.*, 50:1217.

Poliak, B. (1925) Anatomische Veranderungen bei der experimentelle Azetonvergiftung, *Arch. Exptl. Pathol. Pharmakol.* 105:220.

Price, T. O. and D. Rittenberg (1950) The Metabolism of Acetone, *J. Biol. Chem.*, 185:449.

Quevauviller, A. (1946) Toxicité et Pouvoir hypnotique de l'Acetophenone et des Theinylcetones, *Compt. Rend. Soc. Biol.*, 140:367.

Quick, A. J. (1928) The Metabolism of conjugated Glycuronic Acids, *J. Biol. Chem.*, 80:535.

Renshaw, P. R. and R. M. Mitchell (1956) Acetone Poisoning following the Application of a light-weight Cast, *Brit. Med. J.*, 1:615.

Rosgen and Mamier (1944) Sind Azeton Gäse blutschädigend? *Der öffentliche Gesundheits Krankedienst*, 10:A 83.

Rowe, V. K. and M. A. Wolf (1963) Ketones; in F. A. Patty (1963) *Industrial Hygiene and Toxicology*, Vol. II. 2nd ed. Interscience Publishers, New York and London.

Sack, G. (1940) Ein Fall von Azetonvergiftung, *Arch. Gewerbepathol. Gewerbehyg.*, 10:80.

Sakami, W. and J. M. Lafaye (1950) Formation of Formate and labile Methyl Groups from Acetone in intact Rat, *J. Biol. Chem.*, 187:369.

Sakami, W. and J. M. Lafaye (1951) The Metabolism of Acetone in intact Rat, *J. Biol. Chem.*, 193:199.

Salant, W. and N. Kleitman (1922) Pharmacological Studies on Acetone, *J. Pharmacol. Exptl. Therap.*, 19:293.

Sanderson, J. McE. (1933) Solvents used in Surface Coatings, *Paint, Oil, Chem. Rev.*, 95 No. 2, 10.

Sanoyeshi, S. (1911) Über Zwei-Butanolglycosäure, *Biochem. Z.*, 36:22.

Sax, N. Irving (1957) *Dangerous Properties of Industrial Materials*, Rheinhold, New York.

Scheiner, H. (1945) Recherches sur la Contraction musculaire, *Compt. Rend. Soc. Biol.*, 139:1091.

Schrenk, H. H., W. P. Yant and F. A. Patty (1936) Acute Response of Guinea pigs to vapors of some new commercial organic Compounds – Hexanone (Methyl Butyl Ketone), *U.S. Treas. Dept. Publ. Hlth. Rep.*, 51:624.

Schultze, D. (1932). Dissertation, Wurzburg (cited by Flury and Wirth, 1934).

Schwartz, L. (1898) Über die Oxydation des Acetons und homologer Ketone der Fettsäurereihe, *Arch. Exptl. Pathol. Pharmakol.*, 40:168.

Schwartz, L., L. Tulipan and S. M. Peck (1947) *Occupational Diseases of the Skin*, Kempton, London.

Sessa, F. and F. M. Troisi (1947) Sulla Patologica professionale dei Verniciatori; Osservazione cliniche, *Folia Med. Nap.*, 30:129.

Shell Chemical Corporation (1957) Methyl Isobutyl Ketone, *Ind. Hyg. Bull.*, *Toxicity Data Sheet S.C.*, 57–113. Cited by Rowe and Wolf (1963).

Shell Chemical Corporation (1949) Cited by Rowe and Wolf (1963) in F. A. Patty (Ed.), *Industrial Hygiene and Toxicology*, Vol. 2. 2nd ed. Interscience Publishers, New York.

Silverman, L., H. F. Schulte and W. W. First (1946) Further Studies in Sensory Response to certain industrial solvent Vapors, *J. Ind. Hyg. Toxicol.*, 28:262.

Sklianskaya, R. M., F. E. Urieva and L. M. Mashbitz (1936) Relative Toxicity of Acetone, Methyl Alcohol and their Mixtures, *J. Ind. Hyg. Tocicol.*, 18:106.

Smith, A. R. and M. R. Mayers (1944) Poisoning and Fire Hazards of Butanone and Acetone, *Ind. Bull. New York, State Dept. Labor.*, 23:174.

Smith, J. N., R. H. Smithies and R. T. Williams (1954) Stereochemical Aspects of the biological Hydroxylation of Ethyl Benzene to Methyl Phenyl Carbinol, *Biochem. J.*, 56:320.

Smith, J. N., R. H. Smithies and R. T. Williams (1954) The Metabolism of Alkyl Benzenes; The biological Reduction of Ketones derived from Alkyl Benzenes, *Biochem. J.*, 57:74.

Smoley, E. R. and W. W. Kraft (1935) Production of Lubricating Oils, *Ind. Eng. Chem.*, 27:1418.

Smyth, H. F. Jr. (1956) Hygienic Standards for Daily Inhalation, *Am. Ind. Hyg. Ass. Quart.*, 17:129.

Smyth, H. F. Jr. and C. P. Carpenter (1944) Further Experience with the Range Finding Test in the Industrial Toxicology Laboratory, *J. Ind. Hyg. Toxicol.*, 26:269.

Smyth, H. F. Jr. and C. P. Carpenter (1948) Further Experience with the Range Finding Test in the Industrial Toxicology Laboratory, *J. Ind. Hyg. Toxicol.*, 30:63.

Smyth, H. F. Jr., C. P. Carpenter and C. S. Weil (1949) Range-finding Toxicity Data. List III, *J. Ind. Hyg. Toxicol.*, 31:60.

Smyth, H. F. Jr., C. P. Carpenter, C. S. Weil and V. C. Pozzani (1954) Range Finding Toxicity Data. List V, *Arch. Ind. Hyg. Occ. Med.*, 10:61.

Smyth, H. F. Jr., and J. Seaton (1940) Acute Response of Guinea Pigs and Rats to Inhalation of the Vapours of Isophorone, *J. Ind. Hyg. Toxicol.*, 22:477.

Smyth, H. F. Jr., J. Seaton and L. Fischer (1942) Response of Guinea pigs and Rats to repeated Inhalation of Mesityl Oxide and Isophorone, *J. Ind. Hyg. Toxicol.*, 24:46.

Specht, H. (1938) Acute Response of Guinea Pigs to Inhalation of Methyl Isobutyl Ketone, *U.S. Treas. Dept. Publ. Hlth. Rep.*, 53:292.

Specht, H., J. W. Miller and P. J. Valaer (1939) Acute Response of Guinea pigs to Inhalation of Dimethyl Ketone (Acetone) Vapour, *U.S. Publ. Hlth. Rep. Wash.*, 54:944.

Specht, H., J. W. Miller, P. J. Valaer and R. R. Sayers (1940) Acute Response of Guinea pigs to Inhalation of Ketone Vapours, *U.S. Publ. Hlth. Serv., Nat. Inst. Hlth Bull.* No. 176.

Tersand, R. (1935) Les Proprionates et l'Oxide de Mésityle, Solvants de la Nitrocellulose, *Rev. Prod. Chim.*, 38:97.

Thierfelder, H. and K. Daiba (1923) Zur Kenntnis der Verhaltens fettaromatischer Ketone in Tierkörper, *Z. Physiol. Chem.*, 130:380.

Thierfelder, H. and E. Klenke (1924) Zur Kenntniss des Verhaltens des Acetophenons und Benzols in Tierkörper, *Z. Physiol. Chem.*, 141:219.

Thomson, T. (1946) *Specificity of the salicylaldehyde Reaction for the Detection of Acetone.*

Threshold Limit Values for 1962, *Am. Ind. Hyg. Ass. J.*, 23:419.

Threshold Limit Values for 1963, *J. Occ. Med.*, 1963, 5:491.

Treon, J. F., W. E. Crutchfield Jr., and K. V. Kitzmiller (1943) The physiological Response of Rabbits to Cyclohexane, Methylcyclohexane and certain Derivatives of these Compounds, *J. Ind. Hyg. Toxicol.*, 25:199, 323.

Tsao, M. V. and E. L. Pfeiffer (1957) Isolation and Identification of a new Ketone Body in normal Urine, *Proc. Soc. Exptl. Biol.*, 94:628.

Walton, D. C., E. F. Kehr and A. S. Loevenhart (1928) Comparison of the pharmacological Actions of Diacetone Alcohol and Acetone, *J. Pharmacol. Exptl. Therap.*, 33:175.

Williams, R. T. (1959) *Detoxication Mechanisms*, Chapman & Hall, London.

Yant, W. P., F. A. Patty and H. H. Schrenk (1936) Acute Response of Guinea pigs to Vapours of some new commercial organic Compounds (Pentanone), *U.S. Treas. Publ. Hlth. Rep.*, 51:392.

Yarsley, V. E. (1934) Solvents and Plasticisers, *Synth. Appl. Finish.*, 5:37:57.

Zangger, H. (1930) Über die modernen organischen Lösungsmittel, *Arch. Gewerbepathol. Gewerbehyg.*, 1:77.

Chapter 9

ALDEHYDES AND ACETALS

The aldehydes, only a few of which have assumed some importance as industrial solvents, are used chiefly in the manufacture of various types of resins – in this respect formaldehyde and furfural are the most outstanding. Acetaldehyde is used to some extent in the rubber and tanning industries, and paraldehyde, better known as a medicinal sedative, and furfural, are used in the plastics, paint and varnish industries. Their main toxic effect is that of irritation of skin and mucous membranes, but some, such as acetaldehyde and paraldehyde, have a narcotic action, while formaldehyde, in addition to being a potent irritant, is also a protoplasmic poison, and furfural, at least in animals, a central nervous poison.

In spite of these toxic potentialities, there have been, except for dermatitis, few reports of injury from their industrial use. One reason for this may be found in their metabolic characteristics; their metabolism is so rapid that a cumulative effect, sufficient to cause systemic injury, is scarcely to be expected.

The acetals, produced by reactions of alcohols with aldehydes, have been examined for their possible value as anaesthetics, but none of them have been found to have the efficiency of paraldehyde as a hypnotic (Knoeffel, 1934, 1935), possibly because paraldehyde is more resistant to acid hydrolysis in the stomach when given by mouth.

In animals, inhalation of high concentrations, particularly of methylal, have been found to cause bronchopneumonia and some fatty degeneration of the liver and kidney; most of them are to some extent irritants but less so than the aldehydes.

Few investigations of their industrial effects have been carried out, but in view of their fairly extensive use in the plastics and varnish industries, and the paucity of adverse reports, it appears unlikely that they represent a serious toxic hazard if they are handled with ordinary care.

64. Formaldehyde

Synonyms: methanol formic aldehyde, formalin

Structural formula: $\begin{matrix} H \\ H \end{matrix} {>} C {=} O$

Molecular formula: CH_2O

Molecular weight: 30.0 (gas)

Properties: a colourless gas with an irritating odour; also, as used commercially, as a 35–40% solution in water, known as formalin, and as a crystalline solid by condensation with ammonia.

Extremely reactive and capable of combining with practically all other classes of chemicals, especially alcohol and ether, so that it is of wide industrial application.

boiling point: −19.5 °C (in aqueous solution: 98.18 °C)

melting point: −92° C

vapour pressure: 10 mm Hg

vapour density (air = 1): 1.075

specific gravity (liquid density): 0.815

flash point: 572 °F (ignition temperature)

conversion factors: 1 p.p.m. $= 1.2$ mg/m²

  1 mg/l $= 815$ p.p.m.

solubility: very soluble in water

maximum allowable concentration: 5 p.p.m.

ECONOMY, SOURCES AND USES

Production

(1) By oxidation of methanol, with copper, silver or iron-molybdenum as catalyst.
(2) From petroleum gases as starting material.

Industrial uses

(1) In the manufacture of various resins, e.g. phenolformaldehyde; ureaformaldehyde, and in the plastics industry (Malten and Zielhuis, 1964).
(2) In leather tanning.
(3) In the paper industry, as a water-resistant coating.
(4) In the textile industry, as a crease-preventing agent (Schwartz, 1941; Bourne *et al.*, 1959; Malten, 1963).

(5) In the glass fibre industry (McKenna *et al.*, 1958).
(6) In the production of the urinary antiseptic, urotropin, and of hexamethylene tetramine, used as an accelerator in the rubber industry.
(7) As a disinfectant and fumigating agent (of limited application, Henson, 1949).
(8) As a hardening agent for photographic films.
(9) As an embalming fluid and preservative of anatomical specimens.

BIOCHEMISTRY

Estimation

In the atmosphere
   (a) The bisulphite method (Goldman and Yagoda, 1943; Parker, 1949). – This method, recommended by the A.C.G.I.H., and by Elkins (1959), depends on a non-volatile sodium formaldehyde compound with bisulphite, which can be fixed in an alkaline solution. The excess bisulphite is titrated with a standard iodine solution.
   (b) Chromotropic acid reaction (McDonald, 1954). – This method, described by Bricker and Johnson in 1945, in which the reaction of formaldehyde with chromotropic acid gives a purple colour, is stated to be specific for formaldehyde, rapid and accurate; it has been adapted by McDonald (1954) as a field test, and modified to enable atmospheric formaldehyde to be determined in the range of 0.5 to 30 μg.

Metabolism

Formaldehyde is known to be the most toxic of the metabolites of methanol, and at least 150 times more toxic than methanol itself (Gilger *et al.*, 1952); it has been held responsible for the amblyopia due to methanol, by inhibiting retinal respiration and glycolysis (Leaf and Zatman, 1952).
   It is absorbed rapidly by all routes of administration, and following inhalation disappears rapidly from the blood (McGuignan, 1914). It is oxidised to formic acid, and partly excreted as formate in the urine. The formic acid may be further oxidised to CO_2 and water (Simon, 1914).

TOXICOLOGY

Formaldehyde vapour is primarily a powerful irritant of mucous membranes. It is also a protoplasmic poison, forming irreversibly coagulated protein products possibly including a haeme-linked group of haemoglobin (histidine; Guthe, 1959). Ingestion of the liquid causes initial stimulation of respiration, followed by depression and while small doses have a stimulating effect on the heart, large doses

Bibliography on p. 489

cause a marked fall of blood pressure. Small doses also cause a slight increase in kidney function, with little or no irritation of the digestive tract, but large amounts may cause severe inflammation leading in some cases to death; if death is delayed uraemia may develop. Inhalation of the vapour by animals, even in low concentrations, causes inflammation of the upper respiratory tract and congestion and emphysema of the lungs.

In industry the chief toxic effect is that of irritation of the skin and mucous membranes, though there have been some reports of systemic effects.

Dermatitis may arise from contact with various resins and adhesives, especially in uncured forms which may contain small amounts of formaldehyde, and it is a potent sensitiser.

Toxicity to animals

Acute

Lethal dose. – (i) By oral administration LD_{50} for rats, 0.1 to 0.2 g/kg (Fassett 1963). – (ii) By subcutaneous injection, for rabbits, 0.24 g/kg (McGuignan, 1914), 0.30 g/kg (Skog, 1950). – (iii) By intraperitoneal injection, for mice, 0.07 g/kg (Gilger et al., 1952). – (iv) By inhalation, for rats, 815 p.p.m. (Skog, 1950).

SYMPTOMS OF INTOXICATION

Oral or subcutaneous administration of a toxic dose is followed in rabbits by depression, clonic tetanus, opisthotonus and irregular respiration leading to early death. Inhalation causes lacrimation, increased nasal secretion, difficult noisy breathing. Death, usually from pneumonia (McGuignan, 1914), may be delayed up to 15 days. Corrosion of the cornea following exposure to 4000 p.p.m. was observed in cats by Iwanoff (1911), and local application may, it is stated by Meyer (1893) and Fischer (1905), cause severe conjunctivitis, keratitis, corneal ulcers and iritis.

The blood

A decrease in the haemolytic power of the serum of a dog following intravenous injection, at the rate of about 11 ml/min, of a 1% solution of formaldehyde in 0.9% NaCl was observed by Guthrie in 1905.

CHANGES IN THE ORGANISM

(1) The kidneys

These may show tubular degeneration, vacuolisation and necrosis.

(2) The gastro-intestinal tract

This is markedly hyperaemic, with hardening or necrosis.

(3) The respiratory tract

The larynx and lungs may be oedematous and there may be emphysema of the lungs and bronchopneumonia.

(4) The nervous system

The brain may show oedema (Böhmer, 1934) and destruction of ganglionic cells (Scheidegger, 1936).

Toxicity to human beings

(1) By ingestion

Most of the severe or fatal systemic effects of formaldehyde reported in human beings have been due to ingestion, accidental or suicidal. In 1934 Böhmer had collected 25 such cases from the literature and 4 more have been recorded by Frenkel (1936) and Scheidegger (1936).

The essential symptoms are those of gastro-intestinal inflammation, with severe pain, loss of consciousness and collapse. If, with smaller doses, death is delayed for several days, uraemia may develop.

According to Yonkman *et al.* (1941) no significant effects other than mild pharyngeal and gastric discomfort were caused by the daily ingestion by two male subjects of 22 to 200 mg of pure formaldehyde in water over a period of 13 weeks.

(2) The skin

Primary formaldehyde dermatitis. Dermatitis is the best known industrial injury due to formaldehyde, which is both a primary irritant and also a potent sensitiser.

(a) Urticaria. – In an outbreak of dermatitis in a New Zealand factory making formaldehyde resins (Glass, 1961) the chief manifestation was an itching erythematous rash, with or without scattered macules and papules, generally on the wrists and forearms and between the fingers, sometimes on the face and accompanied by oedema of the eyelids. The atmospheric concentration of formaldehyde vapour was always greater than 5 p.p.m. and in the vicinity of the more severe cases reached 16 to 30 p.p.m.

A similar manifestation was described by Markuson *et al.* (1943) as a result of contact with formaldehyde resins, in some cases with the fine dust emanated during sanding and polishing. These observers state that some workers develop a tolerance or immunity, but this later may be lost.

(b) Contact eczema has been reported from handling fabrics on which urea formaldehyde has been used (Schwartz, 1941; Malten, 1962, 1963), and in cobblers, due to the use of a new additive (a polycondensate made from *p-tert.* butyl phenol and formaldehyde) (Malten, 1958). In these cases however patch tests for formaldehyde were present in only two of the ten cobblers and in 7 out of 28 of

the textile workers, several of the latter showing a polyvalent sensitivity to various finishing compounds.

(3) Sensitisation

Formaldehyde is formed when hexamethylene tetramine is decomposed by heat and may thus be the cause of allergic urticaria (Key, 1961). Brunner (1962) has reported six cases of sensitivity to formaldehyde occurring from contact with glues, and Quoss (1959) several of allergic dermatoses in textile workers using resin finishes, while Hovding (1961) found 137 cases of formaldehyde contact sensitivity among 2110 routine patch tests; of these 137, 45 appeared to be due to textile-finish contact. A suitable concentration for patch testing for formaldehyde recommended by Malten and Zielhuis (1964) is a 1% water solution.

(4) The nails

In 3 of the cases described by Glass (1961) severe fissuring dermatitis of the palms was associated with paronychia and softening of the nails.

(5) The eyes

Conjunctivitis, as an effect of formaldehyde vapour, and keratitis, due to flakes of uncured resin, in women employed in sewing textiles to which resins containing formaldehyde have been added to make them crease-resistant, have been described by Ettinger and Jeremias (1955) and by Giel et al. (1956).

Lacrimation (at concentrations of 4 to 5 p.p.m.) has been described by Fassett (1963) and has also been noted by Baader (1932).

(6) Respiratory disturbances

Fassett (1963) states that at about 2–3 p.p.m. a mild tingling sensation occurs in the nose and posterior pharynx, the discomfort increasing at 4–5 p.p.m. At such concentrations some tolerance is usually established, but at 10 and 20 p.p.m. the irritation of the nose and throat becomes more severe and is accompanied by coughing; he believes that a 5 or 10 min exposure to 50–100 p.p.m. might result in serious inflammation of the bronchi and lower respiratory tract. Wyse (1950) gives the frequency of symptoms due to industrial use of formaldehyde as bronchitis, dermatitis, rhinitis, oropharyngitis and conjunctivitis.

(7) Systemic effects

Although most of the toxic effects of formaldehyde encountered in industry and arising from either contact with the liquid or vapour or from inhalation of the dust or vapour appear in the form of dermatitis or respiratory irritation, other symptoms have been observed particularly during the manufacture of phenol-formaldehyde resins in the absence of adequate ventilation.

Weger (1927) described a syndrome which he designated a 'thalamic symptom-complex'. This included headache, weakness, sensory disturbances, irregular perspiration, and changes in body temperature. Baader (1932) also described, in addition to lacrimation, cough and oppression in the chest, a rapid pulse and heaviness in the kidney region.

TREATMENT

(1) By ingestion. – Gastric lavage with water, and administration of small doses of ammonium acetate and demulcents such as starch solution, milk and eggs (U.S. Public Health Rep., 1945).

(2) By inhalation. – The irritation of the respiratory tract may be alleviated by inhalation of dilute ammonia vapour.

(3) By liquid contact. – Contact of the skin with solutions of formaldehyde should be removed immediately by thorough washing with soap and water, and contaminated clothing or gloves removed.

Bibliography on p. 489

65. Acetaldehyde

Structural formula: $CH_3-CH=O$

Molecular formula: C_2H_4O

Molecular weight: 44.05

Properties: a volatile, colourless, markedly reactive liquid.

    boiling point: 21 °C

    melting point: -123.5 °C

    vapour pressure: 740 mm Hg at 20 °C

    vapour density (air = 1): 1.52

    specific gravity (liquid density): 0.788

    flash point: -36 °F

    conversion factors: 1 p.p.m. = 1.8 mg/m³

                           1 mg/l = 556 p.p.m.

    solubility: soluble in water, miscible with ether and alcohol. May react explosively with oxygen (Fassett, 1963)

    maximum allowable concentration: 200 p.p.m.

ECONOMY, SOURCES AND USES

Production

(1) By hydration of acetylene during the manufacture of acetic acid (Fairhall, 1957).

(2) By oxidation of ethyl alcohol (Fassett, 1963).

Industrial uses

While acetaldehyde has its chief application as an intermediate in the manufacture of synthetic chemicals, it is used to some extent as a solvent in the rubber, tanning and paper industries.

BIOCHEMISTRY

Estimation

(1) In the atmosphere

    (a) By absorption in water and reaction with sodium bisulphite, the uncom-

[470]

bined bisulphite being titrated with iodine or with *p*-hydroxylphenyl (Stotz, 1943).

(*b*) *By Schiff's reagent* (a solution of fuchsin decolourised by sulphurous acid).

(*c*) *By reaction with benzidine hydrochloride*, giving a yellow-brown colour (Smitt, 1922).

(2) In blood and tissues

By the method of Stotz (1943) in which the acetaldehyde is collected from the distillation of a tungstic acid filtrate of blood or tissue and passed into sodium bisulphite solution and reacted with *p*-hydroxylphenyl.

Metabolism

It was established as early as 1910 (Battelli and Stern) that acetaldehyde is an intermediate in the oxidation of ethyl alcohol, and this has since been confirmed in animals and human beings (Jacobsen, 1952).

It can be isolated in the breath of human beings after ingestion of ethyl alcohol (Hald and Jacobsen, 1948), and antabuse (tetraethyldiuram disulphide) and similar substances are believed to inhibit the rapid disappearance of acetaldehyde from the blood; in such cases the amount detected may be 2–10 times the level in animals not treated with antabuse.

Ethyl ethers can also undergo cleavage by an enzyme (phenyl etherase) present in the liver, with the formation of acetaldehyde (Williams, 1959). The same factors which accelerate the disappearance of acetaldehyde increase the formation of acetoin (Stotz *et al.*, 1944) which is of no great importance in its natural form, because the isomer synthesised from acetaldehyde *in vivo* is itself very rapidly metabolised. All metabolic investigations point to the fact that though acetaldehyde is toxic at higher levels it is very rapidly metabolised, which may account for its relatively low general toxicity.

TOXICOLOGY

Acetaldehyde is both narcotic and irritant. Very high concentrations produce headache, stupefaction, bronchitis, pulmonary oedema, diarrhoea, albuminuria, fatty degeneration of the liver and of the heart muscle and finally death – a course of intoxication similar to that following an overdosage of paraldehyde. Chronic exposure to lower concentrations is followed by irritation of the eyes, nose and upper respiratory passages, and a symptomatology similar to that of chronic alcoholism, including hallucinations of sight and hearing, loss of intelligence and psychic disturbances. In fact, a death during acute alcoholism was attributed by Romano in 1955 to poisoning by acetaldehyde of metabolic origin. At concentrations liable to occur in atmospheric pollution by Diesel engines how–

Bibliography on p. 489

ever, it has been found to be almost non-irritant (200 p.p.m.)compared with formaldehyde at 12 p.p.m., which caused severe irritation (Pattle and Cullumbine, 1956).

Toxicity to animals

Acute

Lethal dose. – (i) By oral administration, for rats, 1.93 g/kg (Smyth, Carpenter and Weil, 1951). – (ii) By intraperitoneal injection, for rats, 50 mg/100 g, lethal within 10 min (Skog, 1950). – (iii) By inhalation, for rats, 20,000 p.p.m. for 30 min (Skog, 1952).

SYMPTOMS OF INTOXICATION

Excitement, followed by narcosis or anaesthesia after about 15 min. Survivors recover rapidly, explained by the fact that there is a rapid decrease of acetaldehyde from the blood.

CHANGES IN THE ORGANISM

In the experiments of Skog (1950) the chief injury was found in the lungs – evidence of pulmonary oedema.

Hypertension was observed in dogs following intravenous injection of 5 mg/kg by Handovsky (1934). This was stated to be due partly to a reflex mechanism originating in the carotid sinus, partly to a direct action on the blood vessels, and the tachycardia observed to a direct action on the heart, though in 1936 he stated that in small non-toxic doses he had not succeeded in tracing any stimulation of striated muscle to the effect of acetaldehyde. He had found however, that it increased the tone of involuntary muscles, including uterus, intestine and peripheral blood vessels.

Toxicity to human beings

Very few investigations on human beings have been carried out, especially from the industrial point of view, but the effects of intravenous injection of a 5% solution in experimental human subjects were studied by Asmussen *et al.* (1948) with a view to confirming Handovsky's (1934, 1936) results in animals indicating that acetaldehyde produces a stimulation of the respiration, an increase in arterial blood pressure and a dilatation of the bronchial muscles. They confirmed that acetaldehyde, given by injection, did result in a marked increase in pulse rate and ventialtion with a decrease in alveolar CO_2, and symptoms similar to those seen after alcohol intake, especially if preceded by antabuse treatment. If oxygen were inhaled during the injection there was a marked depression of respiratory function. They also noted that an increase of blood acetaldehyde from the normal level of 0.02–0.37 mg% to 0.2 mg% will produce marked vaso-dilatation of the facial blood vessels, giving intense flushing.

No reports of industrial injury from the use of acetaldehyde have been published, and, as Fassett (1963) remarks, acetaldehyde, because of its explosive
hazard, is usually handled in industry in closed systems and exposures are not
apt to be continuous or at high levels. Its irritant properties also give warning of
concentrations above the recommended level of 200 p.p.m. when signs of eye
irritation occur (Silverman, Schulte and First, 1946); these observers state that
it can be readily detected below 50 p.p.m. though as already remarked (see p. 472)
as an atmospheric pollutant irritation is not severe at 200 p.p.m.

Bibliography on p. 489

66. Paraldehyde

Structural formula:

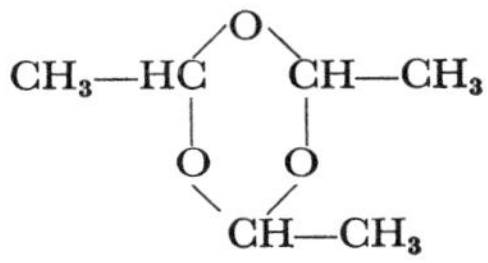

$$CH_3-HC \underset{\underset{CH-CH_3}{\overset{O \quad O}{\diagup}}}{\overset{O}{\diagup \diagdown}} CH-CH_3$$

Molecular formula: $(C_2H_4O)_3$

Molecular weight: 132.2

Properties: a colourless liquid with an odour resembling fusel oil.

boiling point: 124 °C

melting point: 12.6 °C

specific gravity (liquid density): 0.9943

flash point: 111.2 °F (Durrans, 1950 gives 81 °F)

solubility: in water 10.5 g in 100 ml; less soluble in warm water than cold. Not in itself a solvent for nitrocellulose, but when mixed with alcohols exhibits a high dilution ratio (Durrans, 1935).

maximum allowable concentrations: not established

ECONOMY, SOURCES AND USES

Production

By polymerisation of acetaldehyde.

Industrial uses

(1) In the manufacture of pigments and varnishes, as a diluent (Yarsley, 1934),

(2) In the plastics industry (Carrol, 1933).

(3) In high-grade lubricating oils (Hamilton, 1934).

(4) As a combustible and motor fuel (mixed with 40 to 60% of benzene – Baslini, 1924).

BIOCHEMISTRY

Estimation

(1) In the atmosphere

The method developed by Stotz (1943) for the colorimetric estimation of

[474]

acetaldehyde and paraldehyde in blood is based on the coloration with *p*-hydroxy-biphenyl reagent and could be adapted to air contamination (Fairhall, 1957).

(2) In blood and tissues

The method of Hitchcock and Nelson (1943) for estimation of paraldehyde in tissues and expired air is that of depolymerisation of the paraldehyde to acetaldehyde in hot sulphuric acid and absorption of the liberated acetaldehyde in sodium bisulphite solution, followed by iodometric titration.

Metabolism

Practically all authorities, with the exception of Nitzescu *et al.* (1936) who reported that the rat excretes 100% of an injected dose, are agreed that a large part of paraldehyde (70 to 88%, according to Levine *et al.*, 1940) is destroyed in the body, being first depolymerised to acetaldehyde and eventually oxidised through acetic acid to CO_2 and water. According to Levine *et al.* (1939) in dogs 11 to 28% is eliminated by the lungs and only 0.1 to 2.5% excreted in the urine. In mice, about 8% of the dose administered orally is excreted by the lungs (Hitchcock and Nelson, 1943) but if the mice have been subjected to poisoning by carbon tetrachloride, with resultant liver injury, elimination by the lungs may be as much as 26%. From this, and the fact that the time for elimination is prolonged, it is assumed that destruction of paraldehyde takes place chiefly in the liver (Levine *et al.*, 1939, 1940).

TOXICOLOGY

While no industrial poisoning from paraldehyde has been reported, and is in fact unlikely owing to its low volatility, a description of some of its toxic effects when used as a hypnotic and sedative are here given as an indication of its mode of action.

It was first used as an anaesthetic in Italy by Cervello in 1884, and in England by Strahan in 1885, and form 1890 onwards reports of fatal cases following its administration both by mouth and per rectum began to appear. Nevertheless it has been regarded by many authorities as one of the safest of basal anaesthetics. Stewart (1932) for example, stated that it had been so used by rectal injection in 500 cases without any mortality and that the margin between the hypnotic and the toxic dose is wide. Burstein (1943) on the other hand remarks that it exhibits a very low margin of safety between the minimum anaesthetic dose and the minimal lethal dose.

In animals lethal doses appear to cause death by massive pulmonary haemorrhage and in all the reported human fatalities autopsy has shown congestion

Bibliography on p. 489

and oedema of the lungs and dilatation of the right side of the heart. Burstein (1943) believes that the toxic effect is exerted on the capillaries.

Toxicity to animals

(1) Acute

    (a) Lethal dose. – (i) By oral administration, for dogs, 14 g/kg (Schneider, 1929), 3 to 4 g/kg (Spector, 1956). – *(ii) By stomach tube*, for rabbits, 3 g/kg (Cervello, 1884). – *(iii) Per rectum*, for mice, 0.208 ml/100 g (Gage, 1933). – *(iv) By intravenous injection*, LD_{50}, for dogs, 0.5 ml/kg, for cats and rabbits, 0.45 ml/kg (Burstein, 1943).

    (b) Narcotic dose. – (i) By oral administration, for dogs, 1.5 to 2 ml/kg, deep anaesthesia within 18 to 30 min (Kistler and Luckhardt, 1929). – *(ii) Per rectum*, for mice, 0.012 ml/100 g (Gage, 1933). – *(iii) By intravenous injection*, for dogs, 0.8 ml/kg (Nitzescu, 1932), or 0.3 ml/kg (Burstein, 1943).

(2) Chronic

    Animals given repeated doses of paraldehyde show wasting and diarrhoea, albuminuria, lowering of body temperature, respiratory catarrh and finally oedema of the lungs, causing death (Bau, 1929).

SYMPTOMS OF INTOXICATION

Immediate fall of blood pressure to 50% of the initial level; apnoea followed by rapid shallow respiration, coughing and cyanosis; unconsciousness; death in the majority of animals 6 to 24 h after anaesthesia.

CHANGES IN THE ORGANISM

(1) The heart

    Dilatation of the right side, distending the pericardial sac. The heart and liver showed fatty degeneration, with chronic intoxication.

(2) The lungs

    Gross pulmonary haemorrhages and acute oedema. All viscera show congestion and oedema.

Toxicity to human beings

All the fatal cases following administration by mouth or per rectum have shown a similar sequence of events – profound unconsciousness with cyanosis, labored and rapid respiration and a rapid irregular pulse; death occurring from pulmonary oedema and heart failure. Bau (1929) states that the fatal dose is from 50 to 100 g, but according to Burstein (1943) deaths have occurred following ingestion of 25 ml and rectal injection of 12 ml, as in the case described by Shoor (1941).

In the case described by Kotz *et al.* (1938) in which it was suggested that there was some idiosyncrasy to paraldehyde, the blood pressure was decreased from an initial level of 148 systolic and 98 diastolic to 118/58, and a loud blowing murmur over the tricuspid area indicated failure of the right side of the heart.

In only one (suicidal) case, that of McDougall (1932) in which death occurred 50 h after ingestion of 4 oz. has it been reported that the liver and kidneys showed fatty degeneration, but some parenchymatous degeneration of the kidneys was observed in a fatal case described by Bau (1929).

RESIDUAL SYMPTOMS

Epileptic attacks, first described by Kraft Ebbing in 1897 as a residual effect of acute paraldehyde poisoning, were also mentioned by Bau, in one of his cases which survived, after recovery from a comatose condition.

Chronic

The habitual use of paraldehyde may produce symptoms similar to those of chronic alcoholism – hallucinations, delirium and psychic disturbances. Neither acute nor chronic poisoning has been reported from the industrial use of paraldehyde.

Bibliography on p. 489

67. Methylal

Synonyms: formal, dimethoxymethane, methylene dimethyl ether, formaldehyde dimethyl acetal, anesthesyl.

Structural formula: $CH_3-O-CH_2-O-CH_3$

Molecular formula: $C_3H_8O_2$

Molecular weight: 76.1

Properties: a clear thin mobile liquid with a slightly pungent odour and a burning, aromatic taste. Solvent for nitrocellulose, cellulose acetate, ethyl cellulose, vinyls, polystyrene, gums, waxes and resins.

> *boiling point:* 42.3 °C
> *melting point:* −104.8 °C
> *vapour pressure:* 400 mm Hg at 25 °C
> *vapour density (air = 1):* 2.6
> *specific gravity (liquid density):* 0.8630
> *flash point:* 0 °F. The view of Bacq and Dallemagne (1943), contrary to that of other observers, is that its vapour is inflammable, and needs the same care as ether.
> *conversion factors:* 1 p.p.m. = 3.1 mg/m³
>   1 mg/l   = 322 p.p.m.
> *solubility:* soluble in water 1 part in 3. Stable in alkaline and moderately acid media (pH3) (Fairhall, 1957)
> *maximum allowable concentration:* 1000 p.p.m. (Threshold Limit Values, 1962)

ECONOMY, SOURCES AND USES

Production

By interaction of formaldehyde and methanol, catalysed by dry HCl or $CaCl_2$ (Weaver *et al.*, 1951).

Industrial uses

(1) Especially in the plastic and perfume industries.
(2) As an extraction solvent.
(3) As a special fuel in rocket and jet engines.

BIOCHEMISTRY

Estimation

In the atmosphere

The method described by Weaver *et al.* (1951) consisted in adding dilute HCl (1/100) to the atmospheric sample, then diluting to 100 ml with water, making up 10 ml of this solution to 100 ml of water and adding Schiff's reagent; the colour formed is compared with a standard solution prepared by the same method.

Metabolism

It appears that methylal is not hydrolysed in the body but is generally excreted by the respiratory tract. No formaldehyde or formic acid has been detected in the vitreous humour or urine (Weaver *et al.*, 1951) as in the case of methyl alcohol (Keeser, 1931). Nevertheless, Fassett (1963) points out that because of its irritative action when inhaled by animals and the necrosis following subcutaneous injection, it is possible that there is some hydrolysis to formaldehyde, which is readily metabolised and therefore difficult to detect.

TOXICOLOGY

Methylal is narcotic, less powerful than chloroform but stronger than diethyl ether (Meyer and Gottlieb–Billroth, 1921). Although anaesthesia can be produced in both animals and human beings, its onset is slower than with ether and its effect more transitory. Bacq and Dallemagne (1943) quote Dujardin–Beaumetz (1885–1889) as stating that methylal is a powerful hypnotic producing profound tranquil and immediate sleep, lasting only a short time owing to its rapid elimination, and leaving no organic disturbance, but slightly increasing the heart rate, lowering the blood pressure and deepening and slowing the respiration. They themselves (Bacq and Dallemagne) on the basis of experiments with dogs, consider methylal a less toxic anaesthetic than ether, while Dallemagne and Bacq (1943) point out that the pure methylal (Anesthesyl) used as an anaesthetic is devoid of traces of methanol or formaldehyde, in contrast to that used in animal experiments, which contained 0.2–3% of methanol.

Very high concentrations can be fatal to animals. It has a marked irritant effect on mucous membranes and prolonged exposure has resulted in animals in fatty degeneration of the liver and kidneys and bronchopneumonia.

No toxic effects from its industrial use have been reported.

Toxicity to animals

Acute

(a) *Lethal dose.* – By inhalation *(single)*, for guinea pigs after about 2 h (Weaver

Bibliography on p. 489

et al., 1951), 153,000 p.p.m.; for mice, LD_{50}, 18,000 p.p.m. during a 7 h exposure; (repeated), for mice, 11,000 p.p.m. killed 6 out of 50 during 22 days of 7 h exposure, and 14,000 p.p.m. about 30% during 17 days' exposure.

(b) Narcotic dose. – By inhalation, for mice, 2.8% compared with 0.5% for chloroform and 3.4% for diethyl ether (Meyer and Gottlieb–Billroth, 1921; Meyer and Hemmi, 1935). Lack of coordination appeared (Weaver *et al.*, 1951) after 3 to 4 h exposure to 11,000 p.p.m.

SYMPTOMS OF INTOXICATION

Irritation of eyes, nose and mouth and respiratory tract followed inhalation of concentrations below the lethal dose in guinea pigs, and subcutaneous injection of 0.3 to 1.0 g caused severe inflammation at the site, with swelling and serious exudate (Lewin, 1929), together with general weakness and incontinence of urine, but no evidence of a toxic effect upon the heart (Weaver *et al.*, 1951). In dogs, Bacq and Dallemagne (1943) found a marked reduction in diuresis, even complete anuria, if administration was prolonged at high temperatures.

Fall of blood pressure occurred in the anaesthetised dogs, but not to such an extent as with ether.

CHANGES IN THE ORGANISM

Following high exposure (above 45,000 p.p.m.) guinea pigs showed moderate to severe fatty degeneration of liver and kidneys and extensive bronchopneumonia, but no significant changes of this kind after 5 daily exposures for 7 h to concentrations up to this level. Mice exposed repeatedly to 14,000 p.p.m. showed slighter changes – slight fatty degeneration of the kidney and occasional pulmonary oedema; no ocular changes similar to those of methyl alcohol were detected.

Toxicity to human beings

No toxic effects from its industrial use have been reported, nor, in spite of the fact that during the period 1886 to 1888 methylal had a wide application as a hypnotic, analgesic and even general anaesthetic was it regarded as highly toxic to human beings (Kobert, 1906).

68. Furfural

Synonyms: furan-2-dialdehyde, pyromucic aldehyde

Structural formula:

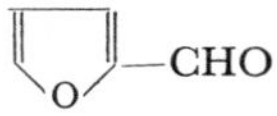

$$\text{O}\!\!\!-\!\!\!\text{CHO}$$

Molecular formula: $C_5H_4O_2$

Molecular weight: 96.09

Properties: an oily colourless liquid with a penetrating odour, turning brown on standing. According to Jeffroy and Servaux (1896) the discoloration is a result not of furfural itself but of an impurity, probably methyl furfural.

    boiling point: 162 °C
    melting point: −37 °C
    vapour pressure: 1 mm Hg at 19 °C; 14 mm Hg at 60 °C
    vapour density (air = 1): 3.30
    specific gravity (liquid density): 1.1563
    flash point: 155 °F
    conversion factors: 1 p.p.m. = 3.9 mg/m³
                       1 mg/l = 255 p.p.m.
    solubility: slightly soluble in water (8.3–11%), readily soluble in alcohol (Korenmann and Reznik, 1930), and is present in crude alcohol (Jeffroy and Servaux, 1896).
    maximum allowable concentration: 5 p.p.m. (Threshold Limit Values, 1962).

ECONOMY, SOURCES AND USES

Production

From the pentosans present in straws and bran, by hydrolysis and dehydration with sulphuric acid (Fassett, 1963).

Industrial uses

(1) Especially in the lacquer industry, as a solvent for various types of resins and cellulose derivatives.
(2) In the refining of mineral oil.
(3) In the rubber industry, as a vulcanising accelerator.
(4) As a chemical intermediate.

BIOCHEMISTRY

Estimation

In the atmosphere

The method described by Korenmann and Reznik (1930) depends on the production of a red colour, proportional to the amount of furfural present, caused by the reaction of furfural vapour drawn into distilled water with a mixture of equal parts of pure aniline and 68% acetic acid.

Metabolism

Furfural is unique among aromatic aldehydes in forming a derivative of furyl acrylic acid (Williams, 1959). It is readily metabolised in animals by oxidation to furoic acid (pyromucic acid), and in dogs and rabbits, but not in rats (Paul *et al.*, 1949); three metabolites are excreted: α furoic acid, furoylglycine and furylacryloylglycine (Jaffe and Cohn, 1887).

TOXICOLOGY

Furfural is primarily a central nervous poison, causing cramps and convulsions but by oral administration to animals relatively high doses are required to cause significant symptoms of poisoning. By subcutaneous and intravenous injection it acts as a convulsant and also affects the gastro-intestinal tract. In man, however, Jeffroy and Servaux (1896) have stated that it would require 10 g of furfural in the blood stream to kill a 70 kg man; they noted that a litre of rum or cognac might contain 15–40 mg, but a litre of kirsch only 5 mg and cider only traces. It is an irritant of mucous membranes, including the digestive system, but owing to its relatively low volatility, exposure to its vapour is not likely to involve a serious hazard in this respect. Handling of the liquid does carry a risk of dermatitis, and Korenmann and Reznik, having observed instances where relatively low levels of atmospheric concentration have led to complaints of headache, and irritation of eyes and throat, insist that owing to its increasing use in industry it must be regarded as a potential hazard.

Toxicity to animals

Acute

Lethal dose. – (i) By oral administration, for rats, 50–100 mg/kg (Fassett, 1963). – (ii) By subcutaneous injection, for dogs, 0.214 g/kg to 0.85, increasing with the speed of injection (Jeffroy and Servaux, 1896). These observers noted that with slower injection the amount of urine, faeces and saliva excreted was much greater than when given rapidly, an effect which they suggested was due to elimination of the poison, preventing it from exerting its full toxic effect. For guinea pigs, Lépine (1887) has found about 1 g/kg rapidly fatal; 0.1 g/kg lethal after 24–48 h. – *(iii) By intramuscular injection*, for dogs, all survived 0.33 g/kg; for rabbits, 0.078–0.156 g/kg (Jeffroy and Servaux, 1896). – *(iv) By intraperitoneal injection*, for rats, 20–50 mg/kg (Fassett, 1963). – *(v) By intravenous injection*, for dogs, 0.29 g/kg, (Jeffroy and Servaux, 1896), 0.25 g/kg (Lépine). – *(vi) By inhalation*, for cats 2800 p.p.m. for half an hour caused death from pulmonary oedema (Fassett, 1963), 3000 p.p.m. for one hour caused death after three days (Wand, 1932).

SYMPTOMS OF INTOXICATION

Respiration slow, difficult and deep at first, but with a fatal dose becoming more and more superficial; pulse increased at first but then decreased, but less affected than the respiration. Epileptiform convulsions, more marked with the commercial than the pure product; lowering of the rectal temperature; diarrhoea and haematemesis, followed by bronchopneumonia; muscular incoordination; disappearance first of corneal then of other reflexes; depression leading to coma and finally death. According to McGuignan (1923) respiration is paralysed before the heart stops.

CHANGES IN THE ORGANISM

(1) The liver

According to Gander (1932), following repeated subcutaneous injection of 0.3–0.35 ml of pure furfural, the liver showed in some animals isolated areas of fatty degeneration, occasionally small haemorrhages and necrotic foci.

(2) The central nervous system

After a lethal subcutaneous injection of 0.6 ml, severe degenerative changes were found in the medulla and spinal cord. Less severe but similar changes occurred after repeated injection of 0.2 ml. Single injections of 0.3 ml produced in rabbits no such lesions in the central nervous system.

Toxicity to human beings

Lépine (1887), having administered furfural to human subjects suffering from various convulsive nervous disorders such as paralysis agitans, found it not only completely ineffective in a dosage of 6 g per day, but also a marked irritant of the digestive mucous membrane.

In industrial use, the only record of a possible toxic effect is that of Korenmann and Reznik (1930) who state that workers in a Russian factory where the atmospheric concentration varied from 1.9–13.5 p.p.m. complained of headache and irritation of eyes and throat. No details of the actual process are given.

Bibliography on p. 489

69. Acetal

Synonyms: ethylidene diethyl ether, diethyl acetal, 1,1-diethoxyethane

Structural formula: $CH_2OH-CHOH-CH{\overset{\textstyle OCH_2CH_3}{\underset{\textstyle OCH_2CH_3}{}}}$

Molecular formula: $C_7H_{16}O_4$

Molecular weight: 118.2

Properties: a liquid with a bitter pungent taste and an odour resembling ether.
  boiling point: 107–112 °C
  vapour pressure: 20 mm Hg at 20 °C
  vapour density (air = 1): 4.1
  specific gravity (liquid density): 0.825
  flash point: −5 °F
  conversion factors: 1 p.p.m. = 4.8 mg/m³
              1 mg/l = 207 p.p.m.
  solubility: soluble in water to the extent of 5.5 g/100 ml. Miscible with alcohol in all proportions. Forms a constant boiling mixture (79 °C) with 67% of ethyl alcohol (Durrans, 1944).
  maximum allowable concentration: not established.

ECONOMY, SOURCES AND USES

Production

By condensation of acetaldehyde with alcohol.

Industrial uses

In the paint and varnish industry as a 'latent' solvent for nitrocellulose, mixed with other substances such as alcohols (Durrans, 1935).

BIOCHEMISTRY

Metabolism

According to Knoefel (1934) acetal is probably rapidly hydrolysed in the stomach, giving rise to either a hemiacetal or to acetaldehyde and ethyl alcohol, hence the

[484]

necessity for large doses if it is desired to use it as a narcotic, and the uncertainty of its effect; this allows the presumption that it is destroyed before being absorbed.

TOXICOLOGY

Acetal is a narcotic, more toxic and less efficient than paraldehyde. When given by mouth it causes drowsiness and some analgesia, but no anaesthesia (Von Mering, 1882). It is also a skin irritant (Schwartz, Tulipan and Peck, 1947) but no injuries from its industrial use have been recorded.

Toxicity to animals

Acute
(a) *Lethal dose.* – (i) *By oral administration,* for rats, 4.6 g/kg (Knoefel, 1934). – (ii) *By intraperitoneal injection,* for rats, 0.9 g/kg (Fassett, 1963); 0.8 g/kg (Lehmann and Flury, 1943). – (iii) *By inhalation,* for rats, 4000 p.p.m. killed 2 out of 6 (Fassett, 1963).
(b) *Narcotic dose.* – (i) *By oral administration,* for dogs, 10 g (Von Mering, 1882). – (ii) *By subcutaneous injection,* for rabbits, 2.4 g (von Mering, 1882).

SYMPTOMS OF INTOXICATION

According to von Mering, animals pass from sleep into narcosis with little change in blood pressure and very slight slowing of the heart, indicating that acetal is a central nervous depressant affecting the respiration more strongly than cardiac activity. Death in fatal cases is due to respiratory failure.

Toxicity to human beings

When given by mouth in a dosage of 10–12 g, von Mering observed drowsiness and analgesia, with no after-effects. No industrial injury has been recorded.

Bibliography on p. 489

70. Glyoxal

Structural formula:

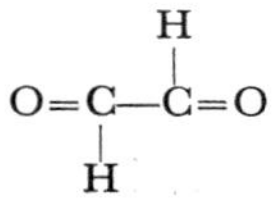

$$O=C-\overset{\displaystyle H}{\underset{\displaystyle H}{C}}=O$$

Molecular formula: $C_2H_2O_2$

Molecular weight: 58.0

Properties: a yellow liquid which tends to polymerise spontaneously.
  boiling point: 51 °C
  melting point: 15 °C
  vapour pressure: 220 mm Hg at 20 °C
  vapour density (air = 1) 2.0
  specific gravity (liquid density): 1.14
  conversion factors: 1 p.p.m. = 2.42 mg/m³
                        1 mg/l = 422 p.p.m.
  solubility: very soluble in water
  maximum allowable concentration: not established.

ECONOMY, SOURCES AND USES

Industrial uses

(1) In the paper industry – for sizing, washable wall paper, treating the glue surface of envelopes (Henson, 1959).
(2) In the textile industry – for preventing shrinking and creasing.
(3) As a substitute for formaldehyde in enbalming fluids.

BIOCHEMISTRY

Metabolism

In vitro glyoxal is oxidised by dilute HNO_3 to glyoxyl acid, and by concentrated HNO_3, to oxalic acid (Pohl, 1896). Doerr (1949) has stated that both diethylene glycol and alloxan pass through glyoxal in their intermediary metabolism, and has suggested that it is glyoxal which is responsible for the toxic effects of diethylene glycol, as it is for the necrosis of the pancreas observed in cats by Pohl (1896).

[486]

TOXICOLOGY

There appears to be some disagreement with regard to the irritant property of glyoxal, at least in human beings, but in animals by oral administration acute poisoning is accompanied by violent vomiting (Pohl, 1896) and application to the skin of guinea pigs has caused severe irritation (Fassett, 1963). Chronic poisoning is followed by injury to the pancreas. No industrial injury from its use has been recorded.

Toxicity to animals

Acute

Lethal dose: – (i) By oral administration, for dogs, it was found impossible by Pohl (1896) to assess quantitatively the lethal dose since glyoxal caused violent vomiting; for rabbits, even when combined with bisulphite (2.5 g), 0.2 g was lethal for a rabbit weighing 1050 g (Pohl, 1896); for rats, (30% in water solution) 2.02 g/kg and for guinea pigs (30% in water solution) 0.76 g/kg (Fassett, 1963). – (ii) By subcutaneous injection, for dogs, 0.2 g for a 7 kg animal (Pohl, 1896). – (iii) By intraperitoneal injection, for rats (30% solution) less than 0.1 g/kg (Fassett, 1963).

SYMPTOMS OF INTOXICATION

(1) Acute

The main effect appears to be of an irritant character – violent vomiting with oral administration (Pohl, 1896) and severe irritation of the skin of guinea pigs following application of a 30% solution (Fassett, 1963). According to Pohl the urine contained oxalic acid the day following oral administration but this disappeared during the two next days.

(2) Chronic

In cats, Doerr (1949) found that repeated administration caused necrosis of the pancreas.

Toxicity to human beings

According to Henson (1959) glyoxal is not an irritant of skin and mucous membranes and does not cause a burn when applied undiluted to the skin, but in the experience of Fassett (1963) its vapour, though less irritant than that of formaldehyde is somewhat irritating to the eyes and nose. No cases of injury from its industrial use have been reported.

Bibliography on p. 489

71. Glycerol Formal

Synonym: Sericosol-N

Properties: a colourless slightly viscous liquid with no appreciable odour. Glycerol formal is a condensation product of glycerol and formaldehyde, and is a mixture of the two materials, 4-hydroxymethyl-1:3 dioxolane and 5-hydroxy-1:3 dioxane, the proportions of the two compounds depending on the temperature reaction.

    boiling point: 194 °C (mixtures: 192.5 °C)
    vapour pressure: 0.22 and 0.25 mm Hg
    specific gravity (liquid density): 1.2113 and 1.2256 at 20 °C
    solubility: miscible with water and chemically stable
    maximum allowable concentration: not established

ECONOMY, SOURCES AND USES

Industrial uses

As a solvent for cellulose acetate (Hannay, 1959).

TOXICOLOGY

The only experiments carried out on the toxicology of glycerol formal are those of Sanderson (1959) in the course of a search for suitable solvents for injection into rats in 'range finding' toxicity tests. No investigations of the effects during industrial exposure have been reported, but these animal tests indicate that glycerol formal is a narcotic, but of low toxicity; it is not irritant to the skin even when 1000 mg/kg is applied undiluted and caused only slight temporary irritation when applied to the eye of a guinea pig. The fact that, according to Hannay, it has been used industrially on the tonscale as a solvent for cellulose acetate without special precautions and with as yet no detected hazards tends to confirm the comparative innocuity shown in the above animal experiments.

Toxicity to animals

(a) Lethal dose. – *(i) By intraperitoneal injection,* for rats, 3000 mg/kg compared with 1500 mg/kg for methyl alcohol. – *(ii) By oral administration,* for rats, greater than 4000 mg/kg (Sanderson, 1959).

    (b) Narcotic dose. – *By oral administration,* 2000 mg/kg (Sanderson, 1959).

Sanderson observed no symptoms at or below 1500 mg/kg; at 2000 mg/kg narcosis supervened, and at 4000 mg/kg weakness persisting until death.

CHANGES IN THE ORGANISM

No macroscopic abnormalities were found in any of the animals; microscopic examinations were apparently not made.

BIBLIOGRAPHY

Asmussen, E., J. Hald and V. Larsen (1948) The pharmacological Action of Acetaldehyde on the human Organism, *Acta Pharmocol.*, 4:311.

Baader, E. W. (1932) Investigation of Health Damages from artificial Resins, *Reichsarbeitsblatt*, 3:173.

Bacq, Z. M. and M. J. Dallemagne (1943) l'Anesthésie au Méthylal; Étude expérimentale, *Arch. Intern. Pharmacodyn.*, 69:127.

Baslini, E. (1924) Impiego della Paraldeide come Combustibile e come Carburante, *Atti Congr. Naz. Chim. Ind. Milan*, p. 240.

Battelli, F. and L. Stern (1910) Production de l'Aldéhyde dans l'Oxidation de l'Alcool par l'Alcoolase des Tissus animaux, *Compt. Rend. Soc. Biol.*, 68:5.

Bau, S. (1929) Über Paraldehydvergiftung, *Deut. Ges. Gerichtl. Med.*, 13:337.

Böhmer, K. (1934) Vergiftung mit Formalin, *Samml. Vergiftungsfall.*, 5:97.

Bourne, H. G. and S. Seferian (1959) Insufficiently polymerised Resins used for wrinkleproofing Clothing may liberate toxic Quantities of Formaldehyde, *Ind. Med. Surg.*, 28:232.

Bricker, C. E. and H. R. Johnson (1945) Spectrophotometric Method for determining Formaldehyde, *Ind. Eng. Chem., Anal. Ed.*, 7:400.

Brunner, L. (1962) Neuerer beruflichbedingte Hauterkrankungen, *Beruf-Dermatosen*, 10:61.

Burstein, C. L. (1943) The Hazard of Paraldehyde Administration, *J. Am. Med. Ass.*, 121:187.

Carroll, S. J. (1933) Use of Paraldehyde as a Plasticiser with Cellulose Acetate, *Chem. Abstr.*, 27:2809.

Cervello, V. (1884) Recherches cliniques et physiologiques sur la Paraldéhyde, *Arch. Ital. Biol.*, 6:113.

Dallemagne, M. J. and Z. M. Bacq (1943) l'Anesthésie en Clinique, *Arch. Intern. Pharmacodyn.*, 69:235.

Doerr, W. (1949) Pathological Anatomy of Glycol Poisoning and Alloxan Diabetes; cited in *Chem. Abstracts*, 1950 44 (III):8456.

Dujardin-Beaumetz (1885–1889) *Dictionnaire de Thérapeutique*, Vol. III, 681. Doin, Paris.

Durrans, T. H. (1935) Review of the technical Aspects of Industrial Solvents, *Chem. Ind.*, 13:585.

Durrans, T. H. (1935) Solvents and Plasticisers, *J. Oil. Col. Ass.*, 18:340.

Durrans, T. H. (1944) *Solvents*, 5th Ed., Chapman and Hall, London.

Elkins, H. B. (1959) *The Chemistry of industrial Toxicology*, Wiley, New York.

Ettinger, J. and M. Jeremias (1955) (cited by Malten and Zielhuis, 1964) A Study of the Health Hazards involved in working with flame-proofed fabrics, *Monthly Rev. Div. Ind. Hyg. N.Y.*, 34:25.

Fairhall, L. T. (1957) *Industrial Toxicology*, Williams and Wilkins, Baltimore.

Fassett, D. W. (1963) *Aldehydes and Acetals*, in F. A. Patty (Ed.), Industrial Hygiene and Toxicology. Vol. II, 2nd. ed., Interscience Publishers, New York, 1963.

Fischer, M. H. (1905) The toxic Effects of Formaldehyde and Formalin, *J. Exptl. Med.*, 6:487.

Frenkel, Y. A. (1936) The question of Formalin Poisoning, *Chem. Zentral.*, 2:1380.

Gage, J. C. (1933) Variations in Susceptibility of Mice to certain Anaesthetics, *Quart. J. Pharmacol.*, 6:418.

Gander, G. (1932) Histologische Befunde an mit Furfural vergifteten Kaninchen, *Arch. Exptl. Pathol. Pharmakol.*, 167:681.

Giel, C. P., J. Jampol and E. Koehler (1956) Health Hazards from flame-proofed Fabrics, *Monthly Rev. Div. Ind. Hyg. N.Y.*, 35:20.

Gilger, A. P., A. M. Potts and L. V. Johnson (1952) Studies on the visual Toxicity of Methanol, *Am. J. Ophthalm.*, 35:113.

Glass, W. I. (1961) Outbreak of Formaldehyde dermatitis, *New Zealand Med. J.*, 60:423.

Goldman, F. H. and Y. Yagoda (1943) Collection and Estimation of Traces of Formaldehyde in Air, *Ind. Eng. Chem. Anal. Ed.*, 15:377.

Guthe, K. F. (1959) The Formaldehyde-haemoglobin Reaction, *J. Biol. Chem.*, 234:3169.

Guthrie, C. C. (1905) Effect of intravenous Injection of Formaldehyde and $CaCl_2$ on haemolytic Power of Serum, *Am. J. Physiol.*, 12:139.

Hald, J. and E. Jacobsen (1948) The Formation of Acetaldehyde after Ingestion of Antabuse and Alcohol, *Acta Pharmacol.*, 4:305.

Hamilton, A. (1934) *Industrial Toxicology*, Harper, New York.

Handovsky, H. (1934) Au Sujet des Propriétés biologiques et pharmacodynamiques de l'Acétaldéhyde, *Compt. Rend. Soc. Biol.*, 117:238.

Handovsky, H. (1936) Au Sujet de l'Effet de L'Acétaldéhyde sur la Rhythmicité et le Tonus des Muscles non volontaires, *Compt. Rend. Soc. Biol.*, 123:1242.

Hannay, R. J. (1959) Personal Observation to and cited by Sanderson (1959).

Henson, E. V. (1959) The Toxicology of some Aliphatic Aldehydes, *J. Occup. Med.*, 1:457.

Hitchcock, P. and F. E. Nelson (1943) The Metabolism of Paraldehyde, *J. Pharmacol. Exptl. Therap.*, 79:286.

Hovding, G. (1961) Contact Eczema due to Formaldehyde in Resin-finished Textiles, *Acta Dermatol. Venereol.*, 41:194.

Iwanoff, N. (1911) On the Toxicity of Aldehydes, *Arch. Hyg.*, 73:307.

Jacobsen, E. (1952) The Metabolism of Ethyl Alcohol, *Pharmacol. Rev.*, 4:107.

Jaffe, M. and R. Cohn (1887) cited by Gander (1932) *Ber. Deut. Chem. Gesellsch.*, 20:2311.

Jeffroy, A. and J. P. Servaux (1896) Mensuration de la Toxicité expérimentale et de la Toxicité vraie du Furfurol, *Arch. Med. Exptl.*, 8:195:473.

Keeser, E. (1931) Ätiologie und therapeutische Beeinflussbarkeit der specifischen toxischen Wirkung des Methylalkohols, *Arch. Exptl. Pathol. Pharmakol.*, 160:687.

Key, M. M. (1961) Some unusual allergic Reactions in Industry, *Arch. Dermatol.*, 83:3.

Kistler, G. A. and A. B. Luckhardt (1929) Pharmacology of some Ethylenehalogen Compounds, *Curr. Res. Anesth.*, 8:65.

Kobert, R. (1906) *Lehrbuch der Intoxikationen*, Enke, Stuttgart.

Korenmann, J. and J. B. Reznik (1930) Furfural als gewerblicher Gift und seiner Bestimmung in der Luft, *Arch. Hyg.*, 104:344.

Kraft-Ebbing, R. von (1897) Arbeiten aus den Gesamtgebiet der Psychiatrie und Neuropathologie, *Barth. Leipzig.*, Hft. 2:186.

Knoefel, P. K. (1934) Narcotic Potency of the aliphatic acyclic Acetals, *J. Pharmacol.*, 50:88.

Knoefel, P. K. (1935) Narcotic Potency of some cyclic Acetals, *J. Pharmacol.*, 53:440.

Kotz, J., G. B. Roth and W. A. Ryon (1938) Idiosyncrasy to Paraldehyde, *J. Am. Med. Ass.*, 110:2145.

Leaf, G. and L. J. Zatman (1952) Study of the Conditions under which Methanol may exert a toxic Hazard in Industry, *Brit. J. Ind. Med.*, 9:19.

Lehmann, K. B. and F. Flury (1943) *Toxicology and Hygiene of Industrial Solvents*, Williams and Wilkins, Baltimore.

Lépine, C. (1887) Sur l'Action du Furfurol, *Compt. Rend. Soc. Biol.*, p. 437.

Levine, H., A. J. Gilbert and M. Bodansky (1939) The Effect of Liver Damage on the Blood Level and Action of Paraldehyde, *J. Pharmacol. Exptl. Therap.*, 67:299.

Levine, H., A. J. Gilbert and M. Bodansky (1940) The pulmonary and urinary Excretion of Paraldehyde in normal Dogs and in Dogs with Liver Damage, *J. Pharmacol. Exptl. Therap.*, 69:316.

Lewin, L. (1929) *Gifte und Vergiftungen*, Springer, Berlin.
Malten, K. E. (1958) Occupational Eczema due to *p-tert.*-Butyl Phenol in a Shoe Adhesive, *Dermatologica*, 117:103.
Malten, K. E. (1962) Dermatological Aspects of Plastics., *Proc. XIIth Intern. Congr. Dermatology*, Washington.
Malten, K. E. (1963) *Textile Finish contact Hypersensitivity*; cited in Malten and Zielhuis (1964).
Malten, K. E. and R. L. Zielhuis (1964) *Industrial Toxicology and Dermatology in the Production and Processing of Plastics*, Elsevier, Amsterdam.
Markuson, K. E., T. F. Mancuso and J. S. Soet (1943) Dermatitis due to Formaldehyde Resins, *Ind. Med. Surg.*, 12:383.
McDonald Jr., W. F. (1954) Formaldehyde in Air – a specific Field Test, *Am. Ind. Hyg. Ass. Quart.*, 15:217.
McDougall, J. (1932) Fatal Case of Paraldehyde Poisoning with *post-mortem* Findings, *J. Ment. Sci.*, 78:374.
McGuignan, H. (1914) Formaldehyde, *J. Am. Med. Ass.*, 62:984.
McGuignan, A. (1923) The Action of Furfural, *J. Pharmacol. Exptl. Therap.*, 21:65.
McKenna, W. B., J. F. F. Smith and D. A. McLean (1958) Dermatoses in the Manufacture of Glass Fibre, *Brit. J. Ind. Med.*, 15:47.
Mering von (1882) Über die hypnotisierende und anästhesierende Wirkung des Acetals, *Klin. Wochschr.*, 19:648.
Meyer, H. A. (1893) On some pharmacological Reactions of the Avian and Reptilian Iris, *Arch. Exptl. Pathol. Pharmakol.*, 32:117.
Meyer, K. H. and H. Gottlieb-Billroth (1921) Théorie der Narkose durch Inhalations-Anästhetika, *Münch. Med. Wochschr.*, 68:8.
Meyer, K. H. and H. Hemmi (1935) Beitrag zur Theorie der Narkose, *Biochem. Zschr.*, 277:52.
Nitzescu, I. I. (1932) Anesthésie générale par Injection intraveineuse de Paraldéhyde et d'Alcool éthylique, *Compt. Rend. Soc. Biol.*, 111:337.
Nitzescu, I. I., I. D. Georgescu and D. Timus (1936) Le Dosage de la Paraldéhyde dans l'Air respiratoire chez les Animaux anesthésiés avec la Paraldéhyde, *Compt. Rend. Soc. Biol.*, 121:1660.
Nitzescu, I. I., I. D. Georgescu and D. Timus (1936) Le Dosage de la Paraldéhyde fixée dans les Tissues et les Humeurs après Injection intraveineuse de cette Substance, *Compt. Rend. Soc. Biol.*, 121:1657.
Parker, A. L. (1949) Determination of Formaldehyde in Air. Bisulphite Method, *Am. Conf. Govt. Ind. Hyg.*
Pattle, R. E. and H. Cullumbine (1956) Toxicity of some atmospheric Pollutants, *Brit. Med. J.*, 2:913.
Paul, H. E., F. L. Austin, M. F. Paul and V. R. Ells (1949) Metabolism of Nitrofurans, *J. Biol. Chem.*, 180:345.
Pohl, J. (1896) Über den oxydativen Abbau der Fettkörper im thierischen Organismus, *Arch. Exptl. Pathol. Pharmakol.*, 37:413.
Quoss, H. (1959) *Gesundheitsgefahren in der Kunststoffindustrie*, Barth, Leipzig.
Romano, C. (1955) Death due to Acetaldehyde Poisoning of metabolic Origin during acute Alcoholism, *Riforma Med.*, 69:211.
Sanderson, D. M. (1959) A note on Glycerol Formal as a Solvent in Toxicity Testing, *J. Pharm. Pharmacol.*, 11:150.
Scheidegger, S. (1936) Akute Formalinvergiftung (Selbstmord), *Samml. Vergiftungsfall.*, 7:153.
Schneider, P. (1929) *Einiges über Paraldehydevergiftung*, Wien. Klin. Wochschr., 42:357.
Schwartz, L. (1941) Dermatitis from new synthetic Resin Fabric Finishes, *J. Invest Dermatol.*, 4:459.
Schwartz, L., L. Tulipan and S. M. Peck (1947) *Occupational Diseases of the Skin*, Kimpton, London.
Shoor, M. (1941) Paraldehyde Poisoning; Report of a Fatality, *J. Am. Med. Ass.*, 117:1534.
Silverman, L., H. F. Schulte and W. W. First (1946) Further Studies on sensory Response to certain industrial Solvent Vapours, *J. Ind. Hyg. Toxicol.*, 28:262.
Simon, F. (1914) On the Behaviour of Formaldehyde Sulphite in the Organism, *Biochem. Zschr.*, 65:71.
Skog, E. (1950) A toxicological Investigation of lower aliphatic Aldehydes, *Acta Pharmacol.*, 6:299.

Skog, E. (1952) Anaesthetic and hemolytic Action of lower aliphatic Aldehydes and their Effect on Respiration and Blood Pressure, *Acta Pharmacol.*, 8:275.

Smitt, N. K. (1922) A rapid Method for the Estimation of Acetaldehyde (cited by Fairhall, 1957), *Bull. Bur. Biotechnicol.*, 5:117.

Smyth, H. F. Jr., C. P. Carpenter and C. S. Weil (1949) Range Finding Toxicity Data, List III, *J. Ind. Hyg. Toxicol.*, 31:60.

Spector, W. (1956) *Handbook of Toxicology*, Vol. I, Saunders, Philadelphia.

Stewart, J. D. (1932) Rectal Paraldehyde before Operation, *Brit. Med. J.*, 2:1139.

Stotz, E. (1943) A colorimetric Determination of Acetaldehyde in Blood, *J. Biol. Chem.*, 148:585.

Stotz, E., W. W. Westerfield and R. L. Berg (1944) The Metabolism of Acetaldehyde with Acetoin Formation, *J. Biol. Chem.*, 152:41.

Strahan, S. A. K. (1885) Paraldehyde Administration, *Lancet*, 2:243.

Threshold Limit Values for 1962, *Am. Ind. Hyg. Ass. J.*, 1963, 23:419.

U.S. Publ. Hlth. Serv., Formaldehyde; its Toxicity and potential Dangers, *P. H. Rep.* (1945) *No. 181 Suppl.*

Wand, H. (1932) Cited by K. N. Lehmann and F. Flury (1943), in *Tocicology and Hygiene of Industrial Solvents*, Williams and Wilkins, Baltimore.

Weaver, F. L., A. R. Hough, B. Highman and L. T. Fairhall (1951) The Toxicity of Methylal, *Brit. J. Ind. Med.*, 8:279.

Weger, A. (1927) Thalamic Symptom Complex in Formaldehyde Poisoning, *Zschr. Ges. Neurol.*, 111:370.

Williams, R. T. (1959) *Detoxication Mechanisms*, Chapman and Hall, London.

Wyse, V. (1950) Pathological Symptoms caused by Formaldehyde, *Rass. Med. Ind.*, 19:200 (*Ind. Hyg. Digest*, 1951; 994).

Yarsley, V. E. (1934) Solvents and Plasticisers, *Synth. Appl. Finish.*, 5:37, 57.

Yonkman, F. F., A. J. Lehman, C. C. Pfeiffer and H. F. Chase (1941) A Study of the possible toxic Effects of prolonged Formaldehyde Ingestion, *J. Pharmacol. Exptl. Therap.*, 72:46.

Chapter 10

ETHERS

72. Diethyl Ether

Synonyms: ethyl ether, sulphuric ether, diethyl oxide

Structural formula: $CH_3-CH_2-O-CH_2-CH_3$

Molecular formula: $C_4H_{10}O$

Molecular weight: 74.12

Properties: a transparent volatile liquid, extremely flammable, with a characteristic odour. It forms explosive peroxides on standing in air, especially in sunlight. These may be removed by shaking with a 5% aqueous solution of ferrous sulphate (Green and Schietzow, 1933). Other impurities likely to occur are acetaldehyde, ethyl sulphide and ethyl mercaptan, and ketones. Bourne (1926) showed that in dogs acetaldehyde in a concentration of more than 1% in an admixture with pure ether, and ether peroxide in concentrations of more than 0.5%, caused respiratory embarrassment and fall in blood pressure, and that ethyl sulphide caused also gastro-enteritis. In presence of an open flame or metal catalysts ether may decompose with the formation of formaldehyde, but according to Kärber (1930) this is not likely to occur in any but small unventilated rooms.

   boiling point: 34.6 °C

   melting point: −116.3 °C (stable crystals)

   vapour pressure: 438.9 mm Hg at 20 °C

   vapour density (air = 1): 2.55

   specific gravity (liquid density): 0.7146

   flash point: −40 °F

   conversion factors: 1 p.p.m. = 3.03 mg/m³

                1 mg/l   = 330 p.p.m.

   solubility: in water 8.43% at 15 °C; miscible with benzene, chloroform, petroleum, some alcohols, fat solvents and oils.

   maximum allowable concentration: 400 p.p.m.

ECONOMY, SOURCES AND USES

Production

By the dehydration of ethanol or the hydration of ethylene in the presence of sulphuric acid.

Industrial uses

(1) As a solvent for waxes, fats, oils, gums, resins and alkaloids.
(2) As a cleaning and spotting agent, especially in the shoe industry (Elkins, 1959).
(3) In the textile industry as a solvent in the manufacture of cellulose acetate rayon and of dyes.
(4) In the perfume industry.
(5) In the plastics industry, mixed with ethanol.
(6) In the manufacture of photographic films.
(7) In the rubber industry (Fairhall, 1957).
(8) As a surgical anaesthetic.

BIOCHEMISTRY

Estimation

(1) In the atmosphere
   (a) By absorption in a solution of potassium dichromate in sulphuric acid, followed by iodometric titration (Silverman, 1947).
   (b) By adsorption on activated charcoal or silica gel.

(2) In blood
   (a) By infra-red analysis. – This method, originally devised by Stewart *et al.* (1959) was used, with a slight modification, by Chenoweth *et al.* (1962) for determining the ether content of arterial and venous blood. The sample of blood is added to carbon disulphide and centrifuged. The separated solvent, after refrigeration, is scanned in a special microcell on an infra-red spectrometer.
   (b) The iodine pentoxide method. – For both air and blood (Haggard, 1924), in which ether vapour is drawn through iodine pentoxide and the liberated iodine titrated with thiosulphate with starch as an indicator. Haggard stated that his method has a maximum accuracy of ±0.04 mg of ether in 1 ml of blood.

Metabolism

Absorption by inhalation is rapid, with equally rapid passage from the blood stream to the brain, due primarily to the rich blood supply of the brain. About 87% of an absorbed dose is expired unchanged (Haggard, 1924) and 1 to 2% excreted in the urine, so that it is unlikely that it is metabolised or utilised in the body to any extent (Williams, 1959). In dogs however, and in human beings suffering from certain metabolic diseases, such as cirrhosis, it has been shown (Bunker, 1962) that metabolic acidosis, with impaired lactic acid utilisation and a rise in serum lactate may occur; this, according to Bunker, presumably reflects release of epinephrine which occurs in the dog but not in the normally healthy human being.

The ratio of alveolar concentration to that of the blood has been variously estimated as 1/10, 1/14 and 1/15. Robbins (1935) states that very rarely does the ether in the blood reach equilibrium with that of the inspired air, and that when this does occur the ratio is 1/15, the lag being due, as shown by Haggard (1924) to the great capacity of blood to take up ether.

In animals, ether also passes rapidly into fatty tissue, reaching a maximum in omental fat after 30 min, at a higher level than in the blood at this time. Dybing and Skovlund (1957) found that the ether level of the blood of a rat weighing 345 g exposed to 100,000 p.p.m. (300 mg/l) was 0.98 mg/g compared with 3.42 for omental fat and 1.28 for perirenal fat. Elimination from fatty tissue begins only when the concentration in the blood has become relatively low, and practically ceases at the end of 8 h. In rabbits, subcutaneous fat takes up ether only a little more slowly than abdominal fat. Chenoweth et al. (1962) also found high levels of ether in the fatty depots of the dog after $2\frac{1}{2}$ h of anaesthesia, and an unexplainable high concentration in the adrenals during anaesthesia.

TOXICOLOGY

As shown by its widespread use as a surgical anaesthetic, the primary action of ether is exerted on the central nervous system, the body during anaesthesia containing a much lower concentration than the brain. It is considered a safer anaesthetic than chloroform, but if the rise in the concentration in the central nervous system is too high and too sudden it may cause respiratory arrest and if this occurs after the body has absorbed a considerable amount, spontaneous re-establishment is not easily achieved.

It is not a severe skin irritant, though cracking and dryness may result from prolonged contact, and there have been a few cases of a slight rash in workers in a smokeless powder factory (Hamilton and Minot, 1920).

Whether it can cause nephritis is doubtful, though there have been cases of albuminuria and one regarded definitely as nephritis due to prolonged inhalation (Hamilton, 1925). No kidney injury has been observed in animals.

Toxicity to animals

Acute

(a) Lethal dose. – By inhalation lethal concentrations have differed greatly in the hands of various investigators, partly due to differences in the induction mixtures used, the duration of exposure and the species of animals (Robbins, 1935). Robbins himself gave the lethal concentration for dogs as 670,000 to

800,000 p.p.m., but a more recent value for mice is that of Mörch (1956) – 180,000 p.p.m. – with rapid induction and shorter duration. For a continuous 3 h exposure for mice Molitor (1936) give the LD_{50} as 420,000 p.p.m. Molitor found in mice, but not in rats, a high percentage of delayed deaths for which no pathological cause could be ascertained.

(b) *Narcotic dose.* – A similar discrepancy exists in the narcotic dose given by various authorities. Knoefel *et al.* (1935) for example giving a much lower figure (4.7 vol% for 10 min) as compared with 14 vol% by Mörch *et al.* (1956). The lower figure, according to Mörch *et al.*, may be due to the fact that the absence in Knoefel's experiment of an effective device for mixing air and anaesthetic in the bell jar may have caused the calculated concentration to be lower than the actual.

SYMPTOMS OF INTOXICATION

After preliminary irritation narcosis sets in rapidly, and with lethal concentrations death is due to respiratory paralysis. Acidosis during the phase of anaesthesia and a compensatory tendency to alkalosis during recovery has been stated to occur (Chabanier *et al.*, 1932).

CHANGES IN THE ORGANISM

The only lesions reported are those of Sand (1910) – haemorrhage and emphysema of the lungs, congestion of all organs and fatty degeneration of the liver and kidneys in dogs kept for some weeks in a chamber in which 500 g of a mixture of alcohol and ether had been evaporated. Sand himself stated that it could not be definitely concluded whether these effects were due to ether or alcohol.

Toxicity to human beings

The anaesthetic effect of ether, causing complete unconsciousness, has generally been recorded from its use as a surgical anaesthetic, and in such cases there is usually no serious or lasting ill-effect. Acute toxic effects from its industrial use are very rare and fatalities practically unknown. One case was described by Hayhurst (1930) – a man who was employed in the manufacture of perfumery where ether was used as an extraction agent, and who developed acute mania and uraemic convulsions. The most frequent manifestation of less severe acute industrial poisoning has occurred in workers in the smokeless powder industry during the first World War, in the form of 'ether jag', a condition observed more often in women than in men, and consisting of hysterical singing and weeping, nausea, dizziness, mental confusion and sometimes unconsciousness. Men who had these attacks in the early days of their employment apparently developed tolerance later (Hamilton and Minot, 1920). Similar effects were noted by the Home Office in Great Britain in 1922 in workers using ether as an extractive in conditions of poor ventilation. They complained also of after-effects of the acute attacks – nausea, headache, irritability, mental confusion, lack of appetite, vomiting and excessive perspiration.

Chronic effects

In the explosives industry Hamilton and Minot (1920) observed many cases of apathy, drowsiness, depression, loss of appetite and weight, constipation, and in a few cases albuminuria. In women, gastro-intestinal disturbance was also shown by a variation in appetite from a complete distaste for food to a ravenous desire for it, constipation, nausea and actual vomiting, while the narcotic effect was manifested by extreme drowsiness and disturbed sleep.

SYMPTOMS OF INTOXICATION

(1) The skin

Some of the women observed by Hamilton and Minot showed an itching rash on the side of the face nearest to the cutting machine, and in the case of the man suffering from chronic nephritis (Hamilton, 1925) who also had pemphigus, it was stated that this was closely related to the nephritis stated to be due to this exposure to ether. In cases of 'ether habit' from drinking and from long-continued inhalation, redness of the skin is a frequent manifestation, but is believed to be due to cardiac irregularity and dilatation of blood vessels (Flury and Zernik, 1931).

(2) The blood

The chief abnormality observed by Hamilton and Minot (1920) among the women was polycythaemia, with counts in some cases up to or over 6 millions; others showed slight anaemia; of the men the latter condition was more marked than polycythaemia, only 2 showing counts over 6 millions.

CHANGES IN THE ORGANISM

The kidneys

Nephritis has not been a frequent manifestation, but Hamilton (1916), citing the results of an investigation by the U.S. Bureau of Labor Statistics, stated that 'it may occur'. It was revealed that one man had symptoms of nephritis, another had albuminuria and swelling of the eyelids, while among the women 3 out of 55 had slight albuminuria, 2 without accompanying symptoms.

The most definite case of nephritis is that described by Hamilton (1925), a man who had worked continuously for 7 years and intermittently for 5 years in a smokeless powder factory; he developed severe chronic interstitial nephritis, and though death was finally due to pulmonary oedema and pemphigus, the medical examiners were of the opinion that the true cause of death was chronic nephritis caused by long exposure to ether.

Bibliography on p. 519

Ether addiction

Ether addiction, though not common, should be mentioned as a not too remote possibility in industries where access to ether, either liquid or vapour, is not impossible. In earlier times both drinking and 'sniffing' ether were not uncommon and had the result of either acute intoxication or, following prolonged abuse, a psychosis similar to that of chronic alcoholism. It has been shown that addiction by sniffing is more specific than by drinking, in that in the former case there is usually no additional addiction to drugs or alcohol. Bartholomew (1962) described a case of this kind in a man who was described as a psychopathic personality, not certifiable, who sniffed ether from a pad soaked in it to the point of unconsciousness. In another case, also described by Bartholomew the addiction was to drinking ether. This man was a laboratory assistant who had access to ether and who had heard that it was as good as, or even better than alcohol for producing intoxication and who also developed psychotic symptoms.

73. Divinyl Ether

Synonyms: vinyl ether, divinyl oxide, ethenyloxyethene, vinethene.

Structural formula: $CH_2=CH—O—CH=CH_2$

Molecular formula: C_4H_6O

Molecular weight: 70.09

Properties: a colourless, volatile, flammable liquid, as flammable as ethyl ether, with a disagreeable odour (Ruigh and Major, 1931).

Polymerises readily to a solid, transparent mass in the absence of an inhibitor such as 0.01% of phenyl-α-naphthylamine (Molitor, 1936). Decomposes on exposure to light, air or acid fumes, with the formation of formaldehyde, formic acid and peroxide (Hake and Rowe, 1963).

   boiling point: 28.3 °C

   vapour pressure: 430 mm Hg at 20 °C

   vapour density (air = 1): 2.4

   specific gravity (liquid density): 0.774

   flash point: > −22 °F

   conversion factors: 1 p.p.m. = 2.86 mg/m³

              1 mg/l = > 349 p.p.m.

   solubility: only slightly soluble in water (0.4% as compared with 6.9% for ethyl ether at 20 °C; Molitor, 1936).

ECONOMY, SOURCES AND USES

Production

By the action of caustic on dichloroethyl ether in the presence of ammonia (Ruigh and Major, 1931).

Industrial uses

Almost exclusively confined to preparation for its use as an anaesthetic.

BIOCHEMISTRY

Metabolism

Divinyl ether is not metabolised in the body, and, like ethyl ether is mainly eliminated in the expired air (Williams, 1959).

Bibliography on p. 519   [499]

TOXICOLOGY

Most of the information regarding the toxic properties of divinyl ether have been based on its use as an anaesthetic since it was first recommended for this purpose by Leake and Chen in 1930. In this respect it is less potent than ethyl ether (8 vols % being required to produce surgical anaesthesia as compared with 6 vols % for ethyl ether), but it is more potent in producing respiratory arrest, and therefore more hazardous as an anaesthetic, though recovery is more rapid than with ethyl ether (Mörch *et al.*, 1958).

Toxicity to animals

Acute

(a) *Lethal dose.* – 12 vols % (Mörch *et al.*, 1958) for mice; 0.24 mg/l (von Brandis, 1935).

(b) *Narcotic dose.* – There is some discrepancy between the results of Mörch *et al.* (1958) (6 vols % for mice) and those of Knoefel *et al.* (1931) (3.0–3.9 vols % in 10 min). Mörch *et al.* suggest that this descrepancy may be due to the fact that in the experiments of Knoefel *et al.* the heavy anaesthetic vapour was allowed to collect at the bottom of the bell jar.

SYMPTOMS OF INTOXICATION

Staggering, twitching, irregular respiration, followed by little or no movement with regular respiration, then slow gasping diaphragmatic respiration and finally death from respiratory arrest. Occasional delayed deaths occurred in mice even from non-anaesthetic concentrations, but not in rats or other species (Molitor, 1936).

CHANGES IN THE ORGANISM

A potential toxic effect on the liver is suggested by the experiments of Cavalieri *et al.* (1958) in dogs receiving a low dosage of divinyl ether; these animals showed a sharp increase and a qualitative alteration of bile products. This effect, possibly similar to that of chloroform, was not however observed by von Brandis (1935) in mice; he noted only a slight increase of fat in the liver and heart such as frequently occurs in normal mice. Liver lesions have been found in dogs where anoxaemia was likely to occur (Bourne and Raginsky, 1935), who remarked that when cyanosis is a feature of the anaesthesia moderate impairment of liver function occurs, but is due to the associated anoxaemia rather than to a direct action of the divinyl ether.

The acid-base balance does not appear to be caused in dogs as in the case of ethyl ether (Knoefel *et al.*, 1931).

Toxicity to human beings

The disadvantage of divinyl ether compared with ethyl ether as an anaesthetic have already been mentioned – a higher potentiality for respiratory arrest.

Apart from these effects of which none have been reported from industrial contact, the potential hazard of fire and explosion must be taken into account.

Bibliography on p. 519

74. Isopropyl Ether

Synonyms: diisopropyl ether, 2-isopropoxypropane

Structural formula:
$$\text{CH}_3\text{—CH—O—CH—CH}_3$$
with CH_3 groups

Molecular formula: $C_6H_{14}O$

Molecular weight: 102.17

Properties: a colourless flammable liquid with an odour resembling that of a mixture of camphor and ethyl ether. It forms explosive oxides on standing in air; this can be inhibited by the addition of oxidation inhibitors (α- and β-naphthol, hydroquinone, 0.5%) or even water, 1%.

The commercial variety may contain approximately 3% of isopropyl alcohol, less than 0.01% of sulphur and less than 0.04% of peroxide.

It is an excellent solvent for oils, fats, waxes and ethyl cellulose.

boiling point: 68.3 °C

melting point: −60 °C

vapour pressure: 119 mm Hg at 20 °C (Durrans, 1950)

vapour density (air = 1): 3.5

specific gravity (liquid density): 0.7258

flash point: 15 °F

conversion factors: 1 p.p.m. = 4.18 mg/m³
                 1 mg/l   = 240 p.p.m.

solubility: soluble in water 0.2–0.9% at 20 °C. miscible with alcohol, ether and most organic solvents and with acetic acid.

maximum allowable concentration: according to Hake and Rowe (1963) established by the A.C.G.H.I. (1960) 500 p.p.m., but not included in the list of Threshold Limit Values for 1962.

ECONOMY, SOURCES AND USES

Production

(1) By action of sulphuric acid on isopropyl alcohol.

(2) As a by-product of the production of isopropyl alcohol from cracked gasoline.

Industrial uses

(1) For extraction purposes *e.g.* nicotine from tobacco.

(2) In the manufacture of pharmaceuticals.

(3) In the paint and varnish industry as a remover.

(4) In the rubber industry.

(5) In the manufacture of smokeless powder.

(6) As a fuel in internal combustion engines.

(7) As an intermediate in alkylation reactions (Hake and Rowe, 1963).

BIOCHEMISTRY

Estimation

In the atmosphere

(1) High combustion method. – Machle *et al.* (1939) describe a method in which samples are subjected to combustion in a specially constructed furnace which avoids incomplete combustion with tarry residues; this is followed by estimation with a Zeiss Interferometer.

(2) Oxidation with standard bichromate, as for diethyl ether (Association of Official Agricultural Chemists, 1935).

Metabolism

No specific investigations have been carried out, but it appears probable that like ethyl ether it is chiefly eliminated by the lungs without any metabolic change in the body. Its elimination is however relatively slow (Jackson, 1933).

TOXICOLOGY

Isopropyl ether is primarily an anaesthetic, considered, on the basis of animal experiments, to be $1\frac{1}{2}$ to 2 times as toxic as ethyl ether. It has not been considered to be suitable for surgical anaesthesia on account of its pronounced depressant action, its unpleasant odour, and the narrow margin between anaesthetic and dangerous concentrations which are followed by a rapid fall in blood pressure and respiratory arrest. Animal experiments have shown however that animals dying from lethal concentrations show few lesions of internal organs other than general visceral and cerebral congestion, but those surviving for some weeks after exposure have shown severe toxic changes in the liver. Its vapour is not highly irritant to the skin, though repeated application to the skin of animals has produced some evidence of dermatitis. It is not absorbed by the skin in amounts sufficient to cause intoxication.

In high concentrations it is somewhat irritating to the eyes, nose and respiratory tract. No cases of injury from its industrial use have been recorded, but Jackson

Bibliography on p. 519

(1933) draws attention to the possibility that workmen using lacquers and varnishes prepared from it might readily be overcome if confined in small rooms or closed spaces.

Toxicity to animals

(1) Acute

Lethal dose. – (i) By oral administration, for rabbits, 5–6.5 mg/kg (Machle et al., 1939). – (ii) By inhalation, for monkeys, rabbits and guinea pigs, 6 vols % in air.

(2) Chronic

Repeated exposures (10 in number) to 3 vols % were not lethal, but the animals, especially monkeys, showed some signs of narcosis, and at 1% daily for 20 days some signs of intoxication and depression, but with shorter exposures (2 h daily) to 0.3%, and for 3 h daily to 0.1% there was no detectable ill-effect.

SYMPTOMS OF INTOXICATION

With a minimum oral lethal dose rapid intense anaesthesia was followed by death from respiratory failure (Machle et al., 1939). According to Jackson (1933) exposure to dangerous concentrations is followed by a rapid fall in blood pressure and respiratory depression, and the fact that it produces a lighter anaesthesia than ethyl ether leads to some spasticity, tremors, slight convulsive movements and some disturbance of respiration. Salivation is present for some time after recovery from the anaesthesia.

CHANGES IN THE ORGANISM

Animals dying from lethal concentrations showed, according to Machle et al. (1939) only general visceral and cerebral congestion.

The liver in animals surviving for some weeks after exposure to 3 vols % showed severe toxic changes.

The blood picture was that of lowered red cell and haemoglobin levels.

Toxicity to human beings

Attempts to introduce isopropyl ether as a surgical anaesthetic have proved impracticable owing partly to its unpleasant odour and partly to its depressant effect, with a narrow margin of safety. Jackson (1933) noted that in addition to its unpleasant odour it is apparently excreted by the saliva, so that the odour is noticeable 12 to 24 h after inhaling a small amount.

Amiot (1932) assaying its possible advantages over ethyl ether as an anaesthetic, found that induction was rapid (6–7 min) with no disturbance of respiration, no vaso-dilatation and no rise of blood pressure, and that in rabbits it caused none of the toxic lesions characteristic of chloroform and no micro-haemorrhagic lesions similar to those caused by ethyl ether.

In the observations of Silverman *et al.* (1946) on human subjects exposure to 300 p.p.m. was found to be unpleasant, but at this level and at 500 p.p.m. not irritating. At 800 p.p.m. for 5 min it was irritating to the eyes and nose and caused some respiratory discomfort.

No cases of injury from its industrial use have been recorded, but Jackson (1933) has issued a warning that workmen using lacquers and varnishes prepared from it might possibly be overcome if confined to small rooms or confined spaces.

Bibliography on p. 519

75. n-Butyl Ether

Synonyms: n-dibutyl ether, 1-butoxybutane

Structural formula: $CH_3-CH_2-CH_2-CH_2-O-CH_2-CH_2-CH_2-CH_3$

Molecular formula: $C_8H_{18}O$

Molecular weight: 130.22

Properties: a colourless liquid with a mild odour. Solvent for fats, oils, ester gum, resins, rubber and hydrocarbons, but not for cellulose esters or benzyl cellulose (Durrans, 1950). Tends to form explosive peroxides.

> *boiling point:* 142.4 °C
> *melting point:* −95.2 °C
> *vapour pressure:* 4.8 mm Hg at 20 °C
> *vapour density (air = 1)* 4.48
> *specific gravity (liquid density):* 0.7704 (Vogel, 1948)
> *flash point:* 100 °F
> *conversion factors:* 1 p.p.m. = 5.33 mg/m³
>   1 mg/l = 188 p.p.m.
> *solubility:* soluble in water to the extent of 0.3–0.5% at 20 °C. Miscible with benzene, alcohol, acetone and most organic solvents.
> *maximum allowable concentration:* not established; 100 p.p.m. has been suggested by Silverman *et al.* (1946) on the basis of sensory response.

ECONOMY, SOURCES AND USES

Production

(1) From dibutyl alcohol and concentrated H_2SO_4, excess of alcohol being removed by repeated washing with water or 50% H_2SO_4 (Vogel, 1948).

(2) As a by-product in the manufacture of butyl esters (Hake and Rowe, 1963).

Industrial uses

(1) As an extracting agent.

(2) As a solvent for ester gums, resins, rubber, alkaloids and hydrocarbons.

BIOCHEMISTRY

Estimation

In the atmosphere (Hake and Rowe, 1963)
(1) By absorption on silica gel.
(2) By gas chromatography of the eluate with ethanol.
(3) By infra red analysis.

Metabolism

No metabolic studies have been undertaken.

TOXICOLOGY

From the results of animal studies butyl ether is considered more toxic by inhalation, but less toxic by oral administration than isopropyl ether. It is also more irritating to the skin, but not severely irritating to the eyes of animals; in human beings it is more irritating to mucous membranes than isopropyl ether, but no reports of any serious injury have been recorded.

Toxicity to animals

In the range-finding toxicity tests carried out by Smyth *et al.* (1954) no report on the symptoms of intoxication or of lesions of internal organs are given.

   Lethal dose. – (i) By oral administration, for rats (LD_{50}), 7.40 g/kg compared with 5 to 6.5 for isopropyl ether. – *(ii) By inhalation* (LD_{50}), 4000 p.p.m. (compared with 6 vols % for isopropyl ether.

SYMPTOMS OF INTOXICATION

(1) Skin irritation – By rabbits, undiluted application as Grade 4 – moderately severe but no necrosis (Smyth and Carpenter, 1946).
(2) Corneal injury – Very slight; only capillary injury from application of the undiluted compound.

Toxicity to human beings

The only report of its effects on human beings is that of Silverman *et al.* (1946), based on the sensory response to its vapour. They found 200 p.p.m. irritating to the eyes and nose, though the odour was not objectional even at 300 p.p.m. They suggested 100 p.p.m. as the maximum level for an eight hour daily exposure.

Bibliography on p. 519

76. Ethylene Oxide

Synonyms: 1,2-epoxyethane, dimethylene oxide, oxirane

Structural formula: $\begin{matrix} CH_2 \\ | \\ CH_2 \end{matrix} \diagdown_{\displaystyle O}$

Molecular formula: C_2H_4O

Molecular weight: 44.05

Properties: at room temperature ethylene is a gas; below its boiling point a colourless hygroscopic liquid with a characteristic sweetish ether-like odour. It is flammable and forms an explosive mixture with air; soluble in water and most solvents. It tends to undergo slow spontaneous polymerisation which can be inhibited by keeping at 10 °C in cold-isolated containers under nitrogen pressure with exclusion of air (Thiess, 1963). Polymerisation is specially likely to occur with catalysts, some chemicals (including monoethanolamine and acrylonitrile (Curme and Johnston, 1952) and copper and copper alloys (Hine and Rowe, 1963).

  boiling point: 10.5 °C
  vapour pressure: 1.49 mm Hg at 40 °C
  specific gravity (liquid density): 0.8711 at 20 °C
  flash point: −4 °F
  conversion factors: 1 p.p.m. = 1.80 mg/m³
        1 mg/l = 556 p.p.m.
  solubility: soluble in water and most solvents
  maximum allowable concentration: 50 p.p.m.

ECONOMY, SOURCES AND USES

Production

By synthesis from ethylene, either through the intermediate ethylene chlorohydrin or by direct oxidation with oxygen or air.

Industrial uses

(1) Chiefly in the manufacture of ethylene glycol and its derivatives, and of other chemicals.
(2) As a solvent and plasticiser in combination with other chemicals.
(3) In the production of high-energy fuels (Johnstone and Miller, 1960).

(4) As a fumigant, to a limited extent, mixed with CO_2.

(5) As a sterilising agent for surgical instruments and thermolabile materials (Thiess, 1963).

BIOCHEMISTRY

Estimation

In the atmosphere

Hine and Rowe (1953) state that most methods of estimation of ethylene oxide in air are not entirely precise or reliable; they describe in detail a colorimetric method with which Gage (1953) has reported success. This method is based on removal of ethylene oxide from the air sample by scrubbing with silica gel, removal of the oxide from the gel by water, oxidation with periodic acid, and reaction with sodium arsenite and acetylacetone.

Metabolism

Elimination by the lungs is not a major route, owing to its high chemical reactivity (Hake and Rowe, 1963). It has been suggested but not generally confirmed, that it is absorbed into the cell, where it undergoes hydrolysis to ethylene glycol, thus causing cellular dysfunction.

TOXICOLOGY

Ethylene oxide has anaesthetic properties similar to those of ether and chloroform but with undesirable side effects. It is a respiratory and severe skin irritant (Royce and Moore, 1955), and, being a protoplasmic poison, can cause systemic effects (Hess and Tilton, 1950). Prolonged slight exposure leads to increasing intolerance, so that symptoms appear after several minor intoxications, with nausea, uncontrollable vomiting, mental dulness, somnolence, inco-ordination and cyanosis (von Oettingen, 1949), and slight blood changes, mostly lymphocytosis (Sexton and Henson, 1949).

Toxicity to animals

(1) Acute

Lethal dose. – *(i) By oral administration*, LD_{50}, for rats, as a 1% aqueous solution, 0.33 g/kg (Smyth *et al.*, 1941); for guinea pigs, 0.27 g/kg; for rats, in cold olive oil 10% solution, 0.2 g/kg (Hollingsworth *et al.*, 1956). – *(ii) By inhalation*, for guinea pigs, 50,000–100,000 p.p.m., in a few minutes (Waite *et al.* 1930).

Bibliography on p. 519

Dangerous in 30–60 min: 3000–6000 p.p.m. Maximum for 60 min without serious disturbance: 3000 p.p.m. Very slight symptoms after several hours: 250 p.p.m.

(2) Chronic

(i) By oral administration, for rats: repeated dosage of 0.1/kg in cold olive oil solution 5 times a week caused marked loss of body weight, gastric irritation and slight liver damage (Hollingsworth *et al.*, 1956). No evidence of injury from a dosage of 0.03, 0.01 and 0.003 g/kg for 30 days. – *(ii) By inhalation*, lethal dose, for rats, guinea pigs, rabbits, mice and one monkey, 841 p.p.m., 8 exposures in 10 days. Mice were the most susceptible.

SYMPTOMS OF INTOXICATION

Nasal irritation, with blood-tinged exudation from the nostrils, lacrimation, unsteadiness and staggering, dyspnoea, progressing to gasping.

Impairment of motor and sensory function; paralysis and atrophy of hind limbs with repeated exposure to 357 p.p.m., and in some animals at 204 p.p.m.

CHANGES IN THE ORGANISM

Congestion and oedema of the lungs; hyperaemia of liver and kidneys.

Slight haemorrhage and congestion of lungs, slight fatty degeneration of liver; slight congestion and cloudy swelling of convoluted tubules of kidney; fat vacuoles in the adrenal cortex.

Toxicity to human beings

There have been several reports of severe, even fatal, poisoning by ethylene oxide owing to heavy exposure following accidental escape of the liquid and/or vapour from defective apparatus during its manufacture.

A recent extensive report on the injurious effect of exposure to high concentrations of ethylene oxide is that of Thiess (1963); this describes cases occurring as the result of an accidental exposure following the breakage of a ventilator in a storage tank where ethylene oxide was kept under nitrogen pressure. This resulted in the liberation of 3 ml of ethylene oxide.

SYMPTOMS OF INTOXICATION

All the cases complained of nausea, heaviness in the stomach and vomiting recurring every 15 to 20 min, except the workman who attempted to close the defective opening in the tank. He was covered from head to foot with a layer of crystalline ethylene oxide, but after the clothing was immediately removed and his body washed with a strong stream of water he had only two attacks of vomiting and was not incapacitated. Some cases experienced diarrhoea immediately after the accident, others complained of headache, irritation of the nose and skin affections, similar to those described by Sexton and Henson (1949). Two firemen who had

had their feet immersed in liquid ethylene oxide suffered from severe bullous dermatitis; another, who perspired excessively, developed severe lesions of both feet 5 h after contact; these healed only after 8½ weeks of hospital treatment and left a brown pigmentation.

One case only was unconscious for 30 min, and there was no case of corneal injury. Among 41 cases investigated between 1956 and 1963 there was no case of severe lung injury, though there was some evidence of upper respiratory irritation in those whose gas masks were defective.

Another account of severe poisoning in which ethylene oxide was involved, though not considered solely responsible, was that of Marchand et al. (1957). During the manufacture of ethylene oxide a distillation apparatus broke, and workmen were exposed to the vapours not only of ethylene oxide but also to those of glycol chlorohydrin and dichloroethane. Of five who were hospitalised, three were only slightly affected (vomiting, diarrhoea, abdominal pain and head-ache) but two died with symptoms of severe central nervous injury – torpor, coma and circulatory and respiratory failure. In a third fatal case autopsy revealed acute pulmonary oedema and cerebral and meningeal congestion. It was con-cluded however that the poisoning was due rather to the glycol chlorohydrin and the dichloroethane than to the ethylene oxide itself.

(1) The eyes

One case of a human corneal burn following contact with ethylene oxyde during an industrial accident during chemical manufacture was reported by McLaughlin (1946), but he listed it among those compounds which, with suitable treatment, show healing within 48 h and cause no subsequent loss of vision.

The absence of any cases of corneal injury among the total number of cases of exposure to ethylene oxide investigated by Thiess (1963) would appear to confirm the relative innocuousness of ethylene oxide in this respect.

(2) The skin

There has been some difference of opinion as to the capacity of ethylene oxide for injuring the skin. Walker and Greeson (1932) for example were unable to produce any injury, but a controlled experiment by Sexton and Henson (1950) on human volunteers indicated that the decisive factor is intimate contact with the liquid or its aqueous solution, especially if there is impediment to evaporation. Thus, a 10 min contact with a 65% solution produced on the forearm blebs varying from small vesicles to large hemispheres filled with serum. The first symptoms were a chilling and tingling sensation, followed in 1 to 5 h by oedema and erythema with tenderness on pressure, and after 6 to 12 h by vesiculation. With spraying on the skin and rapid evaporation, frosting occurred, similar to that caused by ethyl chloride, with pain and urticaria. Absorption by shoe leather of the liquid or a 50% water solution can cause severe dermatitis of the feet

Bibliography on p. 519

either immediately or several hours later with blisters which later burst and become crusted, leaving areas of pigmentation (Beard and Dumire, 1957).

(3) Sensitisation

Some authorities believe that contact with ethylene oxide can lead to skin sensitisation, but others, such as Thiess (1963) consider ethylene oxide dermatitis to be of the primary toxic variety. Thiess found no evidence of any allergic manifestation in persons subjected to patch tests who had worked in contact with ethylene oxide for periods up to 28 years, 3 of whom had suffered from disturbances of health presumed to be due to ethylene oxide.

Sexton and Henson found that sensitivity occurred only at points of previous contact, with symptoms of pruritus and erythema.

TREATMENT

Warmth, rest and fresh air, with removal of soaked clothes and if possible a thorough bath; for severe cases transportation to hospital. Cardiac stimulants may be necessary if vomiting is profuse and prolonged, and anti-acidosis remedies may be advisable. For skin injuries, if severe, the treatment should be the same as that for burns.

77. Dichloroethyl Ether

Synonyms: 1-chloro-2(β-chloroethoxy)ethane, chlorex

Structural formula: $CH_2Cl–CH_2–O–CH_2–CH_2Cl$

Molecular formula: $C_4H_8Cl_2O$

Molecular weight: 143.02

Properties: a colourless liquid with an odour resembling ethylene dichloride. Solvent for many resins, including glyceryl phthalate resins (Durrans, 1950), ester gums, paraffin wax, gum camphor, castor, linseed and other fatty oils, turpentine, polyvinyl acetate and ethyl cellulose, but not for rubber, or cellulose esters except in the presence of 10–30% alcohol.

    boiling point: 178 °C
    melting point: −51.7 °C
    vapour pressure: 0.73 mm Hg at 20 °C
    vapour density (air = 1): 4.93
    specific gravity (liquid density): 1.22
    flash point: 131 °F
    conversion factors: 1 p.p.m. = 5.85 mg/m³
                      1 mg/l = 171 p.p.m.
    solubility: soluble in water to the extent of 1.1% at 20 °C. Miscible with aromatic but not paraffin hydrocarbons
    maximum allowable concentration: 15 p.p.m. (Threshold Limit Values, 1962)

ECONOMY, SOURCES AND USES

Production

(1) By treating β-chloroethyl alcohol with H_2SO_4 (Durrans, 1950).
(2) As a by-product in the production of ethylene glycol from ethylene chlorohydrin (Hake and Rowe, 1963).

Industrial uses

(1) In the paint and varnish industry, as a solvent for special lacquers, resins and oils.
(2) In the textile industry, for grease-spotting and the removal of paint and tar

brand marks from raw wool (Fife and Reid, 1930; Elkins, 1959), and incorporated in scouring and fulling soaps.

(3) In the petroleum industry, as an extractive for lubricating oils (Fairhall, 1957).

(4) In chemical synthesis.

(5) As a soil insecticide.

BIOCHEMISTRY

Estimation

In the atmosphere

(a) By passage through alcoholic KOH, and, after hydrolysis, determination by chloride titration (Allen, 1956).

(b) By silica gel absorption followed by warming, combustion and chloride titration (Hake and Rowe, 1963).

(c) By infra-red or interferometer methods.

Metabolism

No specific investigations of the metabolic fate of dichloroethyl ether have been made. Since its chemical constitution is similar to that of mustard gas (β-β'-dichloro-diethyl sulphide) the sulphur atom of the latter being replaced by an oxygen atom, and since dichloroethyl ether has some of the vesicant properties of mustard gas with regard to the respiratory system, it might be assumed that it shares with mustard gas the capacity for being rapidly distributed throughout the body tissues, the kidney and lung taking up the greatest amounts (Williams, 1959). The substitution of the O atom for the S atom of mustard gas deprives it of the blistering action on the skin and of the toxic action on cells by oxidation to sulphoxides and sulphones, an action suggested by Flury and Wieland (1921) as being due to these oxidation products.

TOXICOLOGY

Dichloroethyl ether is primarily a severe respiratory irritant; it can also be narcotic in high concentrations, but the extreme irritation from non-narcotic concentrations makes the occurrence of narcosis unlikely. Animal experiments have indicated that it is a highly toxic compound, but death, even when delayed, has been considered to be due to respiratory injury: accompanying congestion of other organs is apparently a secondary phenomenon.

It is not acutely irritant to the skin, but can be absorbed rapidly with lethal effect. In human beings the vapour is highly irritant to the eyes, nose and respiratory passages. One fatal case in a fulling mill, where it was presumably used warm, is briefly mentioned, without details, by Elkins (1959).

Toxicity to animals

(1) Acute

Lethal dose. – *(i) By oral administration*, for rats, 75 mg/kg (Smyth and Carpenter, 1948); for mice, 136 mg/kg (Smyth, unpublished, cited by Spector, 1956); for rabbits, 126 mg/kg; LD_{50} for rats, 110–210 mg/kg (Hake and Rowe, 1963). – *(ii) By skin application*, LD_{50}, for rabbits, 90 mg/kg in 10% solution in propylene glycol (Hake and Rowe, 1963). By 'poulticing' method (guinea pig) 0.3 ml/kg (Smyth and Carpenter, 1948). – *(iii) By inhalation*, for guinea pigs, 500–1000 p.p.m. for 30–60 min; 105–260 p.p.m. for 10–15 h (Schrenk *et al.*, 1933); LD_{50}, for rats, 1000 p.p.m. for 45 min, death within 14 days (Smyth and Carpenter, 1948); 250 p.p.m. for 4 h (Carpenter *et al.*, 1949).

(2) Chronic

By inhalation, for rats and guinea pigs, repeated exposures to 69 p.p.m., 5 per week over a period of 130 days caused no injury other than depression of growth. Appearance, behaviour, mortality and haematological values were unaffected (Hake and Rowe, 1963).

SYMPTOMS OF INTOXICATION

Intense irritation of conjunctiva with lacrimation, and of nose; unsteadiness or vertigo, slow respiration at first, becoming shallow and rapid, slight retching, unconsciousness leading to death. Lower concentrations (100 p.p.m.) caused no lacrimation, and unconsciousness only after 13 h.

(1) The eyes

Application to the cornea of rabbits caused injury which was graded by Carpenter and Smyth (1946) as of moderate severity; Hake and Rowe (1963) state that both the pure compound and also a 10% solution in propylene glycol cause moderate pain, conjunctival irritation and corneal injury which generally heals within a short time.

(2) The skin

Although toxic amounts were rapidly absorbed from the skin, the skin itself showed no marked irritative effect (Allen, 1956).

CHANGES IN THE ORGANISM

The respiratory tract was the chief site of injury; the lungs showed emphysema, oedema and haemorrhages, sometimes complete consolidation. These lesions were

Bibliography on p. 519

more severe if death were delayed 24 hours. The nasal passages, trachea and bronchi showed congestion, as also did the brain, liver and kidney. No abnormalities were observed following the above repeated exposures.

Toxicity to human beings

Irritation, considered intolerable, to the eyes and nose, with coughing, retching and nausea, was noted by Schrenk, Patty and Yant (1933) in human beings voluntarily exposed to concentrations above 500 p.p.m. At 260 and 100 p.p.m. there was some irritation, but not so severe, and at 35 p.p.m. none. Corneal injury generally heals within 24 hours (McLaughlin, 1946).

No cases of injury from its industrial use have been reported.

78. Dichloroisopropyl Ether

Synonym: bis(β-chloropropyl)ether

Structural formula:

$$\begin{array}{ccc} CH_2Cl & & CH_2Cl \\ | & & | \\ CH & -O- & CH \\ | & & | \\ CH_3 & & CH_3 \end{array}$$

Molecular formula: $C_6H_{12}Cl_2O$

Molecular weight: 171.07

Properties: a colourless liquid, soluble in water to the extent of 0.17 g in 100 ml.

    boiling point: 187.3 °C

    melting point: −96.8 to −108 °C

    vapour pressure: 0.71–0.85 mm Hg at 20 °C

    vapour density (air = 1): 5.9

    specific gravity: 1.1122 at 20 °C

    flash point: 185 °F

    conversion factors: 1 p.p.m. = 7 mg/m³

                     1 mg/l   = 143 p.p.m.

    solubility: 0.79 mg/100 ml water; miscible with most organic solvents and oils

    maximum allowable concentration: not established.

ECONOMY, SOURCES AND USES

Production

As a by-product in commercial production of propylene glycol.

Industrial uses

(1) As a solvent for fats, oils and waxes.

(2) In the textile industry, as a cleaning and spotting agent and as an ingredient of soap solutions for preventing excessive loss by evaporation.

(3) In the paint and varnish industry, as a paint remover.

(4) As an intermediate in the manufacture of dyes, resins and pharmaceuticals (Hake and Rowe, 1963).

BIOCHEMISTRY

Estimation

In the atmosphere
By methods used for estimation of dichloroethyl ether (*q.v.*).

Metabolism

Except for the observation (Smyth, Carpenter and Weil, 1951) that it is rapidl·
absorbed from the skin with possibly lethal results, no details of its metabolic fat·
are available.

TOXICOLOGY

Dichloroisopropyl ether is less toxic to animals, both by mouth and by inhalatio·
than dichloroethyl ether with regard to lung irritation, but with exposure fo·
some hours it causes in animals liver damage, occasionally necrosis. It is moderatel·
irritating to eyes and nose in high concentrations.

No reports of injury to human beings have been recorded.

Toxicity to animals

(1) Acute
Lethal dose. – (i) By oral administration, for rats, 0.8 g/kg; LD_{50} 0.24 g/k·
(Smyth *et al.*, 1951). – *(ii) By skin application*, 3.0 ml/kg. – *(iii) By inhalation*, fo·
rats, 700 p.p.m. for 6 h (Hake and Rowe, 1963); 1000 p.p.m. for 4 h caused onl·
1/6 deaths; 350 p.p.m. for 8 h 2/5, and 175 for 8 h 1/4.

(2) Chronic
By oral administration, repeated doses (22 over 31 days) of 0.2 g/kg caused a·
increase in weight of the liver and kidneys; 0.01 g/kg only a decrease in growth
weight. No abnormality of the blood picture was indicated even at the highes·
repeated oral dosage (Hake and Rowe).

SYMPTOMS OF INTOXICATION
With lethal dosage by inhalation some eye irritation and inco-ordination.

(1) The eyes
Application of the liquid to the eyes of rabbits caused moderate irritation,
more marked with exposure to the concentrated vapour (Carpenter and Smyth,
1946).

(2) The skin

No primary irritation of the skin after 20 applications to the ear of rabbits was noted by Smyth *et al.*, and only scaliness after the same number of applications by the poultice method to the skin of the abdomen (Hake and Rowe, 1963).

CHANGES IN THE ORGANISM

The lungs showed slight to moderate congestion depending on the duration of exposure. The liver injury also varied with the duration of exposure, necrosi being observed after 8 h exposure to 175 and 350 p.p.m. (Hake and Rowe, 1963).

Toxicity to human beings

No investigations have been carried out and no reports of injury from its industrial use have been recorded.

BIBLIOGRAPHY

Allen, H. (1956) cited by Hake and Rowe (1963), *Chem. Prod.*, 19:482.

Amiot, L. G. (1932) Contribution à l'Étude des Propriétés anaesthésiques de la Fonction Ether-oxyde, *Presse. Méd.*, 40:300.

Assoc. Official Agric. Chemists (1935) *Methods of Analysis*, 4th ed. Washington (cited by Hake and Rowe, 1963).

Bartholomew, R. A. (1962) Two Cases of Ether Addiciton/Habituation, *Med. J. Australia*, 49:550.

Beard, H. C. and K. B. Dumire (1957) Retention of Ethylene Oxide Fumigant by Shoes, *Arch. Ind. Hlth.*, 15:167.

Bourne, W. (1926) On the Effects of Acetaldehyde, Ether Peroxide, Ethyl Mercaptan, Ethyl Sulphide and several Ketones, when added to anaesthetic Ether, *J. Pharmacol. Exptl. Therap.*, 28:409.

Bourne, W. and B. B. Raginsky (1935) Vinyl Ether (Vinethene) Anaesthesia in Dogs; Effects upon normal and impaired Liver, *Brit. J. Anaesthesia*, 12:62.

Brandis von (1935) (cited by Molitor, 1936), Schweiz, *Narkose, Anesthesie*, 8:84.

Bunker, J. P. (1962) Metabolic Acidosis during Anesthesia and Surgery, *Anaesthesiology*, 23:107.

Cage, J. C. (1957) Determination of Ethylene Oxide in the Atmosphere, *Analyst.*, 82:587.

Carpenter, C. P. and H. F. Smyth Jr. (1946) Chemical Burns of the Rabbit Cornea, *Am. J. Ophthalm.* 29:1355.

Carpenter, C. P., H. F. Smyth Jr. and U. C. Pozzani (1949) Assay of acute vapor Toxicity and Grading and Interpretation of Results on 90 Chemical Compounds, *J. Ind. Hyg. Toxicol.*, 31:343.

Cavaliere, R., B. Giovanella and G. Moricea (1958) Influence of some anaesthetic Drugs on the Liver as determined by electrophoretic examination of Bile Proteins, *Chem. Abstr.*, 52:12228.

Chabanier, H., C. Libo-Onell and E. Lelu (1932) Modifications del'Équilibre acide-base au cours de l'Anésthésie générale par l'Éther, *Compt. Rend. Soc. Biol.*, 110:1282.

Chenoweth, M. B., D. N. Robertson, D. S. Erley and R. Goleke (1962) Blood and Tissue Levels of Ether, Chloroform, Halothane and Methoxyflurane in Dogs, *Anaesthesiology*, 23:101.

Curme, G. O. Jr. and F. Johnston (1952) *Glycols*, Am. Chem. Soc. Monograph Series 114, Reinhold, New York.

Durrans, T. H. (1950) *Solvents*, 6th ed. Chapman and Hall, London.

Dybing, O. and K. Skovlund (1957) Ether in fatty Tissue during Ether Absorption and Elimination, *Acta Pharmacol. Toxicol.*, 13:252.

Elkins, H. B. (1959) *The Chemistry of Industrial Toxicology*, Wiley and Sons, New York, Chapman and Hall, London.

Fairhall, L. T. (1957) *Industrial Toxicology*, Williams and Wilkins Co., Baltimore.

Flury, F. and H. Wieland (1921) Die pharmakologische Wirkung des Dichloräthylsulfids, *Z. Ges. Exper. Med.*, 13:367.

Fife, H. R. and E. W. Reid (1930) New industrial Solvents; Ethylene Dichloride, Dichlorethyl Ether and Isopropyl Ether, *Ind. Eng. Chem.*, 22:513.

Green, L. W. and P. E. Schietzow (1933) Method for Determination of minute Amounts of Peroxides in Ether, *J. Am. Pharmacol. Ass.*, 22:412.

Haggard, H. W. (1924) The Absorption, Distribution and Elimination of Ethyl Ether, *J. Biol. Chem.*, 59:737.

Hake, C. L. and V. K. Rowe (1963) *Ethers*; in F. A. Patty: *Industrial Hygiene and Toxicology*, Vol. II, 2nd ed., Interscience Publishers, New York.

Hamilton, A. (1916) *U.S. Dept. Labor Statist. Bull.*, 219:54.

Hamilton, A. (1925 and 1929) *Industrial Poisons in the U.S.*, Macmillan, New York.

Hamilton, A. and G. R. Minot (1920) Ether Poisoning in the Manufacture of Smokeless Powder, *J. Ind. Hyg. Toxicol.*, 2:41.

Hayhurst, E. K. (1930) *Ether*, I.L.O. Brochure No. 186.

Hess, L. G. and V. V. Tilton (1950) Ethylene Oxide; Hazards and Methods of Handling, *Ind. Eng. Chem.*, 42:1251.

Hine, C. H. and V. K. Rowe (1963) *Epoxy Compounds*, in F. A. Patty (1963), *Industrial Hygiene and Toxicology*, Vol. II, 2nd ed., Interscience Publishers, New York.

Hollingsworth, R. L., V. K. Rowe, D. D. McCollister and H. C. Spencer (1956) Toxicity of Ethylene Oxide determined on experimental Animals, *Arch. Ind. Hlth.*, 13:217.

Jackson, W. E. (1933) The pharmacological Action of Isopropyl Ether, *J. Pharmacol. Exptl. Ther.*, 48:278.

Johnstone, R. T. and S. E. Miller (1960) *Occupational Diseases and industrial Medicine*, W. B. Saunders Co., Philadelphia and London.

Kärber, G. (1930) Beitrage zur Toxikologie bei den Gegenwart brennender Flammen auftretenden Zersetzungsprodukte des Äthers, *Klin. Wschr.*, 9:1130.

Knoefel, P. K., A. E. Guedel and C. D. Leake (1931) Experimental Observations on the anaesthetic Properties of Divinyl Ether, *Proc. Soc. Exptl. Biol. Med.*, 29:139.

Knoefel, P. K. and F. C. Murrell (1935) The Rate of Production of Anaesthesia in Mice by Ether containing Aldehyde and Peroxide. *J. Pharmacol. Exptl. Therap.*, 55:235.

Leake, C. D. and M. Y. Chen (1930) The anaesthetic Properties of certain unsaturated Ethers, *Proc. Soc. Exptl. Biol. Med.*, 28:151.

Machle, W., E. W. Scott and J. Treon (1939) The physiological Response to Isopropyl Ether and to a Mixture of Isopropyl Ether and Gasoline, *J. Ind. Hyg. Tocicol.*, 21:72.

Marchand, M., R. Delesvaux, C. Claeys and F. Lejeune (1957) The Toxicity of Ethylene Oxide and a Report on 3 fatal cases of poisoning, *Rev. Med. Minière*, 10:5.

McLaughlin, R. S. (1946) Chemical Burns of the Human Cornea, *Am. J. Ophthalm.*, 29:1355.

Molitor, H. (1936) Some pharmacological and toxicological Properties of Vinyl Ether, *J. Pharmacol. Exptl. Ther.*, 53:274.

Mörch, E. T., J. B. Aycrigg and M. S. Berger (1956) The anaesthetic Effects of Ethyl vinyl Ether, Divinyl Ether and Diethyl Ether on Mice, *J. Pharmacol. Exptl. Ther.*, 117:184.

Nelson, K. W., J. F. Ege Jr., L. E. Woodman and L. Silverman (1943) Sensory Response to certain industrial Solvent Vapours. *J. Ind. Hyg. Toxicol.*, 25:282.

Oettigen, W. E. von (1949) cited by Hine and Rowe (1963) *Encyclopaedia of Hygiene, Pathology and Social Welfare*, I.L.O. Geneva.

Robbins, B. J. (1935) Ether Anaesthesia – Concentrations in inspired Air and in Blood required for anaesthesia, loss of Reflexes and Death, *J. Pharmacol. Exptl. Therap.*, 53:251.

Royce, A. and W. K. S. Moore (1955) Occupational Dermatitis caused by Ethylene Oxide, *Brit. J. Ind. Med.*, 12:169.

Ruigh, W. L. and R. T. Major (1931) The preparation and Properties of pure Divinyl Ether, *J. Am. Chem. Soc.*, 53:2662.

Sand, R. (1910) Intoxication expérimentale par l'Alcool-Éther. *Rep. 2nd Congr. Internat. Malad. Prof.*, Brussels.

Schrenk, H. H., F. A. Patty and W. P. Yant (1933) Acute Response of Guinea Pigs to Vapours of some new commercial organic Compounds. Dichloroethyl Ether, *U.S. Publ. Hlth. Rep.*, 48:1389.

Sexton, R. J. and E. V. Henson (1949) Dermatological Injuries by Ethylene Oxide, *J. Ind. Hyg. Tocicol.*, 31:297.

Sexton, R. J. and E. V. Henson (1950) Experimental Ethylene Oxide Human Skin Injuries, *Arch. Ind. Hyg.*, 2:549.

Silverman, L. (1947) *Industrial Air Sampling and Analysis* (cited by Hake and Rowe, 1963), Industrial Hygiene Foundation, Pittsburg.

Silverman, L., H. F. Schulte and W. W. First (1946) Further Studies on sensory Response to certain industrial Solvents Vapours, *J. Ind. Hyg. Toxicol.*, 28:262.

Smyth, H. F., Jr. and C. P. Carpenter (1948) Further Experience with the Range-Finding Test in the Industrial Toxicological Laboratory, *J. Ind. Hyg. Toxicol.*, 30:1.

Smyth, H. F., Jr., C. P. Carpenter and C. S. Weil (1951) Range-Finding Toxicity Data. List IV, *Arch. Ind. Hyg.*, 4:119.

Smyth, H. F., Jr., C. P. Carpenter, C. S. Weil and U. C. Pozzani (1954) Range-Finding Toxicity Tests, Data List 5, *Arch. Ind. Hyg.* 10:61.

Smyth H. F., Jr., J. Seaton and L. Fischer (1941) Single Dose Toxicity of Some Glycols and Derivatives, *J. Ind. Hyg. Toxicol.*, 23:259.

Spector, W. S. (1956) *Handbook of Toxicology*. Vol. I, Saunders, Philadelphia.

Stewart, R. D., D. S. Erley, D. R. Torkelson and C. L. Hake (1959) Post-exposure Analysis of organic Compounds in Blood by a rapid Infra-red Technique, *Nature*, 184:192.

Thiess, A. M. (1963) Beobachtungen über Gesundheitsschädigen durch Einwirkung von Äthylendioxyd, *Arch. Toxikol.*, 29:127.

Threshold Limit Values for 1962, *Am. Ind. Hyg. Ass. J.*, 23:419.

Vogel, A. I. (1948) Physical Properties and Chemical Constitution. Ethers and Acetals, *J. Chem. Soc.*, 616.

Waite, C. P., F. A. Patty and W. P. Yant (1930) Acute Response of Guinea Pigs to Vapours of some new commercial organic Compounds – Ethylene Oxide, *U.S. Treas. Publ. Hlth. Rep.*, No. 45:1832.

Walker, W. J. C. and C. E. Greeson (1932) The Toxicity of Ethylene Oxide, *J. Hyg.*, 32:409.

Williams, R. T. (1959) *Detoxication Mechanisms*, Chapman and Hall, London.

Chapter 11

ESTERS

79. Ethyl Acetate

Synonym: acetic ether

Structural formula:

$$CH_3-\overset{\overset{\textstyle O}{\|}}{C}-O-CH_2-CH_3$$

Molecular formula: $C_4H_8O_2$

Molecular weight: 88.1

Properties: a colourless liquid with a pleasant odour. There are several grades of ethyl acetate, differing slightly in their boiling ranges, acidity and ester content. A widely used variety is 'technical 99–100%'. Boiling range 76–78 °C. Acidity 0.1% max. Ester content 99–100%.

Pure ethyl acetate:
   boiling point: 77.15 °C
   vapour pressure: 73 mm Hg at 20 °C
   vapour density (air = 1): 3.04
   specific gravity (liquid density): 0.901
   flash point: 28 °F
   conversion factors: 1 p.p.m. = 3.60 mg/m³
                       1 mg/l = 278 p.p.m.
   solubility: ethyl acetate is a good solvent for cellulose nitrate, but not for cellulose acetate except with addition of 5–30% of alcohol, for ethyl cellulose, rubber chloride, wholly or partially for many resins, cumarone and mastic but not hard copals or polyvinyl chloride (Durrans, 1950).
   maximum allowable concentration: 400 p.p.m. (Threshold Limit Values, 1962).

ECONOMY, SOURCES AND USES

Production

(1) By direct continuous esterification.
(2) By catalytic condensation of acetaldehyde by means of alkoxide.

Industrial uses

(1) In the lacquer industry, chiefly in the manufacture of cellulose nitrate lacquer as a substitute for acetone; also as a constituent of bronze cellulose lacquer (Weingand, 1931).

(2) In the straw hat industry as a constituent of the lacquer (Kruger, 1932).

(3) In the celluloid industry, for 'joining'.

(4) In the artificial leather industry.

(5) In the shoe industry.

(6) As a constituent of paint and rust removers.

(7) As an extracting agent.

(8) In the pharmaceutical industry (Lloyd, Oswald and Fuller, 1930).

BIOCHEMISTRY

Estimation

In the atmosphere

The method described by Hestrin (1949) depends on the reaction with alkaline hydroxylamine and addition of ferric chloride to form a purple colour. This method has been used as a basis for the reaction as described by Strafford *et al.* (1956) and Fassett (1963).

Metabolism

Although no detailed investigations of the metabolic fate of ethyl acetate have been made, Fassett (1963) includes ethyl acetate in his statement that the acetates, on account of their solubility in plasma, are readily hydrolysed either by simple chemical hydrolysis or by esterases present in liver or plasma.

In the case of ethyl acetate further metabolism produces the corresponding ethyl alcohol and is partly excreted in the exhaled air and urine and partly metabolised.

TOXICOLOGY

Ethyl acetate is an irritant of mucous membranes; in general less so than other acetates (propyl, butyl and amyl) but, according to Lehmann and Flury (1943) temporary corneal opacity has been observed. It has been stated to cause hypersensitivity to skin and mucous membranes, and that a tendency to eczematous conditions of the skin may thus develop. A tendency also to the loss of smell after

Bibliography on p. 591

prolonged exposure has been described by Barrios and Devoto (1931). It is also narcotic, to a greater extent than methyl acetate, and one fatal case due to inhalation of the vapour from a paint containing 80% of it has been reported (Althof, 1931).

Nevertheless it is generally regarded as a less toxic solvent for industrial use than methyl acetate, and there is no evidence that it has a cumulative effect, though Durrans (1950), without amplifying his statement, states that it can cause pulmonary oedema and may have a tendency to cause habituation.

It should be mentioned that all these alleged ill-effects of ethyl acetate have occurred during its intensive use during earlier years, when impurities may have been present or it may have been used without due care and often in combination with other solvents.

Toxicity to animals

(1) Acute

(a) Lethal dose. – For mice, 8000 p.p.m. for 3 h (Flury and Zernik, 1931); for cats, 43,000 p.p.m. for 15 min (Fassett, 1963).

(b) Narcotic dose. – For mice, 5000 p.p.m.; for cats, 12,000 p.p.m.

(2) Chronic

Repeated inhalation by mice 6 h per day for 7 days of 4200–4400 p.p.m. was found by Flury and Neumann (1927) and by guinea pigs of 2000 p.p.m. by Smyth and Smyth (1928) to cause no definite narcotic symptoms, but Flury and Wirth noted an increase in erythrocytes with no corresponding increase in haemoglobin, and some increase in polymorphs. Recovery was delayed and there was loss of appetite, but no changes in the urine indicating liver or kidney injury.

SYMPTOMS OF INTOXICATION

Irritation of eyes, salivation, coughing, followed by narcosis with loss of the corneal reflex before those of skin and pain, and followed by death of 25% of the animals during the period of deep narcosis.

CHANGES IN THE ORGANISM

Flury and Wirth (1934) observed hyperaemia of the respiratory tract, with oedema and haemorrhage of the lungs, but they did not consider these lesions severe enough to have been the cause of death, which they believed to be due to the narcotic effect.

Toxicity to human beings

The narcotic effect of ethyl acetate, though greater than that of methyl acetate, has not, according to Fassett (1963) been observed with concentrations of 400–600 p.p.m. after 2–3 h of exposure.

The one fatal case reported by Althoff (1931) was that of a workman who was found dead in the interior of a tank in which he was using a paint containing ethyl acetate but also other constituents. It was stated that at autopsy all the organs and tissues smelt strongly of ethyl acetate, as did those of a guinea pig subjected to similar conditions. Of the internal organs of the man, the spleen and kidneys showed congestion and the lungs also punctiform haemorrhages. Evidence for its acute irritative effect is further somewhat discounted by the fact that, as in the cases of conjunctivitis reported by Kruger (1932) in workers in a straw hat factory, where ethyl acetate was only occasionally a constituent of the lacquer used, but Nelson *et al.* (1943) state that concentrations of 400 p.p.m. cause considerable irritation of the nose and throat. It has a strong odour at 200 p.p.m. and Barrios and Devoto (1931) suggested that such an exposure may lead to the loss of the sense of smell for other odours.

With regard to skin irritation, Engelhardt (1933) on the evidence of patch tests postulated a special sensitivity reaction of skin and mucous membranes to prolonged exposure, and such a special sensitivity of mucous membranes was alleged by Beintke (1928) on the grounds of a severe case of gingivitis in a man exposed to a lacquer containing ethyl acetate, but also butyl acetate and butyl alcohol. Fassett (1963) has noted only minor dryness of the skin and no sensitisation.

Bibliography on p. 591

80. Methyl Acetate

Structural formula:
$$CH_3-\overset{\overset{\textstyle O}{\|}}{C}-O-CH_3$$

Molecular formula: $C_3H_6O_2$

Molecular weight: 74.08

Properties: a colourless, volatile inflammable liquid with a fragrant odour. The technical product used by Flury and Wirth (1934) was stated to contain traces of acetone.

> *boiling point:* 57.8 °C
> *melting point:* —98.7 °C
> *vapour pressure:* 100 mm Hg at 9.4 °C (Sax, 1957); 235 mm Hg at 25 °C (Fassett, 1963)
> *vapour density (air = 1):* 2.55
> *specific gravity (liquid density):* 0.927
> *flash point:* 14 °F
> *conversion factors:* 1 p.p.m. = 3.03 mg/m³
> $\qquad\qquad\qquad$ 1 mg/l $\quad$ = 330 p.p.m.
> *solubility:* in water 32 g/100 ml. Readily soluble in most organic solvents. Explosive when exposed to heat or flame. Good solvent for nitrocellulose and cellulose esters.
> *maximum allowable concentration:* 200 p.p.m.

ECONOMY, SOURCES AND USES

Production

By acetylation of methyl alcohol in the presence of H_2SO_4 followed by distillation.

Industrial uses

Methyl acetate is frequently used as a component of a mixture with acetone and methyl alcohol (methyl acetone).

(1) In the manufacture of artificial leather and plastics.

(2) In the paint, lacquer and varnish industry, but when used as a substitute for

acetone in cellulose coating lacquers it has the disadvantage of too ready hydrolysis.

(3) In the perfume industry.

BIOCHEMISTRY

Estimation

(1) In the atmosphere

No specific method has been described, but Fairhall (1957) suggests: (a) that
methyl acetate be absorbed in alcohol and the acetate content determined by
refluxing with standard NaOH followed by titration; (b) that samples may be
drawn over activated charcoal or silica gel and the increase in weight measured.

(2) In urine

In the urine of subjects exposed to methyl acetate estimation of the amount
of methyl alcohol indicates a harmful exposure if present in amounts greater than
5 mg/l (Henderson and Haggard, 1943).

Metabolism

Little is known of the actual fate of methyl acetate in the body, but it has been
suggested (Duquenois and Revel, 1934; Lund, 1944) that possibly its conversion
to methyl alcohol is related to its toxic action especially on the eyes, as well as its
tendency to cause acidosis (Flury and Wirth, 1934).

TOXICOLOGY

Methyl acetate is irritant to mucous membranes and moderately narcotic (less so
than ethyl acetate) but with deep narcosis animals do not recover and die with
symptoms of general poisoning. They also show some changes in the blood picture. In human beings no fatalities, but some ocular and nervous disorders have
been recorded.

Toxicity to animals

(1) Acute

(a) Lethal dose. – *(i) By subcutaneous injection*, for cats, 3 g/kg after 32 min; for
guinea pigs, 3–5 g/kg from 11–30 min (Flury and Wirth, 1934). – *(ii) By inhala-*
tion, for cats, 22,000–31,000 p.p.m. (Flury and Zernik, 1931); for mice, 11,000
p.p.m. for 10 h (Browning, 1953).

Bibliography on p. 591

(b) Narcotic dose. – By inhalation, for mice, 8000 p.p.m. after 4 h; for cats, 19,000 p.p.m. (Fassett, 1963).

(2) Chronic

Inhalation, repeated, of concentrations one-half to one-third of the narcotic dose caused some loss of weight, apathy and some changes in the blood picture – a preliminary increase in total leucocytes followed by a fall a week later in some of the animals, and an increase in red cells and haemoglobin, falling a week later to the pre-experimental level. One animal showed a relative lymphocytosis.

SYMPTOMS OF INTOXICATION

Irritation of eyes and salivation, followed (in cats) by vomiting, clonic cramps, dyspnoea; respiration at first increased, then decreased. At 11,000–12,000 p.p.m. drowsiness with recovery after one hour and no significant after-effects (Flury and Wirth, 1934).

CHANGES IN THE ORGANISM

Congestion and marginal emphysema of the lungs, in one animal lung oedema. Hyperaemia of trachea, bronchi and kidneys (Flury and Wirth).

Toxicity to human beings

It was stated by Reus (1933) that personal accidental inhalation after 45 min caused severe headache and somnolence lasting several hours, while Flury and Wirth (1934) also observed drowsiness and persistent headache in men subjected to inhalation.

Among the few accounts of an alleged industrial effect are those of Duquenois and Revel (1934) and Lund (1944).

The former described symptoms of visual disturbance, nervous instability, dyspnoea, tightness of the chest, palpitation and exhaustion, but methyl acetate was only one constituent of a mixture of solvents which included ethyl acetate and ethyl and methyl formate, and no actual atmospheric concentrations were given. Lund's case was one of eye injury. This man had had occasional attacks of vertigo, headache, unsteady gait and sudden blindness in both eyes. He later developed bilateral optic atrophy, a central scotoma in one eye and narrowing of the visual field in the other. Lund suggested that this might be due to the formation of methyl alcohol and formaldehyde during the metabolism of methyl acetate.

81. Butyl Acetate

Structural formula:

$$CH_3-\overset{\overset{\displaystyle O}{\|}}{C}-O-CH_2-CH_2-CH_2-CH_3$$

Molecular formula: $C_6H_{12}O_2$

Molecular weight: 116.16

Properties: commercial butyl acetate consists of three isomers: n-, iso- and sec.

n-Butyl Acetate. – A colourless inflammable liquid with an agreeable fruity odour in low concentrations, disagreeable in higher concentrations.

boiling point: 124.8–126.5 °C (Baldi, 1953)
melting point: —77 °F
vapour pressure: 15 mm Hg at 25 °C
vapour density (air = 1): 4
specific gravity (liquid density): 0.877 at 15.6 °C
flash point: 102 °F (Durrans, 1950); 84° F (Fassett, 1963)
conversion factors: 1 p.p.m. = 4.75
      1 mg/l = 211 p.p.m.
solubility: miscible with alcohols, ketones, other esters and most organic solvents. Solubility in water 1 g in 100 ml. Good solvent for nitrocellulose, oils fats, resins, waxes and camphor.
evaporation rate (ether = 1): 12
maximum allowable concentration: 200 p.p.m. (ACGIH, 1965, tentative revision, 150 p.p.m.)

ECONOMY, SOURCES AND USES

Production

By esterification of butyl alcohol with acetic acid in presence of H_2SO_4

Isobutyl acetate. – Similar to those of n-butyl acetate but with a less pungent and more pleasant odour and a lower boiling point (117.2 °C).

sec.-Isobutyl acetate.

> *boiling point:* 116.16 °C
> *melting point:* —99 °C (Durrans, 1950)
> *vapour pressure:* 13 mm Hg at 20 °C
> *vapour density (air = 1):* 4
> *specific gravity (liquid density):* 0.872 at 20 °C
> *flash point:* 66 °F
> *conversion factors:* 1 p.p.m. = 4.75 mg/m³
>   1 mg/l = 211 p.p.m.
> *solubility:* in water 3%
> *evaporation rate(ether = 1):* greater than that of *n*-butyl acetate
> *maximum allowable concentration:* ACGIH, 1965 recommend 150 p.p.m.

ECONOMY, SOURCES AND USES

Industrial uses

(1) In the lacquer industry, chiefly for nitrocellulose lacquers, but also in combination with lacquers containing drying oils, and in many high polish lacquers and varnishes.

(2) In manufacture of patent leather (Enna, 1930).

(3) In the motor industry as a constituent of a protective vehicle coating of low viscosity.

(4) In perfumery and food preservation.

(5) In other industries where amyl acetate is widely used, including shoe cleaning polishes, and stain-removing agents (Zangger, 1930).

BIOCHEMISTRY

Estimation

In the atmosphere

(1) By a method similar to that used for amyl acetate (Patty, Yant, and Schrenk, 1936).

(2) By the colorimetric method described by Hestrin (1949) depending on the reaction with hydroxylamine and addition of $FeCl_3$ to form a purple colour.

TOXICOLOGY

Butyl acetate is primarily an irritant, but also a narcotic to a slightly greater extent than ethyl or methyl acetate (Fassett, 1963). Concentrations causing acute irritation of eyes and nose in human beings have however caused no marked symptoms in guinea pigs even after several hours (Sayers *et al.*, 1936).

In industrial use the only reported effects of alleged injury due to butyl acetate have never been related to its sole application, but always in cases where other solvents have been present.

Toxicity to animals

(1) Acute

(a) *Lethal dose.* – (i) *By oral administration*, for mice, LD_{50} – 7056 mg/kg (McOmie, 1942). – (ii) *By inhalation*, for guinea pigs, Sayers *et al.* (1936) found no concentrations obtainable in the conditions used, the highest being 14,000 p.p.m., immediately lethal, but 10,000–14,000 p.p.m. were dangerous to life after several hours. The maximum for one hour without serious disturbance was 7000 p.p.m.

(b) *Narcotic dose.* – For guinea pigs, 10,000–14,000 p.p.m. for 15–30 min.

(2) Chronic

With repeated inhalation of 3100–4200 p.p.m. 6 h a day for 6 days, mice became habituated to the irritation but showed some fatigue and loss of weight and the blood picture showed an increase in the formed elements and haemoglobin (Sayers, *et al.*, 1936).

SYMPTOMS OF INTOXICATION

Irritation of conjunctivae followed by incoordination and narcosis. With lethal doses progressive narcosis led to death, which was apparently not due to irritation of the lungs (Sayers *et al.*, 1936). In one animal in the experiments of Flury and Wirth (1934) narcosis was preceded by cramps, bouts of excitation and vomiting.

CHANGES IN THE ORGANISM

Congestion of lungs, brain, liver and kidneys were observed by Sayers *et al* (1936). According to Cavalazzi (1938) even in animals which have shown no marked symptoms during life autopsy reveals slight pulmonary emphysema and significant congestion of the renal tubules.

Toxicity to human beings

Sayers *et al.* (1936) stated that men exposed to 14,000, 7000 and 3300 p.p.m. for a short time found the atmosphere extremely disagreeable because of its strong odour and irritation of eyes and nose. In the experience of Fassett (1963), while butyl acetate may produce slight irritation at 200–300 p.p.m. it does not appear to cause the temporary corneal oedema caused by butyl alcohol at these levels, and an eye splashed by butyl acetate has healed within 48 hours. He also found that no anaesthetic symptoms result from 2–3 hours' exposure to 400–600 p.p.m.

In industrial use, alleged injuries from butyl acetate have usually been found to be more probably due to other solvents used in combination with it. Among such reports are those of Kruger (1932), Burger and Stockman (1932), Weber and Gueffroy (1932), Fuhner and Pietrusky (1934) and Schutz (1937).

Kruger reported eye lesions from the use of a lacquer which contained not only butyl acetate but also butyl alcohol; in the report of Burger and Stockman the suggestion of liver injury, as indicated by urobilinuria, is rendered improbable by the fact that the wall-paper paint contained amyl and butyl alcohol, amyl acetate and acetone; in the cases of anaemia, cough, bronchial catarrh and nervous symptoms which, according to Weber and Gueffroy, followed exposure to a nitrocellulose lacquer, this lacquer contained not only a mixture of acetates and alcohols but also aromatic hydrocarbons, chiefly toluol, while in the cases of headache, stupor and gastrointestinal disturbance described by Fuhner and Pietrusky, benzol, xylol and toluol were all present in the lacquers used.

Similar symptoms, with in addition either slight leucopenia or relative lymphocytosis were noted in a group of women exposed to a mixture of xylene and butyl acetate (Schutz, 1937) but it was not stated whether the xylene was pure; if it contained any benzene, this may well have been the cause of the slight blood changes, while xylene itself can produce considerable nausea and vomiting.

A more recent account of suspected injury by butyl acetate, particularly with reference to the eyes, is that of Busing (1952). A group of workers using lacquers ('Diosyn Lack 50,000' and 'Kaltlack 103 AE') during the summer of 1950 complained of burning eyes, throat irritation and loss of appetite and weight. Some showed actual injury of the cornea with vacuolation; this recovered in 9–10 days, but in two cases there was a recurrence on further exposure. These lacquers contained in addition to butyl acetate, benzol, toluol and xylol; butyl alcohol, which is the solvent most likely to have caused the corneal injury, was also present.

82. Propyl Acetate

82a. n-Propyl Acetate

Structural formula:

$$CH_3-\overset{\displaystyle O}{\overset{\|}{C}}-O-CH_2-CH_2-CH_3$$

Molecular formula: $C_5H_{10}O_2$

Molecular weight: 102.13

Properties: a colourless liquid with an odour like pears. It is a major constituent of amyl acetate and is seldom used in a state of purity. Good solvent for cellulose nitrate, celluloid, colophony and many resins (Gnamm, 1943) and for ethyl cellulose when mixed with other substances such as camphor, cyclohexanol and ethyl benzene (Durrans, 1950).

> *boiling point:* 101.6 °C
> *melting point:* —92.5 °C
> *vapour pressure:* 35 mm Hg at 25 °C
> *vapour density (air = 1):* 3.5
> *specific gravity (liquid density):* 0.897
> *flash point:* 58 °F
> *conversion factors:* 1 p.p.m. = 4.17 mg/m³
> 1 mg/l = 240 p.p.m.
> *solubility:* in water 1.89% at 20 °C. Miscible with castor and linseed oil and hydrocarbons.
> *evaporation rate (ether = 1):* 6.1
> *maximum allowable concentration:* 200 p.p.m.

ECONOMY, SOURCES AND USES

Production

From esterification of fusel oil together with other homologues.

Industrial uses

(1) To some extent in the lacquer industry (Alinari, 1930).
(2) In the manufacture of flavoring agents and perfumes (von Oettingen, 1960).

BIOCHEMISTRY

Metabolism

Little is known beyond the fact that it is absorbed through the lungs and gastro-intestinal tract; it is not known whether it is absorbed by the intact skin. According to Fassett (1963), like most of the simple aliphatic esters it is converted in the body to 'normal metabolic products'.

TOXICOLOGY

n-Propyl acetate is irritant to mucous membranes, to a slightly less extent than ethyl acetate (Flury and Wirth, 1934). It is also narcotic, but better tolerated and with more rapid recovery than methyl or ethyl acetate. No cases of systemic injury from its industrial use have been recorded, but it has been suggested that exposure to high concentrations will cause irritative symptoms, nausea and narcotic effects.

Toxicity to animals

(1) Acute

(*a*) *Lethal dose.* – (*i*) *By subcutaneous injection*, for cats and guinea pigs 3 g/kg. – (*ii*) *By inhalation*, for cats, 9400 p.p.m. after $5\frac{1}{2}$ h; 24,500 p.p.m. after $\frac{1}{2}$ h (Flury and Zernik, 1931).

(*b*) *Narcotic dose.* – (*i*) *By intravenous injection*, 4.5–5 ml of a 5% aqueous solution (Wachtel, 1920). – (*ii*) *By inhalation*, for cats, 9100 p.p.m., for mice, 5900 p.p.m. (Flury and Wirth, 1934).

(2) Chronic

Respiratory irritation and some injury to the liver following long-continued exposure to non-narcotic concentrations were observed by Flury and Wirth. Tolerance was greater and more rapidly established than with the lower homologues.

SYMPTOMS OF INTOXICATION

Eye irritation and salivation, followed by stupor and deep narcosis leading to death. The effect of intravenous injection on the circulation was stated by Wachtel (1920) to be a transient fall of blood pressure and slowing of respiration and very weak reflexes.

CHANGES IN THE ORGANISM

In Flury and Wirth's (1934) experiments cats exposed to lethal concentrations showed tracheitis, bronchitis and fatty changes in the liver.

Toxicity to human beings

No actual injury has been reported but Lehmann and Flury (1943) suggest that high concentrations may cause nausea, burning of the eyes, oppression in the fatigue, lassitude and narcosis, while von Oettingen (1960) states that "it is to be expected that exposure to high concentrations will cause narcotic effects characterised by fatigue and lassitude, and with higher concentrations narcosis".

82b. Isopropyl Acetate

Synonym: paracetat

Structural formula:
$$CH_3-\overset{O}{\overset{\|}{C}}-O-\overset{CH_3}{\underset{H}{\overset{|}{\underset{|}{C}}}}-CH_3$$

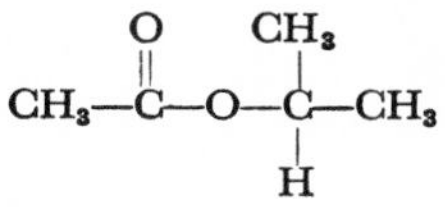

Molecular formula: $C_5H_{10}O_2$

Molecular weight: 102.13

Properties: a liquid similar to *n*-propyl acetate. Good solvent for cellulose nitrate, some gums and resins; partly for shellac; not for cellulose acetate and hard copals (Durrans, 1950).

  boiling point: 88.9 °C
  melting point: —73.4 °C
  vapour pressure: 73 mm Hg at 25 °C
  vapour density (air = 1): 3.5
  specific gravity (liquid density): 0.874
  flash point: 40 °F
  conversion factors: 1 p.p.m. = 4.17 mg/m³
             1 mg/l   = 240 p.p.m.
  solubility: in water 3 parts per 100. Miscible with alcohol, ether, castor oil, linseed oil and hydrocarbons.
  evaporation rate (ether = 1): about $^1/_3$ that of ethyl acetate
  maximum allowable concentration: 250 p.p.m., ACGIH, 1965.

ECONOMY, SOURCES AND USES

Industrial uses

Chiefly in the lacquer industry (Hackett, 1932).

Bibliography on p. 591

BIOCHEMISTRY

Metabolism

It is absorbed through the lungs, gastro-intestinal tract and the skin of animals.

TOXICOLOGY

Isopropyl acetate is an irritant of mucous membranes but only to a slight extent; it is also narcotic, but less so than the *n*-isomer. From experiments on the isolated frog's heart (Fuhner, 1921) it appears to be more toxic in this respect than ethyl or methyl acetate.

No systemic injury has been reported but it has been stated to cause some degree of eye irritation in certain individuals.

Toxicity to animals

Lethal dose. (LD$_{50}$, rabbits). – *(i) By skin penetration*, 20,000 p.p.m. (Smyth *et al.*, 1954). – *(ii) By oral administration*, for rats, 6.5 g/kg. – *(iii) By inhalation*, for rats, 32,000 p.p.m. for 4 h (compared with 9100 p.p.m. for the *n*-isomer for cats (Flury and Zernik, 1931).

SYMPTOMS OF INTOXICATION

Moderate eye irritation; no skin irritation; narcosis preceding death (Smyth *et al.*, 1954).

Toxicity to human beings

According to Silverman, Schulte and First (1946) some irritation of the eyes is caused by exposure to 200 p.p.m. Otherwise no toxic effects have been recorded.

83. Amyl Acetate

Synonym: banana oil

Structural formula:

$$CH_3-\overset{\displaystyle O}{\overset{\|}{C}}-O-CH_2-CH_2-CH_2-CH_2-CH_3$$

Molecular formula: $C_7H_{14}O_2$

Molecular weight: 130.18

Properties: The commercial product is largely a mixture of isoamyl and *n*-amyl acetate, the former predominating, but according to Baldi (1953) there are 8 possible isomers which may be present. The three most important are the iso-, the *n*- and the secondary acetate, the secondary being the least toxic of the three.

The pure amyl acetate is a clear colourless liquid with a pleasant banana-like odour in low concentrations.

The commercial variety is a yellow liquid with a more pronounced odour.

It is a solvent for nitrocellulose, celluloid, camphor, formaldehyde, synthetic resins and waxes.

Isoamyl acetate.
   boiling point: 143 °C
   vapour pressure: 6 mm Hg at 25 °C
   vapour density (air = 1): 4.5
   specific gravity (liquid density): 0.876
   flash point: 92 °F
   conversion factors: 1 p.p.m. = 5.32 mg/m³
                         1 mg/l = 199 p.p.m.
   solubility: in water 0.25 g/100 ml
   maximum allowable concentration: 200 p.p.m. (ACGIH, 1965 recommend 100 p.p.m.)

n-Amyl acetate.
   boiling point: 148.8 °C
   melting point: —71 °C
   vapour pressure: 5 mm Hg at 25 °C
   vapour density (air = 1): 4.5
   specific gravity (liquid density): 0.8756
   flash point: 77 °F

conversion factors: 1 p.p.m. = 5.32 mg/m³
           1 mg/l = 188 p.p.m.
solubility: in water 0.18 g/100 ml
maximum allowable concentration: ACGIH, 1965 recommend 100 p.p.m.

sec.-Amyl acetate.
    boiling point: 133 °C
    vapour pressure: 9 mm Hg at 25 °C
    vapour density (air = 1): 4.5
    specific gravity (liquid density): 0.86
    flash point: 89 °F
    conversion factors: 1 p.p.m. = 5.32 mg/m³
                 1 mg/l = 188 p.p.m.
    solubility: slightly soluble in water
    maximum allowable concentration: ACGIH, 1965 recommend 125 p.p.m.

ECONOMY, SOURCES AND USES

Production

(1) By acetylation of amyl alcohols distilled from fusel oil.
(2) Synthetically from *n*-pentane and isopentane.

Industrial uses

(1) In the lacquer and varnish industry.
(2) In the manufacture of artificial leather, silk, pearls, celluloid cements and bronzing liquids.
(3) In the photographic industry, for films and as fuel for the lamp used as a photometric standard.
(4) In the manufacture of artificial glass.
(5) In the straw hat industry as a constituent of the lacquer and of the stiffening solutions (Kruger, 1932).
(6) In furniture polishes, for improving the odour (Zangger, 1930).
(7) As a flavouring for fruit essences etc.
(8) In the textile industry for dry printing.

BIOCHEMISTRY

Estimation

In the atmosphere

(*1*) *By the colorimetric method* of Korenmann (1932), based on the production of a pink-violet-red colour on addition of furfural and concentrated H_2SO_4.

(*2*) *By reaction with p-dimethyl amino benzaldehyde* (Custance and Higgins, 1949). This method is stated to be accurate up to 10 p.p.m.

TOXICOLOGY

Amyl acetate is primarily an irritant, but also to some extent a narcotic, and though some cumulative systemic effect has been indicated in animal experiments in the form of liver injury, such experience has not of recent years been reported in human beings. This fact tends to confirm the statement by Fassett (1963) that many of these earlier reports of systemic injury may have been due to impurities in the amyl acetate which are no longer present, and also, especially in the lacquer trade, to the improvement in methods of spray painting in ventilated booths. It is also more than possible that some of the slighter disorders of health occasionally reported in industrial workers are due to exposure to other constituents of the solvent of which amyl acetate is only one. The only fatal case alleged to have occurred during the use of amyl acetate was a case in point (Crecelius, 1930); exposure to amyl acetate was certainly not exclusive.

Toxicity to animals

(1) Acute

(a) Lethal dose. – Most investigators from Koelsch (1912), Lehmann (1913), Smyth (1925) to Flury and Wirth (1934) have considered that even high concentrations of amyl acetate are not immediately fatal to animals. Smyth and Smyth found that mice tolerated inhalation of 1000 p.p.m. for 2 to 3 h without ill-effects, and Flury and Wirth that they recovered a day following exposure to concentrations which they calculated to be about 10,500 p.p.m., while Lehmann observed no deaths in animals even after exposure to 5000 p.p.m., Patty, Yant and Schrenk (1936) however considered it dangerous to life after 5 h exposure to 10,000 p.p.m.

(b) Narcotic dose. – Flury and Wirth (1934) found amyl acetate more strongly narcotic to mice than did Lehmann (1913); they found that deep narcosis was produced by exposure for 4–6 h to 3800 p.p.m., while Lehmann found 9 hours' exposure to 4600 p.p.m. necessary. Koelsch (1912) observed that 4000 p.p.m. produced complete loss of reflexes in rabbits, within an hour.

Bibliography on p. 591

(2) Chronic

Reports of the effects of repeated inhalation of concentrations too low to cause narcosis have not been in complete agreement by different observers. According to Lehmann, guinea pigs and one rabbit, after 237 and 340 days' exposure respectively, to doses which he calculated might be as high as 7000 p.p.m. and which did eventually produce narcosis, showed loss of weight and appetite; at 1900 p.p.m. only lassitude, and no marked cerebral disturbance.

In an investigation by the Pennsylvania Department of Labor and Industry in 1926, 36 3-hourly exposures to 500 and 1000 p.p.m. were followed by albuminuria which was interpreted as damage to the kidneys.

During a recent investigation of the possible effect on the heart of rabbits, as estimated by electrocardiogram (see below), Inserra et al. (1962) found no modifications significant of poisoning and no pathological abnormalities of the heart after exposure 3 h daily for 2 months to 7500 p.p.m.

SYMPTOMS OF INTOXICATION

With maximal doses (actual concentrations not estimated) Koelsch (1912) found that after 5 min the animals showed spasmodic movements, slow respiration and salivation, and Lehmann (1913) noted in cats and rabbits at 900 p.p.m. some irritation of eyes and nose and at 5000 p.p.m. lassitude but no cerebral disturbance. In some animals Flury and Wirth noted diarrhoea and albuminuria.

CHANGES IN THE ORGANISM

The lungs, brain, liver and kidneys, in the investigation of Patty, Schrenk and Yant (1936) showed congestion, and Koelsch (1912), using high but not quantitatively estimated concentrations, observed oedema of the lungs and pneumonia, also some fatty degeneration of the liver. Injury of the liver has also been reported by Vernetti Blina (1933) in guinea pigs exposed to lethal concentrations – diffuse hepatosis. In rabbits with subacute poisoning similar changes in the liver were present as well as congestion and hypertrophy of the spleen and congestion of the kidney, with degenerative and reparative changes in the tubular epithelium.

Effect on the heart

As noted above (Chronic effects), there was no significant evidence of injury to the heart in animals subjected to repeated inhalation of 7500 p.p.m. by Inserra et al. (1962).

When the amyl acetate was administered on a mask in a dosage of 5 ml which caused somnolence, bradycardia was observed after a few minutes, the pulse rate falling from 170 to 47, but becoming normal rapidly when exposure ceased. The electrocardiogram indicated a sinus block similar to that caused by other solvents such as trichloroethylene, and the rapid recovery suggested that the disturbance was functional, due to stimulation of and inhibition by the vagus.

A further investigation by Inserra *et al.* which included injection of adrenalin before administration of amyl acetate and also section of the vagus, led them to conclude that the apparent parasympathetic action of amyl acetate is due to vagal stimulation most probably of central origin.

Inflammation of the trachea, bronchi and lungs and an increased fat content of the liver were reported by Flury and Wirth (1934).

Toxicity to human beings

Irritation of mucous membranes has been the chief effect observed from personal or voluntary exposure. Koelsch (1912) noted in himself a sensation of heat, giddiness, slight drowsiness, fatigue, rapid breathing and increased pulse rate, and a cough which was still present a month after a short inhalation.

Lehmann (1913) examined the results of inhalation by two healthy men of 900 p.p.m. for half an hour. The initial effect was irritation of the throat, causing cough, later, irritation of the conjuctiva and marked nasal secretion with dryness of the throat. Apart from slight fatigue, no other symptoms were observed – there was no headache and the pulse rate was normal.

In industrial use reports of ill-effect have been variable, but the evidence for a systemic effect of amyl acetate alone is slight; most of the symptoms complained of by workers have arisen where amyl acetate was used in conjuntion with other solvents. Only one fatal case of 'injury due to amyl acetate' has been recorded (Crecelius, 1930) in a worker using a lacquer consisting of a solution of cellulose in acetone, amyl acetate and ether; death was stated to be due to oedema of the glottis caused by injury of the laryngeal mucous membrane.

Relatively slight disturbances of health have been reported by a number of observers, but denied by others.

Nervous disturbances, in the form of headache, drowsiness, palpitation and excessive fatigue were reported by Koelsch (1912) in workers in a hat factory, and headache was one of the symptoms, as well as eye injury, described by Kruger (1932) in the same industry, while Hamilton (1925) noted occasional drowsiness, fatigue and vague nervousness in aeroplane doping during the First World War, but she did not believe that any organic disturbance was caused by the exposure to amyl acetate. One complaint of headache was made to Home Office of Great Britain in 1931 – a girl employed in lacquering fountain pens.

On the other hand Dr. Bridge, Senior Medical Inspector of Factories, in 1929 examined a large number of workers in a cold lacquer factory where there was a smell of amyl acetate and found no injury to health beyond occasional complaints of sore throat and eye irritation when beginning work.

Gastro-intestinal disturbance. – Symptoms of loss of appetite, loss of weight, a sensation of fulness, eructations and dyspepsia were described by Baader (1933) as

Bibliography on p. 591

the chief manifestation in men using a lacquer of which amyl acetate was the chief constituent, and Holstein (1935) has also stated that gastro-intestinal disturbance does occur.

Liver injury. – The only report incriminating amyl acetate as the cause of liver injury during its industrial use is that of Burger and Stockman (1932). This was a girl who had been working with amyl acetate for 3 months and who showed urobilinuria which decreased considerably after removal from exposure. These observers also noted urobilinuria in workers using mixtures of alcohols and acetates.

Anaemia. – Hamilton (1925) did not consider anaemia a consequence of exposure to amyl acetate but Baader (1933) did record secondary anaemia as one of his findings in a group of Zaponlack workers.

Effect on the skin. – Amyl acetate is not a predominant producer of dermatitis, but Baldi (1953) states that contact with the liquid has a degreasing effect, with a drying action which diminishes the defence reaction and predisposes to dermatitis.

Effect of high environmental temperatures. – While at ordinary temperatures amyl acetate has no effect on the vaso-motor system, it has been suggested (Dautrebande *et al.*, 1935) that if the temperature of the workshop is raised, as in spray painting where rapid drying is essential, vaso-motor paralysis may occur within a very short time. On the other hand, no evidence of ill-health was observed in an investigation in 1931 by the Home Office of Great Britain of a workshop where artificial pearls were being made and where the temperature was 67 °F (19 °C).

84. Benzyl Acetate

Structural formula:
$$CH_3-\overset{\overset{\displaystyle O}{\|}}{C}-O-CH_2-\bigcirc$$

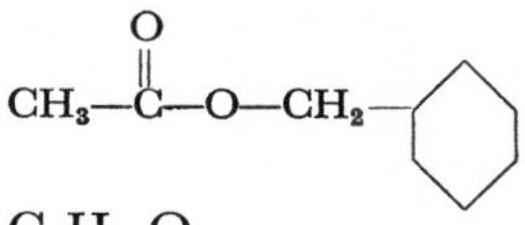

Molecular formula: $C_9H_{10}O_2$

Molecular weight: 150.17

Properties: a colourless liquid with a strong pleasant odour reminiscent of jasmine.

boiling point: 216 °C

melting point: —51.5 °C

vapour pressure: 1.9 mm Hg at 60 °C

vapour density (air = 1): 5.2

specific gravity (liquid density): 1.057

flash point: 216 °F

conversion factors: 1 p.p.m. = 6.13 mg/m³

   1 mg/l = 163 p.p.m.

solubility: insoluble in water. Miscible with aromatic and petroleum hydrocarbons and most other solvents. Excellent solvent for ester gums, copal esters, benzyl abietate, cumarone, mastic, castor and linseed oils, and, with alcohols, for glyceryl phthalate resins.

evaporation rate (ether = 1): 393

maximum allowable concentration: not established.

The commercial preparation used by Flury and Wirth (1934) in their animal experiments had a boiling point of 212–214 °C.

ECONOMY, SOURCES AND USES

Production

(1) By esterification of benzyl alcohol with acetic acid.

(2) By the action of anhydrous sodium acetate on benzyl chloride (Durrans, 1950).

Industrial uses

(1) In the lacquer industry.

(2) In the perfume industry (Herold, 1931).

BIOCHEMISTRY

Metabolism

Benzyl acetate is absorbed by the lungs, the gastro-intestinal tract and the skin, as shown by the fact that application to the skin of animals has caused death. According to Snapper et al. (1925) it is hydrolysed in the body, the benzyl radical being rapidly oxidised to benzoic acid, then conjugated with glycine and excreted almost entirely as hippuric acid.

TOXICOLOGY

The vapour is irritant, more so, according to Lehmann and Flury (1943) than ethyl, propyl, n-butyl, or isoamyl acetate, and moderately narcotic to animals, but repeated inhalation of a saturated air mixture has proved highly toxic to mice, though cats tolerated it well. Oral, subcutaneous and intraperitoneal administration has caused central nervous paralysis in rabbits, and oral administration diuresis. Repeated exposure to its vapour has caused albuminuria, which Flury and Wirth (1934) and Gruber (1924) considered to be an indication of kidney injury.

Toxicity to animals

(1) Acute

Lethal dose. – (i) By oral administration, for rabbits, 4–5 g/kg; for rats, 3.69 g/kg (Graham and Kuizenger, 1945). – (ii) By subcutaneous injection, for guinea pigs, 3.5 g/kg. – (iii) By inhalation, for mice, 212 p.p.m. (von Oettingen, 1960). Cats, rabbits and guinea pigs withstood exposure to 163 p.p.m. without any ill-effects.

(2) Chronic

Cats exposed for $7\frac{1}{2}$ to 10 h for 7 days to 80–245 p.p.m. showed immediate irritation of eyes, and nose with diarrhoea, but soon developed tolerance. Towards the end of the exposure time they became drowsy and apathetic with slight tremor and slow superficial respiration. The urine contained albumen.

CHANGES IN THE ORGANISM

Animals subjected to lethal oral dosage showed slight oedema of the lungs.

Animals killed after repeated inhalation showed slight tracheitis and bronchitis, the kidneys some hyperaemia (Müller, 1932). The blood picture was that of a shift to the left.

Toxicity to human beings

No injury, either accidental or industrial, as been reported, but Zernik (1933) has suggested that care should be taken if a spray process is used, since the concentration of benzyl acetate in such a form is liable to cause more severe irritation.

85. Hexyl Acetate

Structural formula:

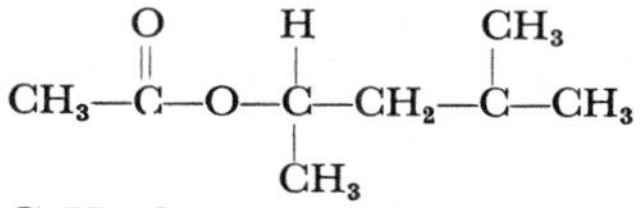

$$CH_3-\underset{\underset{O}{\parallel}}{C}-O-\underset{\underset{CH_3}{\mid}}{\overset{\overset{H}{\mid}}{C}}-CH_2-\underset{\overset{CH_3}{\mid}}{C}-CH_3$$

Molecular formula: $C_8H_{15}O_2$

Molecular weight: 144

Properties: Hexyl acetate exists in the form of several isomers (*sec.*–4-methyl pentyl; 2-methyl amyl, 1.3-dimethyl butyl(methyl) with boiling points ranging from 146–156 °C.

    melting point: 140–147 °C

    vapour pressure: approximately 3.8 mm Hg

    specific gravity (liquid density): 0.857–0.881

    flash point: 110–113 °F

The commercial product has a boiling range of 136–146 °C; specific gravity: 0.875–0.881 and flash point: 113 °F. They are colourless mobile liquids with a characteristic pleasant odour.

    conversion factors: 1 p.p.m. = 5.9 mg/m³

                 1 mg/l = 170 p.p.m.

    solubility: soluble in water 0.08%. Solvents for cellulose nitrate and most gums, but not for cellulose acetate or shellac (Durrans, 1950).

    maximum allowable concentration: not established. (ACGIH, 1965 recommend 50 p.p.m. for *sec.*-hexylacetate.)

ECONOMY, SOURCES AND USES

Industrial uses

In the lacquer industry (Park and Hopkins, 1930).

TOXICOLOGY

None of the isomers is highly toxic; animals tolerate relatively large doses both by mouth and by inhalation of the vapour. There appears to be some absorption from the skin (Smyth *et al.*, 1954) but direct application to the skin and eyes causes only moderate irritation. Nor does *sec*.-hexyl acetate affect the throat of human beings as severely as do other acetates, and there are no reports of systemic injury by any of the compounds (von Oettingen, 1960).

Toxicity to animals

Two of the isomers tested for toxicity to rats by Smyth *et al.* (1954), the 1,3-dimethyl butyl (methyl amyl acetate) and the 2-methyl amyl, have an oral LD_{50} of 6.16 and 7.40 g/kg respectively and the latter an inhalation lethal dose of 4000 p.p.m. for 4 h in 2 out of 6 animals.

Cutaneous application to rabbits greater than 20,000 mg/kg caused death after 14 days in half the animals.

Toxicity to human beings

There are no reports of systemic injury by any of the compounds (von Oettingen, 1960) and, according to Park and Hopkins (1930) *sec*.–hexyl acetate is not so severely irritant to the throat as other acetates.

86. Vinyl Acetate

Structural formula: $CH_3-\overset{\overset{\text{O}}{\|}}{C}-O-\overset{\overset{\text{H}}{}}{C}=CH_2$

Molecular formula: $C_4H_6O_2$

Molecular weight: 86.09

Properties: A colourless liquid which polymerises on exposure to light, forming a solid resin.

    boiling point: 73 °C
    melting point: < —84 °C
    vapour pressure: 115 mm at 25 °C
    vapour density (air = 1): 3.0
    specific gravity (liquid density): 0.9342
    flash point: —8 °F
    conversion factors: 1 p.p.m. = 3.5 mg/m³
                       1 mg/l = 284 p.p.m.
    solubility: in water, 2 parts per 100 at 20 °C. Miscible with alcohol and ether.
    maximum allowable concentration: not established.

ECONOMY, SOURCES AND USES

Production

By reaction of acetic acid with acetylene in presence of a catalyst such as salts of mercury, cadmium, lead or zinc.

Industrial uses

In the plastics industry vinyl acetate resins are important in films and coatings and as binders in lacquers (Malten and Zielhuis, 1964).

TOXICOLOGY

Vinyl acetate is to some extent a skin irritant and sensitiser, and from experiments on animals appears to be absorbed by application to the skin. There are no reports of any systemic intoxication in human beings (von Oettingen, 1960), but skin sensitisation and actual dermatoses from vinyl acetate resins, especially if not fully polymerised, have been observed.

Toxicity to animals

Acute

   Lethal dose. LD$_{50}$. – *(i) By oral administration*, for rats, 2920 mg/kg (Carpenter *et al.*, 1949). – *(ii) By skin application*, for rabbits, 2500 ml/kg. – *(iii) By inhalation*, for rats, 4000 p.p.m. for 4 h (Carpenter *et al.*, 1949).

SYMPTOMS OF INTOXICATION

Slight skin irritation, similar to that of acetone. Slight eye irritation.

Toxicity to human beings

Skin sensitisation due to garters, suspenders and a wrist watch strap with a coating of vinyl acetate resin has been described by Zeisler (1940) and to adhesives used in the construction of parquet floors by Raymond (1959). Dermatoses due to the use of these resins especially if not fully polymerised have been observed by Gunther (1956). Otherwise, no toxic effects of vinyl acetate have ever been reported. It is apparently a relatively non-toxic material.

87. Cyclohexyl Acetate

Synonyms: Adronal acetate; Hexalin acetate

Structural formula:

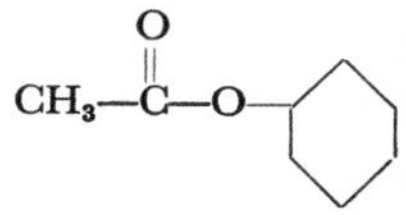

$$CH_3-\overset{\overset{\textstyle O}{\|}}{C}-O-\bigcirc$$

Molecular formula: $C_8H_{14}O_2$

Molecular weight: 142.1

Properties: a neutral colourless oily liquid with a strong fruity odour resembling amyl acetate.

Technical product:
    boiling point: 170–177 °C
    vapour pressure: 7 mm Hg at 30 °C
    vapour density (air = 1): 4.9
    specific gravity (liquid density): approx. 0.96
    flash point: 136 °F
    conversion factors: 1 p.p.m. = 5.8 mg/m³
                       1 mg/l   = 172 p.p.m.
    solubility: a powerful solvent for cellulose nitrate, other cellulose esters and many resins and gums and collodion cotton.
    evaporation rate (ether = 1): 77
    maximum allowable concentration: not established.

ECONOMY, SOURCES AND USES

Production
By direct esterification of cyclohexanol (Durrans, 1950).

Industrial uses
(1) In the lacquer industry, sometimes in combination with lacquers of collodion cotton and drying oils.

(2) In the textile industry, as a substitute for amyl acetate (Clayton and Clark, 1931).

(3) In the leather industry, for improving the adhesion of leather varnishes.
(4) In the waterproof industry.

TOXICOLOGY

Cyclohexyl acetate is more narcotic (3 times more potent than amyl acetate) and more lethal to animals at lower concentrations than other acetates, but being of lower volatility it is less hazardous from the industrial point of view. It is also an irritant; animals acutely intoxicated have shown severe irritation of the respiratory tract and congestion of liver and kidneys.

Some irritation of the eyes has been experienced by human subjects, but there are no reports of injury from its industrial use.

Toxicity to animals

(1) Acute
(a) Lethal dose. – (i) By subcutaneous injection, for cats, 7.5 g/kg. – (ii) By inhalation, 9461 p.p.m. (Flury, Klimmer and Rösser, 1937).
(b) Narcotic dose. – (i) Light narcosis, for cats, 1550 p.p.m. (Lehmann, 1913). – (ii) Deep narcosis, 1700 p.p.m. after 10 h.

(2) Chronic
In cats and dogs low exposures (up to 516–637 p.p.m.) 8 h daily for 30 days caused no toxic symptoms; 1020–1630 p.p.m. for 5 consecutive days caused moderate irritation of mucous membranes, fatigue and drowsiness but with complete recovery.

SYMPTOMS OF INTOXICATION

Irritation of eyes and nose, restlessness, tremors, convulsions, incoordination followed by narcosis, if deep usually fatal. In mice, subcutaneous injection was followed by dyspnoea and paralysis (Flury et al., 1937).

CHANGES IN THE ORGANISM

Tracheitis, bronchitis, oedema of the lungs, hyperaemia of liver and kidneys.

Toxicity to human beings

Exposure to 516 p.p.m. (Lehmann, 1913) caused some irritation of pharynx, larynx and conjunctiva, and, as the only after-effect, a sweetish taste. There are no reports of injury from its industrial use (von Oettingen, 1960).

88. Methyl Cyclohexyl Acetate

Synonyms: sextate, methyl hexalin acetate

Structural formula:

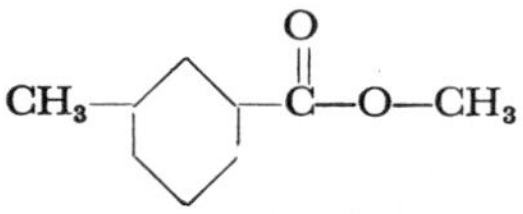

$$CH_3-\overset{}{\bigcirc}-\overset{\displaystyle O}{\overset{\displaystyle \|}{C}}-O-CH_3$$

Molecular formula: $C_9H_{16}O_2$

Molecular weight: 156.11

Properties: a colourless neutral liquid with a strong long-lasting odour. A mixture of three isomeric esters.

According to Clayton and Clark (1931) its evaporation rate is slower than that of cyclohexyl acetate and its action slower; otherwise it is similar in solvent properties, *i.e.* a good solvent for cellulose nitrate, some resins, waxes and bitumen.

Technical product:
  boiling point: 167–171 °C
  vapour density (air = 1): 5.37
  specific gravity (liquid density): 0.941
  flash point: 140 °F
  conversion factors: 1 p.p.m. = 6.4 mg/m³
                    1 mg/l = 156 p.p.m.
  solubility: it is insoluble in water (Lehmann and Flury, (1943)
  maximum allowable concentration: not established

ECONOMY, SOURCES AND USES

Chiefly in the lacquer industry, for automobile lacquers (Deschiens, 1928).

TOXICOLOGY

No animal experiments appear to have been carried out.

The only allusion to any toxic effect from its industrial use is that of Browning (1953) in which workers employed in printing on plastic materials complained of slight drowsiness and irritation of the throat, but in this case, sextate was only one of several constituents of the paint used.

Bibliography on p. 591   [551]

89. Octyl Acetate

Synonym: 2-ethyl hexyl acetate

Structural formula:

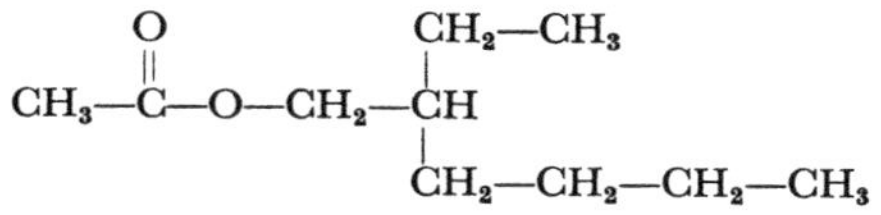

$$CH_3-\overset{\overset{O}{\|}}{C}-O-CH_2-\underset{\underset{CH_2-CH_2-CH_2-CH_3}{|}}{\overset{\overset{CH_2-CH_3}{|}}{CH}}$$

Molecular formula: $C_{10}H_{20}O_2$

Molecular weight: 172.3

Properties: a colourless liquid. Solvent for cellulose nitrate and resins (von Oettingen, 1960).

> *boiling point:* 199 °C
> *melting point:* —93 °C
> *vapour pressure:* 0.4 mm Hg at 20 °C
> *vapour density (air = 1):* 6.0
> *specific gravity (liquid density):* 0.872
> *flash point:* 180 °F
> *conversion factors:* 1 p.p.m. = 7.0 mg/m³
> 1 mg/l = 142 p.p.m.
> *solubility:* in water 0.55 g/100 ml (Fassett, 1963). Miscible with alcohol and ether.
> *maximum allowable concentration:* not established.

ECONOMY, SOURCES AND USES

Industrial uses

In the lacquer industry.

TOXICOLOGY

Octyl acetate is moderately irritant and can be absorbed by the skin of animals. It can be fatal with oral administration but not by inhalation of saturated air-vapour mixtures. No ill effects on human beings have been reported.

Toxicity to animals

Acute

   Lethal dose. – (i) By oral administration, for rats, 3 g/kg. – (ii) By skin application, for guinea pigs, greater than 20,000 µl/kg (Smyth *et al.*, 1954).

   Inhalation of saturated air-vapour mixtures for 15 min was non-lethal to rats (Smyth *et al.*, 1954).

SYMPTOMS OF INTOXICATION

Moderate irritation of skin and eyes (von Oettingen, 1960).

Toxicity to human beings

None have been reported. Von Oettingen (1960) remarks that "in view of its high boiling point and low vapour pressure dangers from inhalation of its vapour are quite remote".

Bibliography on p. 591

90. Ethyl Formate

Synonyms: formic ether, formic acid ethyl ester

Structural formula:

$$\begin{array}{c} \quad\quad O \\ \quad\quad \parallel \\ H-C-O-CH_2-CH_3 \end{array}$$

Molecular formula: $C_3H_6O_2$

Molecular weight: 74.08

Properties: a volatile liquid with an odour resembling acetone. Readily develops acidity in presence of moisture (Durrans, 1950). Rapid solvent for cellulose nitrate and cellulose acetate, giving solutions of low viscosity.

  boiling point: 53–57 °C
  melting point: —80.5 °C
  vapour pressure: 200 mm Hg
  vapour density (air = 1): 2.56
  specific gravity (liquid density): 0.925–0.930
  flash point: —4 °F
  conversion factors: 1 p.p.m. = 3.03 mg/m³
               1 mg/l   = 330 p.p.m.
  solubility: soluble in water to the extent of 9 parts per 100 at 18 °C, with some hydrolysis. Miscible with benzene, alcohol and ether.
  maximum allowable concentration: 100 p.p.m.

ECONOMY, SOURCES AND USES

Produced by esterification of formic acid and ethyl alcohol.

Industrial uses

(1) In the lacquer industry, but not suitable for metal lacquers on account of its tendency to develop acidity in presence of moisture.
(2) In artificial silk manufacture as a solvent for cellulose acetate (Cazeneuve *et al.*, 1932).
(3) In the shoe industry as a constituent of the mixture used to dissolve celluloid for covering heels; according to Duquénois and Revel (1934) the mixture is used boiling.

(4) In the manufacture of safety glass.
(5) As a flavouring agent for lemonade and essences.
(6) As a fungicide and larvicide.

BIOCHEMISTRY

Estimation

In the atmosphere and in tissues as for methyl formate *(q.v.)*.

Metabolism

Ethyl formate is absorbed by the lungs and the gastro-intestinal tract; slight penetration of the skin is said to occur (more than 20 ml/kg is necessary for LD_{50}, Smyth *et al.*, 1954). No investigations of its fate in the body appear to have been carried out.

TOXICOLOGY

While ethyl formate is an irritant of mucous membranes, it has been considered by most authorities as less irritating and less apt to cause respiratory disturbance than methyl formate (Duquénois and Revel, 1934). It is however more strongly narcotic, causing depression of the central nervous system leading to death from circulatory and respiratory failure without the convulsions and coma produced by a lethal dose of methyl formate. There are no reports of toxic effects on human beings except slight irritation of the eyes and nose (Flury and Zernik, 1931) and none from its industrial use, except that of Duquénois and Revel (1934) in which ethyl formate was not the only solvent present in the mixture used.

Toxicity to animals

Acute

Lethal dose. – (i) By oral administration, for rats, 4.29 g/kg (Smyth *et al.*, 1954). – *(ii) By subcutaneous injection*, for rabbits, according to the earlier investigations of Weber (1902) 1 ml/kg was lethal, but Gross (1943) observed no local or general injury from 1.0 ml/kg (Lehmann and Flury, 1943). – *(iii) By inhalation*, for cats, 100,560 p.p.m. after 90 min; for rats, 8000 p.p.m. within 4 h (Smyth *et al.*, 1954). – *(iv) By penetration of skin*, for rabbits, LD_{50} after 14 days, more than 20 ml/kg (Smyth *et al.*, 1954).

SYMPTOMS OF INTOXICATION

Irritation of mucous membranes, severe dyspnoea, staggering, depression of central nervous system, sometimes pneumonia (von Oettingen, 1959). Application

Bibliography on p. 591

to the skin caused only slight irritation, and to the eyes moderate injury of the cornea (Smyth *et al.*, 1954).

CHANGES IN THE ORGANISM

The lungs showed oedema in dogs and in cats exposed to a 'flowing' mixture of air and ethyl formate (concentration 14,000 p.p.m.) (Flury and Zernik, 1931).

Toxicity to human beings

According to Flury and Neumann (1927), 10,500 p.p.m. causes moderate but progressive irritation of the eyes and nose, remaining 4 h after the exposure.

91. Methyl Formate

Synonym: methyl methanoate

Structural formula:

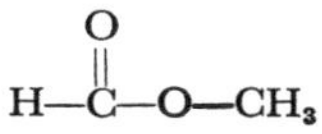

$$H-\overset{\overset{\textstyle O}{\|}}{C}-O-CH_3$$

Molecular formula: $C_2H_4O_2$

Molecular weight: 60.05

Properties: a colourless inflammable liquid with a pleasant ethereal odour.

    boiling point: (pure compound) 31.8 °C

    melting point: —100.4 °C

    vapour pressure: 476.4 mm Hg at 20 °C

    vapour density (air = 1): 2.07

    specific gravity (liquid density): 0.975

    flash point: —2 °F

    conversion factors: 1 p.p.m. = 2.55 mg/m³

                   1 mg/l   = 408 p.p.m.

    solubility: soluble in water 30 parts per 100 at 20 °C. Miscible with ethanol; soluble in methanol. Good solvent for fats, oils, fatty acids, acetyl cellulose, collodion and celluloid (Gnamm, 1943).

    maximum allowable concentration: 100 p.p.m.

ECONOMY, SOURCES AND USES

Production

By esterification of formic acid and ethyl alcohol.

Industrial uses

(1) As a solvent for ethyl cellulose.

(2) As an insecticide and fumigant.

(3) As an chemical intermediate.

(4) As a high-boiling refrigerant for household appliances (Jacobs, 1941).

BIOCHEMISTRY

Estimation

(1) In the atmosphere

(a) By means of air-equilibrated charcoal to absorb the vapour from a measured volume of the vapour-air mixture and determination of the gain in weight, the soda lime being removed from the adsorption train since this would cause hydrolysis of the methyl formate (Schrenk *et al.*, 1936).

(b) By absorption on silica gel, with hydrolysis with standard alkali and titration with standard acid (Fairhall, 1957).

(c) By hydrolysis and precipitation of silver formate from a neutral solution of silver nitrate (Fairhall, 1957).

(2) In tissues

Gettler and Siegel (1955) described a method by means of a specially constructed distillation apparatus and a micro-rectification flask; the isolated volatile liquids were identified by micro-determination of their boiling points. Gettler (1940) applied this method to the distillate from 600 g of brain from a child fatally poisoned by methyl formate applied to the scalp. The total quantity of methyl formate in the brain and liver was calculated from the methyl alcohol content after hydrolysis.

Metabolism

Absorption takes place usually through the lungs but it can be absorbed also by the gastro-intestinal tract and the skin. It hydrolyses appreciably in body fluids, producing methyl alcohol and formic acid (Gettler, 1940). Ciaranfi (1940) showed that the formic acid fraction is oxidised by liver and striated muscle, but not by slices of kidney; the methanol fraction remained intact.

According to Duquénois and Revel (1934) small amounts of methyl formate itself may be found in the blood of animals killed by inhalation of its vapour, and Kendal and Ramanathan (1952) found that methyl formate can be formed in the body from methanol and formaldehyde by the action of liver alcohol dehydrogenase, and suggested that because of the preferential fat solubility of methyl formate it might be responsible for the toxic effects of methanol in the eye.

Since animals killed by methyl formate present a symptomatic picture similar to that of formic acid (convulsions and coma) rather than that of the central nervous depressant action of the higher homologues, it appears that the greater tendency to hydrolysis of the molecule of methyl formate may be responsible for its more toxic effects than, for example, ethyl formate.

TOXICOLOGY

Methyl formate is an irritant, and gives some warning of its presence, but owing to its pleasant odour and the occurrence of olfactory fatigue Schrenk et al. (1936) state that it is doubtful whether the odour will serve as an effective warning of harmful conditions of exposure, and that the possibility of an explosive hazard should be recognised – the lower limit of inflammability is about 5% (Jones et al., 1933).

It is also to some extent narcotic, but according to Elkins (1959) this action is less than that of some other esters owing to its readier hydrolysis. Von Oettingen (1959) is of the opinion that methyl formate is definitely the most hazardous of the aliphatic esters. Nevertheless there have been no reports of injury from its industrial use as the sole solvent, and only one fatal case from its use as a skin application against pediculosis.

Toxicity to animals

Acute

Lethal dose. – By inhalation, for guinea pigs (Schrenk et al., 1936), 50,000 p.p.m. for 30 min; 25,000 p.p.m. for 60 min; 10,000 p.p.m. for 2 to 3 h. Lehmann and Flury (1943) give 10,200 for 2–3 h. Maximum concentration without disturbance, for one hour 2000 p.p.m., for 2–3 h 1500–2000 p.p.m.

SYMPTOMS OF INTOXICATION

Irritation of eyes and nose, retching movements, incoordination, convulsions and coma followed by death.

CHANGES IN THE ORGANISM

Following lethal dosage the lungs showed the most marked toxic effects – congestion and oedema. The liver, kidneys and surface vessels of the brain and adrenals also showed congestion. With non-lethal concentrations these findings were present but to a much less extent; they were not found in animals exposed for 30 to 60 min to 3500 p.p.m. nor for 3 to 8 hours to 1500 p.p.m.

Toxicity to human beings

According to Schrenk et al. (1936) men exposed for 1 min to 1500 p.p.m. of the vapour in air noticed the odour of methyl formate but no irritation of the eyes and nose and no other symptoms.

The only report of a possible industrial effect is that of Duquenois and Revel (1934) who noted central nervous symptoms, including some temporary visual disturbance in workers using a mixture of formates and acetates. Since no concentrations were determined and since ethyl formate, ethyl acetate and methyl acetate were also constituents of the solvent mixture, these effects cannot be interpreted as specifically due to methyl formate. It may be noted that Jacobs (1941) states that ethyl, butyl and amyl formate all have a paralysing effect on the central nervous system, and ethyl acetate is known to have a more powerful narcotic action than methyl formate.

An unusual case of death from application of methyl formate to the skin was reported by Gettler in 1940. This was a child aged 19 months who had had one ounce of a liquid insecticide applied to the scalp on a sponge which was left on for 20 min, covered with a tightly fitting cap. When it was removed the child was collapsed, cyanotic and with slow respiration. The pupils were contracted and did not react to light; knee jerks, Babinski and abdominal reflexes were absent and death occurred from circulatory and respiratory failure. At autopsy the internal organs, brain and meninges all showed congestion; the lungs some oedema but no pneumonia.

Analysis of portions of the brain, liver and stomach contents revealed very small amounts of methyl alcohol, but micro-distillation of 600 g of brain substance resulted in the isolation of a volatile liquid with a boiling point of 47.5 °C, and when this was distilled fractionally by means of the special distillation apparatus capillary fractions were obtained with a boiling point and molecular weight corresponding to methyl formate. Two other fractions were evidently mixtures of methyl formate and methyl alcohol, and formic acid was later identified by typical mercurous formate crystals. The total quantity of methyl formate (hydrolysed and unhydrolysed) present in the brain was calculated to be 246.5 mg in 1050 g, and in the liver 97.2 mg in 440 g.

TREATMENT

Cases of acute poisoning by inhalation should be treated by removal to fresh air and rest. Respiratory irritation may be reduced by inhalation of a mist of sodium bicarbonate, 5% solution (von Oettingen, 1959). If pulmonary oedema should develop oxygen should be administered. Contaminated skin should be thoroughly washed with soap and water.

92. n-Butyl Formate

Synonyms: formic acid n-butyl ester, butyl methanate

Structural formula:

$$H-\overset{\overset{\displaystyle O}{\|}}{C}-O-CH_2-CH_2-CH_2-CH_3$$

Molecular formula: $C_5H_{10}O_2$

Molecular weight: 102.13

Properties: a colourless liquid, very slightly soluble in water but miscible with alcohol and ether, castor and linseed oils and hydrocarbons. Solvent for cellulose nitrate and acetate, ester gums, copal ester but not hard copals, coumarone and mastic and partly for shellac (Durrans, 1950).

Commercial product:

    boiling point: 96–110 °C

    melting point: —90 °C

    vapour pressure: 30 mm Hg at 25 °C

    vapour density (air = 1): 3.5

    specific gravity (liquid density): 0.8885

    flash point: 64 °F

    conversion factors: 1 p.p.m. = 4.17 mg/m³

                        1 mg/l = 240 p.p.m.

    maximum allowable concentration: not established

ECONOMY, SOURCES AND USES

Industrial uses

In the lacquer industry, giving a film of high strength but not so efficient as either butyl or amyl acetate in preventing water blush (Durrans, 1950). It may replace methyl acetate or acetone in the proportion of about 3 to 8 (Deschiens, 1930).

BIOCHEMISTRY

Metabolism

It can be absorbed by the lungs and gastro-intestinal tract, but no details of its fate in the body are available.

Bibliography on p. 591

TOXICOLOGY

Butyl formate is primarily an irritant of mucous membranes, including the respiratory tract, but has also some narcotic action in animals; deep narcosis has been produced after one hour's exposure to 10,300 p.p.m. (Flury and Neumann, 1927). This concentration is extremely irritating to the eyes of human beings, but no reports of injury from its industrial use have been reported.

Toxicity to animals

Acute

   (a) *Lethal dose.* – For cats, 10,418 p.p.m. after 70 min (Flury and Neumann, 1927).

   (b) *Narcotic dose.* – For dogs, 10,000 p.p.m. after 20–60 min (Flury and Zernik, 1931).

SYMPTOMS OF INTOXICATION

Irritation of eyes, salivation, vomiting, staggering, somnolence; death from pulmonary oedema.

CHANGES IN THE ORGANISM

In cats following lethal dosage the lungs showed oedema and haemorrhage (Flury and Zernik, 1931).

Toxicity to human beings

According to Flury and Neumann (1927) concentrations of 10,300 p.p.m. cause immediate severe irritation of the eyes, with blepharospasm, becoming intolerable within one minute.

93. Amyl Formate

Synonym: formic acid amyl ester

Structural formula:

$$\underset{\text{H}-\text{C}-\text{O}-\text{CH}_2-\text{CH}_2-\text{CH}_2-\text{CH}_2-\text{CH}_3}{\overset{\overset{\text{O}}{\|}}{}}$$

Molecular formula: $C_6H_{12}O_2$

Molecular weight: 116.16

Properties: a colourless liquid with an odour suggestive of leather. It consists chiefly of two isomers, *n*-amyl and isoamyl, the latter being the main constituent of the technical product. It is slightly soluble in water; miscible with alcohol and ether.

n-Amyl formate
    boiling point: 130.4 °C
    melting point: —73.5 °C
    vapour pressure: 9.6 mm Hg at 25 °C
    vapour density (air = 1): 4.0
    specific gravity (liquid density): 0.8926
    flash point: 79 °F
    conversion factors: 1 p.p.m. = 4.74 mg/m³
                       1 mg/l = 211 p.p.m.
    solubility: soluble in water 3 parts per 100 at 22 °C (von Oettingen, 1959).
    maximum allowable concentration: not established

Isoamyl formate
    boiling point: 123–124 °C
    specific gravity: 0.882 (Durrans, 1950).

The technical product is a good solvent for cellulose nitrate, colophony, ester gums, copal gums, raw rubber and mastic, and, in the presence of alcohol, glycerylphthalate. Solutions of cellulose nitrate in amyl formate are slightly less viscous than those of corresponding concentrations in butyl acetate.

ECONOMY, SOURCES AND USES

(1) In the manufacture of leather cloth, as a substitute for butyl acetate. It has been suggested as a substitute for amyl acetate, but according to Lehmann (1913)

it should not be so regarded on account of its greater narcotic potency and higher volatility.

(2) In the manufacture of safety glass.

TOXICOLOGY

According to Lehmann (1913) amyl formate is about twice as volatile as amyl acetate, and has a narcotic effect at a concentration of about one-third that of amyl acetate, while Flury and Zernik (1931) considered that its irritant effect is similar to that of amyl acetate.

Toxicity to animals

The only experiments on its toxic effects in animals are those carried out by Lehmann in 1913 and he gives no detailed description of the concentrations used, but, as mentioned above considered its narcotic effects more potent than that of amyl acetate.

Toxicity to human beings

There are no reports, either accidental or industrial, of any injury to human beings.

94. Cyclohexyl Formate

Structural formula:

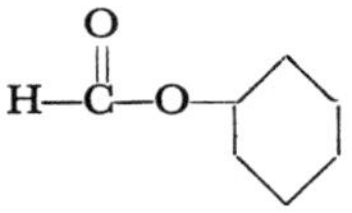

$$\underset{\text{H}}{\text{H}}-\overset{\displaystyle \text{O}}{\underset{\displaystyle \|}{\text{C}}}-\text{O}-\bigcirc$$

Molecular formula: $C_7H_{12}O_2$

Molecular weight: 128.10

Properties: a colourless liquid.
  boiling point: 162.5 °C
  vapour density (air = 1): 4.4
  specific gravity (liquid density): 1.010
  flash point: 123.8 °F
  conversion factors: 1 p.p.m. = 5.24 mg/m³
              1 mg/l = 191 p.p.m.
  solubility: a high boiling solvent for nitrocellulose
  maximum allowable concentration: not established

ECONOMY, SOURCES AND USES

Industrial uses

Cyclohexyl formate is not of great industrial importance except for its use as a solvent of nitrocellulose (Gnamm, 1943).

TOXICOLOGY

Although no detailed investigations of its toxicity to animals have been carried out, Lehmann (1913) stated that it has approximately the same degree of toxicity as cyclohexyl acetate, and Gross (cited by Lehmann and Flury, 1943) that it has a nature and intensity of effect similar to that of amyl acetate.

There have been no reports of any injury in human beings from its use (von Oettingen, 1959).

Bibliography on p. 591   [565]

95. Methyl Cyclohexyl Formate

Structural formula:

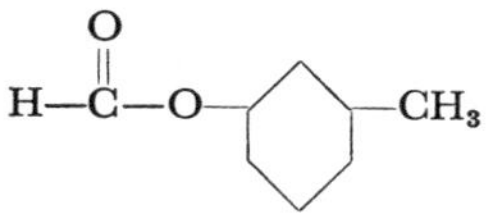

$$H-\overset{\displaystyle O}{\overset{\|}{C}}-O-\langle\text{cyclohexyl}\rangle-CH_3$$

Molecular formula: $C_7H_{14}O_2$

Molecular weight: 142.12

Properties: a colourless liquid. Solvent for nitrocellulose.
    boiling point: 176–180 °C
    vapour density (air = 1): 4.9
    specific gravity (liquid density): 0.957
    flash point: 64 °F
    conversion factors: 1 p.p.m. = 5.81 mg/m³
                      1 mg/l = 172 p.p.m.
    maximum allowable concentration: not established

TOXICOLOGY

Few details are available, but according to Lehmann and Flury (1943) its toxicity is about the same as that of amyl acetate. No cases of injury from its industrial use are known. It is of only moderate industrial importance.

96. Benzyl Formate

Structural formula:

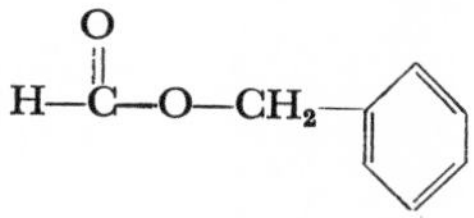

$$H-\overset{\overset{\textstyle O}{\|}}{C}-O-CH_2-\bigcirc$$

Molecular formula: $C_8H_8O_2$

Molecular weight: 136.14

Properties: a colourless liquid with an odour less pronounced than that of benzyl acetate, but suggestive of leather.

    boiling point: 203.4 °C

    melting point: 3.6 °C

    vapour pressure: 10 mm Hg at 84 °C (Fassett, 1963)

    vapour density (air = 1): 4.7

    specific gravity (liquid density): 1.081

    conversion factors: 1 p.p.m. = 5.56 mg/m³

                      1 mg/l = 180 p.p.m.

    solubility: very slightly soluble in water, miscible with castor and linseed oils, and aromatic and petroleum hydrocarbons (Durrans, 1950). Good solvent for cellulose acetate and nitrate, ester gum, copal ester, benzyl abietate, glyceryl phthalate resins and cumarone.

ECONOMY, SOURCES AND USES

Industrial uses

To a small extent in the lacquer industry.

TOXICOLOGY

No studies of its toxic effects in animals have been made and there have been no reports of any injurous effects in human beings (von Oettingen, 1959). Durrans (1950) states that it is non-toxic, but gives no evidence in support of his statement.

97. Ethyl Lactate

Synonyms: eusolvan, actylol, solactol

Structural formula:

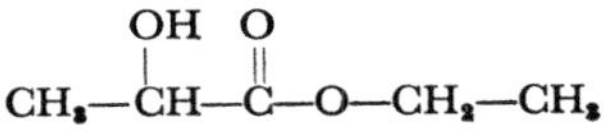

$$\underset{\text{CH}_3-\text{CH}-\text{C}-\text{O}-\text{CH}_2-\text{CH}_3}{\overset{\overset{\displaystyle\text{OH}\ \ \text{O}}{|\ \ \ \ \ \|}}{}}$$

Molecular formula: $C_5H_{10}O_2$

Molecular weight: 118.13

Properties: an almost colourless liquid when pure; the technical product has a faint odour resembling that of ethyl butyrate. An exceptionally good solvent for cellulose nitrate and acetate, also for many resins, basic dyes and for hard copals with prolonged boiling.

    boiling point: 154 °C
    melting point: —25 °C
    vapour pressure: 5 mm Hg at 30 °C
    vapour density (air = 1): 4.1
    specific gravity (liquid density): 1.031
    flash point: 115 °F
    conversion factors: 1 p.p.m. = 4.8 mg/m³
                        1 mg/l = 207 p.p.m.
    solubility: very soluble in water, miscible with gasoline
    maximum allowable concentration: not established

ECONOMY, SOURCES AND USES

Production

(1) By esterification of lactic acid obtained from fermentation of sugar solutions with *Bacterium acidi-lactici*.

(2) Synthetically, by combination of acetaldehyde with hydrocyanic acid to form acetaldehyde cyanhydrin, followed by treatment with alcohol and HCl or H_2SO_4, and purified by fractional distillation (Durrans, 1950).

Industrial uses

(1) In the lacquer industry, especially where large amounts of diluent are desired,

and, in conjunction with phthalic anhydride, for producing frosted effects in lacquers.

(2) In the manufacture of safety glass.

TOXICOLOGY

Although ethyl lactate is generally considered a relatively harmless solvent in industrial use, it has been shown to have a potent narcotic effect in animals, leading with large doses to respiratory failure.

Toxicity to animals

According to Lewin (1929) ethyl lactate is narcotic and lethal to animals in high concentrations (actual levels not stated) causing respiratory paralysis.

Toxicity to human beings

Lewin (1929) states that it is narcotic to human beings in high concentrations but other authorities, including Yarsley (1933) and Zangger (1930) emphasise its relative harmlessness. Zangger includes it in his Group I of solvents described as 'relatively non-toxic'.

Bibliography on p. 591

98. Butyl Lactate

Synonym: Butacol

Structural formula:

$$CH_3—\overset{\overset{\displaystyle OH}{|}}{CH}—\overset{\overset{\displaystyle O}{\|}}{C}—O—CH_2—CH_2—CH_2—CH_3$$

Molecular formula: $C_7H_{14}O_3$

Molecular weight: 146.15

Properties: Butyl lactate exists in three isomers: *n-,* iso-and *sec-. n-*Butyl lactate is a colourless odourless liquid when pure; the technical product is often slightly brown. It has a low volatility – ten times less than amyl acetate, according to Lehmann and Flury (1943). A good solvent for ester gum, cellulose nitrate, ethyl cellulose and cumarone; less so for cellulose acetate, rubber chloride, copal ester, benzyl abietate, shellac and mastic (Durrans, 1950).

> *boiling point:* 155–195 °C
> *melting point:* —43.0 °C
> *vapour pressure:* 0.4 mm Hg at 20 °C
> *vapour density (air = 1):* 5.04
> *specific gravity (liquid density):* 0.980
> *flash point:* 160 °F
> *conversion factors:* 1 p.p.m. = 5.9 mg/m³
>   1 mg/l = 168 p.p.m.
> *solubility:* in water 3.4 g/100 ml. Miscible with castor and linseed oils and hydrocarbons.
> *evaporation rate (ether = 1):* 443
> *maximum allowable concentration:* not established.

Isobutyl lactate evaporates somewhat more rapidly and has a boiling point of 168–200 °C.

*sec.–*Butyl lactate has a faint fruity odour, is almost insoluble in water and has a boiling point of 180 °C and specific gravity of 0.974.

ECONOMY, SOURCES AND USES

Production

By direct esterification of lactic acid with butyl alcohol.

Industrial uses

In the paint and varnish industry; it tends to prevent the formation of a skin on oil varnishes and paints (Durrans, 1950).

TOXICOLOGY

By subcutaneous injection butyl lactate is narcotic to animals, with severe, even fatal effects, causing death delayed for 24 hours, but its toxicity by this route (the only one tested) is stated to be less than that of most alcohols and glycol ethers (Lehmann and Flury, 1943).

There are no reports of injury from its industrial use.

Toxicity to animals

Acute

Lethal dose. – By subcutaneous injection, for mice, 11–12 mg/g (Lehmann and Flury, 1943).

SYMPTOMS OF INTOXICATION

At 5 mg/g no toxic effects; at 10 mg/g giddiness, dyspnoea and prostration after 18 min followed by recovery. At 11 mg/g giddiness and prostration after 1 hour and eath after 25 hours. At 12 mg/g dyspnoea, paralysis of hind limbs and prostration after 25 min, loss of reflexes and death after $3\frac{1}{2}$ h.

There are no reports of ill-effects from its industrial use.

Bibliography on p. 591

99. Ethyl Propionate

Synonym: propionic ether

Structural formula:

$$CH_3-CH_2-\overset{\overset{\displaystyle O}{\|}}{C}-O-CH_2-CH_3$$

Molecular formula: $C_5H_{10}O_2$

Molecular weight: 102.13

Properties: a colourless liquid with a pineapple-like odour. Will react vigorously with oxidising materials and with heat or flame (Sax, 1957).

    boiling point: 99 °C
    melting point: —73.1 °C
    vapour pressure: 40 mm Hg at 27 °C
    vapour density (air = 1): 3.5
    specific gravity (liquid density): 0.891
    flash point: 12 °F (Fassett, 1963)
    conversion factors: 1 p.p.m. = 4.1 mg/m³
                      1 mg/l = 246 p.p.m.
    solubility: in water 2.4 g/100 ml
    maximum allowable concentration: not established

ECONOMY, SOURCES AND USES

Industrial uses

In the lacquer and perfume industries.

BIOCHEMISTRY

According to Fasset (1963) ethyl propionate may be converted in the body to propionic acid in amounts tending to produce acidosis.

TOXICOLOGY

In animals large oral doses may be lethal, with symptoms which may represent acidosis. No industrial injury has been reported.

Toxicity to animals

Acute

    Lethal dose. – By oral administration, for rabbits, LD_{50}, 3.2–3.95 g/kg, according to Treon *et al.* (1949) who state that it has only one-tenth to one-thirteenth the toxicity of the corresponding acrylate.

SYMPTOMS OF INTOXICATION

Ataxia, gasping respiration, hypothermia.

CHANGES IN THE ORGANISM

Essentially similar to those caused by acrylates *viz.* irritation of the gastro-intestinal tract, and degenerative changes in the heart, liver and kidneys.

Bibliography on p. 591

100. Methyl Propionate

Structural formula:

$$CH_3-CH_2-\overset{\displaystyle O}{\overset{\|}{C}}-O-CH_3$$

Molecular formula: $C_4H_8O_2$

Molecular weight: 85.10

Properties: a colourless liquid. Can react vigorously when exposed to heat or flame or with oxidising materials.

    boiling point: 80 °C
    melting point: —87 °C
    vapour pressure: 100 mm Hg at 29 °C
    vapour density (air = 1): 3.0
    specific gravity (liquid density): 0.915
    flash point: —2 °F
    conversion factors: 1 p.p.m. = 3.5 mg/m³
                      1 mg/l = 284 p.p.m.
    solubility: in water 6 g/100 ml
    maximum allowable concentration: not established

ECONOMY, SOURCES AND USES

Industrial uses

To a small extent in the lacquer industry.

BIOCHEMISTRY

Metabolism

According to Fassett (1963) there may be some production of propionic acid during metabolic conversion, leading to acidosis.

TOXICOLOGY

By oral administration to animals methyl propionate appears to be slightly more toxic than ethyl propionate, but no toxic effects in human beings have been reported.

Toxicity to animals

Lethal dose. – By oral administration, for rabbits, LD_{50}, 2.5–3.2 g/kg (Treon *et al.*, 1949).

SYMPTOMS OF INTOXICATION

Ataxia, gasping respiration, hypothermia.

Bibliography on p. 591

101. n-Butyl Propionate

Structural formula:

$$CH_3-CH_2-\overset{\displaystyle O}{\overset{\displaystyle \|}{C}}-O-CH_2-CH_2-CH_2-CH_3$$

Molecular formula: $C_7H_{14}O_2$

Molecular weight: 130.18

Properties: a colourless liquid with a apple-like odour, less disagreeable than that of amyl acetate. Good solvent for cellulose nitrate, ester gum, copal ester, cumarone and rubber chloride; not cellulose acetate, and only partly for shellac (Durrans, 1950).

The pure ester:
  boiling point: 145.5 °C
  specific gravity (liquid density): 0.883
  flash point: 110 °F
  vapour density (air = 1): 4.5

The technical product:
  boiling point: 135–155 °C
  specific gravity (liquid density): 0.878–0.883
  solubility: very slightly soluble in water. Miscible with oils and hydrocarbons but not with water (Durrans, 1950).
  conversion factors: 1 p.p.m. = 5.3 mg/m³
                      1 mg/l   = 188 p.p.m.
  maximum allowable concentration: not established.

ECONOMY, SOURCES AND USES

Produced from the residue arising from the manufacture of acetone by fermentation of seaweed; this residue consists largely of calcium propionate.
Chiefly used in the lacquer industry as a substitute for amyl acetate when lacquer is to be applied under excessively humid conditions.

TOXICOLOGY

No animal experiments appear to have been carried out, and there are no reports of injury to human beings.

102. Amyl Propionate

Structural formula:

$$CH_3-CH_2-\overset{\displaystyle O}{\overset{\|}{C}}-O-CH_2-CH_2-CH_2-CH_2-CH_3$$

Molecular formula: $C_8H_{16}O_2$

Molecular weight: 144.12

Properties: a stable colourless liquid with an apple-like odour (Lange, 1955).
   boiling point: 160 °C
   melting point: —73.1 °C
   vapour pressure: 10 mm Hg at 46.3 °C (Sax, 1957)
   vapour density (air = 1): 5.0
   specific gravity (liquid density): 0.870
   flash point: 105 °F
   conversion factors: 1 p.p.m. = 5.9 mg/m³
                        1 mg/l   = 170 p.p.m.
   solubility: insoluble in water; miscible with castor and linseed oils and hydro-carbons but not with water. Solvent properties similar to those of amyl acetate but slower and giving more viscous solutions.
   maximum allowable concentration: not established.

ECONOMY, SOURCES AND USES

Industrial uses

In the lacquer industry, especially for brushing lacquers where a slower rate of evaporation than that of amyl acetate is required.

TOXICOLOGY

No animal experiments have been carried out and there are no reports of injury to human beings. Durrans states that it is non-toxic.

103. Ethyl ß-Ethoxy-propionate

Structural formula:

$$CH_3-CH_2-O-CH_2-CH_2-\overset{\overset{\textstyle O}{\|}}{C}-O-CH_2-CH_3$$

Molecular formula: $C_7H_{14}O_3$

Molecular weight: 146.0

Properties: a liquid.

    boiling point: 165–172 °C

    melting point: —100 °C

    vapour density (air = 1): 5.0

    specific gravity (liquid density): 0.948 (Scheflan and Jacobs, 1953)

    flash point: 180 °F (Sax, 1957)

    conversion factors: 1 p.p.m. = 5.9 mg/m³

                     1 mg/l = 168 p.p.m.

    maximum allowable concentration: not established.

ECONOMY, SOURCES AND USES

Industrial uses

To a small extent in the lacquer industry.

TOXICOLOGY

As judged by the results of animal experiments ethyl ethoxy propionate is of very low toxicity; even the inhalation of saturated air-vapour mixture for 8 h caused no deaths (Smyth *et al.*, 1951), though it has caused death by oral administration and application to the skin. It is very slightly irritant to the skin and moderately so to the eyes by direct instillation.

No injury to human beings has been reported.

Toxicity to animals

Lethal dose. – *(i) By oral administration,* for rats, LD_{50}, 5 g/kg. – *(ii) By skin application* 10 ml/kg (Smyth *et al.*, 1951).

[578]

104. Ethyl Butyrate

Synonyms: butyric ether, ethyl butanoate

Structural formula:

$$CH_3—CH_2—CH_2—\overset{\overset{\textstyle O}{\|}}{C}—O—CH_2—CH_3$$

Molecular formula: $C_6H_{12}O_2$

Molecular weight: 116.16

Properties: a liquid with a strong pineapple odour. A rapid solvent for cellulose nitrate, and solvent properties for other materials, including ethyl cellulose, ester gum and mastic; intermediate between those of ethyl- and *n*-butyl acetate (Durrans, 1950; Gnamm, 1943).

    boiling point: 121.3 °C

    melting point: —93.3 °C

    vapour pressure: 20 mm Hg at 28 °C

    vapour density (air = 1): 4.0

    specific gravity (liquid density): 0.879

    flash point: 85 °F

    conversion factors: 1 p.p.m. = 4.7 mg/m³

                      1 mg/l = 211 p.p.m.

    solubility: in water 0.75 g in 100 ml (Fassett, 1963). Miscible with alcohol and ether.

    maximum allowable concentration: not established.

ECONOMY, SOURCES AND USES

Industrial uses

In the lacquer industry and as a flavouring agent (Durrans, 1950).

TOXICOLOGY

Ethyl butyrate is of low toxicity, having produced no toxic effects in animals by oral or intravenous administration of large doses, though in birds large oral doses have caused irritation, and in rabbits an increase in respiratory volume. There are no reports of injury in human beings.

Bibliography on p. 591

It vitro it has been shown to have a haemolytic effect slightly greater than that of methyl butyrate (Fühner and Neubauer, 1907).

Toxicity to animals

Acute

Lethal dose. – *(i) Oral administration* to dogs of 3 g in 60 ml of water caused no toxic effects (Albertoni and Lussana, 1874), nor to birds that of 300 mg but doses larger than this caused marked irritation, and in rabbits administration of 2.14 ml/kg caused only an increase in respiratory volume (Vogel, 1897). – *(ii) Intravenous injection,* for dogs, 177–222 mg/kg also had no injurious effect (von Oettingen, 1960).

CHANGES IN THE ORGANISM

According to Vogel (1897) rabbits which had shown an increase in respiratory volume showed no abnormality of lungs or stomach.

105. Methyl Butyrate

105a. Methyl n-Butyrate

Structural formula:

$$CH_3-CH_2-CH_2-\overset{\displaystyle O}{\overset{\|}{C}}-O-CH_3$$

Molecular formula: $C_5H_{10}O_2$

Molecular weight: 102.13

Properties: a liquid with solvent properties similar to those of ethyl butyrate.
  boiling point: 102.8 °C
  melting point: < —95 °C
  vapour pressure: 40 mm Hg at 30 °C
  vapour density (air = 1): 3.52
  specific gravity (liquid density): 0.8721
  flash point: 57 °F (Fassett, 1963)
  conversion factors: 1 p.p.m. = 4.2 mg/m³
        1 mg/l   = 240 p.p.m.
  solubility: in water 1.56 g/100 ml. Miscible with alcohol and ether.
  maximum allowable concentration: not established.

ECONOMY, SOURCES AND USES

Used in lacquers and perfumes.

TOXICOLOGY

No experiments on animals have been carried out, but *in vitro* tests for its haemo-lytic action (Fühner and Neubauer, 1907) have shown it to be slightly less effective in this respect than ethyl butyrate. There are no reports of its toxicity to human beings.

105b. Methyl Isobutyrate

Structural formula:

$$CH_3-\overset{\displaystyle CH_3}{\overset{|}{CH}}-\overset{\displaystyle O}{\overset{\|}{C}}-O-CH_3$$

Bibliography on p. 591   [581]

Molecular formula: $C_5H_{10}O_2$

Molecular weight: 102.13

Properties: a colourless liquid
    boiling point: 92 °C
    melting point: —84.0 °C
    vapour pressure: 50 mm Hg at 24 °C
    vapour density (air = 1): 3.5
    specific gravity (liquid density): 0.890
    flash point: 60 °F
    conversion factors: 1 p.p.m. = 4.1 mg/m³
                      1 mg/l = 240 p.p.m.
    solubility: in water slight
    maximum allowable concentration: not established

ECONOMY, SOURCES AND USES

Used in the lacquer industry to a slight extent; also in perfumes and flavourings (Fassett, 1963).

TOXICOLOGY

From the only animal experiments which appear to have been carried out (those of Fassett, 1963), methyl isobutyrate is apparently of low toxicity.

Lethal dose. – (i) By oral administration, for rats, 1600 mg/kg. – *(ii) By intraperitoneal injection,* 3200 mg/kg. – *(iii) By inhalation,* 42,000 p.p.m. for 63 min killed 2 out of 3 rats.

SYMPTOMS OF INTOXICATION

Labored respiration, vasodilatation, slight roughening of the coat, muscular twitching, death delayed up to 2 days. With lower concentrations (6400 p.p.m. for 6 h) loss of coordination and prostration, but recovery after 14 days and no apparent residual effects.
    There are no reports of injury to human beings.

106. Butyl Butyrate

Synonym: butol

Structural formula:

$$CH_3—CH_2—CH_2—\overset{\overset{\displaystyle O}{\|}}{C}—O—CH_2—CH_2—CH_2—CH_3$$

Molecular formula: $C_8H_{16}O_2$

Molecular weight: 144.2

Properties: butyl butyrate usually consits of a mixture of *n-* and isobutyl butyrate, the former preponderating (Durrans, 1950). A liquid of strong apple-like odour.

Pure n-butyl butyrate:
  boiling point: 165 °C
  specific gravity (liquid density): 0.869
  flash point: 124 °F
  solubility: in water 0.574% at 33 °C. Solvent for cellulose nitrate, ester gum, cumarone and shellac; not for cellulose acetate or hard copals.

Isobutyl isobutyrate:
  boiling point: 147 °C
  vapour pressure: 10 mm Hg at 38 °C
  specific gravity (liquid density): 0.855
  flash point: 120 °F
  conversion factors: 1 p.p.m. = 5.8 mg/m³
             1 mg/l = 174 p.p.m.
  solubility: in water 0.5 g/100 ml
  maximum allowable concentration: not established.

ECONOMY, SOURCES AND USES

Industrial uses

In the lacquer and perfume industries.

Durrans (1950) states that *n*-butyl butyrate is useful when a solvent with a slower evaporation rate than amyl acetate is desired, and that it imparts a good brushing flow and gloss to lacquers.

TOXICOLOGY

Only isobutyl butyrate appears to have been investigated by animal experiment (Fassett, 1963; Parish and Knipling, 1942; Jacobs, 1949).

It is stated by these observers to be practically non-toxic by oral administration and only slightly toxic when given intraperitoneally.

Lethal dose. – (i) By oral administration, for rats and mice, 12,800 mg/kg. – *(ii) By intraperitoneal injection,* for rats, 6300 mg/kg; for mice 1600 mg/kg. – *(iii) By inhalation,* for rats, 5000 p.p.m. for 6 h killed 2 out of 3.

SYMPTOMS OF INTOXICATION

Prostration and complete narcosis.

Skin application

That this solvent can be absorbed through the skin was indicated by the fact that 10 ml/kg, while not lethal, and causing only slight skin irritation, produced some interference with normal growth during a two-week recovery period.

There are no reports of injury to human beings. Durrans (1950) remarks that *n*-butyl butyrate is non-toxic.

107. Ethyl Hydroxy-isobutyrate

Synonym: ethyl oxybutyrate

Structural formula:

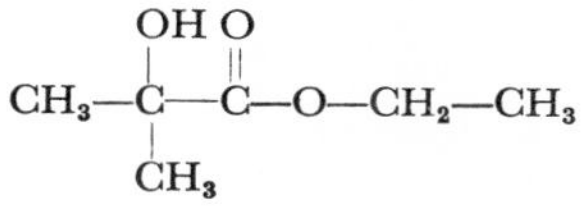

$$CH_3-\underset{\underset{CH_3}{|}}{\overset{\overset{OH}{|}}{C}}-\overset{\overset{O}{||}}{C}-O-CH_2-CH_3$$

Molecular formula: $C_6H_{12}O_3$

Properties: a colourless liquid with a mild pleasant odour; resists hydrolysis. Slow solvent for cellulose nitrate and acetate, forming viscous solutions, but of less viscosity than with amyl acetate and greater than with ethyl acetate. Its low rate of evaporation tends to leave films soft for a considerable time but imparts a high gloss (Durrans, 1950).

> *boiling point:* 142–146 °C
> *specific gravity (liquid density):* 0.978–0.986
> *maximum allowable concentration:* not established.

ECONOMY, SOURCES AND USES

Production

Synthetically by condensing acetone with hydrocyanic acid, forming acetone cyanhydrin, which is then hydrolysed and esterified with ethyl alcohol and HCl.

Industrial uses

Chiefly in the lacquer industry.

TOXICOLOGY

No animal experiments appear to have been carried out, but from comparisons of its haemolytic action *in vitro* with that of ethyl alcohol, its 'toxicity' in this respect was stated by Vandervelde (1906) to be slightly greater than that of isobutyl acetate and less than ethyl acetate.

No cases of actual injury from its industrial use have been reported, but Hamilton *et al.* (1929) state that though it is advertised as 'non-toxic', painters using it have complained of dryness of the throat, tightness of the chest and 'dopiness'.

108. Methyl 3-Hydroxybutyrate

Structural formula:

$$CH_3-\overset{\displaystyle OH}{\underset{\displaystyle |}{CH}}-CH_2-CH_2-\overset{\displaystyle O}{\overset{\displaystyle ||}{C}}-O-CH_3$$

Molecular formula: $C_6H_{12}O_3$

Molecular weight: 118.1

Properties: a colourless liquid.
    boiling point: 174.9 °C
    vapour pressure: 0.85 at 20 °C
    vapour density (air = 1): 4.1
    specific gravity (liquid density): 1.0559
    flash point: 180 °F
    conversion factors: 1 p.p.m. = 4.8 mg/m³
                    1 mg/l = 207 p.p.m.
    solubility: very soluble in water
    maximum allowable concentration: not established.

ECONOMY, SOURCES AND USES

Industrial uses

Chiefly in the perfume industry.

TOXICOLOGY

No investigations of a possible systemic injury have been made; but there are two reports of its effect on the eyes of both animals and human beings.

Effect on the eyes of rabbits

    Carpenter *et al.* (1946) examined the effect of direct application to the eyes of rabbits which had been previously treated with a 5% aqueous solution of fluorescein sodium, and later stained with fluorescein, and classified the corneal injury following application of 0.2 ml of the compound as Grade V, *i.e.* causing necrosis in 63–87% of the animals.

Effect on the human cornea

    Methyl hydroxybutyrate is not included by McLaughlin (1946) in his tabulation of chemicals which have produced corneal injury in human beings.

109. Ethyl Benzoate

Synonym: benzoic ether

Structural formula:

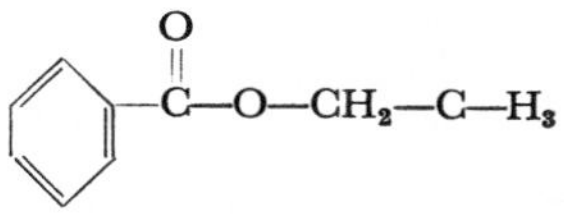

$$\text{C}_6\text{H}_5-\overset{\displaystyle \overset{\text{O}}{\|}}{\text{C}}-\text{O}-\text{CH}_2-\text{C}-\text{H}_3$$

Molecular formula: $C_9H_{10}O_2$

Molecular weight: 150.17

Properties: a liquid with a powerful but pleasant odour, stable to light. Solvent for cellulose nitrate and acetate, ethyl cellulose, ester gum, mastic shellac, but not for hard copals exept on prolonged boiling (Durrans, 1950).

> *boiling point:* 212.6 °C
> *melting point:* —34.6 °C
> *vapour pressure:* 1 mm Hg at 44 °C
> *vapour density (air = 1):* 5.2
> *specific gravity (liquid density):* 1.0509
> *flash point:* 200 °F
> *solubility:* in water 0.8% at 20 °C (Fassett, 1963). Miscible with castor and linseed oils and hydrocarbons, but not with water.
> *maximum allowable concentration:* not established.

ECONOMY, SOURCES AND USES

Industrial uses

(1) In the lacquer industry, especially for imparting good brushing properties to cellulose lacquers.

(2) It can be used as a plasticiser (Durrans, 1950).

TOXICOLOGY

The only animal experiments recorded are based on the Range Finding Toxicity Tests of Smyth *et al.* (1954), which show that it is slightly less systemically toxic than methyl benzoate but slightly more irritant to skin and mucous membranes.

Lethal dose. LD$_{50}$. – *(i) By oral administration*, for rats, 6.48 g/kg after 14 days. – *(ii) By inhalation* of saturated vapour, 8 h was the maximum for no deaths.

Effect of skin application. – Moderate irritation.

Effect on eyes. – A very small area of corneal necrosis from application of 0.5 ml undiluted.

There are no reports of injury from its industrial use.

110. Methyl Benzoate

Synonym: oil of Niobe

Structural formula:

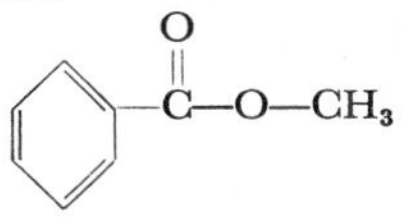

$$\text{C}_6\text{H}_5-\overset{\displaystyle O}{\overset{\|}{\text{C}}}-\text{O}-\text{CH}_3$$

Molecular formula: $C_8H_8O_2$

Molecular weight: 136.14

Properties: a liquid with a less pronounced odour than ethyl benzoate. Solvent for cellulose nitrate and acetate, rubber and ester gum but not for ethyl cellulose, shellac, hard copals or mastic.

    boiling point: 199.6 °C

    melting point: —12.5 °C

    vapour pressure: 1 mm Hg at 39 °C

    vapour density (air = 1): 4.7

    specific gravity (liquid density): 1.0937

    flash point: 181 °F

    solubility: in water 0.0157% at 30 °C. Miscible with oil.

    maximum allowable concentration: not established.

ECONOMY, SOURCES AND USES

Industrial uses

(1) To some extent in the lacquer industry.

(2) In flavors and perfumes.

TOXICOLOGY

On the basis of Range Finding tests for acute toxicity (Smyth *et al.*, 1954) methyl benzoate has a lower LD_{50} oral dose for rats (3.43 g/kg) than ethyl benzoate and therefore a slightly higher systemic toxicity. By inhalation of saturated vapour these two solvents rank as equivalent in toxicity, both being low on account of their low volatility.

    As an irritant of skin and mucous membranes, methyl benzoate is slightly more irritant to the skin, but slightly less irritant to the eyes.

    There are no reports of any injury from its industrial use.

Bibliography on p. 591   [589]

111. Butyl Benzoate

Structural formula:

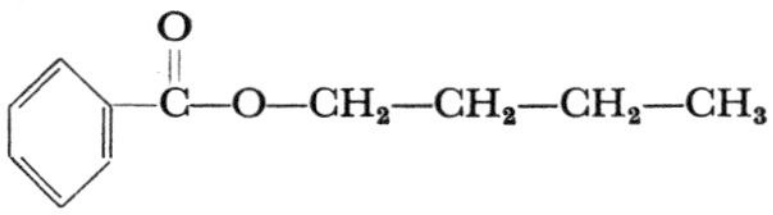

$$\text{C}_6\text{H}_5\!-\!\overset{\displaystyle \text{O}}{\overset{\displaystyle \|}{\text{C}}}\!-\!\text{O}\!-\!\text{CH}_2\!-\!\text{CH}_2\!-\!\text{CH}_2\!-\!\text{CH}_3$$

Molecular formula: $C_{11}H_{14}O_2$

Molecular weight: 178.22

Properties: a colourless liquid with a mild odour. A good solvent for ester gum, copal ester, cumarone, but a poor solvent for cellulose nitrate and acetate, shellac and copals, and not for glyceryl phthalate resins.

boiling point: 250.3 °C
melting point: —21.5 °C
vapour pressure: 0.01 mm Hg at 20 °C
vapour density (air = 1): 6.2
specific gravity (liquid density): 1.009
flash point: 225 °F
solubility: insoluble in water, but miscible with oils and hydrocarbons
maximum allowable concentration: not established.

ECONOMY, SOURCES AND USES

Industrial uses

To a slight extent in the lacquer industry and also as a plasticiser.

TOXICOLOGY

Butyl benzoate has a lower oral toxicity than methyl benzoate but slightly greater than ethyl benzoate.

The LD_{50} for the rat, in the Range Finding Toxicity Tests of Smyth *et al.* (1954) was 5.1 g/kg as compared with 3.43 for methyl and 6.48 for ethyl.

By inhalation there appeared to be no difference. There was no penetration of the skin, but application caused fairly severe irritation. The eyes showed only slight irritation.

There are no reports of any injury from its industrial use. Fassett (1963) attributes the low toxicity of these benzoic acid esters to the probability that they may be excreted as glucuronide or sulphate ester, as well as to their low volatility.

BIBLIOGRAPHY

Albertoni, P. and F. Lussana (1874) (cited by von Oettingen, 1960), *Lo Sperimentale*, 67:141.

Alinari, E. (1930) Miscele entettiche fra Alcooli ed Eteri acetica, *Ann. Chim. Appl. Roma*, 20:159.

Althoff, E. (1931) Tod durch Einatmung von Essigäther, *Z. Med. Beamte*, 15:420.

Baader, E. W. (1933) Gewerbemedizinische Erfahrungen, *Verhandl. Deut. ges. inn. Med.*, 45:318.

Baldi, G. (1953) Patologia professionale da Acetato di Amile, di Butile e di Propile, *Med. Lavoro*, 44:469.

Barrios, D. L. and J. S. Devoto (1931) Commentarios sobre l'Accion toxica del 'Barniz', 'Tini' y 'Pomada', *Sem. Med. B. Aires*, 1:252.

Beintke, R. (1928 Überempfindlichheit gegen Äthylazetat, *Deut. Med. Wochschr.*, 54:528.

Browning, E. (1953) *Toxicity of Industrial Organic Solvents*, Chemical Publishing Co. Inc. New York.

Burger, G. E. C. and R. H. Stockman (1932) Über Urobilinuria als Folge der Einatmung von organischen Lösungsmitteln in geringer Konzentration, *Z. Gewerbehyg. Unfallverhüt.*, 19:29.

Busing, K. H. (1952) Augenschädigung durch Butylazetat und Isobutylalcohol in einen Kabelwerk, *Z. Arbeitsmed. Arbeitsschutz.*, 2:13.

Carpenter, C. P. and H. F. Smyth Jr. (1946) Chemical Burns of the Rabbit Cornea, *Am. J. Ophthalm.*, 29:1363.

Carpenter, C. P., H. F. Smyth and U. C. Pozzani (1949) The Assay of acute Vapour Toxicity and Grading and Interpretation of Results on 96 chemical Compounds, *J. Ind. Hyg. Toxicol.*, 31:343.

Cavalazzi, I. (1938) Acetati di Butile e sua Azione tossica, *Rass. Med. Ind.*, 9:272.

Cazaneuve, P., A. Morel and H. de Leeuw (1932) l'Hygiéne et l'Industrie de Soie artificielle, *Chim. et Ind.*, 28:473.

Ciaranfi, E. (1940) Sulle Ossidazione biologica del Formiato di Metile, *Enzymologia*, 9:187.

Clayton, E. and C. O. Clark (1931) Modern Organic Solvents, *J. Soc. Dy. Col. Bradford*, 47:183, 247.

Crecelius, A. (1930) Schädigung durch Amylazetat, *Klin. Wochschr.*, 9:452.

Custance, H. M. and M. Higgins (1949) Colorimetric Method for Estimation of Amyl Acetate Vapours in Air, *Analyst.*, 74:316.

Dautrebande, L., J. H. Feced, E. Philippot, T. Charlier and M. Th. Bodson (1935) Paralysie du Système vaso-moteur par les Vapeurs d'Acétate d'Amyle et de Vernis dit cellulosique, *Compt. Rend. Soc. Biol.*, 119:314.

Deschiens, M. (1928) *Les Vernis et Peintures cellulosiques pour Automobiles*, 7me. Cong. Paris, Chim. et Ind. Spécial No. p. 673.

Deschiens, M. (1930) *Mélanges solvants et Vernis cellulosiques*, 10me. Cong. Paris, Chim. et Ind. Spécial no. p. 692.

Duquénois, R. and P. Revel (1934) Occupational Poisoning caused by Vapours of certain Esters used as Solvents, *J. Pharm. Chim.*, 19:590.

Durrans, T. H. (1950) *Solvents*, 6th ed., Chapman and Hall, London.

Elkins, H. B. (1959) *The Chemistry of Industrial Toxicology*, Wiley and Sons, New York; Chapman and Hall, London.

Engelhardt, W. E. (1933) Überempfindlichkeitserkrankungen der Haut durch Alkoholesterverbindungen der aliphatischen Alkoholreihe im Lackerberuf, *Arch. Derm. Syph.*, 169:236.

Enna, F. G. A. (1930) Processes of Patent Leather Manufacture, *Leather World*, 22:412.

Fairhall, L. T. (1957) *Industrial Toxicology*, Interscience Publishers, New York.

Fassett, D. W. (1963) *Esters*, in F. A. Patty, *Industrial Hygiene and Toxicology*, Vol. II, 2nd ed., Interscience Publishers, New York.

Flury, F., O. Klimmer and E. Rösser (1937) cited by Lehmann and Flury (1943).

Flury, F. and W. Neumann, cited by K. N. Lehmann and F. Flury (1943).

Flury, F. and W. Wirth (1934) Zur Toxikologie der Lösungsmittel, *Arch. Gewerbepathol. Gewerbehyg.*, 5:1.

Flury, F. and F. Zernik (1931) *Schädliche Gäse. Dämpfe, Nebel, Rauch- und Staubarten*, Springer, Berlin.

Fühner, H. (1921) Die Wirkungsstarke der Narcotica, *Biochem. Z.*, 120:143.

Fühner, H. and E. Neubauer (1907) Hämolyse durch Substanzen homologer Reihen, *Arch. Exptl. Pathol. Pharmacol.*, 56:333.

Fühner, H. and F. Pietrusky (1934) Butylazetatvergiftung, chronische, berufliche Spätfolgung, *Samml. Vergiftungsf.*, 5:1:B40.

Gettler, A. O. (1940) The Detection, Identification and quantitative Determination of Methyl Formate in Tissues, *Am. J. Clin. Pathol.*, 10:188.

Gettler, A. O. and H. Siegel (1935) Isolation from human Tissues of easily volatile organic Liquids and their Identification, *Arch. Pathol.*, 19:208.

Gnamm, H. (1943) *Die Lösungsmittel und Weichmachungsmittel*, Wissenschaftl. Verlags G.m.b.H., Stuttgart.

Graham, B. E. and M. H. Kuizenger (1945) Toxicity Studies on Benzyl Benzoate and related Compounds, *J. Pharmacol. Exptl. Therap.*, 84:358.

Gross, E. (1932) cited by Lehmann and Flury (1943).

Gruber, C. M. (1924) The Effect of Benzyl Alcohol and its Esters, Benzyl Benzoate and Benzyl Acetate upon Kidney Function, *J. Pharmacol. Exptl. Therap.*, 23: Proc. 149.

Gunther, O. (1956) Die Kunststoffe und ihre arbeitsmedizinische Bedeutung, *Z. Arbeitsmed.*, 6:156.

Hackett, J. D. (1932) Lacquers and their Hazards, *Ind. Hyg. Bull.*, 11:223.

Hamilton, A. (1925) *Industrial Poisons in the United States*, Macmillan, New York.

Hamilton, A., E. B. Bricker and H. F. Smyth (1929) Volatile Solvents used in Industry, *Am. J. Publ. Hlth.*, 19:523.

Henderson, V. and H. W. Haggard (1943) *Noxious Gases*, Reinhold Corp., New York.

Herold, I. (1931) Benzyl Azetat und Homolog, *Deut. Parfüm Z.*, 17:362.

Hestrin, J. (1949) The Reaction of Acetylcholine and other Carboxylic Derivatives with Hydroxylamine, *J. Biol. Chem.*, 180:249.

Holstein, E. (1935) Die Gesundheitsgefähren des Malerberufes. Binde-, Lösungsmittel und Lacke, *Med. Welt.*, 9:302.

Inserra, A., C. Spagna and G. B. Petrillo (1962) Reperti elettrocardiographici nelle Intossicazione sperimentale da Acetato di Amile, *Bol. Soc. Ital. Biol. Sper.*, 38:457.

Inserra, A., C. Spagna and C. Spogliano (1962) Reperti elettrocardiographica in Conigli intossicati con Acetato di Amile dopo trattamento con Atropine e Taglio dei Vaghi, *Bol. Soc. Ital. Biol. Sper.*, 38:460.

Jacobs, M. B. (1941) *The analytical Chemistry of industrial Poisons, Hazards and Solvents*, Interscience, New York.

Jacobs, M. B. (1949) cited by Fassett (1963) *Am. Perfum. Essent. Oil. Rev.*, 54:303.

Jones, G. W., W. E. Miller and H. Seaman (1933) Explosive Properties of Methyl-Formate-Air Mixtures, *Ind. Eng. Chem.*, 25:694.

Kendal, L. P. and A. N. Ramanathan (1952) Liver Alcohol Dehydrogenase and Ester Formation, *Biochem. J.*, 52:430.

Koelsch, F. (1912) Gesundheitschädigungen durch Amylazetat, *Concordia*, 19:246.

Korenmann, I. M. (1932) Kolorimetrische Bestimmung von Amylalkohol und Amylazetatdämpfen in der Luft, *Arch. Hyg. Bacteriol.*, 109:108.

Kruger, E. (1932) Augenerkrankungen bei Verwendung von Nitrolacken in der Strohut Industrie, *Arch. Gewerbepathol. Gewerbehyg.*, 3:798.

Lange, N. A. (1956) *Handbook of Chemistry*, 9th. ed., Handbook Publ. Sandusky, Ohio.

Lehmann, K. B. (1913) Experimentelle Studien über den Einfluss technisch wichtiger Gäse und Dämpfe auf den Organismus, *Arch. Hyg.*, 78:260.

Lehmann, K. B. and F. Flury (1943) *Toxicology and Hygiene of Industrial Solvents*, Williams and Wilkins, Baltimore.

Lewin, L. (1929) *Gifte und Vergiftungen*, 4th ed., Springer, Berlin.

Lloyd, J. V., W. Ostwald and W. Haller (1930) A Study in Pharmacy, *J. Am. Pharmacol. Ass.*, 19:1076.

Lund, A. (1944) cited by von Oettingen (1960), *Ugesk. Laeger*, 106:308.

Malten, K. E. and R. L. Zielhuis (1964) *Industrial Toxicology and Dermatology in Production and Processing of Plastics*, Elsevier Publishing Co., Amsterdam.

McLaughlin, R. S. (1946) Chemical Burns of the human Cornea, *Am. J. Ophthalm.*, 29:1355.

McOmie, W. A. (1949) cited by W. S. Spector (1956), *Univ. Calif. Bull Pharmacol.*, 2:231.

Müller, W. (1932) cited by von Oettingen (1960). Diss. Würzburg.

Nelson, K. W., J. F. Ege, M. Ross, L. E. Woodman and L. Silverman (1943) Sensory Response to certain industrial Solvent Vapours, *J. Ind. Hyg. Toxicol.*, 25:282.

Von Oettingen, W. F. (1959) The aliphatic Acids and their Esters, Toxicity and potential dangers, *Arch. Ind. Hyg.*, 20:517.

Von Oettingen, W. F. (1960) The aliphatic Acids and their Esters, Toxicity and potential Dangers, *Arch. Ind. Hlth.*, 21:28.

Parish, H. E. and E. F. Knipling (1942) cited by Fassett (1963), *J. Econ. Entomol.*, 35:70.

Park, J. G. and M. B. Hopkins (1930) Secondary Esters and their Use in Lacquers, *Ind. Eng. Eng. Chem.*, 22:826.

Patty, F. A., H. H. Schrenk and W. P. Yant (1936) Acute Response of Guinea Pigs to Vapours of some new commercial Organic Compounds, *sec.*-Amyl Acetate, *U.S.P.H. Serv. P. H. Rep.*, 51:811.

Pennsylvania Dept. Lab. Ind. (1926) Spray Painting in Pennsylvania, *Dept. Lab. Ind. Special Bull.*, no. 16.

Raymond, V. (1959) Les Dermatoses des Parquetiers, *Travail et Securité*. 5:186.

Reus, R. J. (1933) cited by von Oettingen (1960), Inaug. Diss. Würzburg.

Sax, N. Irving (1957) *Dangerous Properties of Industrial Materials*, Reinhold, New York.

Sayers, R. R., H. H. Schrenk and F. A. Patty (1936) Acute Response of Guinea Pigs to Vapours of some new commercial organic Solvents. *n*-Butyl Acetate, *U.S. Treas. Publ. Hlth. Rep.* 51:1229.

Scheflan, L. and M. Jacobs (1953) *Handbook of Solvents*, Van Norstrand, New York.

Schrenk, H. H., W. P. Yant, J. Chornyak and F. A. Patty (1936) Acute Response of Guinea Pigs to Vapours of some new commercial organic Compounds – Methyl Formate, *U.S. Treas. Publ. Hlth. Rep.*, 51:1329.

Schutz, H. (1937) Über akute kombinierte Lösungsmittelvergiftungen, *Arch. Gewerbepathol. Gewerbeshyg.*, 7:459.

Silverman, L., H. F. Schulte and W. W. First (1946) Further studies on sensory Response to certain industrial Solvent Vapours, *J. Ind. Hyg. Toxicol.*, 28:262.

Smyth, H. F., Jr., C. P. Carpenter and C. S. Weil (1951) Range Finding Toxicity Data. List IV, *Arch. Ind. Hlth.*, 4:119.

Smyth, H. F., C. P. Carpenter, C. S. Weil and U. C. Pozzani (1954) Range Finding Toxicity Tests. List V, *Arch. Ind. Hlth.*, 10:61.

Smyth, H. F. and H. F. Smyth Jr. (1928) Inhalation Experiments with certain Lacquer Solvents, *J. Ind. Hyg. Toxicol.*, 10:261.

Snapper, I., A. Grunbaum and S. Sturkop (1925) Über die Spaltung und die Oxidation von Benzylalkohol und Benzylestern im menschlichen Organismus, *Biochem. Z.*, 155:163.

Spector, W. S. (1956) *Handbook of Toxicology*, Vol. I, Saunders, Philadelphia and London.

Strafford, N., C. R. N. Strouts and W. V. Stubbings (1956) *The determination of toxic substances in air*, Heffer, Cambridge, England.

Threshold Limit Values for 1962, (1963), *Am. Ind. Hyg. Ass.*, 23:419.

Treon, J. R., H. Sigmon, H. Wright and K. V. Kitzmiller (1949) The Toxicity of Ethyl and Methyl Acrylate, *J. Ind. Hyg. Toxicol.*, 31:317.

Vandevelde, A. J. J. (1906) Über die Anwendung von biologischen Methoden zur Analyse von Nährungsstoffen, *Biochem. Z.*, 1:5.

Vernetti Blina, L. (1933) Experimental Investigation of toxic Action of Acetic Acid Esters (Amyl Acetate), *Med. Lavoro*, 24:166.

Vogel, G. (1897) Untersuchungen über die Wirkung einiger Saureäther, *Arch. ges. Physiol.*, 67:141.

Wachtel, C. (1920) Über die Wirkung ätzender Ester, *Z. ges. Exptl. Pathol. Therap.*, 21:1.

Weber, H. H. and W. Gueffroy (1932) Über einige Beiz-lackier- und Poliermittel; ihre Zusammensetzung und physiologische Wirkung, *Z. ges. Geb. Gew. Hyg.*, 40:38.

Weber, S. (1902) Über die Giftigkeit des Schwefelsäuredimethylesters; Dimethylsäure und einiger verwandte Ester der Fettreihe, *Arch. Exptl. Pathol. Pharmacol.*, 47:113.

Weingand, R. (1931) Neuer Celluloseesterbronzelack, *Farbe und Lack*, p. 28.

Yarsley, V. E. (1933) Health Hazards in the Lacquer and Finishing Industries, *Synth. appl. Finish.*, 3:80.

Zangger, H. (1930) Über die modernen Lösungsmittel, *Arch. Gewerbepathol. Gewerbehyg.*, 1:77.

Zeisler, E. P. (1940) Dermatitis from elastiglass Garters, and wrist watch straps, *J. Am. Med. Ass.*, 114:2540.

Zernik, F. (1933) Neuere Erkenntnisse auf dem Gebiete der schädlichen Gäse und Dämpfe. *Ergebn. Hyg. Bakteriol.*, 14:139, 220.

Chapter 12

GLYCOLS AND DERIVATIVES

113. Ethylene Glycol

Synonyms: glycol alcohol; 1,2-ethanediol; Glysantin

Structural formula:
$$\begin{array}{l} CH_2-OH \\ | \\ CH_2-OH \end{array}$$

Molecular formula: $C_2H_6O_2$

Molecular weight: 62.07

Properties: a clear colourless hygroscopic liquid with a sweet taste, somewhat less viscous than glycerol. Solvent for some dyes and gelatinised cellulose nitrate, but does not dissolve cellulose acetate, hydrocarbons, vegetable oils, ester gum, vinyl resins and rubber.

>   *boiling point:* 197.6 °C
>   *melting point:* about —14 °C
>   *vapour pressure:* 0.06 mm Hg at 20 °C
>   *vapour density (air = 1):* 2.14 (Sara, 1957).
>   *specific gravity (liquid density):* 1.1136
>   *flash point:* 240 °F
>   *conversion factors:* 1 p.p.m. = 2.74 mg/m³
>   1 mg/l = 394 p.p.m.
>   *solubility:* miscible with water, some alcohols, aldehydes and ketones; practically insoluble in hydrocarbons. It evolves heat when mixed with water.
>   *evaporation rate (ether = 1):* 2625 times less.
>   *maximum allowable concentration:* not established.

ECONOMY, SOURCES AND USES

Production

(1) From ethylene bromide by heating with Na-formate in presence of methyl alcohol.
(2) By heating ethylene chlorohydrin with Na-bicarbonate, with subsequent recovery by fractional distillation.
(3) By hydrolysis of ethylene oxide prepared from ethylene by direct oxidation with oxygen or air (Curme and Johnstone, 1952).

Industrial uses

(1) As an antifreeze agent for automobiles.
(2) As a solvent for dyes.
(3) As an electrolyte for electrolytic condensers.
(4) As a vehicle for pharmaceutical preparations, food extracts and flavouring essences.
(5) As a component of skin lotions, added to various powders.
(6) As a substitute for glycerin (Mendel, 1917).

BIOCHEMISTRY

Estimation in the atmosphere

The method stated by Rowe (1963) to be the most useful is by oxidation with periodate and colorimetric determination by Na-chromotropate in conc. H_2SO_4.

Metabolism

In spite of a more or less general opinion that the main toxic effect of ethylene glycol on the kidney is related to the metabolic production of oxalic acid, there is not universal agreement as to how far oxalic acid itself, as compared with some of the intermediate metabolites, may be responsible. Bachem (1917), following self-administration of 25 and 45 g diluted with water within two days did observe an increased elimination of oxalic acid in the urine but von Oettingen (1943) reported that only about 2% or less of the dose administered to the dog, rabbit or man is excreted as oxalic acid and Williams (1959) found that while, in the rabbit, 60% of a 350 g dose of ^{14}C-labelled ethylene glycol was eliminated in the expired air as CO_2 within 3 days, and nearly 25% as such in the urine, oxalic acid excretion was negligible. The fact that intravenous single sublethal dosage results in deposition of Ca-oxalate in the renal tubules of rats and rabbits (Mulinos *et al.*, 1943) while lethal doses do not so affect the kidneys, and that oral administration of sodium oxalate does not cause deposition of Ca-oxalate, has raised the question whether some other metabolic product is the toxic agent. Among the potential metabolic toxins suggested is glyoxal, since in some cases of ethylene glycol poisoning and in all cases of glyoxal poisoning in cats, pancreatic necrosis has been observed (Doerr, 1949).

Neither glyoxal nor the other possible intermediates, glycollic aldehyde and glyoxyllic acid have been detected in the urine, but according to Mayer (1903) glycollic acid, in units corresponding to 25% of the dose, has been isolated from the urine of rabbits. Williams (1959) concludes that the chronic toxicity of ethylene glycol is in part due to its oxidation to oxalic acid and possibly also to

Bibliography on p. 686

intermediates in this oxidation, which is now believed to be enzymatic, by means of liver alcohol dehydrogenase, a reaction which can be inhibited by ethanol (Peterson *et al.*, 1963).

Bornmann (1955) distinguishes between the early and late manifestations of the toxic action of ethylene glycol and explains the difference on the grounds that within two hours of the toxic dose excretion begins, followed by disappearance of some of the symptoms, while the late symptoms are caused by the presence of metabolic products.

Gershoff and Andrus (1962) have examined the relation between vitamin B_6 and magnesium with the metabolism of ethylene glycol and have concluded that vitamin B_6 has a marked effect in accelerating its oxidation and that deficiency of the vitamin is associated with inhibition of its oxidation to CO_2. Magnesium has a different mechanism of action in providing a greater degree of resistance to chronic toxicity of ethylene glycol, possibly by altering the solvent characteristics of urine and thus preventing the renal deposition of Ca-oxalate (see 'Treatment of ethylene glycol poisoning').

TOXICOLOGY

From the industrial point of view the chief hazard of ethylene glycol lies in the possibility of its being ingested either accidentally or as a substitute for alcohol. Its low volatility at ordinary temperatures practically rules out an inhalation risk, though there is one report of symptoms indicating a chronic toxic effect in a process where the ethylene glycol was heated. When ingested it has a powerful effect on the central nervous system, and with a sublethal dose, especially if repeated, a highly injurious effect on the kidneys, causing an acute nephrosis with deposition of Ca-oxalate crystals in the tubules.

It is not in animals a severe irritant of mucous membranes (Hanzlik *et al.*, 1931) but in human cases of acute poisoning (Pons and Custer, 1946) the lungs have shown pulmonary oedema and early bronchopneumonia, and according to Sykowski (1951) contamination of the eyes can cause severe conjunctivitis and chemosis, but Carpenter and Smyth (1946) reported that instillation into the eyes of rabbits failed to cause appreciable irritation.

Toxicity to animals

The lethal dose given by various authorities differs to some extent. This variation is explained by Laug *et al.* (1939) as due to three factors – the number of animals used, the dosage levels chosen and the percentage mortality selected.

Lethal dose. – By oral administration, LD_{50}, for rats, 5.5 ml/kg (Laug *et al.*, 1939), 5.8 ml/kg (Peterson *et al.*, 1963), 8.54 ml/kg (Smyth *et al.*, 1941), for mice, 13.1

ml/kg (Laug *et al.*, 1939), 13.8 ml/kg (Bornmann, 1955), for guinea pigs, 7.35 ml/kg (Laug *et al.*, 1939), 6.61 ml/kg (Smyth *et al.*, 1941).

SYMPTOMS OF INTOXICATION

Narcosis after 20–60 min, incoordination, coldness, pallor of mucous membranes, spastic contraction of muscles, loss of reflexes, coma and finally death from central nervous paralysis.

Intravenous injection is followed by a rapid lowering of blood pressure with a marked increase of amplitude of the heart beat (Page, 1927).

Repeated dosage. – *(i) By oral administration (gastric sound)*, for mice, 2% in drinking water within a few days (Bornmann, 1955). – *(ii) By subcataneous injection*, for mice, 2.5 ml/kg (von Oettingen and Jirouch, 1931). – *(iii) By intraperitoneal injection*, for rats, 3.5 ml/kg (Page, 1927).

Symptoms. – Rapid loss of weight, weakened reflexes, diuresis, and, by intraperitoneal injection, haemoglobinuria. According to von Oettingen and Jirouch the haemolytic action of ethylene glycol is less than that of most of its derivatives.

CHANGES IN THE ORGANISM

The kidneys are the organs chiefly affected, especially by repeated non-lethal dosage, though acute nephrosis in rats was observed by von Oettingen and Jirouch by subcutaneous injection of 2.5 to 5.0 ml/kg of a 50% solution and haemorrhage of the kidneys by 10 ml/kg. Severe renal injury, especially of the tubules, and calcium oxalate stones in the bladder were observed by Morris, Nelson and Calvery (1942) in rats maintained for 2 years on diets containing 2% of ethylene glycol, and animals investigated by Wiley *et al.* (1938) showed a high incidence of degenerative changes in the pyramidal tissue. No such changes were observed in the kidneys of mice and rats subjected to repeated inhalations of the vapour from ethylene glycol heated to 62 °C giving a concentration of 0.398 mg/l. It may be noted that Flury and Wirth (1934) found that a concentration of 0.5 mg/l for 28 h during 5 days caused only slight narcosis in rats.

Toxicity to human beings

There have been many reports of fatal injury from the drinking of ethylene glycol. Haggerty (1959) estimates that 40 to 60 deaths occur from accidental ingestion or as a substitute for alcohol each year in U.S.A.

The fatal dose by this route is stated to be about 100 ml (1.4 ml/kg) indicating that human beings are more susceptible to its toxic effect than animals. In the report by Pons and Custer (1946) of 18 fatal cases following the drinking of anti-freeze solution the amount consumed in one case was 200 ml while in a recent report by Friedmann *et al.* (1962) the average amount in two fatal cases was 4 ozs.

Bibliography on p. 686

In 93% of fatal cases death occurs within 72 h from cerebral damage and oedema of the lungs; in a few, following recovery from the initial phase, death occurs after 1 to 2 weeks from renal failure (Ross, 1956).

(1) Fatal cases

The early symptoms are not unlike those of alcoholic intoxication, relating chiefly to the central nervous system, sometimes with vomiting and signs of cardiopulmonary disease. Coma occurs usually after 10 to 12 h, sometimes, as in one of Pons and Custer's cases, later, after a period of restlessness and delirium. Symptoms of pulmonary oedema, with cyanosis and early bronchopneumonia may also be present with cramps and failure of respiration. Later symptoms are focussed on the kidneys, with albuminuria, oliguria and other sings of renal failure.

In the two fatal cases described by Friedmann *et al.* (1962), one, a girl aged 17 died within 47 h in spite of having been treated by haemodialysis and vasopressor agents; the other, an athletic boy of 17, survived the acute phase but succumbed to the subacute phase of renal failure and died, in spite of renal decapsulation, on the 17th day.

(2) Acute non-fatal cases

Two cases, typical of acute non-fatal intoxication, were among the four described by Friedmann *et al.* (1962). Each had drunk about 1 oz. of anti-freeze. One, a 16 year old boy, complained some hours later of dizziness, confusion and dysuria, then of nausea, abdominal pain and vomiting. His blood picture showed a polymorphonuclear leucocytosis ($11,900/\mu l$ with 70% polymorphs) and the urine contained many Ca-oxalate crystals, granular casts and some albumen. Liver function tests indicated some disturbance, and blood urea nitrogen was constantly elevated (88 mg% on the 8th day). The volume of urine rose from 370 ml on the first day to 2400 on the 7th, and later convalescence was uneventful.

The second boy, aged 17, had drunk 2 ozs. Several hours later he became disorientated with signs of central nervous disturbance and a daily output of urine of only 7 ozs. The urine contained albumen and numerous Ca-oxalate crystals in the sediment. The blood urea was 80 mg%, rising to 116 mg% on the third day, and the blood picture was that of leucocytosis ($13,550/\mu l$). All his abnormal findings had practically disappeared after 19 days.

The post mortem appearances in fatal cases have been described by Boemke (1943) and more recently by Patscheider and Hetzel (1961); the latter lay special emphasis on the lesions of the central nervous system.

In this case the man had drunk a Chianti flask full of 'Glysantin' – about

1 litre – and became rapidly delirous and finally unconscious, in deep coma with loss of reflexes. A few hours later lung oedema was suspected but yielded to cortisone administration. Death occurred 33 h after drinking the Glysantin.

The heart showed no abnormality, the liver slight fatty infiltration, the stomach lymphocytes and leucocytes in the submucosa, but no crystals. The kidneys contained many crystals readily visible in unstained sections treated with 1% aus tic soda solution; these were resistant to acetic acid but disappeared on addition of HCl.

In other rapidly fatal cases the kidneys have shown no reaction to the presence of these crystals, but in one, described by Pons and Custer (1946), who survived 120 h there was degeneration of the tubular epithelium.

The spinal cord showed hyperaemia of the meningeal vessels and leucocytosis of the arterioles supplying the spinal nerves; perivascular infiltration was most noticeable in the lumbosacral and cauda equina regions.

The medulla oblongata showed toxic changes in the nerve cells similar to those of anoxia, as also did those of the thalamus with perivascular oedema and leucocytic infiltration, and crystals, similar to those observed in the kidneys, were present in some of the walls of the vessels. The cortex also showed injury of the ganglion cells, and the cerebellum leucocytic infiltration and eosiniphils in the plasma. These lesions are considered to correspond with the description of Pons and Custer as a 'chemical meningo-encephalitis', the result of a primary injury of the vessels, with disturbance of permeability resulting in oxygen deficiency of the nerve tissue, and not a direct consequence of the presence of oxalic acid, though a direct toxic action on the ganglion cells of ethylene glycol itself or its metabolites cannot be excluded.

In the pancreas a subacute local pancreatitis was observed by Smith (1951) and a subperitoneal haemorrhage in the region of the pancreas by Ross (1956) who suggested that this might be related to injury of the pancreas.

The blood picture has in several cases, notably those of Ross (1956) and Patscheider and Hetzel (1961) been that of leucocytosis – 28,000 and 17,000/μl respectively.

The urine before death was slightly opaque and contained some erythrocytes, and post mortem the sediment contained crystals of calcium oxalate.

Chronic poisoning

The report by Troisi (1950) of the chronic toxic affects of inhalation of ethylene glycol related to the manufacture of electrolytic condensers, of which one phase involved spreading a mixture, heated to 105 °C, of 40% ethylene glycol, 55% boric acid and 5% ammonia, on a strip of paper placed on another strip of aluminium. About 40 women were thus exposed to the vapour of the heated ethylene glycol. Nine of them suffered from recurrent attacks of periods of unconsciousness lasting 5–10 min and followed by a rapid return to normality. When removed to other work the attacks ceased. Five other women showed nystagmus but no other signs of abnormality; in two cases the nystagmus was rotatory, suggesting a central nervous lesion. – Nystagmus has also been reported in cases of poisoning by diethylene glycol (Zehrer, 1948).

Troisi (1950) suggests that nystagmus may be regarded as an early sign of more severe intoxication.

TREATMENT

Emergency treatment consists in induction of emesis, followed by gastric lavage with 1:5000 potassium permanganate.

For acidosis, bicarbonate or molar lactate parenteral infusions.

For indication of severe kidney injury, peritoneal dialysis or haemodialysis by artificial kidney (Friedmann *et al.*, 1962).

Among the more recent methods suggested are two which are based on the principle of preventing or inhibiting the formation of metabolic products more toxic than ethylene glycol itself.

(1) Administration of ethyl alcohol (Peterson *et al.*, 1963).

This has not yet apparently been tried in human poisoning, but in animals it has been found that those given a lethal dose of ethylene glycol alone died 14–30 h after receiving an injection, while those receiving a subsequent injection of ethyl alcohol survived. The ethanol-treated animals excreted more ethylene glycol in the urine than those not so treated. It is therefore suggested that in persons who have accidentally ingested ethylene glycol, early administration of ethanol may prevent its lethal effects by inhibiting oxidation and allowing the toxic ethylene glycol to be excreted, without formation of the more toxic metabolites.

(2) Administration of vitamin B$_6$ and magnesium (Gershoff and Andrus, 1962)

In more chronic cases, also on the basis only of animal studies, it is suggested that large amounts of vitamin B$_6$ (pyridoxine) may give partial protection against renal deposition of Ca oxalate by inhibiting the oxidation of ethylene glycol, and that magnesium may give further protection by altering the solvent characteristics of the urine.

114. Ethylene Glycol Derivatives

There are three monoalkyl derivatives of ethylene glycol which are mainly used in industry – the monoethyl ether (Cellosolve), the monomethyl (methyl Cellosolve) and the monobutyl (butyl Cellosolve).

114a. Ethylene Glycol Monoethyl Ether

Synonyms: Cellosolve, ethyl ethylene glycol, 2-ethoxy ethanol, Solvulose
Structural formula: $CH_3-CH_2-O-CH_2-CH_2-OH$
Molecular formula: $C_4H_{10}O_2$
Molecular weight: 90.1
Properties: a colourless, nearly odourless, liquid with a slightly bitter taste. A more powerful solvent for nitrocellulose than any other solvent of similar boiling range, but develops a haze when certain clear solutions of resins are mixed with clear solutions of cellulose nitrate; this haze can often be removed by addition of benzyl alcohol, amyl acetate and ethyl lactate. It is miscible with water in all proportions, also with hydrocarbons and castor oil. It tends to decompose on exposure to sunlight (Durrans, 1950).

> *boiling point:* 135.1 °C
> *vapour pressure:* 5.3 mm Hg at 25 °C
> *vapour density (air = 1):* 3.0
> *specific gravity (liquid density):* 0.931
> *flash point:* 115 °F
> *conversion factors:* 1 p.p.m. = 3.68 mg/m³
>   1 mg/l = 272 p.p.m.
> *solubility:* soluble in water, alcohol and ether
> *maximum allowable concentration:* 200 p.p.m.

ECONOMY, SOURCES AND USES

Production

(1) By reacting ethylene chlorohydrin or glycol with sodium hydroxide and a dialkyl sulphate such as diethyl sulphate.
(2) By reaction of ethylene glycol with an alcohol in the presence of normal metallic sulphates (Curme and Johnston, 1952).

Industrial uses

(1) Chiefly in the lacquer industry, especially for cellulose lacquers for domestic articles.

(2) In the printing industry, as a solvent for inks and printing pastes.

BIOCHEMISTRY

Few details of the fate in the body of cellosolve are available, but according to Shaffer *et al.* (1948) glycol ethers of low molecular weight undergo a limited amount of destruction and do not appear to be distributed in the extracellular fluids of the body; they are cleared from the plasma at a rate identical with that of creatinine in the normal lightly anaesthetised animal. It can be readily absorbed by the skin (Draize *et al.*, 1944).

TOXICOLOGY

The monoethyl ether is the least toxic of the three ethers, and causes less depression of the central nervous system than any other ethylene glycol derivative. In animals large doses are relatively weak as a narcotic; they cause some injury to the kidneys and to a small extent to the liver, but even with subcutaneous injection it appears less toxic than ethylene glycol itself or butyl cellosolve. By inhalation serious injury can only be produced at room temperatures by long exposure to saturated air, though at this level it has a disagreeable odour, and causes some irritation of the eyes.

In human beings, from its industrial use, only slight indefinite symptoms, in the form of eye irritation, a trace of albuminuria and a slight increase in the blood bilirubin have been reported.

Toxicity to animals

(1) Acute. – By oral administration, – MLD, for rats, 5.5 g/kg; for rabbits, 3.1 g/kg; for guinea pigs, 1.4 g/kg (Carpenter *et al.*, 1956).

LD_{50}. – *(i) By oral administration*, for rats, 3.46 g/kg; for mice, 4.31 g/kg; for guinea pigs, 2.79 g/kg (Laug *et al.*, 1939). – *(ii) By subcutaneous injection*, for mice, 5.0 ml/kg (Von Oettingen and Jirouch, 1931). – *(iii) By intravenous injection*, for rats, 2.4 g/kg (Carpenter *et al.*, 1956). – *(iv) By intraperitoneal injection*, for rats, 2.14 g/kg (Carpenter *et al.*, 1956). – *(v) By inhalation*, for mice, 1820 p.p.m. for 7 h (Werner *et al.*, 1943); for guinea pigs, above 6000 p.p.m. for 1 h (Waite, Patty and Yant, 1930; Lehmann and Flury, 1943); for mice, some deaths at 1400 p.p.m. for 7 h (Starrek, 1938).

(2) Chronic

MLD. – *(i) By oral administration*, for rats, 1.89 g/kg after 90 days (in drinking water; Smyth *et al.*, 1951). No deaths at 0.9 g/kg daily in the diet for 2 years (Morris, Nelson and Calvery, 1942). For rabbits, 2.0 ml/kg after 2 daily feedings (Lehmann and Flury, 1943). – *(ii) By inhalation*, for mice, 5 mg/l for 8 h daily for 9 days; for rabbits after 12 days; for cats after 4 or 5 days.

SYMPTOMS OF INTOXICATION

(1) Acute

No immediate signs of distress (Laug *et al.*, 1939) but later dyspnoea and weakness (Werner *et al.*, 1943; Waite *et al.*, 1930), slight paralysis (von Oettingen and Jirouch, 1931); after 7 h prostration (Starrek, 1938). In a few animals the lens and cornea showed opacities.

(a) The eyes. – Instillation of one drop of the pure material caused hyperaemia and slight oedema (Von Oettingen and Jirouch, 1931).

(b) The blood. – In dogs exposed to inhalation of 840 p.p.m. 7 h per day for 12 weeks a slight decrease in red cells and haemoglobin and an increase in immature white cells were noted by Werner *et al.* (1943). The anaemia was less than in animals exposed to methyl cellosolve but there was a similar degree of microcytosis, hypochromia and polychromatophilia.

(2) Chronic

Exhaustion, refusal to eat, staggering, cramps, slow labored respiration; albumen, cylinders and blood in urine.

Death was believed to be due to kidney injury.

CHANGES IN THE ORGANISM

(1) Acute intoxication

The kidneys, following inhalation, showed severe hyperaemia, but no evidence of interstitial nephritis (Waite *et al.*, 1930); with subcutaneous injection, acute nephrosis, with degenerative processes and haemorrhage into intracapsular spaces and tubules (Von Oettingen and Jirouch, 1931), also haematuria (Laug *et al.*, 1939).

The liver showed no injury, the lungs congestion and oedema; the spleen follicular phagocytosis and some siderosis (Werner *et al.*, 1943); the stomach haemorrhage into the mucosa.

(2) Chronic intoxication

In surviving animals the kidney lesions were only slight, but according to Lehmann and Flury (1943) one cat dying after 4–5 days showed glomerulitis. No oxalate concretions in the kidneys or bladder, such as those found in ethylene glycol poisoning, were observed by Morris *et al.* (1942) but Werner *et al.* (1943) noted an increase in the number of oxalate crystals in the urine.

Bibliography on p. 686

While noting no chronic kidney damage in rats and no liver damage Morris *et al.* observed tubular atrophy and interstitial oedema of the testes in about 2/3 of the rats fed on 0.9 kg per day.

Toxicity to human beings

In only two cases, workmen who had been employed for 13 years in lacquer and pigment factories, using Cellosolve as the solvent, has any injurious effect been reported (Browning, 1953). This consisted in one of a slight yellowish discoloration of the sclerotics, and in the other a trace of albumen in the urine and a slightly increased level of urobilin in the blood, possibly indicating slight injury to both kidneys and liver. Otherwise there has been no evidence of injury from the industrial use of cellosolve. Davidson (1926) states that operatives using Cellosolve with a spray gun can work all day without discomfort or ill-effect.

114b. Ethylene Glycol Monomethyl Ether

Synonyms: methyl Cellosolve, 2-methoxyethanol, methyl glycol
Structural formula: $CH_3-O-CH_2-CH_2-OH$
Molecular formula: $C_3H_8O_2$
Molecular weight: 76.1
Properties: a colourless mobile almost odourless liquid, less viscous than the ethyl- or butylmonoethyl glycols. In certain conditions decomposes rapidly into acetaldehyde and methanol.

    boiling point: 124.5 °C
    vapour pressure: 6.2 mm Hg at 20 °C
    vapour density (air = 1): 2.6   *conversion factors:*
    specific gravity (liquid density): 0.9663   1 p.p.m. = 3.11 mg/m³
    flash point: 107 °F (Durrans, 1950)   1 mg/l = 322 p.p.m.
    solubility: miscible with water and light aromatic and paraffin hydrocarbons. Solvent for low viscosity cellulose acetate and nitrate, some resins and gums and spirit-soluble dyes; has no action on raw rubber.
    maximum allowable concentration: 25 p.p.m.

ECONOMY, SOURCES AND USES

Production

(1) By reacting ethylene oxide with methyl alcohol and various catalysts.
(2) By reacting ethylene chlorohydrin or ethylene glycol with NaOH and a dialkyl sulphate (Curme and Johnston, 1952).

Industrial uses

(1) In the lacquer industry.
(2) For sealing moisture-proof cellophane.
(3) As a solvent for rotogravure inks and leather dyestuffs.
(4) In the 'fused collar' industry as a stiffener.

BIOCHEMISTRY

Estimation in the atmosphere

(1) By potassium dichromate oxidation (Elkins *et al.*, 1942; Werner and Mitchell, 1943).
(2) By the infra-red method of Nawrocki *et al.* (1944).

Metabolism

Methyl cellosolve is absorbable by the skin of animals in toxic amounts (Rowe, 1963). Since acute poisoning following oral dosage in animals causes no increase in urinary oxalic acid, methanol or formic acid (Wiley *et al.*, 1938), or, in the one fatal case by ingestion, of methanol (Young and Woolner, 1946) it is concluded that it is not hydrolysed in the body to ethylene glycol. Its considerable toxic effect must therefore be due to a direct action of methyl cellosolve itself, though the site at which its hemolytic effect occurs has not been elucidated; the studies of Werner, Mitchell *et al.* (1943) on this aspect have not revealed any serious injury to the bone marrow, but Rowe (1963) remarks that they were not sufficiently prolonged to demonstrate that the action was not centred on the bone marrow.

TOXICOLOGY

The vapour of methyl cellosolve is irritant to mucous membranes, but, while not irritant to the skin, it is readily absorbed in toxic amounts. In animals a special manifestation of its toxicity is its effect upon the blood.

In this respect, as in several others, methyl cellosolve is more toxic than cellosolve or butyl cellosolve. Repeated exposure of animals to inhalation of 800 p.p.m. has caused severe anaemia and an increased 'shift to the left'. These disturbances have also been reported from the use of methyl cellosolve in the fused collar industry, together with disorders of the central nervous system.

One fatal case in a human being, following ingestion of about half a pint of methyl cellosolve was reported by Young and Woolner in 1946.

Bibliography on p. 686

Toxicity to animals

(1) Acute

(i) By oral administration, MLD, for rats, 3.4 g/kg; for rabbits, 0.89 g/kg; for guinea pigs, 0.95 g/kg (Carpenter *et al.*, 1956). – *(ii) By subcutaneous injection*, for rabbits, 2.0 ml/kg (Lehmann and Flury, 1943); for mice, 3 mg/kg (Starrek, 1938). – *(iii) By intraperitoneal injection*, for rats (LD$_{50}$), 2.5 g/kg (Carpenter *et al.*, 1956). – *(iv) By intravenous injection*, for rats (LD$_{50}$), undiluted 2.2 g/kg, 25% solution in NaCl, 2.7 g/kg (Carpenter *et al.*, 1956). – *(v) By inhalation*, MLD, for mice, more than 3200 p.p.m. for 7 h (Starrek, 1938). – *(vi) By skin contact*, (LD$_{50}$), for rabbits, 2 g/kg (Rowe, 1963).

(2) Chronic

(i) By subcutaneous injection, MLD, for guinea pigs, 5 daily injections of 1 ml/kg; for rabbits, 7 daily injections of 1 ml/kg (Lehmann and Flury, 1943). – *(ii) By intramuscular injection*, LD$_{50}$, for rabbits, 2 daily injections of 2 ml/kg (Wiley *et al.*, 1938). – *(iii) By inhalation*, one rabbit died after 4 days' exposure to 800 p.p.m., others after 5–10 days to 1600 p.p.m. Mice were resistant to such exposures (Lehmann and Flury, 1943). Rats survived exposure to 310 p.p.m. 7 h a day for 5 weeks and dogs to 750 p.p.m. for 12 weeks (Werner *et al.*, 1943).

SYMPTOMS OF INTOXICATION

(1) Acute

With large doses only slight narcosis, but exhaustion, labored breathing, haematuria and albuminuria. With inhalation death from pneumonia and kidney injury.

(2) Chronic

With the highest dosages Lehmann and Flury (1943) observed staggering, prostration, labored respiration, tetanic spasms; in some animals diarrhoea, and albumen, red cells and casts in urine.

CHANGES IN THE ORGANISM

(1) Acute

(a) The lungs. – Oedema or bronchopneumonia.

(b) The liver. – Slight hyperaemia.

(c) The kidneys. – Severe degenerative changes.

(d) Effect on the eyes. – Instillation into the eyes of rabbits caused immediate pain, conjunctival irritation and transitory cloudiness of the cornea (Rowe, 1963).

(2) Chronic

(a) Trachea and lungs showed inflammation.

(b) Kidneys, glomerulitis. Wiley, Hueper *et al.* (1938) also noted irritation of

the bladder mucosa, gastro-intestinal haemorrhage, and injury to the liver and testes. The spleen did not show significant amounts of siderosis.

(c) *Effect on the blood*. – The most significant manifestation of chronic poisoning in most animals subjected to repeated inhalation of methyl cellulose is its effect on the red corpuscles. Werner *et al.* noted in 1943 a decrease in hemoglobin, cell volume and number of red cells, with hypochromia, polychromatophilia and microcytosis; the leucocytes showed an increase in the number of immature cells. Dogs appeared to be more affected from the point of view of blood disturbance than did other species.

Toxicity to human beings

(1) Acute

In the only reported case of fatal poisoning by methyl cellosolve (Young and Woolner, 1946) a man aged 44 had drunk about half a pint of liquid, presumed to have been alcohol, which was later found to have all the physical and chemical properties of methyl cellosolve. He was comatose when admitted to hospital with deep, rapid labored respiration and rapid pulse, both decreasing within 4 h. Urine taken by catheter contained only a trace of albumen; the blood picture showed 5,500,000 red blood corpuscles, 8100 white blood corpuscles; haemoglobin 84%; urea nitrogen 17.9 mg; non-protein nitrogen 38.5 mg per 100 ml. The man died 5 h later without regaining consciousness.

Autopsy showed injuries chiefly to the kidneys and liver, with acute haemorrhagic gastritis. The kidneys showed marked degenerative and toxic changes, the liver fatty degeneration and the pancreas some early necrosis.

(2) Chronic

In human beings the chronic toxic action of methyl cellulose has been manifested more on the central nervous system and the blood picture than on the kidneys.

A form of 'toxic encephalopathy' – headache, drowsiness, lethargy, general weakness, some ataxia, irregular and unequal pupils and some psychopathic disturbance – was reported by Donley (1936) in a woman employed in the 'fused collar' industry. This involved exposure to methyl cellosolve during the process of dipping collars into a solution of methyl cellosolve, isopropyl alcohol and cellulose acetate, the collar being later subjected to heat and pressure.

In 1938, Parsons and Parsons recorded two somewhat similar cases in young men similarly employed. They complained of fatigue, drowsiness, giddiness, headache and burning of the eyes, and it was noted that they had undergone a complete change of personality, from alertness and intelligence to lethargy and stupidity. Both had moderate ataxia and a positive Romberg reaction, hypersensitivity to light and accomodation of the pupils, and macrocytic anaemia and granul-

Bibliography on p. 686

openia. Both eventually recovered after removal from exposure, but with persistence of the high colour index and relative lymphocytosis.

As a result of these two cases Greenburg *et al.* (1938) re-examined them and 17 other workers employed on the same process though the isopropanol had by that time been replaced by ethanol, and the ventilation had been improved so that the concentration now ranged from 25 to 76 p.p.m. Some of these workers showed nervous disturbance of the same nature as the earlier cases – abnormal reflexes, tremor of the hands and mental retardation – and in all the blood picture was abnormal, showing macrocytic anaemia and general immaturity of the leucocytes (shift to the left) but no actual leucopenia or granulopenia.

The most recent account of a similar action of methyl cellosolve was given by Zavon in 1963. He describes the condition of 4 men who had all worked in the printing department of a plant making plastic materials. The cleaning of the machines, and later of the floor and other equipment was done by methyl cellosolve. Hygienic control, in the matter of clothing and washing facilities was poor, and the work period had recently been increased to 9–10 h a day 6 days a week. The concentration of methyl cellosolve during this period was calculated to be from 61 p.p.m. near small cleaning operations, to 3960 p.p.m. while cleaning a high-boy with 2 gallons of methyl cellosolve. All the 4 men exhibited symptoms which led to a diagnosis of central nervous depression – in one case 'cerebral atrophy' (this man was ataxic, with a positive Romberg test, slurred speech and tremor). In only one was the possibility of industrial poisoning suspected. In all 4 the changes of personality were similar to those described by Donley and Parsons and Parsons; all showed some anaemia and one case a hypocellular bone marrow with decrease of the erythroid elements. All 4 ultimately recovered, but in 2 complete restoration of central nervous system function could not be definitely stated, since their previous mental status was unknown.

114c. Ethylene Glycol Monobutyl Ether

Synonyms: butyl cellosolve; 2-butoxyethanol; butyl oxitol
Structural formula: $CH_3–CH_2–O–CH_2–CH_2–O–CH_2–CH_3$
Molecular formula: $C_6H_{14}O_2$
Molecular weight: 118.2
Properties: A colourless mobile liquid with a slightly rancid odour, an initially bitter taste followed by a burning sensation and numbness of the tongue.
　　boiling point: 170–176 °C
　　vapour pressure: 0.88 mm Hg
　　vapour density (air = 1): 4.0
　　specific gravity (liquid density): 0.9019

flash point: 165 °F

conversion factors: 1 p.p.m. = 4.84 mg/m³

1 mg/l   = 207 p.p.m.

solubility: in water 5% at 20 °C. Solvent for cellulose nitrate and other cellulose esters and ethers, also for resins used in surface coatings, oils and greases.

evaporation rate (ether = 1): more rapid than cellosolve or methyl cellosolve (Fairhall, 1957)

maximum allowable concentration: 50 p.p.m.

ECONOMY, SOURCES AND USES

Production

(1) By reaction of ethylene oxide with the suitable alcohol, with various catalysts.
(2) By reacting ethylene chlorohydrin or ethylene glycol with NaOH and a dialkyl sulphate (Curme and Johnston, 1952).

Industrial uses

(1) Chiefly in the lacquer industry where its advantage results from its high boiling point and slow hardening giving a slight increase of gloss to the film.
(2) In cleaning materials for metals and dry-cleaning soaps.
(3) In the textile industry for dyeing and printing.
(4) In hydraulic fluids.

BIOCHEMISTRY

Estimation

(1) In the atmosphere

    (a) The method of bichromate oxidation described by Werner and Mitchell (1943) in which the air being tested is passed into a mixture of potassium bichromate and concentrated H_2SO_4, heated, then cooled and distilled water and potassium iodide added, and the contents titrated with 0.05 N Na_2SO_4, with starch solution as the end-point. Reading by the interferometer.

    (b) The infrared method described by Nawrocki *et al.* (1944) is suggested by Rowe (1963) as the most practical modern method.

(2) In blood

    After precipitation of the proteins of a 5 ml sample of venous blood, the

Bibliography on p. 686

filtrate is extracted by ether. The extract is washed with ammonia and the alkaline solution evaporated to dryness. The amount of butoxy-acetic acid in a solution of the residue in distilled water is estimated chromatographically.

(3) In urine

By means of the chromatograph following addition of a 10% sodium tungstate solution, acidification with H_2SO_4 ether extraction and washing with ammonia

Metabolism

From the investigations of Carpenter *et al.* (1956) it appears that butyl cellosolve is oxidised in the body to butoxy-acetic acid, most of which is excreted within 24 h even after inhalation, the amount and the correlation with dosage differing in various species of animals.

In dogs inhaling 400 p.p.m. for 4 h the estimated amount in the urine was 55 mg in a 24 h sample; with 200 p.p.m. it was 42 mg in one animal and 100 in another. Rabbits inhaling 400 p.p.m. excreted 89–302 mg and with 200 p.p.m. 12–23 mg while guinea pigs on 200 p.p.m. excreted only 5 mg and rats an average of 14 mg.

No butoxy-acetic acid was found in the blood of animals inhaling butyl cellosolve, but it was present in the blood of rabbits 4 h after intravenous injection, and in the urine during the 24 h following the dose. Carpenter *et al.* suggest that the reason for the failure to identify it in the blood after inhalation is that it is present in too low a concentration to be detected by the method used.

In human beings exposed to 100 p.p.m. for 8 h the excretion of butoxyacetic acid was 100–200 mg within 24 h. Carpenter *et al.* suggest that this metabolite, to a greater extent than butyl cellosolve itself, is responsible for the haemolytic effect in some species of animals.

TOXICOLOGY

Butyl cellosolve is regarded as the most toxic of the glycol monoalkyl ethers used as solvents, and though reports of any injury from its industrial use are few and not altogether convincing, and its relatively low volatility makes the hazard o poisoning from inhalation a rather remote possibility, it is readily absorbed by the skin and could carry a hazard from prolonged contact.

In addition to the irritative effect of high concentrations on the lungs of animals when inhaled, its capacity for kidney injury and its narcotic effect, it has a considerable potentiality for producing haemolysis, whether primarily or by means of its metabolite, butoxyacetic acid.

Toxicity to animals

(1) Acute

LD$_{50}$. – *(i) By oral administration*, for rats, 2.5 mg/kg (Carpenter *et al.*, 1956); 0.47 g/kg (Biochem. Res. Lab., cited by Rowe, 1963); for mice, 1.2 g/kg (Carpenter *et al.*, 1956); for rabbits (the most sensitive species), 0.32 g/kg; for rabbits MLD, 1.0–2.0 ml/kg (Lehmann and Flury, 1943). – *(ii) By subcutaneous injection*, MLD, for rabbits, 0.4 mg/kg (Lehmann and Flury, 1943); for cats, 2 ml/kg (Lehmann and Flury, 1943). – *(iii) By intravenous injection*, LD$_{50}$, for rats, 0.34 ml/kg (Carpenter *et al.* 1956), for rabbits, 0.28 ml/kg – *(iv) By skin absorption*, LD$_{50}$, for rats, 0.43 ml/kg within 48 h; for rabbits, 0.56 ml/kg (Carpenter *et al.*, 1956). – *(v) By inhalation*, MLD, for mice, 700 p.p.m. after 7 h (Werner *et al.*, 1943); for rats, 375 p.p.m. (Carpenter *et al.*, 1956).

(2) Chronic

(i) By oral administration, for rats: addition to the diet of amounts up to 2.0% of butyl cellosolve for 90 days was followed by no deaths directly attributable to the toxic action of the compound, but there was loss of weight in the group receiving 2%, with increase in weight of the liver and kidneys. – *(ii) By inhalation*, MLD, for rats, 432 p.p.m. 7 h a day, 5 days a week for 30 days; for guinea pigs, 494 p.p.m. killed only 2 out of 10; for dogs, 617 p.p.m. after 13½ h exposure in 2 days.

SYMPTOMS OF INTOXICATION

(1) Acute

Sluggishness, rough coat, prostration and narcosis; haemoglobinuria in animals dying from an oral dose; it was concluded by Carpenter *et al.*, that this was caused by *in vivo* haemolysis and not by cellular destruction in the kidney. Death, if early, was due to narcosis; if delayed for several days, to pneumonitis and kidney injury. In mice, inhalation did not cause narcosis, but dyspnoea was a constant sign, and with high concentrations Werner *et al.* (1943) noted corneal or lens opacity.

(2) Chronic

Respiratory irritation, haemoglobinuria, low levels of haemoglobin and red cells and fragility of erythrocytes.

Rats, mice and rabbits are the most susceptible to this haemolytic action of butyl cellosolve or its metabolite in increasing the fragility of the erythrocytes, guinea pigs, dogs and monkeys less so, and human beings (see below) least of all. This action is a slow drain upon the erythrocyteproducing organs, and repeated excessive inhalation, even by dogs, was found to result eventually in anaemia.

Kidney injury, of the same nature as that caused by acute intoxication was reported by Lehmann and Flury (1943) to be caused by repeated inhalation of 500 p.p.m.; 300 p.p.m. caused no severe kidney lesions but a moderate retention of urea in the blood.

Bibliography on p. 686

CHANGES IN THE ORGANISM

The lungs showed slight to moderate congestion; sometimes bronchopneumonia. The spleen, congestion and follicular phagocytosis; the kidneys severe congestion (Carpenter *et al.*, 1956).

Toxicity to human beings

In some investigations by Carpenter *et al.* (1956) on volunteer subjects, those inhaling 113 p.p.m. for 4 h reported nasal and ocular irritation with a slight increase in nasal discharge and occasional eructation. In a second experiment a year later 3 subjects inhaled 195 p.p.m. for two 4-h periods separated by an interval of 30 min. Two of the 3 excreted considerable amounts of butoxyacetic acid during the next 24 h, the third only a trace. They all noted immediate irritation of the nose and throat and later of the eyes, and disturbed taste. Other volunteers inhaled 100 p.p.m. for 8 h; their urinary excretion of butoxyacetic acid was approximately the same as that of the 195 p.p.m. exposures. One subject vomited several times the next day and two others complained of headache. No other objective signs were noted, especially no erythrocyte fragility.

From the industrial point of view, only one case of possible systemic injury was that of a man who was reported to the Factory Inspectorate of Great Britain in 1934 as having had two isolated attacks of haematuria, with 5 months interval. In the second attack casts were present in the urine but no albumen, and a month later the urine was normal. His exposure had included butyl carbitol as well as butyl cellosolve, so that it is not certain that the toxic action could be directly attributed solely to butyl cellosolve.

Symptoms of irritation of the eyes and nose and headache were also complained of by two girls who had been in contact for 2 years with enamel containing butyl cellosolve.

114d. Ethylene Glycol Diethyl Ether

Synonym: diethyl Cellosolve
Structural formula: $CH_3-CH_2-O-CH_2-CH_2-CH_2-O-CH_2-CH_3$
Molecular formula: $C_6H_{14}O_2$
Molecular weight: 118.2
Properties: a colourless liquid with a sweetish odour and bitter taste. Solvent for ester gum, shellac and some resins and oils, but not for cellulose acetate or nitrate or polyvinyl resins.

> *boiling point:* 121.4 °C
> *vapour pressure:* 9.4 mm Hg at 20 °C
> *vapour density (air = 1):* 4.1

specific gravity (liquid density): 0.842

flash point: 95 °F

conversion factors: 1 p.p.m. $= 4.84$ mg/m³

1 mg/l $= 207$ p.p.m.

solubility: in water 21%. Soluble in alcohol, ether and oils.

maximum allowable concentration: not established. Rowe (1963) suggests that it should be somewhat less than 100 p.p.m. since it does not have sufficient warning properties to prevent excessive exposure during repeated and prolonged contact.

ECONOMY, SOURCES AND USES

Production

(1) As a by-product in the reaction of ethylene oxide with a monohydric alcohol.

(2) By reacting dialkyl sulphate with the ethylene glycol monoethyl ether (Curme and Johnston, 1952).

Industrial uses

Chiefly in the lacquer industry, but not to such an extent as the monoethyl ether.

BIOCHEMISTRY

Metabolism

No specific information as to the metabolic fate of this ether is available, but according to Curme and Johnston, there is no reason to believe that it is hydrolysed in the body, and Wiley *et al.* (1936) found no formation of oxalic acid in dogs with oral dosage.

TOXICOLOGY

While possessing the potential toxicity – irritation of mucous membranes, kidney and lung injury – of other glycol derivatives, especially with chronic exposure, it appears to be actually less toxic than the monoethyl, monobutyl and monomethyl ethers by oral dosage to animals, with a LD_{50} of 4.39 g/kg for rats, as compared with 3.0, 1.48 and 2.46 for these respectively.

Lehmann and Flury (1943) remark that it is too expensive to be of practical industrial importance.

Bibliography on p. 686

Toxicity to animals

(1) Acute

(i) By oral administration, LD$_{50}$, for rats, 4.39 g/kg (Smyth *et al.*, 1941); for guinea pigs, 2.44 g/kg (Smyth *et al.*, 1941). – *(ii) By subcutaneous injection*, MLD, for cats, 0.5–1 ml/kg. – *(iii) By inhalation*, 10,000 p.p.m. was not lethal (Gross, 1943).

(2) Chronic

(i) By oral administration, for dogs and rabbits, 1.0 ml/kg 6 times within a week was tolerated without symptoms (Lehmann and Flury, 1943); for cats, 1 ml/kg 4 times was followed by death 30 to 40 h after the last dose. – *(ii) By subcutaneous injection*, for guinea pigs, 1 ml/kg was fatal after 7 injections; for dogs, 9.5 ml daily for 7 days caused no noticeable symptoms (Wiley *et al.*, 1938). – *(iii) By inhalation*, for rabbits and cats, 500 p.p.m. 8 h daily for 12 days caused death; for mice and guinea pigs no evident injury (Lehmann and Flury, 1943).

SYMPTOMS OF INTOXICATION

(1) Acute

Irritation of mucous membranes and a suggestion of narcosis in cats, the most susceptible species (Lehmann and Flury, 1943).

(2) Chronic

Loss of weight, temporary narcosis, followed by prostration prior to death.

CHANGES IN THE ORGANISM

(1) Acute

No characteristic findings.

(2) Chronic

(a) The kidneys. – Parenchymatous and interstitial nephritis.

(b) Trachea. – Purulent inflammation in one cat following repeated inhalation of 500 p.p.m.

(c) Effect on the skin. – According to Lehmann and Flury (1943), diethyl cellosolve does not injure the skin of guinea pigs, rabbits and dogs.

(d) Effect on the eyes. – Slight transitory injury of the cornea, healing within a few days, and irritation of the conjunctiva (Carpenter and Smyth, 1946).

Toxicity to human beings

There are no records of any injury to human beings, industrially or otherwise.

114e. Ethylene Glycol Monoacetate

Synonym: Solvent GC

Structural formula:
$$CH_3-\overset{\overset{\displaystyle O}{\|}}{C}-CH_2-CH_2-OH$$

Molecular formula: $C_4H_8O_3$

Molecular weight: 104.1

Properties: a colourless liquid with a slight fruity odour and somewhat pungent taste. Miscible with water and aromatic hydrocarbons but not with paraffins, linseed oil or benzine. Solvent for cellulose acetate and nitrate, partly for mastic, not for shellac, hard copals, ester gum and cumarone (Durrans, 1950).

    boiling point: 182–195 °C

    vapour density (air = 1): 3.59

    specific gravity (liquid density): 1.106

    flash point: > 102 °F

    conversion factors: 1 p.p.m. = 4.25 mg/m³

                   1 mg/l   = 235 p.p.m.

    maximum allowable concentration: not established

ECONOMY, SOURCES AND USES

Industrial uses

(1) In the lacquer industry to a very slight extent.

(2) In the textile industry, in solutions of cellulose acetate intended for printing on fabrics.

(3) In the manufacture of cosmetics and essences.

BIOCHEMISTRY

Metabolism

The amount excreted in the urine of dogs and rabbits following intravenous injection is less than 0.5% of the amount injected (Wiley *et al.*, 1938). It forms oxalic acid in the body to the same extent as ethylene glycol.

TOXICOLOGY

Solvent GC is low in acute oral toxicity to animals, but repeated dosage or repeated inhalation of the vapour causes injury to the kidneys, testes, lungs and

Bibliography on p. 686

brain. Saturated concentrations are irritating to the mucous membranes of the eyes and nose; it is not appreciably irritating to the skin of animals or human beings, and no injury to human beings has been recorded.

Toxicity to animals

(1) Acute

(i) *By oral administration*, LD_{50}, for rats, 8.25 g/kg; for guinea pigs, 3.80 g/kg (Smyth *et al.*, 1941). – *(ii) By subcutaneous injection*, MLD, for cats, 4.5 g/kg. – *(iii) By inhalation:* Single exposure to 8 mg/l (almost saturated – 1900 p.p.m.) caused no deaths and no after-effects (Lehmann and Flury, 1943).

(2) Chronic

(i) *By oral administration*, dogs tolerated feeding of 0.1 or 0.5 ml 12 times without apparent ill-effect. – *(ii) By subcutaneous injection*, guinea pigs showed no injury from 7 injections of 0.5 or 0.1 ml (Lehmann and Flury, 1943). – *(iii) By inhalation*. One rabbit died after the eleventh inhalation of 1900 p.p.m. for 8 h at a time, but cats, guinea pigs and mice survived 12 such exposures (Lehmann and Flury, 1943). Repeated inhalations of higher concentrations by Flury and Rosser (unpublished, cited by Lehmann and Flury) caused death of cats after several days.

SYMPTOMS OF INTOXICATION

(1) Acute

Lehmann and Flury observed only irritation of eyes and nose of cats, rabbits and guinea pigs subjected to inhalation of almost saturated concentrations; there was no albuminuria and no definite narcosis.

(2) Chronic

Irritation of mucous membranes followed by habituation, apathy, exhaustion and stupor, lack of appetite and emaciation.

CHANGES IN THE ORGANISM

The kidneys show degenerative changes, and there is a substantial increase in the excretion of urinary oxalic acid (Wiley *et al.*, 1938).
The lungs show bronchopneumonia (Lehmann and Flury, 1943). Testes and brain also show degenerative changes.
Effect on the eyes. – Moderate irritation (Carpenter and Smyth, 1946).
Effect on the skin. – No appreciable irritation (Lehmann and Flury, 1943).

114f. Ethylene Glycol Diacetate

Synonym: ethylene diacetate

Structural formula:

$$CH_3-\overset{\overset{\displaystyle O}{\|}}{C}-O-CH_2-CH_2-O-\overset{\overset{\displaystyle O}{\|}}{C}-CH_3$$

Molecular formula: $C_6H_{10}O_4$

Molecular weight: 146.2

Properties: a colourless liquid with a slight odour of ethyl acetate. Solvent for cellulose acetate and nitrate, ethyl cellulose, mastic, colophony and gum camphor, but not for ester gum, hard copal or cumarone (Durrans, 1950).

    boiling point: 186–190.8 °C

    vapour pressure: 0.25 mm Hg

    specific gravity (liquid density): 1.1063

    flash point: 255 °F

    conversion factors: 1 p.p.m. = 5.97 mg/m³

                     1 mg/l = 167 p.p.m.

    solubility: in water 16.4% at 20 °C. Not miscible with petroleum or linseed oil.

    maximum allowable concentration: not established

ECONOMY, SOURCES AND USES

Production

By heating ethylene dichloride with potassium or sodium acetate in the presence of about 5% of ethylene glycol under pressure (Durrans, 1950).

Industrial uses

In 1943 Lehmann and Flury stated that "it is scarcely used at all to-day", but it has apparently a limited application in the lacquer industry and in printing inks, and in the removal of free fatty acids from oils and fats (Curme and Johnston, 1952).

BIOCHEMISTRY

Metabolism

No specific investigations of its fate in the body have been made, but in view of the fact that in animals repeatedly dosed with it in amounts sufficient to cause kidney lesions, these amounts have not been severe enough to be the obvious cause of death; Kesten *et al.* (1939) have suggested that there may possibly have been formation of toxic intermediary products.

Bibliography on p. 686

TOXICOLOGY

Acute oral toxicity to animals is low, and even when given intravenously it does not cause hydropic degeneration of the kidneys. Repeated oral administration does, however, cause deposition of calcium oxalate crystals in the kidneys.

No injurious effects on human beings have been recorded.

Toxicity to animals

(1) Acute

By oral administration, LD$_{50}$, for rats, 6.86 g/kg; for guinea pigs, 4.94 g/kg, when fed as a 50% aqueous solution (Smyth *et al.*, 1941).

(2) Chronic

By oral administration, for rats, the minimal repeated dose to produce kidney damage was 6 g/kg daily, in 5% concentration in drinking water for 7 days. Some animals died in 7–114 days.

SYMPTOMS OF INTOXICATION

(1) Acute

According to Kesten *et al.* (1939) and Mulinos *et al.* (1943) the symptoms are like those of ethylene glycol itself.

(2) Chronic

The cause of death was not always obvious (Kesten *et al.*, 1939).

CHANGES IN THE ORGANISM

(1) Acute

Kesten *et al.* found that neither by intravenous nor oral administration did large doses of ethylene glycol diacetate cause hydropic degeneration of the kidney tubules.

(2) Chronic

Mulinos *et al.* (1943) found that repeated administration of 1–3% solutions over a prolonged period caused deposits of calcium oxalate in the kidneys similar to those produced by ethylene glycol; in one animal receiving a 5% solution the deposits were so large as to cause dilatation of the convoluted tubules and slight nitrogen retention, but in no case was hydropic degeneration observed.

Toxicity to human beings

None have been recorded.

114g. Ethylene Glycol Monoethyl Ether Acetate

Synonyms: Cellosolve acetate; ethyl glycol acetate

Structural formula:
$$CH_3{-}CH_2{-}O{-}CH_2{-}CH_2{-}O{-}\overset{\displaystyle O}{\overset{\|}{C}}{-}CH_3$$

Molecular formula: $C_6H_{12}O_3$

Molecular weight: 132.16

Properties: a colourless slightly volatile liquid with a mild ester-like odour, becoming objectionable in high concentrations, and a bitter acid taste.

  boiling point: 156.4 °C
  vapour pressure: 1.2–1.7 mm Hg at 20 °C
  vapour density (air = 1): 4.72
  specific gravity (liquid density): 0.9748
  flash point: 150 °F
  conversion factors: 1 p.p.m. = 5.4 mg/m³
              1 mg/l   = 185 p.p.m.
  solubility: in water 22% at 20 °C; dissolves 6.5% of water (Durrans, 1950). Miscible with olive oil and alcohol in all proportions.
  maximum allowable concentration: 100 p.p.m.

ECONOMY, SOURCES AND USES

Production

By esterification of the monoethyl ether with acetic acid in presence of a catalyst (Curme and Johnston, 1952).

Industrial uses

As a solvent for nitrocellulose, cellulose ether, low-viscosity cellulose acetate and some resins, but not for raw rubber or hard copal (Durrans, 1950).

BIOCHEMISTRY

Estimation in the atmosphere

By adaptation of the infrared spectrophotometric method of Nawrocki *et al.* (1944).

Metabolism

It is not readily absorbed by the skin, but with intensive prolonged application toxic amounts can be absorbed.

Bibliography on p. 686

According to Rowe (1963) its metabolic product is ethylene glycol monoethyl ether to which its systemic effects may be related.

TOXICOLOGY

This ether-ester is only weakly narcotic to animals and not highly toxic, though in high dosage it can cause depression of the central nervous system and injury to lungs and kidneys. With oral dosage its acute toxicity is less than that of the methyl ether-ester, and with repeated application to the skin it is considerably less toxic. It is somewhat irritating to the eyes but not significantly so to the skin. High dosage by inhalation causes definite injury to the kidneys of animals. No injury to human beings has been reported.

Toxicity to animals

(1) Acute

   (i) By oral administration, LD_{50}, for rats, 5.1 g/kg in a 50% aqueous solution (Smyth *et al.*, 1941), for rabbits, 1.95 g/kg (Carpenter, 1947). – *(ii) By subcutaneous injection*, lethal dose for mice, 5.0 ml/kg (von Oettingen and Jirouch, 1931); 4.6 ml/kg (Rosser, 1938). – *(iii) By inhalation:* guinea pigs and rabbits survived exposure to saturated vapour-air mixtures (4000 p.p.m.) for 1 h, but 2 such exposures for 2–6 h caused delayed death to cats. – *(iv) By skin contact,* LD_{50}, for rabbits, 10.3 g/kg with the 'sleeve' technique of Draize *et al.* (1944) (Carpenter, 1947).

(2) Chronic

   (i) By subcutaneous injection, for guinea pigs, 0.5 or 1 ml repeated 7 times did not cause death (Gross, 1943). – *(ii) By inhalation*, for cats, guinea pigs and one rabbit, 12 exposures to 450 p.p.m. for 8 h did not cause death in all animals, but the rabbit died on the 8th day and 2 cats on the 6th and 7th (Gross, 1943). These results do not agree with those of Carpenter, on dogs, which he states survived exposures of 7 h daily to 600 p.p.m. without apparent injury.

SYMPTOMS OF INTOXICATION

(1) Acute

   Very slight narcosis, vomiting, cramps, paralysis, albuminuria, death from central nervous system paralysis.

(2) Chronic

   With repeated subcutaneous injection of 1 ml, temporary emaciation, exhaustion after each injection. With inhalation, increasing weakness and albuminuria (Gross, 1943).

   Methaemoglobinemia was stated by von Oettingen and Jirouch (1931) to occur but Carpenter found none in rats after inhalation of 1500 p.p.m. for 4 h or in dogs given 1 g/kg by stomach tube.

(1) Acute

Injury of the kidneys was observed by Gross (1938).

(2) Chronic

The findings of Gross and Carpenter again differ considerably in this respect, the former noting definite signs of kidney injury, the latter no histopathological changes in dogs – the discrepancy possibly due to difference in species susceptibiliy.

In industrial use, the low volatility, and the objectionable odour of high concentrations indicate that this compound does not carry a high industrial hazard but the fact that lethal amounts can be absorbed by the skin gives warning that prolonged repeated contact should be avoided.

114h. Ethylene Glycol Monomethyl Ether Acetate

Synonyms: methyl Cellosolve acetate; methyl glycol acetate

Structural formula:
$$CH_3-O-CH_2-CH_2-O-\overset{\overset{\displaystyle O}{\|}}{C}-CH_3$$

Molecular formula: $C_5H_{10}O_3$

Molecular weight: 118.13

Properties: a colourless liquid with a weak pleasant odour, and bitter pungent taste. An outstanding solvent for cellulose acetate and nitrate and vinyl acetate, resins, ester gum, hydrocarbons and vegetable oils, without action on rubber.

   boiling point: 144.5 °C
   vapour pressure: 3.3 mm Hg
   vapour density (air = 1): 4.07
   specific gravity (liquid density): 1.007
   flash point: 140 °F
   conversion factors: 1 p.p.m. = 4.83 mg/m³
         1 mg/l   = 207 p.p.m.
   solubility: miscible with water in all proportions
   maximum allowable concentration: 25 p.p.m.

ECONOMY, SOURCES AND USES

Produced by esterification of ethylene glycol monomethyl ether with acetic acid.

Used (1) in the lacquer industry, (2) in textile printing, (3) in the manufacture of photographic film, (4) in the manufacture of coatings and adhesives.

Bibliography on p. 686

BIOCHEMISTRY

Estimation

By modification of the infra-red method described by Nawrocki *et al.* (1944) for glycol ethers.

Metabolism

Methyl cellosolve acetate can be absorbed by the skin with prolonged contact. Little is known of its specific metabolic fate, but it would appear that like other acid esters of the glycol ethers it is saponified in the body, giving a systemic effect characteristic of the parent glycol ether (methyl cellosolve, Lepkowski *et al.*, 1935). It has also been suggested (Flury and Wirth, 1933) that some formation of acetaldehyde occurs.

TOXICOLOGY

The effects of methyl cellosolve acetate when administered to animals are similar to those of methyl cellosolve itself, the main injury being found in the kidneys and brain; also in some species in some disturbance of the blood picture. It is only slightly narcotic and irritating to mucous membranes. There is no evidence of injury to human beings.

Toxicity to animals

(1) Acute

  (i) By oral administration, LD_{50}, for rats, 3.93 g/kg of a 50% aqueous solution; for guinea pigs, 1.25 g/kg (Smyth *et al.*, 1941). – *(ii) By subcutaneous injection,* MLD, for guinea pigs, 5 g/kg, for cats, 3–4 g/kg (Flury and Wirth, 1933). – *(iii) By inhalation*, for rats, 7000 p.p.m. for 4 h was lethal to 2 out of 6 (Smyth and Carpenter, 1948); for cats, 1500 p.p.m. for 7 h caused delayed death (Flury and Wirth, 1933); for guinea pigs and cats, almost saturated vapour caused death delayed for 36 h to 21 days (Gross, 1943). – *(iv) By skin contact*, LD_{50}, for rabbits, 5.25 ml/kg (Smyth and Carpenter, 1948).

(2) Chronic

  (i) By oral administration, MLD, for rabbits, 3 daily doses of 0.5 or 0.1 ml/kg (Gross, 1943). – *(ii) By subcutaneous injection*, for guinea pigs, 7 daily doses of 0.5 ml caused death 2–5 days after the last injection; 1.0 ml after 1–2 days. – *(iii) By inhalation*, for cats, 8 h exposure to 500 p.p.m. (Gross, 1943); for cats, 4–6 h

exposure to 800 p.p.m. for 5 days caused death in 2 out of 3 (Flury and Wirth, 1933); for guinea pigs and rabbits, 8 h exposure to 1000 p.p.m.

SYMPTOMS OF INTOXICATION

(1) Acute

Irritation of mucous membranes, lack of appetite, disturbance of equilibrium, drowsiness but no definite narcosis, apathy leading to death.

(2) Chronic

Slight narcosis, loss of weight, albumen and casts in urine.

CHANGES IN THE ORGANISM

(1) The brain showed engorgement of the pia mater; the lungs broncho-pneumonia; the blood delayed coagulation (Gross, 1943).

(2) The kidneys showed injury of tubules and formation of casts; in one guinea pig glomerulitis (Gross, 1943).

(2) Effect on the blood. – Decrease in red cells and haemoglobin.

(4) Effect on the eyes. – Only slight irritation (Carpenter and Smythm, 1946).

(5) Effect on the skin. – No significant irritation, but toxic amounts can be absorbed if exposure is prolonged (Smyth and Carpenter, 1948).

Toxicity to human beings

None has been recorded.

Bibliography on p. 686

115. Diethylene Glycol

Synonyms: 2,2'-oxydiethanol, Diglycol, polyglycol

Structural formula:
$$CH_2-CH_2-O-CH_2-CH_2$$
$$\quad\;|\qquad\qquad\qquad\quad|$$
$$\quad OH\qquad\qquad\qquad OH$$

Molecular formula: $C_4H_{10}O_3$

Molecular weight: 106.12

Properties: a colourless, almost odourless liquid, more viscous and more hygroscopic than ethylene glycol. Non-inflammable in air at ordinary temperatures but if heated slowly inflammable at 130 °C (Renkenbach and Aaronson, 1931).

> *boiling point:* 244.5 °C
>
> *vapour pressure:* less than 0.1 mm Hg at 20 °C
>
> *flash point:* 290 °F
>
> *conversion factors:* 1 p.p.m. = 4.35 mg/m³
> $\qquad\qquad\qquad\quad$ 1 mg/l $\;$ = 230.7 p.p.m.

solubility: miscible with water, alcohols, glycols, acetone, furfural, chloroform esters. Non-miscible with ether, benzene, toluene, CCl_4, linseed or castor oil, petroleum. Solvent for cellulose nitrate, colophony and dyes; not for cellulose acetate, ester gum, copals or rubber. Good plasticiser for shellac in proportions up to 25% (Durrans, 1950).

maximum allowable concentration: Rowe (1963) suggests 100 p.p.m.

ECONOMY, SOURCES AND USES

Production

(1) By partial dehydration of ethylene glycol.

(2) By combination of ethylene glycol and ethylene oxide (Durrans, 1950)

Industrial uses

(1) In the motor industry as a constituent of anti-freeze solutions and brake fluids.

(2) In the textile industry as a softening agent for vinyl resins in rayon finishing.

(3) In the plastics industry as an alcohol component for polyester resins (Malten and Zielhuis, 1964).

(4) In the lacquer industry.

(5) As a hygroscopic agent for cigarettes (Flinn, 1935).

(6) As an intermediate in the explosives industry.

(7) As a vehicle for medicinal preparations (Geiling and Cannon, 1938).

(8) In the manufacture of face creams.

[624]

BIOCHEMISTRY

Estimation and metabolism

(1) By the chromatographic method described by Bergner and Sperlich (1953) based on that of Williams and Kirby (1948) using the capillary ascent technique. (2) By the chemical method of Duke and Smith (1940), based on the reaction of alcoholic hydroxyl groups with ammonium hexanitratocerate, but using hexaperchloratocerate to give an intense red colour.

According to Hanzlik et al. (1947) commercial diethylene glycol can be absorbed by the skin of animals in toxic amounts. No detailed results of metabolic investigations are available but the fact that long-continued administration to animals has led to the development of Ca oxalate stones in the bladder has suggested to some observers (Fitzhugh and Nelson, 1946), that it is metabolised to oxalic acid. Earlier observers, however (Wiley et al., 1938) were not able to find oxalic acid in the urine of rabbits and dogs given large doses, and Haag and Ambrose (1937) found that in dogs a large proportion of the diethylene glycol administered was excreted unchanged in the urine. It appears that the discrepancy may lie partly in the difference between acute and chronic poisoning, as in the case of ethylene glycol, or partly, according to Rowe (1964) in the comparative purity of the diethylene glycol used.

TOXICOLOGY

The chief hazard of diethylene glycol, like that of ethylene glycol, is by oral ingestion; this was strongly emphasized by the disaster caused in 1937 by the use of diethylene glycol as a vehicle for a pharmaceutical preparation (see p. 627).

In animals it has a depressant effect on the central nervous system similar to that caused by ethylene glycol and produces similar changes in the kidney and calculi in the urinary tract.

By subcutaneous injection it has proved less toxic than ethylene glycol, but more toxic than triethylene glycol.

It is not highly irritant to mucous membranes or by application to the skin and does not cause sensitisation when used in polyester resins (Malten and Zielhuis, 1964).

A recent examination of the toxicity of diethylene glycol by Loeser (1954) has led him to the conclusion that it is much less toxic than has hitherto been believed; he states that its toxic effect is similar to that of glycerine, and that the difference of opinion among earlier observers is probably due to the differences in elimination of the two compounds. He notes that while there should be no general contra-indication to the use of diethylene glycol, it must be regarded

Bibliography on p. 686

with caution in special conditions of usage, especially when given in combination with other active compounds. In this connection may be mentioned the investigation by Geiling, Coon and Schoeffer in 1937 of the relative toxicities of the components of the elixir sulfanilamide which caused so many deaths in that year. They put forward the suggestion that the sulfanilamide may have had an additive toxic effect, in that if the kidneys and liver are rapidly injured by a large critical dose of diethylene glycol the sulfanilamide may not be eliminated or detoxified and would therefore have an injurious effect on other tissues.

No injuries from industrial exposure to its vapour have been reported, most probably because its vapour pressure at ordinary temperatures is so low, but a potential hazard may exist from contact with the heated compound or in spraying processes where a fine mist is created.

Toxicity to animals

(1) Acute

Lethal dose. – *(i) By oral administration*, for rats, 14.8 ml/kg; for guinea pigs, 7.76 ml/kg; for mice, 23.7 ml/kg (Laug *et al.*, 1939); for rats, 20.76 g/kg; for guinea pigs, 13.21 g/kg (Smyth *et al.*, 1941). – *(ii) By subcutaneous injection*, for mice, 5 ml/kg (von Oettingen and Jirouch, 1931). – *(iii) By intravenous injection*, for rabbits, 2 ml/kg (Haag and Ambrose, 1937); 1–2 ml/kg (Kesten *et al.*, 1937).

(2) Chronic

Repeated dose, LD_{50}, for rats and rabbits, 3% in drinking water daily for 2 months; 5% killed 25% within a week (Kesten *et al.*, 1937); for rats, 5–20% (Loeser *et al.*, 1954); 5% (Holck, 1937).

SYMPTOMS OF INTOXICATION

(1) Acute

With lethal single doses death may occur within 24 h from central nervous depression. In some cases the symptoms are those of acute renal insufficiency, resulting finally in anuria and uraemic coma.

(2) Chronic

After several doses the fur becomes ruffled, there is increased thirst and refusal of food and some diuresis, followed by scanty urinary excretion and anuria.

According to Rowe (1964) some of the symptoms of chronic toxicity may be due to liver damage, such as was observed by Geiling and Cannon (1938) in some of the cases of human poisoning by the elixir of sulfanilamide (see below).

CHANGES IN THE ORGANISM

(1) Acute

Some observers, such as Haag and Ambrose (1937) and Holck (1937) have found no essential abnormality of the internal organs of rats dying of acute oral poisoning by diethylene glycol, though Holck observed considerable irritation of the stomach and intestines. Kesten *et al.* (1937) on the other hand found that rats given a single intravenous injection of 1 or 2 ml/kg of pure diethylene glycol or 2 to 4 ml/kg of a 50% solution showed kidney lesions in half the animals in the form of calcification and degeneration of the convoluted tubules. The discrepancy in these results, particularly with regard to the evidence of the high toxicity of diethylene glycol for human beings suggests that the rat is less susceptible to this compound, as noted by Hunt (1932) with regard to ethylene glycol.

(2) Chronic

The kidneys. – Kesten *et al.* (1937) found that of 25 rats given 3% in their drinking water for 15 to 95 days, 14 died in 5 to 56 days with extensive degeneration of the renal cortex, the remaining 11, killed after 51 to 95 days, were normal. Of 25 animals receiving 5% for 1 to 6 days, 9 died during this time as a result of renal insufficiency, the remainder showed swelling of the kidneys with widespread, sometimes total, destruction of the epithelial cells of the convoluted tubules – a form of hydropic degeneration with necrotic cells in the severe lesions. The collecting tubules sometimes contained hyaline and granular casts.

The liver was less frequently involved, but was sometimes enlarged and pale, with vacuolation of the cytoplasm of many cells but no necrosis.

The adrenals also showed occasionally fat-free vacuolisation of the epithelial cells of the cortex.

These lesions are not exactly comparable with those caused by ethylene and propylene glycol and it is suggested that the ether linkage of the diglycol may be the portion of the molecule responsible for the degeneration of epithelial cells of parenchymatous organs, especially the kidney.

Effect on fertility. – Holck (1937) and Wegener (1953) have reported on the fertility of rats receiving diethylene glycol in their drinking water. Holck observed that pregnancy did not occur when males and females both receiving 0.5% of pure diethylene glycol in their drinking water, were mixed, and that there was some evidence of smaller and fewer litters of females receiving 0.25 and 0.5% when mated with fresh stock males. Wegener however concluded that 1 ml/100 g of a 20% aqueous solution daily for 12 weeks had no influence on the reproductive ability of the animals or their offspring.

Effect on the eyes. – No irritation of the eyes of rabbits was caused by the instillation of diethylene glycol (Carpenter and Smyth, 1940).

Toxicity to human beings

The outstanding experience of the injurious effects of diethylene glycol has been that of the outbreak of poisoning from Elixir of Sulfanilamide-Massengill – a 10%

Bibliography on p. 686

solution of sulfanilamide in about 72% of diethylene glycol, with some colouring and flavouring agents. Each fluid ounce therefore contained approximately 21.5 ml of the glycol and 2.7 g of sulfanilamide (Calvery and Klumpp, 1939).

During September and October 1937, 73 deaths from this 'new medicine' were reported in U.S.A. and by 1939 the number had risen to 105. The ages of the patients ranged from 11 months to 70 years and the dosage from $1\frac{1}{2}$ to 6 ounces.

SYMPTOMS OF INTOXICATION

In most cases the initial symptoms, occurring about 24 h after taking the elixir, were gastrointestinal – heartburn, nausea, abdominal cramps, vomiting and diarrhoea. It is to be noted that 260 persons who had taken the elixir survived, probably on account of the rapid appearance of these gastro-intestinal symptoms.

In fatal cases they were followed by headache, pain in the kidney region and abdomen, transient polyuria, and later by oliguria and anuria, drowsiness, slight oedema of the face, and in some cases slight jaundice. Progressive coma led to death within 2 to 7 days after the onset of anuria. The temperature was subnormal and the pulse slow, and the blood picture that of a moderate leucocytosis. The urine contained albumen, casts and occasional leucocytes. The non-protein nitrogen of the blood rose to 200 mg and the creatinine in some cases to 12 mg/100 ml.

Autopsies showed in several cases generalised oedema (ascites, hydrothorax, hydropericardium and oedema of the lungs) and recent haemorrhages into the gastro-intestinal tract and lungs and bronchopneumonia. The chief lesions were in the kidneys and liver.

The kidneys were enlarged and showed symmetrical cortical necrosis and in children cortical infarcts. Microscopically there was hydropic degeneration of the cells, causing complete obstruction of the lumen, and the collecting tubules contained hyaline casts, erythrocytes and leucocytes.

The liver was enlarged in all but one case of the 12 subjected to post mortem examination and showed a central hydropic degeneration of the hepatic cells.

The stomach and intestines showed congestion and haemorrhages.

Diethylene glycol as a hygroscopic agent

Diethylene glycol is one of the most popular agents for maintaining the moisture content of cigarettes. It was shown by Mulinos and Osborne in 1934 that cigarettes made with this substance as a hygroscopic agent were less irritating than those using glycerine, and in 1935 they made a further investigation, using oedema of the conjunctival sac of rabbits, which confirmed their previous view. A further confirmation was provided by an investigation by Flinn in 1935; he found that such cigarettes produced neither symptoms nor any irritation of mucous membranes; in fact that habitual smokers had found that congestion of the larynx and pharynx disappeared when they transferred to diethylene glycol cigarettes.

116. Diethylene Glycol Derivatives

116a. Diethylene Glycol Monoethyl Ether

Synonym: carbitol

Structural formula: $CH_3—CH_2—O—CH_2—CH_2—O—CH_2—CH_2$
                                                                  $|$
                                                                  OH

Molecular formula: $C_6H_{14}O_3$

Molecular weight: 134.2

Properties: a colourless hygroscopic liquid, with a weakly fruity odour and a somewhat bitter taste.

> *boiling point:* 201.9 °C (pure); 180–200 °C (technical)
>
> *vapour pressure:* 0.13 mm Hg
>
> *vapour density (air = 1):* 4.62
>
> *specific gravity (liquid density):* 0.9898
>
> *flash point:* 205 °F
>
> *conversion factors:* 1 p.p.m. = 5.49 mg/m³
>
>   1 mg/l   = 188.2 p.p.m.
>
> *solubility:* good solvent for cellulose nitrate, many gums, resins and dyes; only partly for ester gum, and not for cellulose acetate, polyvinyl chloride or rubber. Miscible with water and alcohol in all proportions.
>
> *maximum allowable concentration:* not established.

ECONOMY, SOURCES AND USES

Production

By the action of ethylene oxide on the sodium compound of Ethylene Glycol Monoethyl Ether (Cellosolve) (Durrans, 1950).

Industrial uses

(1) In the manufacture of textile soaps and in dye printing.

(2) In the cosmetic industry (Harry, 1940; De Navarre, 1941; Meininger, 1948). Meininger draws attention to the fact that the product used for many years in the cosmetic industry is the commercial grade generally known as 'Carbitol Solvent' or 'Technical Carbitol'. In the U.S.A. a content of not more than 5% of Carbitol in cosmetic substances is permitted by the Food and Drug Act. According to Hanzlik *et al.* (1947) the amount causing no demonstrable injury to rabbit skin

(0.04 ml for 30 days) falls within the permitted range, indicating that the amounts currently used in cosmetics and dermatological formulae appear to be safe. It has the advantage of being an excellent solvent for most perfumes, as well as retarding the drying of ointments and enhancing the emollient effect.

BIOCHEMISTRY

Suitable modification of the infra-red method described by Nawrocki *et al.* (1944) for the determination of monoalkyl ethers of ethylene glycol is suggested by Rowe (1963) as the most practical method.

Metabolism

Carbitol is capable of being absorbed by the skin of animals in toxic amounts, and other observers (Hanzlik *et al.*, 1947) have noted a similar result in human beings, though this was denied by Meininger in 1948.

According to Fellows *et al.* (1947) Carbitol is largely destroyed in the body or conjugated with glucuronic acid and excreted as the glucuronate. In this respect it differs from ethylene and diethylene glycol, but the reason for this difference is not clear.

Williams (1959) remarks that this metabolic peculiarity may explain its lesser toxicity when compared with that of diethyl, methyl and butyl cellosolve. It must be noted however that this relatively low toxicity apparently applies only to the pure product; according to Lehmann and Flury (1943) the industrial product is more toxic to animals, and Rowe (1963) remarks on the possibility that commercial products may contain appreciable amounts of ethylene glycol.

TOXICOLOGY

Carbitol, when pure, is of low oral toxicity to animals and, having a very low volatility its vapour does not constitute an industrial hazard. It can however in large doses cause in animals depression of the central nervous system and injury to the kidneys. No human injuries have been reported.

Toxicity to animals

(1) Acute

  (i) By oral administration, LD$_{50}$, for rats, 5.54 g/kg (Laug *et al.*, 1939); 8.69 g/kg (pure) and 9.05 g/kg (commercial) (Smyth, Seaton and Fischer, 1941). It is suggested by Curme and Johnston (1952) that the difference in absolute values in these results may be due to differences in technique. *By oral administration*, for

mice, 6.58 g/kg; for guinea pigs, 3.8 g/kg (Laug *et al.*, 1939); for cats, 1-2 ml/kg of a 25% solution (Lehmann and Flury, 1943). – *(ii) By subcutaneous injection*, MLD, for cats, 1–2 ml/kg after 2 and 8 days (Lehmann and Flury, 1943); for mice, 2.5–5 ml/kg (Von Oettingen and Jirouch, 1931). – *(iii) By external application*, LD_{50}, for rabbits, 8.5 ml/kg (Hanzlik *et al.*, 1947).

(2) Chronic

(i) *By oral administration*, for rats, no injury to the kidneys or adverse effect on growth from addition to the diet of 2.16% of a purified preparation for 2 years (Morris *et al.*, 1942). Slight if any effect from 1% in the drinking water over 2 years (Hanzlik *et al.*, 1947). For mice, slight if any effect from 5% in the drinking water over 2 years. – *(ii) By external application*, LD_{50}, for rabbits, 0.32 ml/kg daily for 30 days by inunction. – *(iii) Inhalation* of Carbitol is well tolerated by animals. No injury occurred, in the experiments of Lehmann and Flury (1943) from almost saturated concentrations for 12 days.

SYMPTOMS OF INTOXICATION

(1) Acute

Central nervous depression and ataxia, without initial twitching, tremors or convulsions. Some haemoglobinuria. Death usually within one or two days due chiefly to kidney injury (Lehmann and Flury, 1943).

(2) Chronic

Only negligible impairment of health occurred following repeated oral administration, but there was delayed death of some animals probably from uraemia.

CHANGES IN THE ORGANISM

(1) Acute

Kidneys, tubular injury; intestinal tract, inflammation; lungs, pneumonia.

(2) Chronic

With repeated oral doses there was only slight liver damage and no kidney injury (Morris *et al.*, 1942). With external application, in the form of bandaging, of 0.3 ml/kg over 90 days there was transient dermatitis, but severe kidney injury in the form of necrosis of the tubular epithelium (Biochemical Research Laboratory, Dow Chemical Co., 1963) and even some kidney injury from applications above 0.04 ml/kg.

Toxicity to human beings

One severe case of poisoning from ingestion of Carbitol has been recently reported (Brennaas, 1960). This was a man aged 44, an alcoholic, who drank a liquid

Bibliography on p. 686

containing 47% of Carbitol and less than 0.2% of methanol (about 300 ml of Carbitol). He developed severe symptoms of central nervous and respiratory injury (dyspnoea), thirst and acidosis. The urine contained albumen and some casts but there was no oliguria. He recovered after symptomatic treatment with Na bicarbonate, glucose, penicillin and chlorpromazine.

The opinions of Meininger (1948) and Cranch et al. (1942) appear to agree that Carbitol applied to human skin causes neither irritation nor sensitisation and Cranch et al. stated that a 70% aqueous mixture did not retard wound healing, but a warning by the U.S. Food and Drug Administration in 1943 that cosmetic preparations containing more than 5% of Carbitol should not be used even for application to small areas of the body emphasises the fact that the use of Carbitol for this purpose may constitute an unsuspected hazard, especially if applied to broken skin or in persons with renal disorders.

Excessive exposure to inhaled mist or vapour should, in view of its low volatility, be readily controllable by ordinary precautions, but excessive contact with the skin should be strictly avoided.

116b. Diethylene Glycol Monomethyl Ether

Synonym: methyl Carbitol

Structural formula: $CH_3—O—CH_2—CH_2—O—CH_2—CH_2$
$\qquad\qquad\qquad\qquad\qquad\qquad\qquad\qquad\qquad |$
$\qquad\qquad\qquad\qquad\qquad\qquad\qquad\qquad\quad OH$

Molecular formula: $C_5H_{12}O_3$

Molecular weight: 120.1

Properties: a colourless liquid with a mild pleasant odour and a bitter taste.

   boiling point: 194.2 °C

   vapour pressure: 0.18 mm Hg at 25 °C

   vapour density (air = 1): 4.1

   specific gravity (liquid density): 1.018

   flash point: 200 °F

   conversion factors: 1 p.p.m. = 4.91 mg/m³

   $\qquad\qquad\qquad\qquad$ 1 mg/l   = 204 p.p.m.

   solubility: miscible with water in all proportions

   maximum allowable concentration: not established.

ECONOMY, SOURCES AND USES

Industrial uses

The industrial uses are similar to those of other glycol ethers, especially in the lacquer industry for thinners and quick-drying varnishes.

BIOCHEMISTRY

Metabolism

While it is known that methyl carbitol can be absorbed by the skin, no further information on its metabolic fate in the body is available.

TOXICOLOGY

While generally recognised as being relatively low in oral toxicity to animals, it is regarded by some authorities (Smyth and Carpenter, 1948) as being more toxic, from the point of view of subacute poisoning, than carbitol or butyl carbitol; Kesten, Mulinos and Pomerantz (1939) found its effects, when administered over a brief period, similar to those of carbitol and of diethylene glycol itself.

It is not irritating to the skin, and though it can be absorbed by this route in toxic amounts, severe and prolonged contact is necessary to produce this result.

It is somewhat painful when applied to the eyes but does not cause any permanent injury. With high dosage to animals, death occurs either through narcosis or kidney injury. In ordinary conditions hazard from inhalation is improbable on account of its low volatility, but since no animal experiments on the results of exposure to its vapour, even at high temperatures, have been made, it is not possible to state definitely that there is no possibility of hazard when it is heated or inhaled repeatedly.

Toxicity to animals

(1) Acute

Lethal dose, LD_{50}, 50% aqueous solution – *By oral administration*, for rats, 9.21 g/kg (Smyth *et al.*, 1941); for guinea pigs, 4.16 g/kg.

Attempts to administer methyl carbitol by stomach tube were followed by acute bronchitis and pneumonia (Kesten *et al.*, 1939). – *Undiluted material*, LD_{50}, for rats, 5.5–7 ml/kg (Biochemical Research Laboratory, 1963).

(2) Chronic

Oral administration, for rats, repeated administration of methyl carbitol over a long period has not proved lethal in a dosage of 1.83 g/kg (Smyth and Carpenter, 1948), while among rats given drinking water containing 3 to 5% of methyl carbitol for 11 to 64 days only one died at the end of this time (Kesten *et al.*, 1939).

SYMPTOMS OF INTOXICATION

(1) Acute

Death usually occurred within 48 h or not at all, and was believed to be due either to profound narcosis or kidney injury (Rowe, 1963).

Bibliography on p. 686

(2) Chronic

The animals did not tolerate well methyl carbitol in water or in food, and many of them refused food, so that a certain degree of starvation was present. In no case was less than 1 ml/kg effective (Kesten *et al.*, 1939).

CHANGES IN THE ORGANISM

The kidneys of animals killed after 28 and 45 days showed lesions comparable to those caused by diethylene glycol and Carbitol, in the form of hydropic degeneration of the convoluted tubules, but somewhat larger amounts of the methyl carbitol than of Carbitol itself were necessary to produce these effects.

Effect on the eyes. – While contact with the eyes is painful, it does not cause any permanent injury (Carpenter and Smyth, 1946).

Effect on the skin. – Investigations by the Biochemical Research Laboratory, The Dow Chemical Co. (cited by Rowe, 1963) have shown that while methyl carbitol is not appreciably irritating to the skin, it can, with extensive and prolonged contact, be absorbed in toxic and even lethal amounts; the LD_{50}, using the 'sleeve' technique of Draize *et al.* (1944) was found to be about 20 ml/kg for the rabbit.

Toxicity to human beings

No injury to human beings, whether industrial or otherwise has been reported.

116c. Diethylene Glycol Monobutyl Ether

Synonym: butyl carbitol
Structural formula: $CH_3-CH_2-CH_2-CH_2-O-CH_2-CH_2-O-CH_2-CH_2-OH$
Molecular formula: $C_8H_{18}O_3$
Molecular weight: 162.2
Properties: a colourless liquid with a mild odour.
    boiling point: 162–230 °C
    vapour pressure: 0.02 mm Hg
    vapour density (air = 1): 5.58
    specific gravity (liquid density): 0.952
    flash point: 230 °F
    conversion factors: 1 p.p.m. = 6.64 mg/m³
                1 mg/l   = 150.8 p.p.m.
    solubility: solvent for cellulose nitrate but not for cellulose acetate; solvent for some gums and resins.
    maximum allowable concentration: not established.

ECONOMY, SOURCES AND USES

Used in the textile industry as a wetting-out solution.

BIOCHEMISTRY

Butyl carbitol can be absorbed through the skin, but only in toxic amounts if application is prolonged and continuous.

TOXICOLOGY

Butyl carbitol is low in acute oral toxicity to animals and also by single inhalation, but repeated dosage may cause lesions of the kidney, similar to but less extensive than those caused by diethylene glycol and differing in character from those of ethylene glycol and ethylene glycol diacetate. Though slightly irritating to the skin with prolonged contact, and capable of being absorbed, it is only toxic by this route if applied in large amounts and with continuous and prolonged contact. It is moderately irritating and injurious to the eyes. No definite cases of injury to human beings have been recorded.

Toxicity to animals
(1) Acute
Lethal dose – (i) By oral administration, LD_{50}, for rats, 6.56 g/kg; for guinea pigs, 2.0 g/kg (Smyth *et al.*, 1941). – *(ii) By inhalation*, LD_{50}, for rats, single exposure to saturated air heated to 100 °C and then cooled caused no symptoms other than transient loss of weight (Biochem. Research Laboratory).

(2) Chronic
Among rats given 3–5% in drinking water for 5–35 days, 1/3 died on the 5th, 23rd and 35th day. The maximum dosage having no effect was 0.051 g/kg (Kesten *et al.*, 1939); 0.65 g/kg caused kidney lesions.

SYMPTOMS OF INTOXICATION
(1) Acute
Similar to those of carbitol and diethylene glycol when given over a brief period. Its subacute toxicity is 4 times as great as that of pure carbitol (Smyth and Carpenter, 1948).

(2) Chronic
Refusal to eat, with partial hydration and starvation (Kesten *et al.*, 1939). The blood non-protein nitrogen was 162 mg/100 ml.

Bibliography on p. 686

CHANGES IN THE ORGANISM

(1) Acute

No autopsies appear to have been carried out.

(2) Chronic

(a) The kidneys showed injuries similar to those of diethylene glycol but less extensive. The characteristic lesion was hydropic degeneration of the tubules, differing from the deposition of oxalate crystals which are a feature of the injury due to ethylene glycol and ethylene glycol diacetate.

Kesten *et al.* (1939) suggest that the ether linkage between the glycol molecules which exists in carbitol, butyl carbitol and methyl carbitol, may be responsible for the hydropic degeneration characteristic of the effect of these compounds.

(b) Effect on the eyes. – Moderate irritation and moderate corneal injury (Carpenter and Smyth, 1946).

(c) Effect on the skin. – Only slight irritation even with prolonged and repeated contact (Rowe, 1963).

Toxicity to human beings

No injurious effects on human beings have been definitely traced to butyl carbitol; in the one case where haematuria was reported to the British Home Office in 1934, butyl cellosolve was also being used (Browning, 1953).

116d. Diethylene Glycol Monoethyl Ether Acetate

Synonym: carbitol acetate

Structural formula: CH_3—CH_2—O—CH_2—CH_2—O—CH_2—CH_2—O—$\overset{\overset{\text{O}}{\|}}{C}$—$CH_3$

Molecular formula: $C_8H_{16}O_4$

Molecular weight: 176.2

Properties: a colourless liquid of very low volatility with a slight odour and bitter taste.

    boiling point: 217.4 °C
    melting point: −25 °C
    vapour pressure: 0.05 mm Hg at 20 °C
    vapour density (air = 1): 6.07
    specific gravity (liquid density): 1.0114
    flash point: 230 °F

conversion factors: 1 p.p.m. = 7.20 mg/m³
              1 mg/l   = 139 p.p.m.

solubility: soluble in all proportions in water, alcohol and ether

maximum allowable concentration: not established.

ECONOMY, SOURCES AND USES

Produced by esterification of diethylene glycol monoethyl ether.

Used as solvent for lacquers, oils, resins and adhesives.

BIOCHEMISTRY

Estimation in the atmosphere by infra-red absorption spectroscopy.

TOXICOLOGY

Very little detailed investigation has been carried out, except that of oral toxicity to animals, which is low, and of local application to the skin, which shows only slight irritation.

No inhalation effects have been studied and no chronic effects by any route. No human injury has been reported.

Toxicity to animals

By oral administration, for rats, LD_{50}, 11.0 g/kg (Smyth *et al.,* 1941); for guinea pigs, 3.93 g/kg.

The eyes (rabbit).

Only very slight irritation from application of the liquid (Carpenter and Smyth, 1946).

Toxicity to human beings

It would appear that the industrial use of this compound is attended by little or no hazard if reasonable methods of use and handling are observed.

116e. Diethylene Glycol Monomethyl Ether Acetate

Synonym: methyl carbitol acetate

Structural formula:
$$CH_3-O-CH_2-CH_2-O-CH_2-CH_2-O-\overset{\displaystyle O}{\overset{\displaystyle \|}{C}}-CH_3$$

Molecular formula: $C_7H_{14}O_4$

Bibliography on p. 686

Molecular weight: 162.2

Properties: a colourless liquid with a faint odour and bitter taste
    boiling point: 194.2 °C
    vapour pressure: 0.12 mm Hg at 20 °C
    specific gravity (liquid density): 1.04
    flash point: 180 °F
    conversion factors: 1 p.p.m. = 6.63 mg/m³
                   1 mg/l = 151 p.p.m.
    solubility: soluble in water in all proportions
    maximum allowable concentration: not established.

ECONOMY, SOURCES AND USES

Produced by esterification of diethylene glycol monomethyl ether.

Used in industry as other glycol ether-esters.

BIOCHEMISTRY

Estimation in the atmosphere by infra-red absorption spectroscopy.

TOXICOLOGY

As with the monoethyl ether ester of diethylene glycol there is very little information as to its toxicity to animals other than that it is low in acute oral toxicity and
appreciably irritating to the eyes of rabbits. There are no reports of any adverse
effects on human beings.

Toxicity to animals

By oral administration (50% aqueous solution), LD_{50}, for rats, 11.96 g/kg; for guinea
pigs, 3.46 g/kg (Smyth *et al.*, 1941).

SYMPTOMS OF INTOXICATION

The eyes (rabbits). – Appreciably irritating (Carpenter and Smyth, 1946).

Toxicity to human beings

In industrial use, in view of its low volatility and apparent low toxicity to animals
it should present no hazard.

116f. Diethylene Glycol Monobutyl Ether Acetate

Synonym: butyl carbitol acetate

Structural formula: $CH_3-CH_2-CH_2-CH_2-O-CH_2-CH_2-O-CH_2-CH_2-O-\overset{\displaystyle O}{\overset{\|}{C}}-CH_3$

Molecular formula: $C_{10}H_{20}O_4$

Molecular weight: 204.26

Properties: a clear liquid with a mild odour and bitter taste.
   boiling point: 245.8 °C
   melting point: −32 °C
   vapour pressure: < 0.01 mm Hg at 20 °C
   specific gravity (liquid density): 0.9810
   flash point: 240 °F
   conversion factors: 1 p.p.m. = 8.34 mg/m³
                    1 mg/l   = 120 p.p.m.
   solubility: soluble in water 6.5%. Dissolves 3.7% of water at 20 °C. Miscible with many solvents and diluents. Solvent for cellulose acetate, ester gum, polyvinyl acetate, but not for polyvinyl chloride or raw rubber (Durrans, 1950).
   maximum allowable concentration: not established

ECONOMY, SOURCES AND USES

Produced by esterification of diethylene glycol monobutyl ether.

Used in the paint and lacquer industry. Formerly used as an insect repellant.

BIOCHEMISTRY

Estimation in the atmosphere by infra-red absorption spectroscopy.

No information other than that it can be absorbed by the skin in toxic amounts.

TOXICOLOGY

It is low in acute oral toxicity to animals though in high dosage narcotic, and when absorbed by the skin in toxic amounts causes haematuria and degenerative changes in the kidney. It is only slightly irritating to skin and eyes.

Bibliography on p. 686

The only report of injury to human beings arises from its one-time use, now abandoned, as an insect repellant.

Toxicity to animals

(1) Acute

Lethal dose – (i) By oral administration, LD_{50}, for rats, 7.1 g/kg (Draize et al., 1948); (as a 50% suspension), 11.92 g/kg (Smyth et al., 1941); (as an emulsion with 5% gum arabic), 7 ml/kg (Biochemical Research Laboratory, 1963); for guinea pigs, 2.34 g/kg (Smyth et al., 1941); 2.7 g/kg (Draize et al., 1948); for mice, 6.6 g/kg; for rabbits, 2.8 g/kg (Draize et al., 1948). – (ii) By skin contact, for rabbits, LD_{50}, 5.5 ml/kg (Draize et al., 1948). – (iii) By inhalation, no experiments carried out.

(2) Chronic

By skin contact, for rabbits, with repeated inunction for 90 days the LD_{50} was found by Draize et al. (1948) to be 2 ml/kg.

SYMPTOMS OF INTOXICATION

(1) Acute

Marked narcosis.

(2) Chronic

Severe haematuria, mild erythema and exfoliation of the skin.

CHANGES IN THE ORGANISM

Degenerative changes in the kidney.

Toxicity to human beings

Only one report of injury to human beings has been recorded, and this was not from the industrial use of butyl carbitol acetate but from prolonged contact of excessive amounts with the skin during its use as an insect repellant. The subject was a 3 year old child who was stated (Hoehn, 1945) to have developed nephrosis from this cause. The material used was known as Sta-way (which contained 50% of butyl carbitol acetate and 15% of Carbitol), and even at that time, according to Hoehn, information had been received by the mother of the child that Sta-way had been banned for use in the Army, and tests by the Committee on Medical Research and the Office of Scientific Research and Development had shown that it was a severe kidney and liver poison to rabbits (Draize et al., 1948). According to Rowe (1963) it was on account of this case that butyl carbitol acetate was entirely withdrawn from its use as an insect repellant.

In industrial use, no adverse effects have been reported and none would be expected from exposure by inhalation, since its volatility is so low, but prolonged and intensive contact with the skin does present a hazard which could be avoided by strict prevention of such skin contact.

Bibliography on p. 686

117. Propylene Glycol

Synonyms: 1,2-propanediol; methyl ethylene glycol

Structural formula:
$$CH_3-\overset{\overset{\displaystyle OH}{|}}{CH}-CH_2-OH$$

Molecular formula: $C_3H_8O_2$

Molecular weight: 76.10

Properties: a colourless, somewhat viscous hygroscopic liquid with a bitter taste. Miscible with water, alcohol, ether and many organic solvents.

> *boiling point:* 188 °C
> *vapour pressure:* 0.13 mm Hg at 25 °C
> *specific gravity (liquid density):* 1.038
> *conversion factors:* 1 p.p.m. = 3.11 mg/m³
> 1 mg/l = 322 p.p.m.
> *solubility:* solvent for some gums and resins, and partly for shellac, but not for cellulose esters, polyvinyl chloride, rubber, hydrocarbons or vegetable oils.
> *maximum allowable concentration:* not established.

ECONOMY, SOURCES AND USES

Production

By conversion of propylene to the chlorohydrin and hydrolysing to propylene oxide, with further hydrolysation to propylene glycol (Rowe, 1963).

Industrial uses

(1) As an antifreeze agent.
(2) As a solvent in the pharmaceutical industry, for foods and cosmetics.
(3) In the plastics industry as a plasticiser for resins and paper.
(4) In the manufacture of resins and of other glycol derivatives.
(5) As a hygroscopic agent in textiles and tobacco.

BIOCHEMISTRY

Estimated by methods similar to those for ethylene glycol

Propylene glycol is readily absorbed by the gastro-intestinal tract and more rapidly with low concentrations than high.

Approximately one-third is excreted by the kidneys (van Winkle, 1941) at a rate about 75% faster than that of ethylene glycol (Hanzlik *et al.*, 1939). According to Lehmann and Newman (1937) this excretion represents its conjugation with glucuronic acid, where it has been isolated as the barium salt (Miura, 1911). The remainder is partly oxidised to lactic acid and partly excreted unchanged. Hanzlik *et al.* (1939) suggest that it enters into normal carbohydrate metabolism through the intermediate lactic acid. It increases the glycogen content of the liver (Newman *et al.*, 1940), which appears to provide an automatic protection for the liver in its glycogenic function. Bost and Ruckebusch (1962) state that this protective effect has been utilised in cows in milk, 800 g having been administered daily during a month without any ill-effect. It exists in mammalian tissues as the 1-phosphate, is present in rat liver (Rudney, 1954), and is believed to be a possible intermediate in the metabolism of acetone (Williams, 1959).

TOXICOLOGY

Animal experiments have shown that propylene glycol in large doses is a central nervous depressant; it is a less potent systemic toxin than ethylene or diethylene glycol, but according to Lehmann and Flury (1943) it does cause kidney injury.

The results of moderate prolonged dosage have indicated a lack of chronic toxicity, and according to Hanzlik *et al.* (1947) it is the only glycol suitable for internal use with foods and medicinal products without demonstrable hazards to health. The Council on Pharmacy and Chemistry of the American Medical Association (1949) has also considered it a harmless ingredient for pharmaceutical products. No ill-effects from its industrial use have been reported.

Toxicity to animals

(1) Acute

Lethal dose. – *(i) By oral administration*, for rats, 40, 50 or 60% in the diet was lethal after a few days (Whitlock *et al.*, 1944). LD$_{50}$, for rats, 32.5 ml/kg (Weatherby and Haag, 1938); for rabbits, 18.5 ml/kg (Weatherby and Haag, 1938); for mice, 23.9 ml/kg (Laug *et al.*, 1936). – *(ii) By subcutaneous injection*, for rats, 23.1 ml/kg (Braun and Cartland, 1936); for mice, 5 g/kg (Lehmann and Flury, 1943).

(2) Chronic

(i) By oral administration, for rats, a diet containing 48% was followed by death only after one month, while with doses of 25% (8 ml/kg) no mortality in 20 weeks and no evidence of injury except a slightly poor initial growth, later replaced by a greater average increase in body weight (Braun and Cartland, 1936). – *(ii) By inhalation*, for rats, continuous inhalation of 60% saturation (0.10–0.22 mg/l) or supersaturation (0.17–0.35 mg/l) caused no deaths (Robertson, Loosli *et al.*, 1947).

With lethal dosage mice died with dyspnoea and cramps (Lehmann and Flury, 1947). According to Laug *et al.* (1939) loss of equilibrium, depression, analgesia, finally death after a prolonged moribund state.

Intravenous injection of 1–10 ml in rats provoked a transitory fall in blood pressure without significant alteration of the cardiac rhythm; doses of 0.25–0.8 ml/kg were followed by transitory diuresis (Bost and Ruckenbusch, 1962).

According to Whitlock *et al.* (1944) rats fed on rations containing 30% of propylene glycol showed significant abnormality in their reproductive and weaning capacities.

CHANGES IN THE ORGANISM

(1) Acute

Slight degenerative changes in the kidneys of dogs receiving large intravenous and divided gastric doses were observed by Laug *et al.* (1939).

(2) Chronic

Moderate degeneration of liver cells and, in the kidneys, degenerative changes in the cells of the convuluted tubules in rats (Braun and Cartland, 1936).

No such lesions were observed by Robertson, Loosli *et al.* (1947) following continuous inhalation, but the lungs, in only 2 animals out of 26, showed a slight localised infectious process.

Toxicity to human beings

A report by Allbright, Butler and Bloomberg (1937) of a child with severe rickets and resistant to vitamin D therapy, who was treated for $4\frac{1}{2}$ months with crystalline vitamin D in propylene glycol (15–30 ml daily) – a procedure which was much more effective than crystalline vitamin D injected intravenously – confirms the low toxicity of propylene glycol by the oral route for human beings. The boy suffered no injury.

SYMPTOMS OF INTOXICATION

The skin. – An investigation by Warshaw and Herrmann (1952) on the effect of applying propylene glycol to the normal skin of 866 patients showed positive patch tests in 15.7%. Inunction in some of these 15% showed no inflammatory response. It was not decided whether the reactions were allergic or due to primary irritation, but the assumption of primary irritation received some support from the finding that only 5 out of 23 subjects with a positive response to the undiluted material showed a reaction to a 10% dilution. One subject with a positive patch test had cheilitis from a lipstick containing propylene glycol.

118. Propylene Glycol Derivatives

118a. Propylene Glycol Monoethyl Ether

Synonyms: ethyl propylene glycol; Dowanol PE

Structural formula:

$$\underset{OH}{\underset{|}{CH_3-CH-CH_2-O-CH_2-CH_3}}$$

Molecular formula: $C_5H_{12}O_2$

Molecular weight: 104.1

Properties: propylene glycol monoethyl ether exists in two isomers, alpha and beta; the commercial variety, Dowanol PE, is a mixture of both.

It is a colourless volatile liquid with an ester-like odour and a bitter taste. A good solvent for gums, resins and cellulose esters.

   boiling point: 132.2 °C
   vapour pressure: 8.2 mm Hg at 25 °C
   specific gravity (liquid density): 0.895
   flash point: 130 °F
   conversion factors: 1 p.p.m. = 4.25 mg/m³
                          1 mg/l = 235 p.p.m.
   solubility: miscible with water and alcohol in all proportions and with most organic solvents
   maximum allowable concentration: not established.

ECONOMY, SOURCES AND USES

Produced (1) by condensation of propylene oxide with alcohols or phenols; (2) by reaction of propylene glycol with dialkyl sulphate in presence of Na or KOH.

Used (1) in the paint and lacquer industry, (2) as a solvent for resins, dyes, oils and greases, (3) as an adhesive-tape remover.

BIOCHEMISTRY

Estimation in the atmosphere by infra-red spectrophotometry is recommended as the best method (Rowe, (1963). No specific information is available concerning its metabolism.

Bibliography on p. 686

TOXICOLOGY

Both isomers have similar toxicities (Smyth *et al.*, 1941). Oral administration to animals is about 1/3–1/4 as toxic as ethylene glycol monoethyl ether, but considerably greater than that of propylene glycol (Curme and Johnston, 1952).

Large single doses are markedly narcotic and cause injury to the kidneys. No cases of injury from industrial exposure have been reported, and the industrial hazard is not considered to be great since dangerous concentrations give warning by irritation and narcosis. It is not irritating to the skin but can however, be absorbed from it in toxic amounts (Calvery, Draize and Woodard, 1944; Draize *et al.*, 1944).

No cases of intoxication of human beings have been reported.

Toxicity to animals
(1) Acute
Lethal dose – *(i) By oral administration*, LD_{50}, for rats, 8.93 g/kg (Smyth, Seaton and Fischer, 1941). – *(ii) By skin contact*, for rabbits, by the 'sleeve' technique of Draize *et al.* (1948), 9 ml/kg. – *(iii) By inhalation*, for mice, guinea pigs and rabbits, no deaths from inhalation of 7000 p.p.m. for 2 h, but albumen and red blood cells in urine, and some irritation of eyes and respiratory organs (Gross, 1943).

(2) Chronic
(i) By oral administration, for rats, according to Smyth and Carpenter (1948), 0.68 g/kg in the drinking water for 30 days had no effect; 2.14 g/kg caused no deaths but reduced growth and appetite. – *(ii) By subcutaneous injection*, for guinea pigs, 0.1, 0.25, 0.5 and 1.0 ml/kg repeatedly caused no symptoms but transient albuminuria (Gross, 1943). – *(iii) By inhalation*, for cats and guinea pigs, 1180 p.p.m. for 8 h over 12 days caused death in 4 out of 6 animals (Gross, 1943). Death was preceded by no particular symptoms of disease, except that one cat showed respiratory catarrh.

SYMPTOMS OF INTOXICATION
Acute
With large oral dosage marked narcosis and some evidence of kidney and injury, and with skin application central nervous depression followed by death usually within 48 h after treatment. With inhalation some irritation of eyes and respiratory organs with temporary traces of albumen and red corpuscles in the urine of the rabbit.

CHANGES IN THE ORGANISM
(1) Acute
The kidneys showed only slight injury in the form of an increase in the cells of the glomeruli with some formation of cylinders in the tubules.

(2) Chronic

The lungs showed pneumonia; the kidneys showed some injury of the tubular epithelium.

Repeated application of the commercial product on 5 consecutive days caused conjunctival irritation and transient cloudiness of the cornea (Biochemical Research Laboratory).

118b. Propylene Glycol Monomethyl Ether

Synonyms: 1-methoxypropanol; Dowanol PM

Structural formula:

$$CH_3-\underset{\underset{OH}{|}}{CH}-CH_2-O-CH_3$$

Molecular formula: $C_4H_{10}O_2$

Molecular weight: 90.1

Properties: a colourless liquid with a mild pleasant odour, consisting of two isomers, α and β, the former being less toxic than the latter. The commercial product is probably a mixture of the two isomers.

   boiling point: 120 °C
   vapour pressure: 10.9 mm Hg at 25 °C
   specific gravity (liquid density): 0.919
   flash point: 100 °F
   conversion factors: 1 p.p.m. = 3.68 mg/m³
                        1 mg/l = 272 p.p.m.
   solubility: soluble in water in all proportions
   maximum allowable concentration: not established
   Commercial product:
   boiling point: 126–127 °C
   specific gravity (liquid density): 0.926
   conversion factors: 1 p.p.m. = 3.68 mg/m³
                        1 mg/l = 272 p.p.m.
   maximum allowable concentration: not established

ECONOMY, SOURCES AND USES

Production similar to that of the ethyl ether, but using methyl alcohol. Chiefly used in the manufacture of lacquers and paints.

Bibliography on p. 686

BIOCHEMISTRY

Estimation in the atmosphere

(1) Physical and chemical methods as described for the ethers of ethylene glycol (*q.v.*).
(2) Infra-red spectrophotometry.

Metabolism

No specific investigations of the fate in the body of this methyl ether have been made; it can be absorbed in toxic amounts through the skin.

TOXICOLOGY

Propylene glycol monomethyl ether is low in both acute and chronic oral toxicity to animals, and also by inhalation; though high concentrations are anaesthetic to animals and essentially intolerably irritative to human beings, they cause little organic injury to animals. Prolonged skin contact can cause central nervous system depression and increased mortality, but only mild irritation.

Auricular fibrillation has been observed in anaesthetised and artificially respired dogs inhaling high concentrations but not in intact animals. No injury to human beings has been reported.

Toxicity to animals

(1) Acute

LD$_{50}$. – *(i) By oral administration*, for rats, α isomer, 7.51 g/kg (Smyth *et al.*, 1941); commercial product, 6.69 g/kg (Rowe *et al.*, 1954); β isomer, 5.71 g/kg (Smyth *et al.*, 1941). – *(ii) By skin contact*, for rabbits, 13–14 g/kg (Draize *et al.*, 1944). – *(iii) By inhalation*, for rats, 10,000 p.p.m. for 5–6 h; for guinea pigs, 10,000 p.p.m. for more than 7 h (Rowe *et al.*, 1954).

(2) Chronic

(i) By oral administration of 1.0 g/kg repeated for 35 days rats showed no ill-effects (Rowe *et al.*, 1954). – *(ii) By inhalation*, for rabbits and monkeys, no ill-effects from 880 p.p.m. over 186 days; for rats and guinea pigs, no ill-effects from 1500 p.p.m. over 184 days; at 3 000 p.p.m. mild initial central nervous depression but tolerance established after several weeks.

SYMPTOMS OF INTOXICATION

(1) Acute

With oral dosage profound central depression lasting up to 48 h, followed by death from respiratory arrest. If these effects are not lethal there are no residual effects.

With skin contact depression and narcosis. With inhalation death appears to be due to anaesthetic action.

(2) Chronic

Slight depression of growth and of central nervous system. Auricular fibrillation in anaesthetised and artificially respired dogs (Procita and Shideman, 1950).

CHANGES IN THE ORGANISM

(1) Acute

Following prolonged application to the skin a slight increase in the weight of the kidneys was observed (Draize *et al.*, 1944).

(2) Chronic

Very slight injury to liver and lungs was observed by Rowe *et al.* (1954) in animals repeatedly exposed to 800 to 1500 p.p.m.

Toxicity to human beings

No injury to human beings has been recorded and it would appear that the likelyhood of injury from its industrial use is remote, especially since its warning property from irritation of mucous membranes by toxic concentrations makes it improbable that these would be tolerated.

118c. Propylene Glycol Isopropyl Ether

Structural formula:

$$\underset{\substack{|\\CH_3-CH-CH_2-O-CH-CH_3}}{\overset{\substack{OH \qquad\qquad CH_3}}{}}$$

Molecular formula: $C_6H_{14}O_2$

Molecular weight: 118.2

Properties: a colourless volatile liquid with a slight odour and bitter taste.
    boiling point: 139–141 °C
    vapour pressure: 5.3 mm Hg at 25 °C
    specific gravity (liquid density): 0.875
    flash point: 140 °F
    conversion factors: 1 p.p.m. = 4.83 mg/m³
                 1 mg/l = 207 p.p.m.
    solubility: soluble in water in all proportions
    maximum allowable concentration: not established.

Bibliography on p. 686

ECONOMY, SOURCES AND USES

Production

(1) By reacting propylene oxide with propyl alcohol.
(2) By direct alkylation of propylene glycol with a dialkyl sulphate in the presence of alkali.

Industrial uses

Not of wide commercial importance, but to some extent as a solvent for lacquers, paints, resins, dyes, oils and greases.

BIOCHEMISTRY

Estimation in the atmosphere by infra-red spectrophotometry.

Metabolism

No specific information is available, except that it is absorbable by the skin, but not rapidly and not readily in toxic amounts (Rowe, 1963).

TOXICOLOGY

Little is known of its toxic effects. The only considerable investigation (of the commercial product) appears to be that of the Biochemical Research Laboratory, Dow Chemical Co. (cited by Rowe, 1963). This suggests that it is of low oral toxicity to animals, but that by inhalation it can cause slight drowsiness and mild kidney injury. It is irritating to the eyes of rabbits but only slightly irritating to the skin even with prolonged contact. No injury to human beings has been recorded.

Toxicity to animals

Acute (Only acute effects have been investigated).

LD_{50}. – *(i) By oral administration*, for rats, approximately 4 g/kg. – *(ii) By inhalation*, no deaths resulted from exposure for 7 h to a saturated atmosphere.

SYMPTOMS OF INTOXICATION

Acute

Drowsiness, labored breathing, temporary loss of weight.

CHANGES IN THE ORGANISM

Mild injury of the kidneys. Application to the eyes of rabbits caused conjunctival irritation, some corneal injury and iritis which healed within a week.

118d. Propylene Glycol Monobutyl Ether

Structural formula:
$$CH_3-\overset{\displaystyle OH}{\underset{\displaystyle |}{CH}}-CH_2-O-CH_2-CH_2-CH_2-CH_3$$

Molecular formula: $C_7H_{16}O_2$

Molecular weight: 132.2

Properties: a colourless slightly volatile liquid with a slight odour and bitter taste.
  boiling point: 160–172 °C
  vapour pressure: 1.4 mm Hg at 25 °C
  specific gravity (liquid density): 0.879
  flash point: 150 °F
  conversion factors: 1 p.p.m. = 5.40 mg/m³
              1 mg/l = 185 p.p.m.
  solubility: a good low-temperature miscibility with castor oil and most organic solvents. Solubility in water 4.4 g/100 g.
  maximum allowable concentration: not established.

ECONOMY, SOURCES AND USES

Industrial uses

(1) As a coupling and dispersing agent.
(2) As a solvent for paints, lacquers, resins, dyes, oils and greases.
(3) As a hydraulic brake fluid component (Curme and Johnston, 1952).

BIOCHEMISTRY

Estimation in the atmosphere by infra-red spectrophotometry.

Metabolism

No specific information other than it is absorbable by the skin in toxic amounts.

Bibliography on p. 686

TOXICOLOGY

Only oral and skin contact toxicity to animals have been reported (Biochemical Research Laboratory, cited by Rowe, 1963; Draize et al., 1944).

It appears to be low in toxicity by the oral route, but application to the skin in doses of 3 to 5 ml/kg causes narcosis, and with the higher dosage death within 24 h after treatment. No inhalation experiments have been carried out. Repeated applications to the eyes are markedly irritating, and prolonged application to the skin causes severe injury.

No toxic effects on human beings have been reported, but Rowe (1963) suggests that contact with the eyes and prolonged or repeated contact with the skin should be prevented and in the absence of any information as to the effects of inhalation of the vapour such exposure should also be avoided.

Toxicity to animals

(1) Acute

Lethal dose. – (i) By oral administration, LD_{50}, for rats, 2.2 ml/kg. – (ii) By skin contact, for rabbits, 5 ml/kg (Draize et al., 1944).

(2) Chronic

Only repeated applications to skin and eyes of rabbits have been described.

Skin: ten applications in 14 days caused slight simple irritation and some evidence of absorption of toxic amounts (Rowe, 1963).

Eyes: one drop on 5 consecutive days caused marked conjunctival irritation and corneal cloudiness healing within a week.

SYMPTOMS OF INTOXICATION

Acute

Deep narcosis, and with prolonged skin application, severe skin injury.

CHANGES IN THE ORGANISM

No information available.

119. Dipropylene Glycol

Structural formula:

$$CH_3-\overset{\overset{\displaystyle OH}{|}}{CH}-CH_2-O-CH_2-\overset{\overset{\displaystyle OH}{|}}{CH}-CH_3$$

Molecular formula: $C_6H_{14}O_3$

Molecular weight: 134.18

Properties: a colourless, odourless slightly viscous liquid, with a greater solvent power for castor oil and some other organic materials than other glycols.

The commercial product consists of three isomers, whose exact proportions are unknown.

boiling point: 231.8 °C

vapour pressure: < 0.01 mm Hg

specific gravity (liquid density): 1.0252

flash point: 250–280 °F (sets to a glass below −50 °C)

conversion factors: 1 p.p.m. = 5.49 mg/m³

1 mg/l = 182 p.p.m.

solubility: miscible with water, methanol and ether

maximum allowable concentration: not established.

ECONOMY, SOURCES AND USES

Production

By condensation of propylene oxide and propylene glycol (Levene and Walti, 1927).

Industrial uses

(1) In the printing industry, especially as a water-miscible solvent in the 'steam-setting' types of printing ink (Curme and Johnston, 1952).

(2) In extraction of aromatic hydrocarbons, mixed with ethylene glycol in the proportion of 65/35%.

(3) As an antifreeze agent.

(4) For air sanitation, since its vapour is highly germicidal (Robertson *et al.*, 1943), but less so than triethylene glycol, 0.027 mg/l being necessary to kill 95% of

air-borne *Staphylococcus albus* as compared with 0.006 mg/l for triethylene glycol.

BIOCHEMISTRY

Estimation in the atmosphere

As for other glycols, but specifically by spectrographic methods.

Metabolism

Unlike propylene glycol, dipropylene glycol is not utilised by the liver or stored as glycogen (Hanzlik *et al.*, 1939), but the consequence of this in depressing the functional activity of the liver is less evident than with ethylene glycol or diethylene glycol (Newman *et al.*, 1940).

When given to dogs by gastric administration in doses of 5 ml/kg, Newman *et al.* found that the dipropylene glycol disappeared from the blood in approximately 24 h, as compared with 36 h for diethylene glycol, but Hanzlik *et al.*(1939) do not consider that this difference is in itself sufficient to account for the much greater toxicity of diethylene glycol.

TOXICOLOGY

Although more acutely depressant to the central nervous system than ethylene, diethylene or propylene glycol, dipropylene glycol is still low in oral toxicity to animals, especially to the liver. With repeated dosage, relatively large amounts are necessary before it develops the same potential capacity as diethylene glycol for injuring the kidneys and the results are less severe.

It is not irritating to the skin and not absorbed in toxic amounts through the intact skin.

No injurious effects on human beings have been recorded and it would appear to carry practically no industrial hazard, especially from inhalation of its vapour, since its vapour pressure is so low.

Toxicity to animals

(1) Acute

LD$_{50}$. – *(i) By oral administration*, for rats, 14.8 g/kg. – *(ii) By intraperitoneal injection*, 10.3 ml/kg. – *(iii) By intravenous injection*, for dogs, 11.5 ml/kg (Hanzlik *et al.*, 1939).

(2) Chronic

By oral administration, for rats: addition to the drinking water of 5% for 77 days had no injurious effect; 10% was followed by the death of some animals from kidney injury (Kesten *et al.*, 1939).

SYMPTOMS OF INTOXICATION

(1) Acute

Narcosis was produced in dogs by the intravenous injection of 5.9 ml/kg (Hanzlik *et al.*).

(2) Chronic

Depression of running activity occurred in rats given 12% in the diet for 15 weeks (van Winkle and Kennedy, 1940) in contract to the increased activity produced by propylene glycol.

CHANGES IN THE ORGANISM

(1) Acute

Autopsies were not performed.

(2) Chronic

The kidneys of rats showed, in the experiments of Kesten *et al.* (1939) hydropic degeneration of the tubular epithelium, and the liver degeneration of the parenchyma, but these lesions were less severe and less uniformly produced than with diethylene glycol. The dogs examined by Hanzlik *et al.* after survival of repeated gastric dosage of dipropylene glycol showed only moderate degenerative changes in the kidneys and only minimal evidence of liver damage.

Effect on the skin

Repeated and prolonged application to the skin of rabbits had a negligible irritative effect, and gave no indication of absorption of toxic amounts (Biochemical Research Laboratory, Dow Chemical Co., cited by Rowe, 1963).

Toxicity to human beings

None have been reported.

Bibliography on p. 686

120. Dipropylene Glycol Derivatives

120a. Dipropylene Glycol Monoethyl Ether

Structural formula: $CH_3-\underset{\underset{\displaystyle OH}{|}}{CH}-CH_2-O-CH_2-\underset{\underset{\displaystyle CH_2-CH_3}{|}}{\underset{\displaystyle O}{|}}CH-CH_3$

Molecular formula: $C_8H_{18}O_3$

Molecular weight: 162.2

Properties: a colourless slightly volatile liquid with a mild pleasant odour and bitter taste.

> *boiling point:* 193–195 °C
> *vapour pressure:* 0.30 mm Hg at 25 °C
> *specific gravity (liquid density):* 0.927
> *flash point:* 205 °F
> *conversion factors:* 1 p.p.m. = 6.64 mg/m³
>   1 mg/l = 150.7 p.p.m.
> *solubility:* Miscible with water and many organic solvents
> *maximum allowable concentration:* not established.

ECONOMY, SOURCES AND USES

Production

(1) By reaction of propylene oxide with the appropriate alcohol.
(2) By direct alkylation of dipropylene glycol with dialkyl sulphate in presence of alkali.

Industrial uses

(1) As a coupling and dispersing agent.
(2) As a solvent for paints, lacquers, resins, dyes, oils and greases.

BIOCHEMISTRY

Estimation in the atmosphere by infra-red spectrophotometry.

Metabolism

No specific information is available except that it can be absorbed from the skin, but only in toxic amounts by intensive application by the 'sleeve' technique of Draize et al. (1944).

[656]

TOXICOLOGY

According to the only investigations carried out (Biochemical Research Laboratory, Dow Chemical Company, 1963, and Draize *et al.*, 1944) dipropylene glycol monoethyl ether is low in toxicity to animals by oral administration, inhalation and moderate skin application, but narcotic and even lethal by intensive application to the skin, to which it can cause burning. The vapour is somewhat irritating to the mucous membranes of the eyes and nose. No injury to human beings has been reported and none would be expected from its industrial use in ordinary conditions.

Toxicity to animals

(1) Acute

(i) By oral administration, LD_{50}, for rats, 4 ml/kg. – *(ii) By skin contact*, lethal dose, 15 mg/kg. – *(iii) By inhalation*, only 1 out of 12 rats died after 7 h exposure to saturated atmosphere (about 400 p.p.m.).

(2) Chronic

The only investigation of repeated exposure refers to the effect on the eyes of rabbits of introduction of 1 drop of the liquid on 5 consecutive days. This caused slight transitory conjunctival irritation but no corneal injury.

SYMPTOMS OF INTOXICATION

Acute

With intensive skin contact, 5 and 10 ml/kg for 24 h under a cuff (Draize *et al.*, 1944), transient loss of weight and narcosis; with higher dosage (15 ml/kg) profound narcosis, coldness of the body and burning of the skin. With inhalation, transient weight loss and some irritation of the eyes and nose.

120b. Dipropylene Glycol Monomethyl Ether

Synonym : Dowanol 50 B

Structural formula :
$$CH_3-\underset{\underset{}{\overset{|}{OH}}}{CH}-CH_2-O-CH_2-\underset{\underset{O-CH_3}{\overset{|}{}}}{CH}-CH_3$$

Molecular formula : $C_7H_{16}O_3$

Molecular weight : 148.2

Properties : a volatile colourless liquid with a mild ether odour in moderate concentrations but a strong objectionable odour at 1000 p.p.m.

The commercial product is believed to be a mixture of 4 isomeric forms (Rowe, 1963).

Bibliography on p. 686

boiling point: 188.3 °C

vapour pressure: 0.4 mm Hg at 26 °C

specific gravity (liquid density): 0.950

flash point: 185 °F

conversion factors: 1 p.p.m. = 6.06 mg/m³

1 mg/l   = 165 p.p.m.

solubility: miscible with water and many organic solvents

maximum allowable concentration: 100 p.p.m.

ECONOMY, SOURCES AND USES

Production

(1) By reacting propylene oxide with the appropriate alcohol.

(2) By alkylation of dipropylene glycol with a dialkyl sulphate in presence of a catalyst.

Industrial uses

As a solvent and coupling agent for general use, and in manufacture of various cosmetics.

BIOCHEMISTRY

Estimation in the atmosphere

Chiefly by infra-red spectrophotometry.

Metabolism

Apart from the fact that Dowanol 50 B is absorbable by the skin there is no specific information on its metabolic fate.

TOXICOLOGY

A central nervous system depressant of low toxicity to animals, with a specific action, when given intravenously, on the heart in the form of auricular fibrillation.

It is absorbed from the skin but not in dangerous amounts even with high dosage, but sufficiently to produce transient narcosis. No toxic effects on human beings have been reported and Rowe *et al.* (1954) believe that it presents practically no hazard from inhalation of the vapour.

Toxicity to animals

(1) Acute

LD$_{50}$. – *(i) By oral administration*, for rats, 6.6 g/kg (Rowe *et al.*, 1954); for dogs, 10 ml/kg (Shideman and Procita, 1951). – *(ii) By intravenous injection*, for anaesthetised dogs, 0.35–0.5 ml/kg; for artificially respired dogs, 1.3 ml/kg. – *(iii) By skin contact*, for rabbits, 13–14 g/kg (Draize *et al.*, 1944). Not lethal to all animals with single prolonged application of 20 ml/kg. – *(iv) By inhalation*, exposure of rats to 500 p.p.m. for 7 h caused only transient narcosis (Rowe *et al.*, 1954).

(2) Chronic

(i) By oral administration, for rats, repeated dosage of 1.0 g/kg for 35 days caused no ill-effects. – *(ii) By inhalation*, for rabbits and monkeys, 800 p.p.m. for 186 days caused no ill-effects; for rats and guinea pigs, 1500 p.p.m. for 184 days caused only slight depression of growth and very slight injury to liver and lungs, also slight narcosis. – *(iii) By skin contact*, for rabbits, application of 1.0, 3.0, 5.0 and 10.0 ml/kg 5 times a week for 90 days caused no loss of weight; high mortality at the 10 ml level, low at 5 ml and none at levels below these.

SYMPTOMS OF INTOXICATION

(1) Acute

With intravenous administration profound central nervous system depression, with death due to respiratory arrest (Procita and Shideman, 1950). With oral administration (to unanaesthetised dogs) of 5 ml/kg loss of righting reflexes and anaesthesia with recovery in 24 h and no evidence of delayed toxic action.

With intravenous administration to the anaesthetised dog, transient hypotension, slowing of the heart and disturbed respiration; when the dog is artificially respired, ventricular slowing and asystole, followed by auricular fibrillation, uninfluenced by previous dosage with atropine or by bilateral vagotomy (Procita and Shideman, 1950). This effect has not been observed in intact animals.

With inhalation of about 500 p.p.m. for 7 h rats showed only mild transient narcosis with rapid recovery.

This also occurred following skin contact in rabbits, an amount of 20 ml/kg being held in continuous contact for 24 h (Rowe *et al.*, 1954).

(2) Chronic

With repeated inhalation of 300 p.p.m. 7 h a day for 6–8 months only rats showed slight transient narcosis in the initial period; rabbits, guinea pigs and monkeys were unaffected. With skin contact the highest dosage caused narcosis.

CHANGES IN THE ORGANISM

(1) Acute

In animals dying from narcosis only occasional gastric irritation was observed.

(2) Chronic

With prolonged skin contact Draize *et al.* (1944) noted only a slight increase in the weight of the kidneys; Rowe *et al.* (1954) found slight injury to liver, lungs and kidneys (congestion, and some granular and hydropic changes) at the highest dosage level. In animals dying from narcosis the stomach showed distension and occasional small haemorrhages in the gastric mucosa.

Repeated application of 1 drop of undiluted material to the eyes of rabbits caused mild transitory irritation of the conjunctiva but no corneal injury.

Even after several weeks, constant contact with applications of 5 ml/kg and upwards caused only mild irritation.

Toxicity to human beings

While no injuries from the industrial use of Dowanol 50 B have been recorded, high concentrations of the vapour cause marked irritation of the nasal mucous membrane, which is difficult for human beings to tolerate (Rowe, 1963). This warning property is a valuable protection against concentrations which might have toxic effects, and an inhalation hazard is not likely since, as Rowe remarks, "levels that may be toxic on repeated exposure probably will not be tolerated voluntarily". Nor is skin contact likely to be a cause of primary irritation or of toxic absorption in ordinary industrial practice. In 1954 Rowe *et al.* tested the effect of application of the undiluted material to the skin of human subjects. In one group it was allowed to remain in direct contact with the skin for 5 days, and again 3 weeks later for 48 h; in another group the material was applied for 4 to 8 h every other day and again for 24 to 48 h 3 weeks later. None of the subjects experienced any evidence of either irritation or sensitisation.

120c. Dipropylene Glycol Monobutyl Ether

Structural formula:
$$CH_3-\overset{\displaystyle OH}{\underset{\displaystyle |}{CH}}-CH_2-O-CH_2-\underset{\displaystyle \underset{\displaystyle |}{O-CH_2-CH_2-CH_2-CH_3}}{CH}-CH_3$$

Molecular formula: $C_{10}H_{22}O_3$

Molecular weight: 190.2

Properties: a colourless very slightly volatile liquid with a slight odour and bitter taste.

 boiling point: 214–217 °C
 vapour pressure: 0.06 mm Hg at 25 °C
 specific gravity (liquid density): not known
 flash point: 1.418 °F

conversion factors: 1 p.p.m. = 7.77 mg/m³
1 mg/l   = 128.6 p.p.m.

solubility: in water limited, but miscible with most organic solvents
maximum allowable concentration: not established.

ECONOMY, SOURCES AND USES

As for other dipropylene glycol ethers.

BIOCHEMISTRY

Estimation in the atmosphere

Probably best by infra-red spectophotometry.

No information available on metabolism.

TOXICOLOGY

Very little quantitative investigation has been carried out. This indicates that while it is slightly more toxic by single oral administration to animals than either the monoethyl or monomethyl ethers, it is less toxic by skin absorption.

Inhalation experiments have not been carried out.

There have been no reports of ill-effects on human beings and it would appear from the scanty evidence available that it carries little or no industrial hazard.

Toxicity to animals

(1) Acute

By oral administration, LD_{50}, for rats, 2 ml/kg (Biochemical Research Laboratory, 1963).

(2) Chronic

(i) By skin contact: repeated application (amounts not stated) for 10 to 14 days to the skin of rabbits caused only slight temporary irritation. – *(ii) Effect on the eyes:* application of 1 drop of the liquid on 5 consecutive days caused only slight transient conjunctival irriation and no corneal injury.

Symptoms of intoxication and changes in the organism: not described.

Bibliography on p. 686

121. Butylene Glycol

Synonym: butanediol

Structural formula:
$$CH_3-CH_2-\overset{\overset{\displaystyle OH}{\displaystyle |}}{CH}-CH_2-OH$$

Molecular formula: $C_4H_{10}O_2$

Molecular weight: 90.1

Properties: butylene glycol exists in 4 isomers: 1,2-, 1,3-, 1,4-, and 2,3-. The butanediols are syrupy, colourless, odourless liquids, similar in consistency and appearance to ethylene glycol. They are not widely used in industry, but are becoming more important with the increasing use of polyester resins, where they act as intermediates. Owing to their relatively low toxicity, with the exception of the 1,4-isomer, they have been suggested as a substitute for glycerin in cosmetics and pharmaceuticals, but only the 1,3-isomer, the lowest in toxicity as shown by animal experiments, is universally agreed to be innocuous for these purposes.

From the industrial standpoint, owing to their low volatility and, except for the newest isomer, the 1,2, their absence of eye irritation, they are not to be regarded as a serious hazard.

121a. 1,2-Butanediol

A relatively new product of apparently low toxicity. The only report available is that of the Dow Chemical Company's Biological Research Laboratory (unpublished, but cited in detail by Rowe, 1963).

boiling point: 193–195 °C
specific gravity (liquid density): 1.0017
conversion factors: 1 p.p.m. = 3.68 mg/m³
               1 mg/l = 272 p.p.m.
solubility: miscible with water and alcohol
maximum allowable concentration: not established.

ECONOMY, SOURCES AND USES

Produced by hydration of 1,2-butylene oxide.

Used in industry as an intermediate in polyster resins.

BIOCHEMISTRY

No specific investigations on the metabolism of this isomer have been carried out. It is not absorbed by the skin in toxic amounts.

TOXICOLOGY

From the comparatively few animal experiments carried out, 1,2–butanediol appears to be intermediate in toxicity between the 1,3- and 2,3-isomers, and slightly less toxic than ethylene glycol. Although low in oral toxicity to animals, large doses are narcotic, irritative to the gastro-intestinal tract, and cause congestion of the kidneys; the undiluted liquid is highly irritating to the eyes, but not to the skin.

Toxicity to animals

(1) Acute

LD_{50}. – *By oral administration*, for mice, 16 ml/kg, as compared with 23.3 for the 1,3-isomer and 9 for the 2,3-isomer (Fischer *et al.*, 1949).

(2) Chronic

(i) By oral administration, for rats: according to Schlussel (1954), 1,2-butanediol can be tolerated by rats in amounts of 30% of the basic diet but 40% of substitution caused death in 11 to 29 days. – *(ii) By intravenous injection*, for dogs: according to Rowe (1963) no appreciable injury was observed from a dosage of 1 mg/kg daily. – *(iii) By inhalation*, for rats: no effects were observed following. 7 h exposure to an atmosphere saturated at 100 °C and then cooled to room temperature.

SYMPTOMS OF INTOXICATION

Acute

Narcosis, gastro-intestinal irritation, peripheral vasodilatation. Death within a few hours appears to be due to narcosis; delayed death to kidney injury (Rowe, 1963).

CHANGES IN THE ORGANISM

The kidneys show congestion.

121b. 1,3-Butanediol

Properties: a liquid of consistency and appearance similar to that of the other isomers. It has a sweet taste and an odour resembling butter (Kopf *et al.*, 1950).

Bibliography on p. 686

Solvent for shellac and colophony, but not for cellulose esters or ethers, ester gum, vinyl resin or rubber chloride. Plasticiser for rubber latex (Durrans, 1950).

boiling point: 207 °C (pure); 204–208 °C (commercial, Durrans, 1950)

vapour pressure: 0.06 mm Hg

specific gravity (liquid density): 1.0059

flash point: 250 °F (Rowe, 1963).

conversion factors: 1 p.p.m. = 3.68 mg/m³

1 mg/l   = 272 p.p.m.

solubility: soluble in water, acetone, alcohols and ethyl acetate, but not in hydrocarbons, ether or castor oil

maximum allowable concentration: not established.

ECONOMY, SOURCES AND USES

Production

By catalytic reduction of acetaldol, or hydrogenation of aldol (Durrans, 1950).

Industrial uses

(1) As an intermediate in polyester resins.

(2) In cosmetics and pharmaceuticals as a substitute for glycerin (Fischer *et al.*, 1949).

BIOCHEMISTRY

Metabolism

Little is known of its metabolic fate, but according to Williams (1959) it could be expected to be oxidised to hydroxybutyric acid.

TOXICOLOGY

1,3-Butanediol has the lowest oral toxicity to animals of the 4 isomers; according to Kopf *et al.* (1950) it is even slightly less toxic to mice than water-free glycerin.

When given parenterally in large doses it causes narcosis (Bornmann, 1954/55). According to most authorities (Loeser, 1949; Husing *et al.*, 1950; Smyth *et al.*, 1951) it is not irritating to the skin or mucous membranes of animals or human beings, especially not to the eyes of rabbits (Carpenter and Smyth, 1946) though Schneider (1951) states that it is toxic to the skin when not purified. Inhalation of the saturated vapour in air has also been found innocuous to rats (Smyth *et al.*, 1951).

Toxicity to animals

(1) Acute

LD$_{50}$. – *(i) By oral administration*, for mice, 23.3 ml/kg (Fischer *et al.*, 1949; Kopf *et al.*, 1950); for rats, 29.42 g/kg (Fischer *et al.*, 1949; Loeser, 1949). – *(ii) By subcutaneous injection*, for mice, 16.51 ml/kg; for rats, 20.06 ml/kg (Loeser, 1949; Bornmann, 1954). – *(iii) By inhalation:* no adverse effects from saturated air-vapour for 8 h (Smyth *et al.*, 1951).

(2) Chronic

Repeated daily doses of 1 ml/100 g to rats of up to 20% solution for 44 days caused no disorder of health, no pathological changes in liver, kidneys, bladder or blood picture (Fischer *et al.*, 1949). This was confirmed, with administration by gastric sound, continued for 185 days, by Kopf *et al.* (1950), not only in rats but also in dogs given 2 ml/kg of a 50% solution twice weekly for 5–6 months; while Schlussel (1954) found that rats tolerated a substitution of up to 40% of the calories in the diet.

SYMPTOMS OF INTOXICATION

Acute

Deep narcosis when given parenterally (Bornmann, 1954/55), occurring rapidly; by other routes after 10–20 min (Kopf *et al.*, 1950).

121c. 2,3-Butanediol

Properties: in appearance and consistency similar to the other isomers.

    boiling point: 182 °C
    vapour pressure: 0.17 mm Hg
    specific gravity (liquid density): 1.0093
    flash point: 185 °F (Curme and Johnston, 1952)
    conversion factors: 1 p.p.m. = 3.68 mg/m^3
                  1 mg/l = 272 p.p.m.
    maximum allowable concentration: not established.

ECONOMY, SOURCES AND USES

Produced by bacterial fermentation.

Industrial uses similar to those of the other isomers, but is not recommended as a substitute for glycerin either for external or internal use.

Bibliography on p. 686

BIOCHEMISTRY

Metabolism

Little is known of its actual fate in the body, but Gessner et al. (1960) state that most of it appears to be destroyed; Neuberg and Gottschalk (1925) believed that a small amount is excreted partly conjugated with glucuronic acid.

An interesting correlation has been made with the metabolism of acetoin by Dawson and Hullin (1954). They state that it is an excretory product of the metabolism of acetoin. Williams (1959) has drawn attention to the varying level of its presence in the blood in cases of manic-depressive psychosis, a disorder in which, during the depressive phase, the total content of acetoin and 2,3-butanediol in the blood is above normal, while in the manic phase there is an increased level of 2,3-butanediol and a decreased level of acetoin.

TOXICOLOGY

The toxicity of the 2,3-isomer is, on the basis of animal experiments, which are few in number, intermediate between the 1,2- and the 1,3-isomers, being only slightly more toxic than the 1,3. No information as to its actual effect is available, but no injury to human beings has been reported.

Toxicity to animals

LD_{50}. – *By oral administration*, for mice, 9 ml/kg (Fischer *et al.*, 1949; Kopf *et al.*, 1950).

121d. 1,4-Butanediol

Properties: generally similar to those of the other isomers.
  boiling point: 230 °C
  specific gravity (liquid density): 1.020 (Curme and Johnston, 1952).
  conversion factors: 1 p.p.m. = 3.68 mg/m³
                        1 mg/l = 272 p.p.m.
  maximum allowable concentration: not established.

ECONOMY, SOURCES AND USES

Production by hydrogenation of 2-butyne-1,4-diol (Rowe, 1963). Used in industry as an intermediate in polyester resins. It is not suitable as a substitute for glycerin.

BIOCHEMISTRY

According to Williams (1959) one of its metabolites is succinic acid, while Gessner *et al.* (1960) have found small amounts of the corresponding dicarboxylic acid in the urine.

TOXICOLOGY

This isomer is the most toxic of the four – ten times as toxic as the 1,3-isomer when administered to animals – and the only one in which toxic effects in human beings have been attributed, especially by application to the skin, and from internal use.

It is only slightly irritating to the skin and conjunctiva, and Rowe (1963) states that it is not absorbed from the skin in toxic amounts, in conflict with the view of Schneider (1950) who states that it is highly toxic to the skin and should not be used in skin applications. A possible cause of this discrepancy is suggested by Loeser (1949) – the quality of the material used for testing.

Toxicity to animals

Acute

   LD$_{50}$. – *By oral administration*, for mice, 2.14 ml/kg (Fischer *et al.*, 1949); for rats, 1.78 g/kg (Rowe, 1963).

SYMPTOMS OF INTOXICATION

Rapid deep narcosis, constriction of pupils, loss of reflexes; death due to central nervous paralysis (Hinrichs *et al.*, 1948).

Toxicity to human beings

Seven cases of poisoning in human beings were reported in 1948 by Hinrichs *et al.* from its internal use as a substitute for glycerin. Damage to the kidneys was observed.

Bibliography on p. 686

122. Butylene Glycol Derivatives

122a. Butylene Glycol Monoethyl Ether

Synonym: butyl glycol

Structural formula:

$$CH_3—CH_2—\overset{\displaystyle OH}{\overset{|}{CH}}—CH_2—O—CH_2—CH_3$$

Molecular formula: $C_6H_{14}O_2$

Molecular weight: 118.2

Properties: a colourless liquid with a slight pleasant odour.
   boiling point: 147 °C
   vapour pressure: 3.0 mm Hg at 25 °C
   specific gravity (liquid density): 0.888
   flash point: 145 °F
   conversion factors: 1 p.p.m. = 4.83 mg/m³
                 1 mg/l = 207 p.p.m.
   solubility: miscible with water and many organic solvents
   maximum allowable concentration: not established.

ECONOMY, SOURCES AND USES

Production

By reacting the appropriate alcohol with butylene oxide consisting of about 8% of 1,2 isomer and 20% of 2,3 isomer, in presence of a catalyst.

Industrial uses

As a dispersing agent and solvent for lacquers, resins, oils, inks and greases.

BIOCHEMISTRY

Estimation in the atmosphere.

By the same methods as those used for propylene glycol ethers (Rowe, 1963).

TOXICOLOGY

Results of the only investigation published (Biochemical Research Laboratory, Dow Chemical Company, cited by Rowe, 1963) indicate that it is narcotic following exposure to inhalation of supersaturated atmospheres (containing some fog) and in these conditions causing slight injury to lungs, liver and kidneys. It is low in oral toxicity, not appreciably irritating to the skin and not readily absorbed by the skin in toxic amounts. It causes considerable irritation and injury to the eyes of rabbits. Death, when it occurs, appears to be due to its narcotic effect since internal organs show no pathological change considered sufficiently severe to be lethal. There are no reports of injury to human beings.

Toxicity to animals

(1) Acute

(i) *By oral administration*, for rats, LD_{50}, 4 g/kg. 1 out of 3 died following dosage of 2 g/kg. – (ii) *By inhalation*, for rats: exposure to a supersaturated atmosphere (containing some fog) for 7 h was not fatal but was narcotic. Saturated atmosphere (3000–4000 p.p.m.) had no apparent serious effect. – (iii) *By skin contact*: single application caused no appreciable irritation.

(2) Chronic

The only experiments with repeated dosage were those of skin contact. No irritation or evidence of absorption resulted from prolonged and repeated application of the undiluted liquid. It would appear that industrial hazard from its use is slight if contact with the eyes and inhalation of high concentrations over a prolonged period are avoided.

SYMPTOMS OF INTOXICATION

Acute

Inhalation caused irritation of eyes and nose, drowsiness, inco-ordination, and dyspnoea. Eye contact caused pain, marked injury of the conjunctiva and cornea and iritis.

CHANGES IN THE ORGANISM

Both oral dosage, greater than 1 g/kg, and also inhalation of supersaturated vapour caused some injury (nature not described) to lungs, liver and kidneys.

122b. Butylene Glycol Monomethyl Ether

Structural formula:

$$CH_3-CH_2-\overset{\displaystyle OH}{\overset{|}{CH}}-CH_2-O-CH_3$$

Molecular formula: $C_5H_{12}O_2$

Bibliography on p. 686

Molecular weight: 104.1

Properties: a colourless liquid with a slight pleasant odour.
　　boiling point: 136 °C
　　vapour pressure: 5.5 mm Hg at 25 °C
　　specific gravity (liquid density): 0.983
　　flash point: 110 °F
　　conversion factors: 1 p.p.m. =4.25 mg/m³
　　　　　　　　　　　　1 mg/l　= 235 p.p.m.
　　solubility: miscible with water and with many organic solvents and oils.
　　maximum allowable concentration: not established.

ECONOMY, SOURCES AND USES

Production as for butylene glycol monoethyl ether (*q.v.*).

Industrial uses

(1) As a dispersing agent and mutual solvent.
(2) As a solvent for lacquers, resins, inks, oils and greases.

BIOCHEMISTRY

Estimation in the atmosphere as for ethers of propylene glycol.

No information on its metabolism available except that it is not absorbed by the skin.

TOXICOLOGY

This butyl ether is low in oral toxicity to animals, very slightly irritating to the skin but with no evidence of absorption, moderately injurious to the eyes and narcotic on inhalation of high concentrations. There are no reports of injury to human beings.

Toxicity to animals

(1) Acute
　　(i) By oral administration, for rats, lethal dose, 4 g/kg. – *(ii) By inhalation:* 4 out of rats died after exposure for 7 h to supersaturated atmosphere (containing some fog), but none with exposure to 6000–7000 p.p.m. (Biochem. Research Lab., 1963).

(2) Chronic

The only repeated exposure investigated was that of skin contact, which caused only very slight irritation and no evidence of toxic effects from absorption.

No industrial injury has been recorded, nor would be expected if ordinary precautions against eye contact and prolonged inhalation of high concentrations of the vapour are taken.

SYMPTOMS OF INTOXICATION

Acute

Drowsiness, unsteadiness, temporary weight loss, and dyspnoea preceding death from inhalation of supersaturated atmospheres.

CHANGES IN THE ORGANISM

Mild changes in liver and kidneys (nature not described) (Biochem. Research Lab., 1963).

Effect on the eyes

Moderate conjunctival irritation, corneal injury and iritis, disappearing within a week.

122c. Butylene Glycol Monobutyl Ether

Structural formula:
$$CH_3-CH_2-\overset{\overset{\displaystyle OH}{|}}{CH}-CH_2-O-CH_2-CH_2-CH_2-CH_3$$

Molecular formula: $C_8H_{18}O_2$

Molecular weight: 146.2

Properties: a colourless, slightly volatile liquid with a mild pleasant odour.
  boiling point: 180–187 °C
  vapour pressure: 0.62 mm Hg at 25 °C
  specific gravity (liquid density): 0.877
  flash point: 160 °F
  conversion factors: 1 p.p.m. = 5.98 mg/m³
            1 mg/l = 167 p.p.m.
  solubility: miscibility with water limited (3.7 g in 100 g at 25 °C) but miscible with organic solvents.
  maximum allowable concentration: not established.

Bibliography on p. 686

ECONOMY, SOURCES AND USES

Industrial uses similar to those of other butylene glycol ethers.

BIOCHEMISTRY

Estimation in the atmosphere similar to that of propylene glycol ethers.

TOXICOLOGY

Acute oral toxicity about the same as that of the monomethyl ether, but causing some kidney injury with high dosage. Not absorbed by the skin in toxic amounts, but capable of causing a burn. Not highly toxic by inhalation, but causing some kidney injury by this route. Irritating to the eyes and causing some corneal injury and iritis but not of a permanent nature (Biochemical Research Lab., 1963).

No injury to human beings has been reported.

Toxicity to animals

Only acute effects have been investigated.

(i) By oral administration, for rats, lethal dose, 4.0 g/kg of a 20% solution in corn oil. – *(ii) By skin contact*, for rabbits: when applied under a bandage for 48 h caused a burn. – *(iii) By inhalation:* rats exposed for 7 h to an atmosphere saturated at 100 °C and then cooled to room temperature showed no significant disturbance. – *(iv) Effect on the eyes*. Some transient corneal injury and iritis.

SYMPTOMS OF INTOXICATION

Prostration and laboured breathing following high oral dosage.

CHANGES IN THE ORGANISM

Some kidney injury (nature not described).

No injury from its industrial use has been recorded, and it would appear to carry little if any hazard with ordinary handling and precautions.

123. Triethylene Glycol

Synonyms: triglycol; bis(2-hydroxyethoxyethane)

Structural formula:

$$\underset{\underset{\displaystyle CH_2}{|}}{OH}-CH_2-O-CH_2-CH_2-O-CH_2-\underset{\underset{\displaystyle CH_2}{|}}{OH}$$

Molecular formula: $C_6H_{14}O_4$

Molecular weight: 150.17

Properties: a colourless or pale strawcoloured liquid, viscous, hygroscopic and practically odourless.

   boiling point: 287.4 °C
   melting point: —5 °C
   vapour pressure: 0.01 mm Hg at 20 °C
   specific gravity (liquid density): 1.1254
   flash point: 330 °F
   conversion factors: 1 p.p.m. = 6.14 mg/m³
                        1 mg/l = 163.7 p.p.m.
   solubility: completely miscible with water, most alcohols, ketones, esters and some halogenated hydrocarbons of low, molecular weight. Good solvent for nitrocellulose and various gums and resins.
   maximum allowable concentration: not established.

ECONOMY, SOURCES AND USES

Production

As a by-product in the production of ethylene glycol from ethylene oxide.

Industrial uses

(1) In the textile industry as a softening agent.
(2) As a plasticiser, and in the manufacture of phenolic resins.
(3) As an intermediate in the production of resins, plasticisers, emulsifiers, lubricants, inks and explosives (Rowe, 1963).
(4) As a disinfectant in air-conditioning systems.
   Triethylene glycol has been preferred for this purpose to propylene and dipropylene glycol partly because extremely small amounts are required and also because, according to Robertson (1947) it is non-irritating, non toxic, odourless,

tasteless and invisible. It is rapidly bactericidal to streptococcus, pneumococcus and viruses; staphylococcus is somewhat less sensitive. According to Curme and Johnston (1952) an air-vapour concentration of 50–100% of saturation should be maintained at all times; such a mixture, at 70 °F and 40% humidity corresponds to 0.5 p.p.m.

(5) As a humectant in tobacco.

(6) In the formulation of composition corl.

(7) In gas dehydration processes, since the solutions can be concentrated at higher temperatures (Curme and Johnston, 1952).

(8) As a solvent extractor, to separate resin-forming aromatic hydrocarbons such as styrene from mixtures of light oil fractions.

BIOCHEMISTRY

Estimation

(1) In the atmosphere

By the method described by Wise, Puck and Stral in 1943, the vapour is absorbed in water and oxidised with acid potassium dichromate; the green colour so formed is measured colorimetrically.

(2) In urine

The method described by McKennis et al. (1962) depends upon the isolation of its 3,5–dinitrobenzoyl ester, formed when solutions of triethylene glycol in methyl isobutyl ketone have been concentrated to dryness and then treated with 10 times its weight of 3.5 dinitrobenzoyl chloride; the mixture is finally shaken with benzene and the benzene layer concentrated to dryness, to give a residue of triethylene glycol bis(3,5–dinitrobenzoate). This residue is then crystallised by methanol and the final product estimated by chromatography.

Metabolism

A recent study by McKennis et al. (1962) indicates that the metabolic processes of triethylene glycol are compatible with its known low toxicity. They showed by means of the ^{14}C-labelled isotope and also non-radioactive compound that after oral administration of 22.5 mg, the rat and rabbit excrete most of the dose unchanged, the total amount in urine, faeces and expired air amounting to 91–98%; of this amount the expired air contained only 1% and the urine 86–94%. Little or none was excreted as oxalate, but there was a small amount of certain metabolites, the chief one being probably the dicarboxylic acid, ethylene dioxyacetic acid.

TOXICOLOGY

Triethylene glycol has a very low acute and chronic toxicity and is not irritating to eyes or skin, but the commercial variety may contain some diethylene glycol which, though less toxic than ethylene glycol, and, according ot Loeser *et al.* (1954) much less toxic than has hitherto been believed, has certainly a toxic effect on the kidneys in certain conditions of use, espcially in combination with other active compounds.

Toxicity to animals

(1) Acute

LD_{50}. – *(i) By oral administration*, for rats, 22.06 g/kg (Smyth *et al.*, 1941); 16.8 ml/kg (Laug *et al.*, 1939); for guinea pigs, 14.66 g/kg (Smyth *et al.*, 1941); 7.9 ml/kg (Laug *et al.*, 1939); for mice, 18.7 ml/kg (Laug *et al.*, 1939); for rabbits, 8.4 ml/kg (Laug *et al.*, 1939). – *(ii) By intramuscular injection*, for rats, 8.4 g/kg (Lauter and Vrla, 1940). – *(iii) By intraperitoneal injection*, for rats, 8.15 g/kg (Karel *et al.*, 1947).

(2) Chronic

Repeated dosage of 1.2 and 4% (equal to 3–4 g/kg) daily for 2 years in the diet (Fitzhugh and Nelson, 1946) or 3% in the drinking water for 30 days (Lauter and Vrla, 1940) were without any adverse effect, but the latter observers noted that 5% did cause some ill-effect. They were using the commercial variety, possibly containing a percentage of diethylene glycol, which may have been responsible for the toxic effect.

Prolonged inhalation of saturated vapour was also, in the experience of Robertson *et al.* (1947) without any physiological effect on monkeys and rats.

SYMPTOMS OF INTOXICATION

(1) The eyes

Instillation into the eyes of rabbits was stated by Carpenter and Smyth (1946) to cause no appreciable irritation, while Latven and Molitor (1939) found its effect similar to that of glycerin and diethylene glycol and less irritating than that of propylene glycol.

(2) The skin

Although not directly irritant to the skin, Rowe (1963) states that prolonged contact may have a macerating effect. The question of absorption by the skin has not been investigated. Rowe states that with very severe prolonged exposure it is possible that some may be absorbed, but it is extremely doubtful that it would be in an amount large enough to cause a toxic effect.

Bibliography on p. 686

Toxicity to human beings

In experiments on the effect of triethylene glycol as an air steriliser, none of the human beings exposed to air saturated with the vapour (about 0.5–1 p.p.m.) have shown any ill-effects (Jennings *et al.*, 1944; Harris and Stokes, 1945). It is generally believed that its use in air-conditioning systems in hospitals and public buildings is harmless.

No ill-effects from its industrial use have been recorded.

124. Triethylene Glycol Monoethyl Ether

Synonym: ethoxytriglycol

Structural formula:

$$\overset{\text{OH}}{\underset{|}{\text{CH}_2}}-\text{CH}_2-\text{O}-\text{CH}_2-\text{CH}_2-\text{O}-\text{CH}_2-\text{CH}_2-\text{O}-\text{CH}_2-\text{CH}_3$$

Molecular formula: $C_8H_{18}O_4$

Molecular weight: 178.2

Properties: a colourless practically odourless liquid of very low volatility. It may appear in 8 isomeric forms, of which the commercial product is believed to be a mixture.

    boiling point: 255.8 °C

    vapour pressure: 0.01 mm Hg at 25° C

    specific gravity (liquid density): 1.021

    flash point: 275 °F

    conversion factors: 1 p.p.m. = 7.29 mg/m³

                     1 mg/l = 137.2 p.p.m.

    maximum allowable concentration: not established.

ECONOMY, SOURCES AND USES

Production

By direct alkylation of triethylene glycol with an alkylating agent in the presence of alkali.

Industrial uses

As for other glycol ether derivatives.

BIOCHEMISTRY

Estimation in the atmosphere

As for ethers of propylene glycol, *i.e.* by infra-red spectrophotometry.

Bibliography on p. 686

Metabolism

No information available except that it is absorbable by the skin in toxic amounts (Smyth *et al.*, 1948, 1951).

TOXICOLOGY

From the only published results of animal investigations (Laug *et al.*, 1939; Smyth *et al.*, 1948, 1951) triethylene glycol monoethyl ether appears to be of very low acute oral toxicity. With repeated non-lethal dosage it causes no increased mortality, no loss of appetite or growth and no lesions of internal organs. It is not irritating to the skin or eyes. No injury to human beings has been reported.

Toxicity to animals

(1) Acute

   (i) By oral administration, LD_{50}, for rats, 12.1 g/kg (Curme and Johnston, 1952). – *(ii) By skin contact*, LD_{50} 3.6 ml/kg (Laug *et al.*, 1939; Draize *et al.*, 1944).

(2) Chronic

   By oral administration, for rats. Daily dosage in drinking water of 0.18 to 3.30 g/kg for 30 days caused no increased mortality, no loss of weight or appetite and no injury to liver, kidneys, spleen or testes, but Smyth *et al.* state that the maximum intake having no effect was 0.75 g/kg, without giving any description of the nature of any effect at this level of dosage.

SYMPTOMS OF INTOXICATION

None described.

   On the basis of these results it would appear that this compound would present no industrial hazard in ordinary working conditions.

125. Tripropylene Glycol

Structural formula:

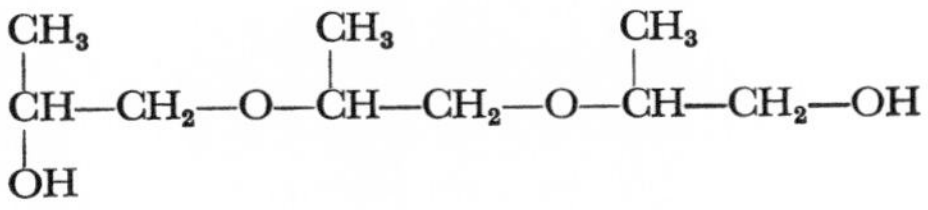

$$\underset{\underset{OH}{|}}{CH}-CH_2-O-\underset{\underset{}{\overset{CH_3}{|}}}{CH}-CH_2-O-\underset{}{\overset{CH_3}{|}}{CH}-CH_2-OH$$

Molecular formula: $C_9H_{20}O_4$

Molecular weight: 192.3

Properties: a colourless, odourless slightly viscous liquid of such low volatility that vapours and mists are encountered only in certain conditions.

    boiling point: 268 °C

    vapour pressure: less than 0.01 mm Hg at 25 °C

    specific gravity (liquid density): 1.019

    flash point: 285 °F

    conversion factors: 1 p.p.m. $= 7.68$ mg/m³

                      1 mg/l $= 128$ p.p.m.

    solubility: miscible with water, alcohol and ether

    maximum allowable concentration: not established.

ECONOMY, SOURCES AND USES

Production

As a by-product of propylene production.

Industrial uses

(1) As a chemical intermediate.

(2) As a non-volatile solvent.

(3) As a humectant and plasticiser.

BIOCHEMISTRY

Metabolism

Nothing is known, except that it is not absorbed by the skin in toxic amounts.

Bibliography on p. 686   [679]

TOXICOLOGY

Practically no information on the potentiality of tripropylene glycol for toxic effects has been published. The results of an investigation by the Biochemical Research Laboratory, Dow Chemical Company, cited by Rowe (1963), indicate that it is low in oral toxicity to rats, is not irritating to the eyes or skin of rabbits and not acutely toxic from skin application even when prolonged and repeated.

Inhalation experiments have not been carried out. No ill-effects on human beings have been reported, and in view of the above results and of its very low volatility and absence of toxic effects from skin absorption it is improbable that it would carry an industrial hazard in ordinary reasonable conditions.

The oral LD_{50} for rats lies between 3 and 10 g/kg.

126. Tripropylene Glycol Derivatives

126a. Tripropylene Glycol Monoethyl Ether

Structural formula:

$$\underset{\displaystyle \overset{|}{\text{OH}}}{\overset{\displaystyle \overset{\text{CH}_3}{|}}{\text{CH}}}-\text{CH}_2-\text{O}-\overset{\displaystyle \overset{\text{CH}_3}{|}}{\text{CH}}-\text{CH}_2-\text{O}-\overset{\displaystyle \overset{\text{CH}_3}{|}}{\text{CH}}-\text{CH}_2-\text{O}-\text{CH}_2-\text{CH}_3$$

Molecular formula: $C_{11}H_{24}O_4$

Molecular weight: 220.3

Properties: a colourless, slightly viscous liquid of very low volatility, with a pleasant ethereal odour and bitter taste.

   boiling point: 250 °C
   vapour pressure: 0.011 mm Hg at 25 °C
   specific gravity (liquid density): not known
   conversion factors: 1 p.p.m. = 9 mg/m³
                        1 mg/l = 111 p.p.m.
   solubility: miscible with water and many organic solvents
   maximum allowable concentration: not established.

ECONOMY, SOURCES AND USES

Production and Industrial uses

Similar to that of other glycol ethers.

BIOCHEMISTRY

No specific information available.

TOXICOLOGY

From the very scanty evidence of animal experiments tripropylene glycol monoethyl ether appears to be of low toxicity (Biochemical Research Laboratory, 1963).

No experiments on inhalation and no quantitative investigations of skin contact have been made, but oral administration to rats gave a LD_{50} of 2 ml/kg and repeated applications to the skin of rabbits for 10 to 14 days resulted in only slight irritation and no evidence of toxic effects from absorption.

Introduction of 1 drop into the eyes on 5 consecutive days caused only very slight conjunctival irritation.

No injury to human beings has been reported and there would seem to be little hazard from its industrial use in ordinary conditions.

126b. Tripropylene Glycol Monomethyl Ether

Synonym: Dowanol TPM

Structural formula:

$$CH_3 \quad\quad CH_3 \quad\quad CH_3$$
$$CH-CH_2-O-CH-CH_2-O-CH-CH_2-O-CH_3$$
$$OH$$

Molecular formula: $C_{10}H_{22}O_4$

Molecular weight: 206.3

Properties: a colourless liquid with an ethereal odour, distinct at about 50 p.p.m. (Rowe *et al.*, 1954).

    boiling point: 242.4 °C

    vapour pressure: 0.022 mm Hg at 25 °C

    specific gravity (liquid density): 0.965

    flash point: 250 °F

    conversion factors: 1 p.p.m. = 8.44 mg/m³

                     1 mg/l = 118.5 p.p.m.

    solubility: miscible with water and a wide variety of organic liquids. Non-corrosive and thermally stable. A powerful solvent for nitrocellulose and synthetic resins.

    maximum allowable concentration: not established.

ECONOMY, SOURCES AND USES

Production

By methods similar to those used for the ethers of propylene and dipropylene glycols (*q.v.*).

Industrial uses

(1) In the paint industry and as a solvent for many domestic products (Shideman and Procita, 1951).

(2) As a chemical intermediate.

BIOCHEMISTRY

Estimation in the atmosphere

By infra-red spectrophotometry.

Metabolism

No information available, apart from the fact that it is readily absorbable by the skin.

TOXICOLOGY

Comparison of tripropylene monomethyl ether (Dowanol TPM) with the methyl ethers of propylene (Dowanol 33B) and dipropylene glycol (Dowanol 50B) by Rowe *et al.* (1954) indicates that the tripropylene methyl ether, whose action is primarily narcotic, has a slightly higher single dose oral toxicity than these, though still low. It can be absorbed more readily by the skin; though it causes no irritation, extensive prolonged application can cause narcosis, though to a less extent than the methyl ether of propylene glycol. Repeated dosage to the skin at slightly lower levels than in the case of Dowanol 33B were found to cause slight liver and kidney damage. It is not significantly irritating to the eyes. No ill-effects on human beings have been reported.

Toxicity to animals

(1) Acute

(i) *By oral administration*, LD_{50}, for rats, 3.3 g/kg (Rowe *et al.*, 1954); for dogs, 5 ml/kg (Shideman and Procita, 1951). – *(ii) By skin contact*, for rabbits, no deaths followed single applications of 20 ml/kg for 24 h (Rowe *et al.*, 1954). – *(iii) By inhalation*, for rats: no ill-effects were observed from single exposures for 7 h to saturated atmosphere.

Bibliography on p. 686

(2) Chronic

    (i) By oral administration, for rats: no deaths attributable to the material and no ill-effects occurred following administration by intubation of 0.1, 0.3, 1.0 and 3.0 ml/kg 5 days a week for 35 days. – *(ii) By skin contact*, for rabbits: 65 applications in 90 days of 10 ml/kg caused 7 deaths out of 8; none at doses below this level. – *(iii) By inhalation*: no experiments were carried out.

SYMPTOMS OF INTOXICATION

(1) Acute

    From oral administration survivors showed only loss of weight.

    With lethal dosage death was due to respiratory failure following narcosis (Shideman and Procita). Narcosis was also the principal symptom of toxic absorption from skin contact.

    Auricular fibrillation was produced by intravenous administration in the anaesthetised artificially respired dog.

(2) Chronic

    Skin application by bandage of 5 ml/kg caused loss of weight greater than that of controls; animals receiving 10 ml/kg showed narcosis with terminal loss of weight probably related to decreased food consumption.

CHANGES IN THE ORGANISM

(1) Acute

    The kidneys showed moderate increase in weight and slight congestion and cloudy swelling (Shideman and Procita, 1951).

(2) Chronic

    The kidneys showed significant increase of weight and slight degeneration and hydropic changes in the rabbits surviving 65 applications to the skin for 90 days, and even at the lowest dosage of 1 ml/kg per day there was some kidney injury (Rowe *et al.*, 1954).

Effect on the eyes

    Mild transitory irritation of the conjunctiva appeared after each application on 5 consecutive days, but there was no cumulative action.

Toxicity to human beings

No ill-effects have been reported, but although this compound is not significantly irritating to the skin, the evidence from animal experiments of its potentiality for toxic absorption suggests that prolonged extensive contact with the skin should be avoided.

126c. Tripropylene Glycol Mono-n-Butyl Ether

Structural formula:

$$\underset{\underset{OH}{|}}{CH}-CH_2-O-\overset{\overset{CH_3}{|}}{CH}-CH_2-O-\overset{\overset{CH_3}{|}}{CH}-CH_2-O-CH_2-CH_2-CH_2-CH_3$$

with CH_3 group also on the first carbon.

Molecular formula: $C_{13}H_{28}O_4$

Molecular weight: 248.3

Properties: a colourless liquid of very low volatility with a slight ethereal odour and bitter taste.

    boiling point: 255 °C

    vapour pressure: 0.008 mm Hg at 25 °C

    conversion factors: 1 p.p.m. = 10.1 mg/m^3

                        1 mg/l = 98.6 p.p.m.

    maximum allowable concentration: not established.

ECONOMY, SOURCES AND USES

Industrial uses

Similar to those of other glycol ethers.

BIOCHEMISTRY

The only information available is that it is possible that toxic amounts may be absorbed by the skin.

TOXICOLOGY

From the results of the only available investigation (Rowe, 1963) this butyl ether appears to be slightly more toxic by oral administration to rats than the ethyl ether of tripropylene glycol (LD_{50}: 1.84 mg/kg compared with 2 ml/kg).

    It is also slightly more toxic by repeated application to the skin of rabbits as evidenced by loss of weight, but it caused no conjunctival irritation when 1 drop was introduced into the eyes on 5 consecutive days.

    No injury to human beings has been reported and apart from the slight risk that might be envisaged from repeated and prolonged skin contact, it appears to carry very little industrial hazard.

Bibliography on p. 686

BIBLIOGRAPHY

Allbright, F., M. Butler and E. Bloomberg (1937) Rickets resistant to vitamin D Therapy. *Am. J. Dis. Child.*, 54:529.

Bachem, C. (1917) Pharmakologische Untersuchungen über Glykol und seine Verwendung in der Pharmazie und Medizin. *Med. Klin.*, 1:7:312.

Bergner, K. G. and H. Sperlich (1953) Detection and determining purity of glycols and similar compounds. *Z. Lebens. Untersuch. Forsch.*, 97:253.

Biochemical Research Laboratory, Dow Chemical Company, cited by Rowe, 1963.

Boemke, F. (1943) Beitrag zur Toxikologie und Pathologie des Äthyleneglykols (Glysantin). *Virchow's Pathol. Anat.*, 310:106.

Bornmann, G. (1954 and 1955) Grundwirkung der Glykole und ihre Bedeutung für die Toxizität. *Arzneim. Forsch.*, 4:643 and 5:38.

Bost, J. and Y. Ruckebusch (1962) Toxicité et Pharmacologie du Propylène glycol. *Thérapie*, 17:83.

Braun, H. A. and G. F. Cartland (1936) The toxicity of propylene glycol. *J. Am. Pharmacol. Ass.*, 25:746.

Brennaas, O. (1960) Poisoning with diethylene glycol monoethyl ether. *Nord. Med.*, 64:1291.

Browning, E. (1953) *Toxicity of industrial organic solvents*. H.M.S.O. London.

Calvery, H. O., J. H. Draize and G. Woodard (1944) Relative acute toxicity of some organic compounds following oral administration and skin application. *Fred. Proc.*, 3:67.

Calvery, H. O., and T. G. Klumpp (1939) The toxicity for human beings of diethylene glycol with sulfanilamide. *Southern Med. J.*, 32:1105.

Carpenter, C. P. (1947) Cellosolve acetate. *J. Am. Med. Ass.*, 135:880.

Carpenter, C. P., U. C. Pozzani and C. S. Weil (1956) The toxicity of butyl cellosolve solvent. *Arch. Ind. Hlth.*, 14:114.

Carpenter, C. P. and H. F. Smyth, Jr. (1946) Chemical Burns of the rabbit cornea. *Am. J. Ophthalm.* 28:1363.

Cranch, A. G., H. F. Smyth Jr. and C. P. Carpenter (1942) External contact with monoethyl ether of diethylene glycol (Carbitol solvent). *Arch. Dermatol. Syph.*, 45:553.

Curme, G. O. and F. Johnston (1952) *Glycols*. Am. Chem. Soc. Monograph. Ser. 114, Reinhold, New York.

Davidson, J. D. (1926) The glycol ethers and their use in the lacquer industry. *Ind. Eng. Chem.*, 18:669.

Dawson, J. and R. P. Hullin (1954) Metabolism of acetoin. *Biochem., J.*, 57:177, 180.

Doerr, W. (1949) cited by Williams R. T. (1959) *Chem. Abstr.*, 1950, 44:8546.

Donley, D. F. (1936) Toxic encephalophathy and volatile solvents in industry. *J. Ind. Hyg. Toxicol.*, 18:571.

Dow Chemical Company; Biochemical Research Laboratory (cited by Rowe (1963)).

Draize, J. H., E. Alvarez, M. F. Whitesell, G. Woodard, E. C. Hagen and A. A. Nelson (1948) Toxicity of insect repellents. *J. Pharmacol. Exptl. Therap.*, 93:26.

Draize, J. H., G. Woodard and H. O. Calvery (1944) Methods for the study of irritation and toxicity of substances applied topically to skin and mucous membranses. *J. Pharmacol. Exptl. Therap.*, 82:377.

Duke, F. R. and G. F. Smith (1940) Rapid qualitative test for alcoholic hydroxyl groups. *Ind. Eng. Chem. Anal. Ed.*, 12:201.

Durrans, T. H. (1950) *Solvents*, 6th ed. Chapman and Hall, London.

Elkins, H. B., D. B. Stortazzi and J. W. Hammond (1942) Determination of atmosphere contaminants. Methyl Cellosolve. *J. Ind. Hyg. Toxicol.*, 24:229.

Fairhall, L. T. (1957) *Industrial Toxicology*, 2nd ed. Williams and Wilkins Co., Baltimore.

Fellows, J. K., F. P. Luduena and P. J. Hanzlik ((1947) Glucuronic excretion after diethylene glycol monoethyl ether (Carbitol) and some other glycols. *J. Pharmacol. Exptl. Therap.*, 89:210.

Fischer, L., R. Kopf, A. Loeser and G. Meyer (1949) Chemische Konstitution und pharmakologische Wirkung der Glykole. *Z. ges. Exp. Med.*, 115:22.

Fitzhugh, O. G. and A. A. Nelson (1946) Comparison of chronic toxicity of triethylene glycol with that of diethylene glycol. *J. Ind. Hyg. Toxicol.*, 28:40.

Flinn, F. B. (1935) Some clinical observations on the influence of certain hygroscopic agents in cigarettes. *Laryngoscope, St. Louis*, 45:149.

Flury, F. and W. Wirth (1934) Zur Toxikologie der Lösungsmittel. *Arch. Gewerbepathol. Gewerbehyg.*, 5:52.

Flury, F. and W. Wirth (1934) Zur Toxikologie der Lösungsmittel. *Arch. Gewerbepathol. Gewerbehyg.*, 5:1.

Friedmann, F. A., J. B. Greenberg, J. P. Merrill and G. J. Dammin (1962) Consequences of Ethylene Glycol Poisoning. *Am. J. Med.*, 32:891.

Geiling, E. M. K. and P. R. Cannon (1938) Pathologic effects of elixir of sulfanilamide (diethylene glycol) poisoning. *J. Am. Med. Ass.*, 111:919.

Geiling, E. M. K., J. M. Coon and E. W. Schoeffel (1937) Preliminary reports of toxicity studies on rats, rabbits and dogs. *J. Am. Med. Ass.*, 109:1532.

Gershoff, S. N. and S. B. Andrus (1962) Effect of vitamin B_6 and magnesium on renal deposition of Ca oxalate induced by ethylene glycol administration. *Proc. Soc. Exptl. Biol. Med.*, 109:99.

Gessner, P. K., D. V. Parkes and R. T. Williams (1960) The metabolism of glycols. *Biochem. J.*, 74:1.

Greenburg, L. M., M. R. Mayers, L. J. Goldwater, W. J. Burke, C. E. Moskowitz and S. Moskowitz (1938) *J. Ind. Hyg.*, 20:138.

Gross, E. (1943) in K. B. Lehmann and F. Flury (1943) *Toxicology and hygiene of industrial solvents.* Williams and Wilkins, Baltimore.

Haag, H. B. and A. M. Ambrose (1937) Studies on the physiological effect of diethylene glycol. *J. Pharmacol. Exptl. Therap.*, 59:93.

Haggerty, R. J. (1959) Toxic hazards: Deaths from permanent antifreeze ingestion. *New. Eng. J. Med.*, 261:1296.

Hanzlik, P. J., W. S. Lawrence, J. K. Fellows, F. P. Luduena and G. L. Laqueur (1947) Epidermal application of diethylene glycol monoethyl ether (carbitol) and some other glycols. *J. Ind. Hyg. Toxicol.*, 29:325.

Hanzlik, P. J., F. P. Luduena, W. S. Lawrence and J. K. Fellows (1947) Toxicity, excretion and fate of diethylene glycol monoethyl ether compared with other glycols applied externally. *Fed. Proc.*, 6:336.

Hanzlik, P. J., H. W. Newman, W. van Winkle, A. J. Lehmann and N. K. Kennedy (1939) Toxicity, fate and excretion of propylene glycol and some other glycols. *J. Pharmacol. Exptl. Therap.*, 67:101, 114.

Hanzlik, P. J., M. A. Seidenfeld and C. C. Johnson (1931) General properties, irritant and toxic actions of ethylene glycol. *J. Pharmacol. Exptl. Therap.*, 41:387.

Harris, T. N. and J. Stokes (1945) Summary of a 3 year study of the clinical application of disinfection of air by glycol vapour. *Am. J. Med. Sci.*, 209:152.

Harry, R. G. (1940) *Modern cosmetology.* Chemical Publishing Co., New York.

Hinricks, A., R. Kopf and A. Loeser (1948) Toxicology of 1–4 butanediol. *Pharmazie*, 3:110; *Chem. Abstr.* (1948) 42:5567.

Hoehn, D. (1945) Nephrosis probably due to excessive use of Sta-way Insect repellant. *J. Am. Med. Ass.*, 128:513.

Holck, H. G. O. (1937) Glycerin, ethylene glycol, prolypene glycol and diethylene glycol. *J. Am. Med. Ass.*, 109:1517.

Hunt, R. (1932) Toxicity of ethylene and propylene glycols. *Ind. Eng. Chem.*, 24:361.

Husing, E. R. Kopf and A. Loeser (1950) Action of 1–3 butylene glycol on the skin. *Fette und Seifen*, 52:45; *Chem. Abstr.* (1950) 44:7999.

Jennings, B. H., E. Biggs and F. C. W. Olson (1944) Cited by Rowe, 1963, *Heating, piping, air conditioning*, 16:538.

Karel, L., B. H. Landing and T. S. Harvey (1947) The intraperitoneal toxicity of some glycols, glycol ethers, glycol esters and phthalates in urine. *J. Pharmacol. Exptl. Therap.*, 90:338.

Kesten, H. D., M. G. Mulinos and L. Pomerantz (1939) Pathologic effects of certain glycols and related compounds. *Arch. Pathol.*, 27:447.

Kesten, H. D., M. G. Mulinos and L. Pomerantz (1937) Renal lesions due to diethylene glycol. *J. Am. Med. Ass.*, 109:1509.

Kopf, R., A. Loeser, G. Meyer and W. Franke (1950) Untersuchungen über die Pharmakologie und Toxikologie mehrwertiger Alkohole (1–3 Butylene Glycol). *Arch. Exptl. Pathol. Pharmakol.*, 210:346.

Latven, H. R. and H. Molitor (1939) Comparison of the hypnotic and irritating properties of 8 organic solvents. *J. Pharmacol. Exptl. Therap.*, 65:89.

Laug, E. P., H. O. Calvery, H. J. Morris and G. Woodard (1939) The toxicology of some glycols and derivatives. *J. Ind. Hyg. Toxicol.*, 21:173.

Lauter, W. M. and V. L. Vrla (1940) Toxicity of triethylene glycol and effect of para-amino-benzoic acid upon this glycol. *J. Am. Pharmacol. Ass. Sci. Ed.*, 29:5.

Lehman, A. J. and H. W. Newman (1937) Propylene glycol; Rate of metabolism, absorption and excretion, with a method for estimation in body fluids. *J. Pharmacol. Exptl. Therap.*, 60:312.

Lehmann, K. B. and F. Flury (1943) *Toxicology and Hygiene of industrial solvents*. Williams and Wilkins Co., Baltimore.

Lepkowski, R., A. Over and H. M. Evans (1935) The nutritive value of the fatty acids of Lard and some of their esters. *J. Biol. Chem.*, 108:431.

Levene, P. A. and A. Walti (1927) On condensation products of propylene oxide and of glycidol. *J. Biol. Chem.*, 74:325.

Loeser, A. (1949) Cited by Rowe, 1963. *Pharmazie*, 4:263.

Loeser, A., G. Bornmann, L. Grossinsky, G. Hess (1954) Diäthylenglykol. *Arch. Exptl. Pathol. Pharmacol.*, 221:14.

Malten, K. E. and R. L. Zielhuis (1964) *Industrial toxicology and dermatology in production and processing of plastics*. Elsevier Publishing Company, Amsterdam.

Mayer, P. (1903) Experimentelle Beitrage zur Frage des intermediären Stoffwechsels der Kohlenhydrate. *Hoppe-Seyler Z.*, 38:135.

McKennis, H., R. A. Turner (1962) The excretion and metabolism of triethylene glycol. *Toxicol. Appl. Pharmacol.*, 4:411.

Meininger, W. M. (1948) External use of 'Carbitol Solvent', Carbitol and other reagents. *Arch. Dermatol. Syph.*, 58:19.

Mendel, F. (1917) Perkaglycerin und Tegoglycol, zwei Glycerin-Ersatzmittel. *Therap. Gegenw.*, 58:49.

Miura, S. (1911) Über das Verhalten von Äthylenglykol, Propylenglykol und Glycerin im Tierkörper. *Biochem. Z.*, 36:25.

Morris, H. J., A. A. Nelson and H. O. Calvery (1942) Observations on the chronic Toxicities of Glycols. *J. Pharmacol. Exptl. Therap.*, 74:266.

Mulinos, M. G. and R. L. Osborne (1934) Influence of hygroscopic agents on irritation from cigarette smoke. *Proc. Soc. Exptl. Biol. Med.*, 32:241.

Mulinos, M. G. and R. L. Osborne (1935) Irritating properties of cigarette smoke as influenced by hygroscopic agents. *N.Y. State J. Med.*, 35:590.

Mulinos, M. G., L. Pomerantz and M. E. Lojkin (1943) Metabolism and toxicology of ethylene glycol and ethylene glycol diacetate. *Am. J. Pharmacol.*, 115:51.

Navarre, M. G. de, (1941) *Chemistry and manufacture of cosmetics*. Van Nostrand, New York.

Nawrocki, C. S., F. S. Brackett and H. W. Werner (1944) Determination of concentration of monoalkyl ethylene glycol ethers in air by infra-red absorption spectroscopy. *J. Ind. Hyg. Toxicol.*, 26:193.

Neuberg, C. and A. Gottschalk (1925) Über das physiologische Verhalten des Acetoins. *Biochem. Z.*, 162:484.

Newman, H. W., W. van Winkle Jr., N. K. Kennedy and M. C. Morton (1940) Comparative effects of propylene glycol, other glycols and alcohol on the liver directly. *J. Pharmacol. Exptl. Therap.*, 68:194.

Oettingen, W. F. von (1943) The aliphatic alcohols. *U.S. Publ. Hlth. Serv. P.H. Bull.*, 281.

Oettingen, W F. von and E. A. Jirouch (1931) Pharmacology of ethylene glycol and some of its derivatives in relation to their chemical properties. *J. Pharmacol. Exptl. Therap.*, 42:355.

Page, I. H. (1927) Ethylene glycol – A Pharmacological study. *J. Pharmacol. Exptl. Therap.*, 30:313.

Parsons, C. E. and M. E. M. Parsons (1938) Toxic encephalopathy and 'Granulopenic Anaemia' due to volatile solvents in industry. *J. Ind. Hyg. Toxicol.*, 20:124.

Patscheider, H. and H. Hetzel (1961) Histologische Befunde bei einem Fall akuter Vergiftung durch Äthylenglykol. *Arch. Toxikol.*, 19:143.

Patty, F. A. (1963) *Industrial Hygiene and Toxicology*, Vol. II, 2nd ed. Interscience, New York.

Peterson, D. I., J. E. Peterson, M. G. Hardinge and W. E. C. Wacker (1963) Experimental treatment of ethylene glycol poisoning. *J. Am. Med. Ass.*, 186:955.

Pons, C. A. and R. P. Custer (1946) Acute ethylene glycol poisoning. A clinicopathologic Report of 18 fatal cases. *Am. J. Med. Sci.*, 211:544.

Procita, L. and F. E. Shideman (1950) Production of auricular fibrillation in the dog by dipropylene glycol methyl ether (Dowanol 50B). *Fed. Proc.*, 9:309.

Renkenbach, W. H. and H. A. Aaronson (1931) Properties of diethylene glycol. *Ind. Eng. Chem.*, 23:160.

Robertson, O. H. (1947) New methods for the control of airborne infection with special reference to the use of triethylene glycol vapour. *Wisconsin Med. J.*, 46:311.

Robertson, O. H., C. G. Loosli, T. T. Puck, H. Wise, H. M. Lemon and W. Lester (1947). Tests for chronic toxicity of propylene glycol and triethylene glycol on monkeys and rats by vapour inhalation and oral administration. *J. Pharmacol. Exptl. Therap.*, 91:52.

Robertson, O. H., T. T. Puck, H. M. Lemon and C. G. Loosli (1943) Lethal effect of triethylene glycol vapour on air-borne bacteria and influenza virus. *Science*, 97:142.

Ross, I. P. (1956) Ethylene glycol poisoning with Meningoencephalitis and Anuria. *Brit. Med. J.*, 1:1340.

Rosser, F. (1938) Diss. Würzburg (unpublished), cited by Lehmann and Flury (1943).

Rowe, V. K. (1963) *Glycols*, in F. A. Patty (1963) *Industrial Hygiene and Toxicology*, Vol. II, 2nd ed. Interscience, New York.

Rowe, V. K., D. D. McCollister, H. C. Spencer, F. Oyen, R. L. Hollingsworth and V. A. Drill (1954) Toxicology of Mono-, Di- and Tripropylene Glycol Methyl Ethers. *Arch. Ind. Hyg.*, 9:509.

Rudney, H. (1954) The synthesis of Propanediol-1-phosphate and C^{14}-labelled Propanediol and their isolation from liver tissue. *J. Biol. Chem.*, 210:3537.

Schlussel, H. (1954) Beitrag zur Verwertung mehrwertiger Alkohole in der Ernährung. *Arch. Exptl. Pathol. Pharmacol.*, 221:67.

Schneider, W. (1950) Dermatological and cosmetic usage of glycols as substitutes for glycerin. *Pharm. Ind.*, 12:226; *Chem. Abstr.* (1951) 45:3998.

Shaffer, C. B., F. H. Critchfield and J. H. Nair (1950) Absorption and excretion of a liquid polyethylene glycol. *J. Am. Pharmacol. Ass. Sci. Ed.*, 39:340.

Shideman, F. E. and L. Procita (1951) Pharmacology of the monomethyl ethers of Mono-, Di- and Tripropylene Glycols in the dog, with observations on the auricular fibrillation produced by these compounds. *J. Pharmacol. Exptl. Therap.*, 102:79.

Smith, D. E. (1951) Morphologic lesions due to acute and subacute poisoning with ethylene glycol (antifreeze). *Arch. Pathol.*, 51:423.

Smyth, Jr., H. F. and C. P. Carpenter (1948) Further Experience with the range finding test in the industrial toxicology laboratory. *J. Ind. Hyg. Toxicol.*, 30:63.

Smyth Jr., H. F., C. P. Carpenter and C. S. Weil (1951) Range Finding Toxicity Data. List IV. *Arch. Ind. Hyg.* 4:119.

Smyth Jr., H. F., J. Seaton and L. Fischer (1941) The signle dose toxicity of some glycols and derivatives. *J. Ind. Hyg. Toxicol.*, 23:259.

Starrek, E. (1938) *Über die Wirkung einiger Alkohole, Glykole und Ester.* Diss. Würzburg, cited by Lehmann and Flury (1943).

Sykowski, P. (1951) Ethylene Glycol Toxicity. *Am. J. Ophthalm.*, 34:1599.

Troisi, F. M. (1950) Chronic Intoxication by Ethylene Glycol Vapour. *Brit. J. Ind. Med.*, 7:65.

Waite, C. P., F. A. Patty and W. P. Yant (1930) Acute Response of Guinea Pigs to Vapours of some new commercial organic compounds – Cellosolve (monoethyl ether of ethylene glycol). *U.S. Publ. Hlth. Rep.*, 45:1459.

Warshaw, T. G. and F. Herrmann (1952) Studies of skin reactions to Propylene Glycol. *J. Invest. Dermatol.*, 19:423.

Weatherby, J. H. and H. B. Haag (1938) Toxicity of Propylene Glycol. *J. Am. Pharmacol. Ass.*, 27:466.

Wegener, H. (1953) Über die Fortpflanzungfähigkeit der Ratte nach Einwirkung von Diäthylen-glykol. *Arch. Exptl. Pathol. Pharmakol.*, 220:414.

Werner, H. W. and J. L. Mitchell (1943) Determination of Monoalkyl Ethers of Ethylene Glycol. *Ind. Eng. Chem. Anal. Ed.*, 15:3775.

Werner, H. W., J. L. Mitchell, J. W. Miller and W. F. von Oettingen (1943) Acute toxicity of vapours of several Monoalkyl Ethers of Ethylene Glycol. *J. Ind. Hyg.*, 25:157.

Werner, H. W., C. Z. Nawrocki, J. L. Mitchell, J. W. Miller and W. F. van Oettingen (1943) Effect of repeated exposure of rats to vapours of Monoalkyl Ethylene Glycol Ethers. *J. Ind. Hyg. Toxicol.*, 25:374.

Werner, H. W., C. Z. Nawrocki and J. L. Mitchell (1943) Effect of repeated exposure of rats to vapours of Monoalkyl Ethylene Glycol Ethers. *J. Ind. Hyg. Toxicol.*, 25:409.

Whitlock, G. P., N. B. Guerrant and R. A. Dutcher (1944) Response of rats to diets containing Propylene Glycol and Glycerine. *Proc. Soc. Exptl. Biol. Med.*, 57:124.

Wiley, F. H., W. C. Hueper, D. S. Bergen and F. R. Blood (1938) Formation of Oxalic Acid from Ethylene glycol and related solvents. *J. Ind. Hyg. Toxicol.*, 20:269.

Wiley, F. H., W. C. Hueper and W. F. von Oettingen (1936) Formation of Oxalic Acid from Ethylene Glycol and related solvents. *J. Ind. Hyg. Toxicol.*, 18:123.

Williams, R. T. (1959) *Detoxication Mechanisms*. Chapman and Hall, London.

Williams, J. W. and H. Kirby (1948) Paper chromatography using capillary ascent. *Chem Abstr.*, 42 11:5494.

Winkle Jr., W. van, (1941) Qualitative Gastro-intestinal Absorption and Renal Excretion of Pro-pylene Glycol. *J. Pharmacol. Exptl. Therap.*, 72:344.

Winkle Jr., W. van, and N. K. Kennedy (1940) Voluntary activity of rats fed Propylene Glycol and other Glycols. *J. Pharmacol. Exptl. Therap.*, 69:140.

Wise, H., T. T. Puck and H. M. Stral (1943) A rapid colorimetric method for the determination of Glycols in air. *J. Biol. Chem.*, 150:61.

Young, E. G. and L. B. Wollner (1946) A case of fatal poisoning by 2-Methoxyethanol. *J. Ind. Hyg. Toxicol.*, 28:267.

Zavon, M. R. (1963) Methyl Cellosolve Intoxication. *Am. Ind. Hyg. Ass. J.*, 24:36.

Zehrer, G. (1948) Tödliche Vergiftung durch Glycerinersatz (Diäthylenglykol). *Med. Klin.*, 43:369

Chapter 13

SILICIUM COMPOUNDS

Many of the silicone compounds which have during the last 20 years assumed considerable industrial importance are not solvents in the strict sense of the word; some of them are in fact resins or rubber-like substances or oils, while others are 'anti-foam' materials. On the whole, as a group, the silicones do not present an appreciable hazard; many of them have been used therapeutically in gastro-intestinal disorders and in pulmonary oedema and also as surgical protheses – a fact which would appear to be a firm indication of the non-toxicity of the solid and resinous varieties. Some of the anti-foam compounds, in view of their many uses in connection with food products have been examined for the possibility that they might remain in these food products and exert a potential toxic effect, while one of the silicone oils (a methyl phenyl polysiloxane) has also been investigated by animal experiments in order to determine whether it is absorbed from the gastro-intestinal tract.

The organic silicates, ethyl silicate (tetraethoxysilane) and methyl silicate (tetramethyl orthosilicate) have on the other hand been found not devoid of toxicity, and another organic silicate, known as MLO 5277, has been found to be an irritant of the eyes and respiratory tract when heated or inhaled, unheated, as an aerosol.

127. Silicone Oils

(Polysiloxanes)

These compounds are viscous fluids which are used widely as anti-foam agents and also in providing 'non-stick' surfaces for domestic utensils. The methyl poly-siloxanes are not lung irritants; they have been found therapeutically active in reducing lung oedema in animals, caused by cardiac disease or experimental administration of epinephrine, but not by irritant gases. Two of them were investigated by Henschler *et al.* (1960), using mice exposed to chlorine and nitrous gases and showing symptoms of intense irritation of the respiratory tract. Administration of these silicone aerosols produced some improvement in 5–7 h, but the condition deteriorated and was followed by death. Autopsy indicated that the silicones encouraged the spread of the irritant gases into the trachea and bronchi and prevented the elimination of the oedematous material. Another anti-foam

[691]

agent (DC Antifoam A) was tested for its therapeutic effect on pulmonary oedema in rats and mice caused by phosgene and chloropicrin and found that it did appear to have some effect on mice exposed to lower concentrations of chloropicrin, but was not effective on chloropicrin or phosgene in rats. In addition to the hazard mentioned by Henschler *et al.* of non-elimination of the oedematous material Smith (1960) has noted the occurrence in dogs of cerebral emboli of silicone antifoam, and silicone embolisation has also been described by Lindberg (1961).

Some Polydimethylsiloxanes have, however, been found effective in preventing the death of rats from pulmonary oedema induced by chlorine and epinephrine (Nickerson and Curry, 1955) and daily administration for 28 days did not produce inflammatory or granulomatous changes in the lungs. Similar results were observed by Princiotto *et al.* (1952), using a product called DC Anti-foam A, on rats with epinephrine-induced oedema, and this indication of very low toxicity of polydimethylsiloxanes, has been generally confirmed by Rowe, Spencer and Bass (1948, 1950) and MacDonald *et al.* (1960). The latter used 5 of these compounds, in a dosage of 1% of the diet of rats for 90 days, and observed no toxic symptoms and no pathological changes which were not present also in many of the control animals, such as varying inflammatory changes in the lungs and fatty changes in the liver.

Hexamethyldisiloxane has been stated (Rowe, 1948) to cause transtitory irritation of the conjunctiva but no corneal damage.

The Methylphenyl polysiloxanes are the only polysiloxanes soluble in oil. Absorption from the intestine is apparently very little when fed to animals dissolved in olive oil. Paul and Pover (1960) found that 85% of a methylphenylsiloxane was recovered from the gastro-intestinal tract after 3 h, and 96% after long-term feeding from the large bowel and the faeces. None was found in the liver, kidneys or fat depots, and no soluble silica in the urine.

Organo-Silicates

128. Ethyl Silicate

Synonyms: tetraethyl ortho silicate; tetraethoxysilane

Molecular formula: $Si(OC_2H_5)_4$

Molecular weight: 208.2

Properties: a colourless liquid with a sharp ester-like odour, slowly hydrolysed by water to form silicic acid.

> *boiling point:* 165–166 °C
> *vapour pressure:* 1.07 mm Hg at 20 °C
> *vapour density (air = 1):* 7.2
> *specific gravity (liquid density):* 0.9356
> *flash point:* 125 °F
> *solubility:* soluble in alcohol and miscible with ether
> *maximum allowable concentration:* 100 p.p.m.

ECONOMY, SOURCES AND USES

Industrial uses

(1) In the building industry as a preservative for stone, brick and concrete, and as a weatherproofing and waterproofing agent.
(2) In the paint industry, for heat- and chemical-restistant paints.
(3) In protective coatings.

BIOCHEMISTRY

Estimation in the atmosphere

(1) By adsorption on equilibrated charcoal and subsequent weight measurement.
(2) By interferometer (Jacobs, 1941).

Metabolism

Ethyl silicate readily undergoes hydrolysis, with formation of ethyl alcohol and hydroxy esters, progressing until the end products are silicic acid or hydrated silicic acid.

TOXICOLOGY

The basic toxic response to ethyl silicate by any route of administration is rupture of the pulmonary capillaries. This leads to haemorrhage into the air sacs with some rupturing of alveolar tissues. In animals, pulmonary haemorrhages, followed by anaemia, haematuria, secondary pneumonia and acute nephritis are followed by narcosis and death.

According to Rowe, Spencer and Bass (1948) ethyl silicate is the most toxic of the silane intermediates, causing, in animals, kidney damage in the form of tubular degeneration and necrosis. It is also a severe irritant of the eyes and respiratory tract.

Smyth and Seaton (1940) however do not consider it a compound of 'high' toxicity since its hazard in industrial use is lessened by its low vapour pressure. They found some indication that atmospheric humidity lessens the acute toxicity of its vapour, probably by partly hydrolysing the ester.

Toxicity to animals

(1) Acute

Lethal dose. – (i) By subcutaneous injection, for rats, 0.09–0.35 ml/100 g (5 out of 9 survived longer than 4 days (Kaspar et al., 1937). – (ii) By intravenous injection, for rats, approximately 0.2 ml/100 g. Death within 5 min. – (iii) By intraperitoneal injection, for rats, 0.56 ml within 60 min; 0.06–0.56 ml within 3 days. – (iv) By inhalation, for rats and guinea pigs, 2530 p.p.m. (approx. saturation at 25 °C) for 120 min. Almost no immediate deaths at 3070 p.p.m. for 30 min but delayed deaths at 48 h, or in a few cases at 13 days (Smyth and Seaton, 1940); for guinea pigs, 1500 to 2300 p.p.m. for 4 h (Rowe et al., 1948).

(2) Chronic

Lethal dose, for rats, by repeated inhalation, 400 p.p.m. for 7 h a day for 30 days (Pozzani and Carpenter, 1951). Exposure to 88 p.p.m., repeatedly, caused no injury.

SYMPTOMS OF INTOXICATION

Acute

Irritation of the eyes and respiratory tract, tremors, weakness, narcosis, leading to death (Smyth and Seaton, 1940).

CHANGES IN THE ORGANISM

The lungs showed general congestion and multiple haemorrhages due to destruction of the capillary walls. Kaspar et al. (1937) state that this lesion may appear within 10 min of intraperitoneal injection of minute quantities of ethyl silicate and without demonstrable local injury within the abdominal cavity. Pulmonary oedema developed in animals which survived 3–4 days.

The kidneys showed acute nephritis following inhalation, with severe necrosis of the tubular epithelium.

The liver also showed necrosis.

The cause of death was believed to be pulmonary oedema, with delayed secondary pneumonia.

In the heart the capillaries of the muscle were injured, and there was dilatation and slight oedema.

In the brain the cerebral capillaries contained vacuoles and globules between collections of red cells – possibly globules of ethyl silicate itself.

The blood showed a temporary fall in red corpuscles, white corpuscles and lymphocytes, with unaltered haemoglobin, later an increase of polymorphs and mononuclears. In fatal cases these changes progressed to profound anaemia.

Toxicity to human beings

While no injurious effects from the industrial use of ethyl silicate have been reported, Fassett (1963) states that 3000 p.p.m. is intolerable to human beings; 250 p.p.m. is irritating to eyes and nose, and 85 p.p.m. can be detected by its odour.

129. Methyl Silicate

Synonym: tetramethylorthosilicate

Molecular formula: $Si(OCH_3)_4$

Molecular weight: 152.2

Properties: a liquid soluble in alcohol.
    boiling point: 121 °C
    vapour pressure: 12 mm Hg at 25 °C
    vapour density (air = 1): 5.2
    specific gravity (liquid density): 1.028
    solubility: soluble in alcohol
    maximum allowable concentration: not established.

ECONOMY, SOURCES AND USES

Industrial uses

Similar to those of ethyl silicate, but also in the ceramic industry; and as a bonding agent for paints and lacquers.

Bibliography on p. 697

TOXICOLOGY

While less toxic than ethyl silicate to animals, it does cause some kidney damage both by inhalation and by intraperitoneal administration. Both the liquid and the vapour may cause necrosis of the cornea.

Toxicity to animals

Lethal dose. – (i) By oral administration, for rats, 700 mg/kg (Fassett, 1963). – *(ii) intraperitoneal injection,* 100 mg/kg. No toxic effects from the industrial use of either ethyl or methyl silicate have been recorded, but according to Fassett (1963) 250 p.p.m. of ethyl silicate is irritating to the eyes and nose, and 3000 p.p.m. is intolerable.

130. Organo Silicate MLO 5277

This compound is used as a hydraulic fluid and comes in contact with heated metal surfaces of engines operating at high temperatures.

Synonym: hexamethyl disiloxane
Molecular formula: $Si_2O(CH_3)_6$
Molecular weight: 162.3
Properties: a fluid which is decomposed at 520 °F forming a fine powder, which, it is suggested, may be silica (Feinsilver *et al.*, 1961).

BIOCHEMISTRY

Estimation in the atmosphere

Its pyrolysis products – CO, and total aldehydes, were estimated as follows:
    CO – by the Mine Safety Appliances CO Tester.
    Total aldehydes, expressed as formaldehyde, by the iodimetric method described by Goldman and Yagoda (1953).

TOXICOLOGY

This compound is a severe irritant of the eyes and respiratory tract, causing in high concentrations, especially when heated, lung oedema and haemorrhage, but also marked inflammation even when unheated and in low concentrations.

Toxicity to animals

Lethal dose. – *(i) By inhalation*, for rats and dogs, 4.0 mg/l at 520 °F pyrolysis; 3.3 mg/l at 1020 °F pyrolysis.

In rats, reddish secretion about the eyes and nose one hour after exposure to 0.3–0.6 mg/l (unheated); respiratory distress one hour after exposure to 0.9–1.3 mg/l, and immediately after exposure to 1.2–2.8 mg/l.

In dogs only eye irritation at 0.6–0.6 mg/l, but anorexia, depression, rhinitis and respiratory distress at 1.3–2.8 mg/l, with an increase in temperature and concentration, salivation, cyanosis and congestion of the eyes.

Lesions were confined to the respiratory tract. At 1.3–2.8 mg/l, the lungs showed pneumonia, oedema, haemorrhage and alveolar collapse, and at lethal concentrations severe necrosis of the epithelial lining of all airways.

BIBLIOGRAPHY

Gogan, H. D. and C. H. Setterström (1946) Properties of ethyl silicate. *Chem. Eng. News*, 24:2499.

Fassett, D. W. (1963) Esters, in F. A. Patty, *Industrial Hygiene and Toxicology*, Vol. II, 2nd ed. p. 1933.

Feinsilver, L., J. Perrigino and M. A. Ross (1961) Acute inhalation toxicity of heated aerosols of 3 hydraulic fluids. *Am. Ind. Hyg. Ass. J.*, 22:14.

Goldman, H. F. and H. Yagoda (1943) Collection and estimation of traces of formaldehyde in air. *Ind. Eng. Chem. Anal. Ed.*, 15:377.

Henschler, D. F., Amend and A. Juettner (1960) Die Wirkung von Siliconaerosoln auf Reizgaslungödeme. *Ardh. Exptl. Pathol. Pharmakol.*, 239:288.

Jacobs, M. B. (1941) *Analytical chemistry of industrial poisons, hazards and solvents*. Interschience, New York.

Kasper, J. A., C. P. Mc Cord and W. G. Frederick (1937) Toxicity of organic silicon compounds. Tetraethyl ortho silicate. *Ind. Med. Surg.*, 6:660.

Lindberg, D. A. (1961) Silicone embolisation. *Southern Med. J.*, 54:654.

MacDonald, W. E., G. E. Lanier and W. B. Deichmann (1960) The subacute oral toxicity to the rat of certain polydimethyl siloxanes. *Arch. Ind. Hlth.*, 21:514.

Nickerson, M. and C. F. Curry (1955) Control of pulmonary oedema with silicone aerosols. *J. Pharmacol., Exptl. Therap.*, 114:138.

Paul, J. and W. F. Pover (1960) The failure of absorption of DC silicone fluid 703 from the gastro-intestinal tract of rats. *Brit. J. Jnd. Med.*, 17:149.

Pozzani, W. C. and P. C. Carpenter (1951) Response of rodents to repeated inhalation of vapours of tetraethylorthosilicate. *Arch. Ind. Hyg.*, 4:465.

Princiotto, J. V., W. L. Howell and C. F. Morgan (1952) Antifoaming effect of a methylpolysiloxane compound in experimental pulmonary oedema. *Am. J. Physiol.*, 171:758.

Rowe, V. K., H. C. Spencer and S. L. Bass (1948) Toxicological studies on certain commercial silicons and hydrolisable silane intermediates. *J. Ind. Hyg. Toxicol.*, 30:332.

Rowe, V. K., H. C. Spencer and S. L. Bass (1950) Toxicological studies on certain commercial silicons – 2-year dietary feeding of DC Antifoam A to rats. *Arch. Ind. Hyg.*, 1:539.

Smith, W. T. (1960) Cerebral lesions due to emboli of silicone antifoam in dogs subjected to cardiopulmonary bypass. *J. Pathol. Bacteriol.*, 80:9.

Smyth, H. F., Jr., and J. Seaton (1940) Acute response of guinea pigs and rats to inhalation of vapours of tetraethylorthosilicate (ethyl silicate). *J. Ind. Hyg. Toxicol.*, 22:288.

Chapter 14

MISCELLANEOUS COMPOUNDS

131. Furan

Synonyms: furfurane, axole

Structural formula:

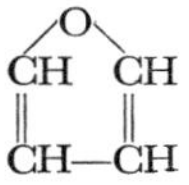

$$\begin{array}{c} \diagup O \diagdown \\ CH \quad CH \\ \| \qquad \| \\ CH{-}CH \end{array}$$

Molecular formula: C_4H_4O

Molecular weight: 68

Properties: a clear liquid. May form unstable peroxides on exposure to air; highly explosive when exposed to heat or flame or on contact with acids or oxidising materials.

> *boiling point:* 30–32 °C
> *melting point:* −85.6 °C
> *vapour density (air = 1):* 2.35
> *specific gravity (liquid density):* 0.944
> *flash point:* −32 °F
> *solubility:* in water 2.3%
> *maximum allowable concentration:* not established by A.C.I.G.H. Sax (1957) suggests 10 p.p.m. and states that this, together with its low boiling point, requires that adequate ventilation be provided in areas where it is handled.

ECONOMY, SOURCES AND USES

Produced by catalytic decarboxylation of furfural, and by synthesis from acetylene (Durrans, 1950).

Industrial uses similar to tetrahydrofurane but not widely used.

BIOCHEMISTRY

It is not known whether furane is hydroxylated *in vivo*, but it appears that the furane ring is stable (Williams, 1959).

TOXICOLOGY

Furane is strongly anaesthetic and analgesic, but highly toxic by inhalation by animals, and readily absorbed by the skin, causing convulsions followed by paralysis of the respiratory centre and asphyxia. It has a corrosive effect on the mucous membrane of the mouth when given orally, and with intravenous injection causes symptoms and post-mortem changes similar to those of acute cyanide poisoning.

It has been suggested, on the basis of its chemical resemblance to divinyl ether, that it might be suitable as a surgical anaesthetic but it has a marked toxic effect on the central nervous system and causes a marked fall in blood pressure and an increase in muscular tonus as anaesthesia deepens (Johnston, 1931).

Toxicity to animals

Acute

Lethal dose. – (i) By oral administration, for dogs and rabbits, 0.25 g/kg. – (ii) By intravenous injection, for dogs, 1½ cc (Williams, 1959). – (iii) By inhalation, no concentrations given but dogs and rabbits collapsed and died after 2 inhalations from a saturated cotton wad (Koch and Cahan, 1925). In the experiments of Johnston (1931) concentrations were expressed as mols/l.

Lethal dose for cats, 0.0020 mols/l.

SYMPTOMS OF INTOXICATION

With oral administration, a copious flow of bloody saliva and watery fluid from the nose. With intravenous injection, convulsions followed rapidly by death. With inhalation, increase of respiratory rate, fall of blood pressure, convulsive movements, complete anaesthesia, death from asphyxia due to paralysis of the medulla.

CHANGES IN THE ORGANISM

(1) *Gastrointestinal tract.* – Haemorrhages, with partial destruction of the mucosa following oral administration.

(2) *Lungs.* – Markedly hyperaemic.

(3) *Blood vessels.* – Much dilated; blood cherry red.

(4) *Kidneys.* – Soft and swollen.

(5) *Liver.* – Resembled the first stages of chloroform poisoning (Koch and Cahan, 1925).

In Johnston's (1931) investigations of mice or cats following death from inhalation no gross post-mortem lesions were found.

No chronic experiments were performed. There is no record of any injury from industrial use.

Bibliography on p. 717

132. Tetrahydrofuran

Synonym: cyclo-tetramethylene oxide

Structural formula:

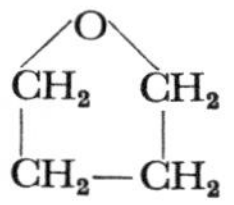

$$\begin{array}{c} O \\ CH_2 \quad CH_2 \\ | \qquad | \\ CH_2 - CH_2 \end{array}$$

Molecular formula: C_4H_8O

Molecular weight: 72.1

Properties: a colourless liquid with a neutral reaction, an odour similar to acetone and a pungent taste. It readily forms explosive peroxides on exposure to air; these can be removed by treatment with strong ferrous sulphate made slightly acidic with sodium bisulphate (Sax, 1957). An explosive hazard is specially possible by contact with lithium-aluminium alloys (Stokinger, 1963).

    boiling point: 65–66 °C

    vapour pressure: 114 mm Hg at 15 °C

    specific gravity (liquid density): 0.891

    flash point: 1 °F

    conversion factors: 1 p.p.m. = 2.94 mg/m³

                   1 mg/l   = 340 p.p.m.

    solubility: soluble in water

    maximum allowable concentration: 200 p.p.m. (Elkins, 1959, suggests 100 p.p.m.).

ECONOMY, SOURCES AND USES

Produced by hydrogenation of furan (Durrans, 1950).

Used in industry as a solvent for resins, and in the formation of lacquers.

TOXICOLOGY

Tetrahydrofuran is a strong narcotic, an irritant of mucous membranes and causes injury to the kidneys in animals. Its narcotic effect is greater than that of any glycol derivatives, but the effects on the kidneys less than those of dioxane.

    Earlier workers believed it to have an irritant and sensitising effect on the skin, but late authorities (Hoffman and Oettel, 1954) attribute these effects to peroxide formation.

    No toxic effects from its industrial use have been recorded.

Toxicity to animals

(1) Acute (Stoughton and Robbins, 1936).

(a) Lethal dose. – (i) By oral administration, for rabbits, 2.5 g/kg of a 20% solution. – *(ii) By inhalation*, for mice, 6.7 vol % in 30 min; 4.9 vol % in 51 min; LD_{50}, 2.2. vol % in 109 min.

(b) Narcotic dose. – By inhalation, for mice, 6.7 vol % in 5 min; 1.1. vol % in 43 min; for dogs, 5.6 vol % (oxygen mixture) for 2 h.

(2) Chronic

Discrepancy in the effects of repeated exposure by Zapp (cited by Fairhall, 1957) and by Lehmann and Flury (1943) are explainable by the difference in the concentrations used. According to Zapp inhalation of 200 p.p.m. by dogs 6 h daily for 3 weeks caused only a fall in pulse pressure; Lehmann and Flury, using much higher dosage (3400 p.p.m. daily for 20 days) observed severe irritation of mucous membranes, cats being especially susceptible, 1 dying after 3 exposures, and 2 after 6.

SYMPTOMS OF INTOXICATION

(i) By oral administration – giddiness, decrease in weight, albuminuria, narcosis. – *(ii) With inhalation* – copious flow of saliva and mucus, fall in blood pressure, unconsciousness with rigidity (Stoughton and Robbins, 1936). Vomiting, loss of corneal reflex, prostration, deep narcosis. One animal died after 12 days from pneumonia and purulent pleurisy (Lehmann and Flury, 1943).

CHANGES IN THE ORGANISM

(1) Acute

Oral administration was found by Lehmann and Flury to cause inflammation, necrosis and haemorrhages of the gastro-intestinal tract. The kidneys showed injury to the tubules. The liver inflammation and the lungs congestion and oedema.

According to Stoughton and Robbins (1936), dogs killed after recovery from a narcotic dose showed no gross abnormalities.

The same discrepancy exists in this regard. Zapp found no demonstrable changes in the principal organs, even after 9 to 12 weeks exposure to 400 p.p.m., while Lehmann and Flury found in the cats which died after repeated exposure, injury to the liver and kidneys.

Toxicity to human beings

According to Stoughton and Robbins (1936), the operators engaged in the animal investigations suffered from severe occipital headache after each experiment.

There are no records of any injury from its industrial use.

Bibliography on p. 717

133. Carbon Disulphide

Synonym: carbon bisulphide

Molecular formula: CS_2

Molecular weight: 76.13

Properties: CS_2 is a highly volatile colourless liquid which becomes yellow with age and exposure to light. Its odour, when impure, is like that of rotten eggs, the impurities consisting chiefly of H_2S, SO_2 and organic sulphur compounds. It has an extremely low auto-ignition temperature (125 °C) so that the vapour may ignite violently on contact with steam pipes or electric light bulbs.

> *boiling point:* 46 °C
>
> *melting point:* —108.6 °C
>
> *vapour pressure:* 360 mm Hg at 20 °C
>
> *vapour density (air = 1):* 2.63
>
> *specific gravity (liquid density):* 1.2661
>
> *flash point:* —22 °F
>
> *conversion factors:* 1 p.p.m. = 3.12 mg/m³
>
> 1 mg/l   = 0.32 p.p.m.

solubility: in water 0.2%. Miscible with alcohols, ether, benzene and fatty oils. Solvent for sulphur, rubber, vegetable oils and ester gum, but not for cellulose acetate or nitrate, vinyl resins or shellac. It forms a gel with ethyl and benzyl cellulose (Durrans, 1950).

maximum allowable concentration: 20 p.p.m.

ECONOMY, SOURCES AND USES

Produced by reaction of sulphur vapours with glowing coke followed by distillation (Lehmann and Flury, 1943).

Industrial uses

(1) In the viscose rayon industry, in the xanthation of cellulose, and in the spinning and washing of the viscose.

(2) In the rubber industry, in the cold vulcanisation process and in the production of rubber accelerators (Brieger, 1961).

(3) In the manufacture of cellophane.

(4) In the chemical industry as a solvent for fats, oils, resins and waxes.

(5) In the manufacture of optical glass (Patty, 1963).

(6) As a pesticide.

[702]

BIOCHEMISTRY

Estimation

(1) In the atmosphere

(a) By the method of McKee (1941), using a solution of 0.5% diethylamine and triethanolamine and 0.001% of cupric acetate in 95% ethyl alcohol, comparing the colour with a prepared standard by means of a photometer.

(b) infra-red photometry.

(c) The method most generally recommended is that described by The Department of Scientific and Industrial Research (1939) and used by McKee (1941).

This consists in bubbling air containing CS_2 through absolute alcohol or isobutanol to which diethylamine and copper acetate are added to form diethyl dithiocarbamate, the colour being compared with a standard by means of a photometer.

(2) In blood and urine

Several methods are recommended by Weist (1959) in addition to his own, which consists in using distilled water, ammonium oxalate and ethyl alcohol to prevent coagulation of the blood and foam formation, and then titrating with 0.001 N iodine solution.

Hunter (1940) used a modification of the method (see above) of that described by the Department of Scientific and Industrial Research for estimation in air.

Zaharadnik, Mansfield and Souček (1955) applied the reaction of CS_2 with histamine and histidine.

Metabolism

CS_2 enters the body chiefly by inhalation of its vapour, but it can also be absorbed by the skin. The proportion absorbed by persons not previously exposed is about 80% during the first 15 min but falls to about 40% after 45 min and remains at that level up to 4 hours (Teisinger and Souček, 1949). In workers previously exposed the absorption is lower (70%) during the first 15 min and falls more rapidly thereafter.

Elimination, both by lungs and urine, is small in previously non-exposed persons (5% of the total amount inhaled by the lungs, 0.06 of the total amount retained in the urine). The remaining 93–95% is retained in the tissues and undergoes metabolic transformation.

In persons previously exposed the excretion by the urine is higher – up to 4 mg/l. These differences in absorption and elimination in previously exposed persons indicate that their tissues are already partially saturated with CS_2 and cannot absorb as much as those with no previous exposure.

Bibliography on p. 717

Retention in the tissues is initially greatest in the blood, but saturation is complete in about 2 h, after which it passes slowly into the tissues. In animals, according to Busing, Sonnenschein *et al.* (1953) saturation of the tissues takes several weeks, and three weeks after inhalation about three times as much CS_2 is found in the brain as in other organs.

The actual mechanism of the metabolic transformation is not yet completely understood in spite of the vast amount of investigation carried out in many countries into its action on bodily enzymes. A suggestion made in 1961 by Simon, for example, is that CS_2 is a universal enzyme inhibitor and cellular poison, injuring first oxidative phosphorylisation, thus causing disturbance of fat metabolism and producing hypercholesterinaemia and hyperlipaemia. In chronic poisoning there has been found an increase in the blood of free cholesterin, phospholipids, neutral fat and β-lipoprotein (Ambrosio *et al.*, 1957; Paterni *et al.*, 1958), which is believed to be due to inhibition of the lipaemia clearing factor (Vigliani and Pernis, 1954; Ruikka, 1959) and from this arises a marked decrease in the lipolytic activity of the vessel wall itself (Simon, 1961), while, since phospholipids show a smaller increase than the other serum lipid fractions, these tend to be deposited in the vessel walls. The portion retained in the tissues also appears to be bound with groups of tissues containing a nitrogen atom-peptide, proteins and amino acids. Enzymic reactions with these substances, especially the amino acids, produce dithiocarbamates, which may be further decomposed by the desulphydrase system, liberating H_2S; this may then be rapidly oxidised to H_2SO_4 and excreted in the urine as sulphate. Some observers, such as Strittmatter, Peters and McKee (1950) and Giovine (1957) have in fact stated that exposure to CS_2 is followed by an increased urinary excretion of inorganic sulphate.

Dithiocarbamate acids contain relatively strong acid sulphydryl groups and guinea pigs exposed to inhalation of CS_2 have shown an increase of these groups; they have also tended to be statistically higher than normal in viscose workers (Souček and Madlo, 1956).

These facts indicate that the intramolecular reaction of CS_2 with albumen causes a marked alteration in the molecule. The liver is undoubtedly an important organ in the metabolism of CS_2, and investigations by Michalova *et al.* (1959) have suggested that signs of its capacity for detoxication of CS_2 are shown by changes which indicate a disturbance of capillary permeability. This endothelial disturbance, present probably in the general arterial system, is not, however, directly its cause. Other factors, especially an increase in blood cholesterol, have been held to be more responsible.

Cholesterinaemia is certainly a feature of CS_2 intoxication in animals, and though, according to Brieger (1961) the findings in this respect are controversial, it is believed by other observers to be another manifestation of altered body metabolism, intricately bound up with the enzyme systems and particularly with the metal complexes (Scheel *et al.*, 1960), associated with them and required as activators. Alkaline phosphatase for example requires Zn and Mg ions as activators, and the urinary excretion of both has been found increased in animals poisoned with CS_2, while the alkaline phosphatase activity is decreased. The chain of events in the metabolic disturbance would in this hypothesis be that of a chelating effect by the dithiocarbamate and thiazolidone, resulting from the reaction of CS_2 with free aminoacid groups in the body. This chelation would result in the formation of non-ionised complexes with the polyvalent metal ions, so that these are prevented from performing their necessary function in normal cell metabolism. In the brain and spinal cord copper is normally present as a structural part of cytochrome oxidase and coenxyme-A dehydrogenase. If it is unavailable the metabolism of the nerve cells may be severely disorganised. Copper is known also to be tightly bound by the thiocarbamate groups. and in animals with severe pathological changes in the spinal cord and cerebral cortex the copper content of these tissues is about half the normal. Thus it appears that the specific toxic action of CS_2 on the nervous system can also be directly associated with its remarkable metabolic behaviour.

TOXICOLOGY

CS_2 poisoning was for many years regarded as predominantly an acute nerve poison with symptoms of mental derangement resembling those of acute alcoholic intoxication – actute mania progressing to depression, apathy, loss of memory, hallucinations and delusions of persecution, these effects being sometimes permanent (Laudenheimer, 1899). Later, chronic poisoning became more widely recognised as a cause of polyneuritis, and later still, attention became focussed on 'chronic carbon disulphide atherosclerosis' (Lewey et al., 1938; Gordy and Trumper, 1938 and 1940; Rubin and Arieff, 1945; Rubin et al., 1950), and its occurrence as a simultaneous occurrence with the earlier types of CS_2 poisoning (Paterni, 1954).

Liver dysfunction, associated with fatty degeneration and haemorrhages has also been emphasised (Lewey, 1941; Saita and Gattoni, 1957; Granati and Candia, 1956; Ciesura, 1956).

Kidney injury, with hypertension, some albuminuria, slight haematuria and raised residual nitrogen has also been observed, a process of nephrosclerosis which is believed (Attinger, 1948) to be not a primary disorder, but a feature of the general atherosclerosis.

Gastro-intestinal disorders have been reported (Weise, 1933; Lewey, 1938; Vigliani, 1954) especially gastric or duodenal ulcer, but according to Blahnik and Tousek (1957) chronic gastritis with achlorhydria is more frequent.

Blood changes, chiefly in the form of hypochromic anaemia, with less significant changes in the leucocyte series, and little abnormality of the bone marrow

Bibliography on p. 717

have been noted by several observers (Maugeri, 1940; Raneletti, 1931; Kiczak and Mrozinski, 1953; Paterni, 1954).

Dermatitis has been stated by Schwartz, Tulipan and Birmingham (1957) to be a frequent effect of CS_2, but according to Brieger (1961) it has been conspicuously absent in the American viscose rayon industry.

Undoubtedly the acute toxic effects of CS_2 in industry have shown a notable decrease since the early years when episodes were described as in the Report of the Departmental Committee on Dangerous Trades of 1899, in which the windows of a vulcanising room had to be barred to keep men from leaping out during attacks of mania.

Even chronic poisoning has been partially overcome, though one severe outbreak occurred in Poland in 1948 (Paluch, 1948). It is now believed in some quarters that at least some of the minor manifestations of nervous disturbance are due to individual susceptibility and are functional in origin.

Toxicity to animals

(1) Acute

(a) *Lethal dose.* – By inhalation, for cats, 1260 p.p.m. after 3 h; 35 000 p.p.m. after 48 min (death after 12 h) (Lehmann, 1894).

(b) *Narcotic dose.* – By inhalation, for mice, 1100 p.p.m. after 20 min; for cats, 23 600 p.p.m. after 30 min (Lehmann and Flury, 1943).

(2) Chronic

Inhalation of lethal or LD_{50} doses does not appear to have been described, the dosage being limited to 37–350 p.p.m. (Wiley, Hueper and von Oettingen, 1936) and to 440 p.p.m. (Raneletti, 1931).

Earlier observers (Delpech, 1856; Lehmann, 1894) had stated that concentrations of about 320 p.p.m. are badly tolerated by animals.

SYMPTOMS OF INTOXICATION

(1) Acute

Giddiness, drowsiness, vomiting, cramp, prostration, death due to respiratory paralysis.

(2) Chronic

Inhalation of 440 p.p.m., 8 h a day for 5 months caused in rabbits after 2 weeks' exposure, restlessness and excitement followed by recovery during intervals of non-exposure, but with further exposure cramps, rapid heart action, loss of weight and dyspnoea.

CHANGES IN THE ORGANISM

(1) Acute

(a) Lungs. – Congestion and slight oedema.

(b) Gastro-intestinal tract. – Acute inflammation (Tomassia, 1882). Punctiform ecchymoses of the mucous membrane (Lehmann, 1894).

(2) Chronic

General engorgement of all organs with punctiform haemorrhages.

(a) Lungs. – Emphysema and atelectasis.

(b) Liver. – Fatty degeneration (Michalova and Fryal, 1957).

(c) Nervous system. – In rabbits, chromatolysis of the cells of the cortex and an increase in neuroglia (Raneletti, 1931). Atrophy of the cerebral cells and dendrites, especially in the striopallidal nuclei (Audo-Gianetti, 1932).

In dogs, swelling of the cytoplasm of the ganglion cells, damage to Purkinje cells and basal ganglia; proliferation of the vascular endothelium, and swelling and fragmentation of the axis cylinders and myelin sheaths of peripheral nerves (Alpers and Lewey, 1940).

Several authorities, cited by Brieger (1961) have emphasised the fact that in animals with a more highly differentiated brain, such as the monkey, the lesions have been found chiefly in the basal ganglia (Richter, 1945) and that the vascular changes are of special importance.

(d) Kidneys. – A condition of 'glomerulonephrosis' and final atherosclerosis has been described in rats exposed intermittently for periods up to 12 months (Isler, 1954), while rabbits exposed for more than 28 weeks to 150–750 p.p.m. showed a high incidence of interstitial nephritis (Cohen *et al.*, 1959).

(e) Blood picture. – There is some discrepancy in the findings of various observers on the blood changes caused by repeated exposure of animals. Lewey (1941) found no significant anaemia even from repeated exposure to 1100 p.p.m., and Brieger (1941 and 1949) observed only pseudoeosinophilia and an increase in granulopoietic activity of the bone marrow following exposure of a prolonged nature to about 300 p.p.m. Binet and Bourlière (1944) on the other hand reported definite anaemia in dogs subjected to daily inhalations of 320–3200 p.p.m., also a slight increase in monocytes.

Injections of large doses of CS_2 were reported by Paterni, Germini and Dotta (1954) to have caused severe changes of a benzene-like character in the bone marrow.

(f) The adrenal glands or rabbits have been stated to show hyperactivity in the form of cortical hyperplasia and adenomata (Cohen *et al.*, 1959).

(g) The eyes. – A decrease in the corneal and pupillary reflexes and retinal angiospasm were observed by Lewey *et al.* (1941).

Bibliography on p. 717

Toxicity to human beings

(1) Acute

   (a) Fatal cases. – Very high exposure to the fumes of CS_2 can cause severe narcosis, followed or preceded by delirium, with loss of reflexes, dilated pupils, loss of consciousness, paralysis and death from respiratory failure. Such cases have been rarely reported since two were reported by Harmsen in 1905; these resulted from cleaning a reservoir and a pump through which CS_2 was delivered.

   (b) Gassing cases. – Most of these cases, especially in Great Britain, have arisen during the process of cleaning tanks which have contained CS_2. Such cases became compulsorily notifiable in 1924. The chief symptoms have been headache, vomiting, general weakness, paralysis of the legs, abdominal pain and loss of consciousness for a short period. In two cases reported to the Factory Department of Great Britain there was mental confusion.

   In Poland (Paluch, 1948) and Italy (Vigliani, 1954) outbreaks have occurred due possibly to the conditions existing during the second World War. In 1946 Vigliani reported several cases of a severe psychotic type, but this type has shown a considerable decrease in number as well as severity in most European countries.

   In France for example, the numbers fell from 252 in 1942 to 62 in 1945.

After-effects of short severe exposures

   In the period when psychotic cases were more common, as in those described by Laudenheimer (1899), some of them developed permanent dementia, but later such an effect became much rarer, as did other severe sequelae, and the prognosis is good if rapid removal from exposure takes place. Even such cases as one described by Floret (cited by Krause in 1931), a man who had inhaled concentrated CS_2 vapour for a short period and later complained of loss of appetite, vomiting, tremor of the hands for more than a year following, are now no longer recorded.

Autopsy findings

   Very little information on this aspect of acute CS_2 poisoning is available. One early observer (Foreman, 1886) noted gross congestion of the cortical veins; a histological investigation of the central nervous system by Quensel in 1904 revealed diffuse lesions of the ganglion cells of the cortex, swelling, of the vascular endothelium and scattered perivascular haemorrhages.

(2) Chronic

   The manifestations of chronic CS_2 poisoning are so numerous and diverse that differing opinions have been expressed as to whether it acts specifically upon the nervous system or as a general vascular poison. In animals the latter has been more commonly observed, and on this basis has arisen the concept of 'CS_2 atherosclerosis' finally causing encephalopathy which is responsible for the nervous symptoms (Vigliani and Pernis, 1954, 1955; Attinger, 1948). This concept has been supported especially by observers in Italy (Nunziante Cesaro and co-workers, 1954), but in France the responsibility is believed to rest more closely on primary lesions of the nerve cells (Garde *et al.*, 1953) and an investigation by Horvath and Michalova in 1956, focusses attention on the cortex-subcortex-suprarenal system. Although no indubitable conclusion can be drawn from these differences of opinion at present, it is certain that the predominant symptoms of chronic poisoning are focussed on the nervous system.

SYMPTOMS OF INTOXICATION

(1) The central nervous system
    (a) The strio-pallidal or Parkinsonian syndrome. – This type of chronic poisoning, believed to be due to the toxic effect of CS_2 on the nerve cells of the corpus striatum and globus pallidus, is characterised by muscular spasticity, tremors, speech disturbance, loss of memory and intense mental depression, evident in the typical 'Parkinson facies'. These cases may progress to complete permanent invalidism and mental disability.
    (b) The 'striate' syndrome. – This rarer manifestation of the central nervous toxic effect was described by Zeglio (1942) as a 'striate' rather than a 'pallidal' effect. It is characterised by intense involuntary muscular movements, choreic or athetotic, rather than by slowness and rigidity.

(2) The peripheral nerves
    In this 'polyneuritic syndrome' the chief symptoms are loss of power in the muscles of the upper and lower limbs, so that the gait becomes unsteady and the grip weak, while paresis of the muscles of the palate may occur causing difficulty in swallowing and a nasal voice (Raneletti, 1931). There may also be loss of sensation, less frequently than loss of motor power, but in one case reported to the Home Office, Great Britain, there was almost complete anaesthesia of the whole body.
    In most cases electrical irritability is decreased (Bashore and Staley, 1938) and though recovery may occur, it is usually slow and often incomplete. Of 20 cases reviewed by Zeglio in 1946 after 4 to 8 years, only 1 had completely recovered and 10 had deteriorated.

Effect on the eyes. – Various ocular disturbances were still being observed in France as recently as 1945, when Auffret (1946) recorded the occurrence of 600 cases. In the earlier literature occasional cases of amblyopia were reported (Constensoux and Heim, 1910; Terrien, 1920; Mattei and Sedan, 1924) and progressive failure of vision due to retrobulbar neuritis in 1031 (Nectoux and Gallois) and 1932 (Baader; Monbrun, Richet and Facquet).

Bibliography on p. 717

(3) The gastro-intestinal syndrome

Symptoms indicating gastro-intestinal disorder are now not dominated by the presence of a gastric or duodenal ulcer as in those observed by Weese in 1933, when he noted these in 14 out of 100 cases of chronic exposure to CS_2.

In those examined by Lewey (1941) 25%, and by Vigliani (1954) 28% complained of gastro-intestinal symptoms, and in 1957 a study by Blahnik and Tousek showed that in 64% chronic gastritis was present, with a low acidity or achlorhydria in many.

Liver injury has been postulated on the basis of an increase in serum cholesterol (Lewey, 1941), or insufficient regeneration of prothrombin (Saiti and Gattoni, 1957) and though microscopic examination of the liver has shown fatty degeneration and haemorrhages, total cholesterol has not shown an increase in workers exposed to 37 p.p.m. of CS_2 over a period of 5–7 years (Soucek, 1960) nor have liver function tests given uniform results (Granati and Candia, 1956; Chiesura, 1956).

(4) The glomerulo-arteriosclerotic syndrome

During the last 12 to 15 years cases of chronic CS_2 poisoning have been described in which the symptoms are very similar to those of cerebral arteriosclerosis of pre-senile origin, occurring at a relatively early age (from 42 to 55 years), after many years of exposure and often associated with renal sclerosis.

Many cases exhibit only one aspect of the atherosclerotic process, others the complete syndrome of cerebral, renal and myocardial sclerosis.

Between 1948 and 1952 seven such cases were described by Attinger; in 1950, 16 by Vigliani and Cazzullo, and further cases by Ambrosio and co-workers (1957) and von Rechenberg (1957). Von Rechenberg called the disorder "a late vascular syndrome of chronic CS_2 poisoning. He found that the first symptom in these workers was pain in the calf of the leg or difficulty in walking, a symptom also frequently observed by Vigliani and Cazzullo, while Vigliani also reported cases with hemiplegia, dementia, pseudobulbar symptoms and signs of cerebral thrombosis.

The pathological lesions in cases which have come to autopsy are those of atheromatous plaque formation, general arteriosclerosis, glomerulosclerosis, changes in the retinal vessels resembling those seen in hypertension, in some cases abnormal electroencephalograms and electrocardiograms suggesting previous myocardial infarction (Nunziante Cesaro, 1953; Ambrosio *et al.*, 1957).

Viscose workers, in the observations of Vigliani and Cazzullo, had been employed for much longer periods of time and with much lower concentrations than animals on which investigations have been carried out. For example, most of these workers had been employed for over 20 years and the concentrations had varied from 30 to 300 p.p.m., whereas the fundamental changes noted by Ferraro *et al.* (1941) in cats – a diffuse vascular proliferation and hypertrophy of vessels, particularly in the brain – were produced by exposure to about 3000 p.p.m. for 2 to 3 hours daily for periods of 24 to 92 days. On the other hand the fundamental changes have been reproduced in animals by Guarino and Arciello (1954) and others in which the concentrations and duration of exposure resemble more closely the working conditions of Vigliani's workers.

The arteriosclerosis occurs especially in the arteries and arterioles of the cerebrum, but also in those of the peripheral muscles, with calcification of the medial layer.

In some cases hypertensive kidney injury with high blood pressure, some albuminuria, slight micro-haematuria and a raised residual nitrogen have also been present, but the whole syndrome of encephalopathy, hypertensive nephropathy and medial sclerosis is not always present in its complete form; individual cases may show only one aspect.

Mechanism of action of CS_2 on the blood vessels

Several hypotheses have been advanced in an attempt to explain the arteriosclerotic effect of CS_2. Most of them are concerned with the behaviour of the blood lipids, especially cholesterol, and a more recent approach to the problem has been suggested by an examination of the serum turbidity of human beings suffering from chronic CS_2 poisoning (Ruikka, 1959).

(a) Cholesterolaemia

The association between a high level of cholesterol in the blood and arteriosclerosis, more especially atherosclerosis, is based on the fact that deposits in aortic plaques consist mainly of esterified cholesterol, and the opinion of Aschoff in 1924 that "from plasma of low cholesterol content no deposition of lipoids will occur even though the mechanical conditions are favourable" remains a strong point in the case for the role of hypercholesterolaemia in the production of atherosclerosis, and it appears to be accepted that the blood cholesterol of hypertensive individuals should be kept at a permanent level as near to the normal as possible, since, according to Snapper (1941) arteriosclerosis begins as a "fatty infiltration of the intima of the vessel walls". The cholesterolaemia of some cases of CS_2 poisoning is regarded by some authorities (e.g. Michalova, Bartonicek and Zastava 1957) as the result of a primary liver disturbance caused by CS_2.

(b) Lipoprotein ratio

An increased ratio of beta- to alpha-lipoproteins in the plasma, similar to that found in arteriosclerotic subjects, has been noted in viscose workers suffering from arteriosclerosis and from severe chronic CS_2 poisoning (Vigliani and Pernis, 1954; Granati, Scavo and Montevino, 1956; Ambrosio et al., 1957).

Bibliography on p. 717

(c) Serum turbidity

After a fatty meal the serum normally becomes turbid, owing to the presence of particles called 'chylomicrons' (Gage and Fish, 1924) which are composed primarily of neutral fat, with 3% of cholesterol, about 8% of phospholipids and 0.2–2% of protein (Bragdon, 1958). Clearing of the turbidity normally takes place within 6 to 10 h; the exact mechanism of the clearing action is not known but it is believed possible that a disturbance of the clearing factor may result in the high lipo-protein values found in atherosclerosis and other disorders where there is abnormal lipid metabolism.

In Ruikka's (1959) investigations of the clearing of semi-turbidity in persons exposed to CS_2, he found that there is a marked retardation of serum clearing only when manifest symptoms of chronic CS_2 poisoning appear; the highest turbidities were found in a group of non-exposed persons suffering from coronary thrombosis. These findings led him to conclude that the disturbance in lipid metabolism in CS_2 poisoning are similar to those occurring in atherosclerosis but that they did not explain the mechanism of its development in CS_2 poisoning.

Kidney injury in the form of 'nephrosclerosis' has been described by Nunziante Cesaro (1952) and Rossi (1955) but is usually regarded (Attinger, 1952) as an involvement of the kidney in the general arteriosclerosis rather than as a direct toxic action of CS_2.

(5) The blood picture

Hypochromic anaemia of varying degree has been reported in viscose workers in Italy (moderate according to Maugeri, 1940; and Paterni, 1956; more severe according to Raneletti, 1931); in Poland by Kiczak and Mronzinski (1953) and in America by Creskoff (1938).

Monocytosis was present in about 25% of the cases examined by Kiczak and Mronzinski, and the most consistent abnormality in those of Creskoff.

The bone marrow is reported to undergo little change (Creskoff) and to be less marked than in animals (Paterni, 1954).

TREATMENT OF CS_2 POISONING

(1) Acute

Removal from exposure and keeping warm. If necessary artificial respiration should be applied.

(2) Chronic

Treatment is mainly symptomatic. For vascular manifestations, cerebral vasodilators and sympathetic stimulants have been advocated by Nunziante Cesaro (1954). For polyneuritic symptoms vitamin B, in view of the hypothesis of Lewey (1939) that thiamine deficiency may be a factor in its causation.

For suspected liver injury, a diet low in fat (Lewey, 1941).

134. Dimethyl Sulphate

Structural formula:
$$CH_3-O \diagdown \quad \diagup O$$
$$S$$
$$CH_3-O \diagup \quad \diagdown O$$

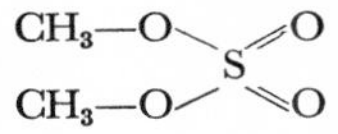

Molecular formula: $(CH_3)_2SO_4$

Molecular weight: 126.14

Properties: a colourless oily liquid vapourising at 50 °C. The vapour has a slight odour of onions and is readily decomposed by moist air, giving methyl alcohol and sulphuric acid. Almost insoluble in water; miscible with alcohol and ether.

> *boiling point:* 188 °C
> *melting point:* —26.8 °C
> *vapour pressure:* 0.1 mm Hg at 25 °C
> *vapour density (air = 1):* 4.35
> *specific gravity (liquid density):* 1.3322
> *flash point:* 182 °F
> *solubility:* almost insoluble in water; miscible with alcohol and ether.
> *maximum allowable concentration:* 1 p.p.m.

ECONOMY, SOURCES AND USES

Production

By interaction of methyl alcohol and chlorosulphonic acid, with distillation under reduced pressure.

Industrial uses

(1) Chiefly in the chemical industry as a methylating agent in the manufacture of many organic chemicals.

(2) In the manufacture of many dyes, colours and perfumes.

(3) As a solvent for the separation of mineral oils (Tara *et al.*, 1954, 1955).

(4) In analysis of automobile fluids (de Grosz, 1937).

(5) Formerly as a war gas (D-Stoff; Rationite).

Bibliography on p. 717

BIOCHEMISTRY

Estimation in the atmosphere

By absorption in alcoholic KOH solution and precipitation as barium sulphate (Fairhall, 1957).

Metabolism

In the tissues, dimethyl sulphate is slowly hydrolysed with formation of methyl alcohol and sulphuric acid. Its toxic effect is apparently dual, related both to the complete molecule and to the separated acid root (Weber, 1902; Wachtel, 1920). The narcotic effect probably differs from that characteristic of the complete unbroken molecule, as in the case of other esters (de Grosz, 1937). According to Gheringhelli *et al.* (1957, 1958), who attempted to assess the role of methanol liberation, the amount of methanol excreted by guinea pigs subjected to inhalation of its vapour is only a relatively small fraction of that which would be expected if all the dimethyl sulphate had been hydrolysed; they believe therefore that while the local effects on skin and eyes are partly due to the liberation of H_2SO_4, the effects on the central nervous system may be due to the intact molecule. They also suggest that the primary toxic action is due to methylation of certain enzymes, but not blood catalase, as judged from *in vitro* as well as *in vivo* experiments; in the latter no changes were found in the blood catalase of guinea pigs exposed to inhalation of 76 p.p.m.

TOXICOLOGY

Dimethyl sulphate is a highly toxic substance, with a powerful vesicant effect. The most frequent cause of poisoning in industrial use is the breakage of a container, or spillage on floor or clothing, and not least of its potential dangers are the absence of a warning odour and the latent period (6 to 8 h) before the onset of symptoms. Several fatal cases have been described.

The most frequent initial injury is to the eyes; this is usually in the form of severe conjunctivitis, with photophobia, and sometimes corneal clouding and loss of visual acuity. Laryngitis, with dysphonia, pharyngitis, tracheobronchitis, and respiratory disturbance comparable with that of phosgene, but with less evidence of pulmonary oedema, and injury of the kidneys, liver and heart have also been described. Contact of the liquid with the skin can cause very severe burns (von Nina, 1947). Minimal doses absorbed for some time have been stated (Wachtel, 1920) to cause, without a local respiratory effect, a toxic cachexia and gradual weakening of the heart.

Toxicity to animals

Acute

   Lethal dose. – (i) By skin application, for rabbits, 5 ml (Weber, 1902). – (ii) By gastric sound, for rabbits, 0.05 g/kg, death after 12 to 15 h; 0.25 g/kg, death after 1 h. – (iii) By intravenous injection, for rabbits, 0.3 g/kg in 45 min. – (iv) By inhalation, for rats, LD_{50}, 75 p.p.m. in 18 min (Ghirenghelli, 1957); for monkeys, 26 p.p.m., death in 1.5 weeks (Flury and Zernik, 1931); for guinea pigs, LD_{50}, 75 p.p.m. (Ghiringhelli, 1957), 30 p.p.m. for 1 h (5 out of 6) (Smyth et al., 1951). Saturated vapour, maximum for no deaths, 2 min.

SYMPTOMS OF INTOXICATION

(1) Skin. – Direct application causes secondary and tertiary burns.

(2) Eyes. – Severe irritation, lacrimation.

(3) Gastric. – Some animals had diarrhoea.

(4) Lungs. – Coughing, dyspoea, cyanosis.

(5) Central nervous system – Convulsions; in some cases nystagmus; coma preceding death.

CHANGES IN THE ORGANISM

Intense congestion of all organs.

(1) The kidneys showed acute parenchymatous degeneration.

(2) The liver parenchymatous and fatty degeneration.

(3) The lungs intense oedema.

(4) The blood showed slight relative lymphocytosis; spectroscopic examination indicated a combination of the poison with the red corpuscles (Mohlau, 1920).

Toxicity to human beings

(1) Fatal cases

   The first report of fatal poisoning occurring in industry was made by Weber in 1902, when two out of three men exposed to dimethyl sulfate died. One of these was a worker occupied with a tank in which there was 'gray fume' of dimethyl sulphate. He was rapidly affected by burning pain in the chest, throat and eyes; 48 h later he developed pneumonia, membranous inflammation of the uvula and wall of the pharynx, and necrotic areas of the conjunctiva. The urine contained traces of albumen and many cylinders. He died the following day. Autopsy showed, in addition to the necrosed membranes of the upper respiratory tract and hepatisation of the lower lobes of both lungs, petechial haemorrhages of the outer surfaces of the lungs and of the endocardium, the left ventricle, duodenum and kidney, and swelling of the liver parenchyma.

   The second fatal case was that of a chemist whose clothes became contaminated by the breaking of a flask containing about 20 g of dimethyl sulphate. In the evening he noticed pain in his limbs, body and eyes and a burning sensation in the respiratory tract. By the next morning there were severe burns of the abdomen and legs, severe pharyngitis, tracheitis and bronchitis and oedema of the eyelids with conjunctivitis and photophobia. The pulse was rapid and irregular but there were no abnormal signs in the heart or lungs. Three days later inflammation of the lungs developed, with fever, icterus and albuminuria; the patient died the following day.

In 1934, Boskowitz (cited by de Grosz, 1937) described the case of a laboratory technician who was accidentally exposed to the vapour of dimethyl sulphate for 3 h. After a latent period of 13 h he developed oedema of the glottis and laryngo-tracheo-bronchitis, followed by cardiac failure and death from pneumonia. Death from oedema of the glottis was reported by von Nida in 1947.

(2) Severe non-fatal cases

In 1920 Mohlau had described two fatal cases similar in origin to those of Weber (1902). Both these men were exposed to both the liquid and the vapour while opening a tank without due care, and both had a latent period of some hours following only slight irritation of throat and eyes. Acute congestion of both lungs developed, with oedema of the throat and larynx and considerable cyanosis. The urine showed an increase in phosphates and sulphates (changes which Mohlau considered evidence of liver involvement) and a faint trace of albumen and an occasional hyaline cast. Both men recovered, but the condition of the eyes and larynx remained troublesome and in one case the field of vision was reduced to one-tenth of its normal range.

Four cases following the breakage of a container, with dyspnoea, restlessness, high fever and pneumonia developing after 6 to 8 hours and gradual weakening of the heart 3 to 4 days later were described by de Grosz (1937). In two cases reported by Brina (1946) there was hypoglycaemia, while Balazs (1934) noted albuminuria and haematuria in two of nine persons involved in the wiping-up of spilt dimethyl sulphate.

A collective intoxication of ten laboratory employees following the accidental escape of the vapour was reported by Roche *et al.* (1962). The symptoms, becoming severe some hours later, included intense conjunctival irritation with, in one case, severe photophobia, inflammation of the pharyngo-laryngeal mucosa, with local burns and dysphonia or transient aphonia, in two cases slight dysphagia; vomiting and diarrhoea; persistent pain and burning on micturition; irritating cough with expectoration, oppression in the chest and dyspnoea. The larynx and sub-glottal region showed congestion and oedema but there were no corneal ulceration and no radiographic signs in the lungs. The symptoms, especially dysphonia and irritative cough, were slow to disappear. Most of the cases which have eventually recovered have shown more or less severe injury of the eyes, but in only a few has the injury had permanent sequelae. In two cases occurring during the manufacture of dimethyl sulphate (Duverneuil, 1957), the first sign was irritation of the eyes, increasing during the next hour to severe lacrimation and chemosis and in one case later desquamation of the corneal epithelium, in the other clouding of vision. Both however ultimately recovered with no corneal scars or diminution of vision. In two cases described by Littler and McConnell (1955) one, a chemistry student, had spilt some of the liquid on his clothing and hands; four hours later his eyes were painful, with gross oedema of the lids and extensive excoriation of the corneal epithelium. This gradually healed with no resulting opacity, but photophobia persisted for more than a week. In the second case, a worker on a chemical process where dimethyl sulphate was used as a methylating agent, the first sign of ocular injury was loss of the upper half of his visual fields. An hour later though he could not see at all, and though the eyelids were swollen and there was excoriation of the cornea he had no symptoms of eye discomfort. Three weeks later the cornea had cleared, but photophobia persisted for several months.

Similar cases have been described by Tara (1955) and Tara and Cavigneaux (1954). These and other observers have attributed the action of the dimethyl sulphate on the eyes to the fact that it is hydrolysed *in situ* forming sulphuric acid and methyl alcohol.

TREATMENT OF POISONING

(1) Acute respiratory symptoms

Ice packs on the neck and chest; oxygen and steam inhalation and antibiotics are recommended by Littler and McConnell (1955).

For the tracheal and pharyngeal oedema, spraying with adrenalin every half hour (de Grosz, 1937).

(2) Eye irritation

Abundant irrigation with water or 3% sodium bicarbonate solution (Duverneuil 1956) of instillation of 1% atropine and liquid paraffin, followed by application of an alkaline eye cream (sodium biborate and bicarbonate in white petroleum).

(3) Skin burns

Application of compresses with sodium bicarbonate.

BIBLIOGRAPHY

Ambrosio, L., F. Marsico and P. Riccioli (1957) Solfocarbonismo professionale. *Folia Med. (Nap.),* 40:544.
Alpers, B. J. and F. H. Lewey (1940) Changes in Nervous System following CS₂ poisoning in Animals and Man. *Arch. Neurol. Psychiatr.,* 44:725.
Aschoff, L. (1924) *Lectures on Pathology,* p. 131. Hoeber, New York.

Attinger, E. (1948) Chronische Schwefelkohlenstoffvergiftung unter dem 'scheinbar ungewöhn-lichen' Bilde einer schweren Gefässkrankheit. *Schweiz. Med. Wschr.*, 78:667.

Attinger, E. (1932) Chronische Schwefelkohlenstoffvergiftung unter dem Bilde einer schweren Gefässkrankheit. *Schweiz. Med. Wschr.*, 82:829.

Audo-Gianotti, G. B. (1952) Le Parkinsonisme sulfocarbone professionel. *Presse Méd.*, 40:1289.

Auffret, J. (1946) l'Industrie des Fibres artificielles et ses Dangers. *Arch. Mal. Profess.*, 7:181.

Baader, E. W. (1932) An Hirntumor erinnernde Vergiftungserscheinen durch Schwefelkohlen-stoff. *Med. Klin.*, 28:1740.

Balazs, J. (1934) Dimethyl sulfat Vergiftung. *Samml. Vergiftungsfäll.*, 5:47. A414.

Bashore, F. and T. Staley (1938) Survey of CS$_2$ and H$_2$S Hazards in Viscose Rayon Industry. *Occup. Disease Prevention Bull.* no. 46. Dept. Labor and Industry, Pennsylvania.

Binet, L. and F. Bourlière (1944) Sur les Modifications du Sang au cours du Sulfocarbonisme chronique. *Arch. Mal. Profess.*, 6:12.

Blahnik, Z. and M. Tousek (1957) Cited by Brieger, 1961. Effect of CS$_2$ on the Gastro-intestinal System. *Pracov Lek.*, 9:18.

Boskowitz, (1934) Cited by de Grosz (1937). *Trans. Hung. Med. Week.*

Bragdon, J. H. (1958) C^{14}-S$_2$ Excretion after intravenous Administration of Chylomicrons in Rat. *Arch. Biochem.*, 75:528.

Brieger, H. (1941) The Effects of CS$_2$ on the Blood Corpuscles. *J. Ind. Hyg. Toxicol.*, 23:388.

Brieger, H. (1949) On Theory and Pathology of CS$_2$ Poisoning. *J. Ind. Hyg. Toxicol.*, 31:98 and 103.

Brieger, H. (1961) Chronic CS$_2$ Poisoning. *J. Occup. Hlth.*, 3:302.

Brina, A. (1946) Due Case di Intossicazione da Solfatodimetilico. *Med. Lavoro*, 37:225.

Büsing, K. H., W. Sonnenschein, E. W. Becker and H. Dreiheller (1953) Tierexperimentelle Untersuchungen mit markierten Schwefelkohlenstoff (C^{35}S$_2$). *Naturforsch.*, 8 b. 495.

Carpenter, C. P. and H. F. Smyth (1946) Chemical Burns of the Rabbit Cornea. *Am. J. Ophthalm.*, 29:1363.

Cesaro, A. N. (1952) La Diagnosi di Solfocarbonismo professionale. *Med. Lavoro*, 43:307.

Cesaro, A. N. (1952) La Pressione arteriosa retinica negli Operai esposti al Rischio Solfocarbonico. *Med. Lavoro*, 43:312.

Cesaro, A. N. (1953) Il Solfocarbonismo cronico quale Encefalovasculopatia primitiva. *Gior. Clin. Med.*, 34:731.

Cesaro, A. N. (1954) Note istiopatologische sul Solfocarbonismo cronico. *Folia Med. (Nap.)*, 37:466.

Chiesura, P. (1956) Valutazione clinica delle Glomerulonefretici proteinuriche con particulare Riferimento alle cosidetta Nefrosi lipoidea. *Minerva Nefrologica*, 3:1.

Cohen, A. E., L. D. Scheel, J. F. Kopp, E. R. Stockell, R. G. Keenan, J. T. Mountain and H. J. Paulus (1959) Biochemical Mechanisms in chronic CS$_2$ Poisoning. *Am. Ind. Hyg. Ass. J.*, 20:303.

Constensoux, M. G. and M. F. Heim (1910) Fréquence relative des Stigmates nerveux dans le Sulfocarbonisme chronique. Question VI. *2me Congr. Internat. Mal. Profess.* Brussels.

Creskoff, A. F. (1938) Survey of CS$_2$ and H$_2$S in the Viscose Rayon Industry. *Pennsylvania Dept. Labor and Industry, Bull.*, no. 46.

Delpech (1856) Accidents produits par l'Inhalation du Sulfre de Carbone en Vapeur; Expériences sur les Animaux. *Gaz. hebd. Med. Chir.*, 1:384.

Departmental Committee on Certain Miscellaneous Dangerous Trades (1899) *H.M. Stationery Office, London.*

Department of Scientific and Industrial Research (1939) Leaflet No. 6. Carbon Disulphide Vapour. *H.M. Stationery Office, London.*

Durrans, T. H. (1950) *Solvents*, 6th ed. Chapman and Hall, London.

Elkins, H. B. (1959) *The Chemistry of Industrial Toxicology*. Chapman and Hall, London.

Fairhall, L. T. (1957) *Industrial Toxicology*. Williams and Wilkins, Baltimore.

Ferraro, A., G. A. Jervis and D. J. Flicker (1941) Neuropathologic Changes in experimental CS$_2$ Poisoning in Cats. *A.M.A. Arch. Pathol.*, 32:723.

Floret, F. Cited by F. Krause (1931) Beitrag zur Frage der Schwefelkohlenstoffvergiftung. *Z. ges Neurol. Psychiatr.*, 134:139.

Flury, F. and F. Zernik (1931) *Schädliche Gäse, Dämpfe, Nebel, Rauch- und Staubarten*. Springer, Berlin.

Foreman, W. (1886) Notes of a fatal Case of Poisoning by Bisulphide of Carbon, with postmortem Appearances and Remarks. *Lancet, ii*: 118.

Gage, S. H. and P. A. Fish (1924) Fat Digestion, Absorption and Assimilation in Man and Animals. *Am. J. Anat.*, 34: 1.

Garde, A., F. Tolot and P. F. Girard (1953) Hémisyndrome cérébelleux par Sulfocarbonisme probable. *Arch. Mal. Profess.*, 14: 67.

Ghiringhelli, G. L., V. Colombo and A. Monteverdi (1957) Osservazione in Animali da Esperimento sulla Tossicita da Dimetilsolfato. *Med. Lavoro*, 48: 634.

Ghiringhelli, G. L. and G. Sironi (1958) Dimetilsolfato e Catalisi. *Med. Lavoro*, 49: 690.

Giovine, G. P. (1957) Cronassia e Curve Intensiti-tempo nella Diagnosi del Sulfocarbonismo. *Med. Lavoro*, 48: 11.

Gordy, S. T. and M. Trumper (1938) CS$_2$ Poisoning with Report of 6 Cases. *J. Am. Med. Ass.*, 110: 1543.

Gordy, S. T. and M. Trumper (1940) CS$_2$ Poisoning; Report of 21 Cases. *Ind. Med. Surg.*, 9: 231.

Granati, A. and L. Candia (1956) Il Comportamento di alcuni Testi di Funzione epatica nel Sulfocarbonismo cronico professionale. *Folio Med. (Nap.)*, 39: 864.

Granati, A., D. Scavo and C. Montervino (1956) Il Ricambio proteitico nel Solfocarbonismo cronico. *Folia Med. (Nap.)*, 39: 763.

Grosz, S. de (1937) Dimethyl Sulphate Poisoning in relation to Ophthalmology. *Am. J. Ophthalm.*, 20: 700.

Guarino, A. and G. Arciello (1954) Richerche istologiche della Coronarie nelle Intossicazione cronica sperimentale da Solfuro di Carbonic. *Folia Med. (Nap.)*, 37: 1021.

Harmsen, E. (1905) Die Schwefelkohlenstoffvergiftung im Fabrikbetriebe und ihre Verhutung. *Z. gerichtl. Med.*, 30: 149.

Hoffman, F. W. and J. A. Oettel (1954) Zur Frage der Toxizität von Tetrahydrofuran. *Arch. Exptl. Pathol. Pharmakol.*, 222: 233.

Hosvath, M. and C. Michalova (1956) Veränderungen des EEG bei experimenteller Exposition im Schwefelkohlenstoff. *Arch. Gewerbepathol. Gewerbehyg.*, 15: 131.

Hunter, R. W. (1940) Determination of CS$_2$ in Blood and Urine. *J. Ind. Hyg. Toxicol.*, 22: 231.

Isler, U. M. (1957) Die Nierenveränderungen bei der chronischen Schwefelkohlenverwendung der Ratte. *Z. ges. exp. Med.* 128: 314.

Johnston, J. F. A. (1931) On the anaesthetic Action of Furan. *J. Pharmacol. Exptl. Therap.*, 43: 85.

Kiczak, J. and S. Mrozinski (1953) Cited by Brieger (1961) *Med. Pracy.*, 4: 245.

Koch, E. M. and M. H. Cahan (1925) Physiological Action of Furane. *J. Pharmacol. Exptl. Therap.*, 26: 281.

Krause, F. (1931) Beitrage zur Frage der Schwefelkohlenstoffvergiftung. *Z. ges. Neurol. Psychiatr.*, 134: 139.

Laudenheimer, R. (1899) *Die Schwefelkohlenstoffvergiftung der Gummiarbeiter unter besonderer Berucksichtigung der psychischen und nervösen Störungen und der Gewerbehygiene.* Veit, Leipzig.

Lehmann, K. B. (1894) Experimentelle Studien über den Einfluss technische und hygienisch wichtiger Gäse und Dämpfe auf den Organisimus. *Arch. Hyg. Berl.*, 67: 93.

Lehmann, K. B. and F. Flury (1943) *Toxicology and Hygiene of industrial Solvents.* Williams and Wilkins, Baltimore.

Lewey, F. H. (1939) Vitamin C Deficiency and nervous Diseases. *J. Nerv. Ment. Dis.*, 89: 1: 174.

Lewey, F. H. (1941) Neurological, medical and biochemical Signs and Symptoms indicating chronic industiral CS$_2$ Absorption. *Ann. Intern. Med.*, 15: 869.

Lewey, F. H., B. J. Alpers and A. C. Creskoff (1941) Experimental chronic CS$_2$ Poisoning in Dogs; a clinical, biochemical and pathological Study. *J. Ind. Hyg. Toxicol.*, 23: 415.

Maugeri, S. (1940) Contributo allo Studio del Sulfocarbonismo; Carrateria e Natura del Anemia. *Gazz. d. Osp. e Clin.*, 61: 563.

McKee, R. W. (1941) Quantitative microchemical colorimetric Determination of CS$_2$ in Air, Water and Biological Fluids, *J. Ind. Hyg. Toxicol.*, 23: 151.

McKee, R. W., C. Kiper, J. H. Fountain, A. M. Riskin and P. Drinker (1943) A Solvent Vapor: CS$_2$. *J. Am. Med. Ass.*, 122: 217.

Mattei, C. and J. Sedan (1924) Contribution à l'Étude de l'Intoxication par le Sulfure de Carbone. *Ann. Hyg. publ. Paris, N.S.*, 2: 385.

Michalova, C., V. Bartoniček and V. Zastava (1959) Organotoxische Wirkung von Schwefel-
    kohlenstoffe nach parenteraler Intoxikation von Kaninchen. *Arch. Gewerbepathol. Gewerbehyg.*,
    16:653.
Michalova, C. and Z. Frydl (1957) Veränderungen der höheren Nerventätigkeit und einiger humo-
    ralen Faktoren nach parenteraler Intoxikation des Kaninchens mit Schwefelkohlenstoff.
    Arch. Gewerbepathol. Gewerbehyg., 15:553.
Mohlau, F. D. (1920) Report of 2 Cases of Dimethyl sulphate Poisoning. *J. Ind. Hyg. Toxicol.*,
    2:238.
Monbrun, A., C. Richet and J. Facquet (1932) La Névrite optique bulbaire par le Sulfure de Car-
    bone. *Arch. Ophthal. Paris*, 49:697.
Nectoux, R. and R. A. Gallois (1931) Quatre Cas de Névrite rétrobulbaire par le Sulfure de Car-
    bone. *Bull. Soc. Ophthal. Paris*, p. 750.
Nida, S. von (1947) Tödliches Glottisödem nach Dimethyl sulphatverätzung der oberen Ver-
    dauungswege. *Klin. Wschr.*, 50:230.
Paluch, A. (1948) Two Outbreaks of Carbon Disulphide Poisoning in Rayon Staple Fibre Plants
    in Poland. *J. Ind. Hyg. Toxicol.*, 30:37.
Paterni, L. (1954) *XI Congresso Internationale di Medicina del Lavoro Naples*, Vol. II, p. 363.
Paterni, L. (1956) l'Arteriosclerosi nella Medicina del Lavoro. *Folia Med. (Nap.)*, 39:573.
Paterni, L., P. Germini and F. Dotta (1954) *XI Congresso Internationale di Medicina del Lavoro Naples*,
    Vol. II, p. 366.
Paterni, L., G. Pusic and S. Teodori (1958) Intossicante lenta da CS₂ e Arteriosclerosi da Dieta
    ipercolersterolica del Coniglio. *Fol. Med.* 41:705.
Patty, F. A. (1963) *Industrial Hygiene and Toxicology*, Vol. II, 2nd ed. Interscience, New York.
Quensel, F. (1904) Neue Erfährungen über Geistesstorungen nach Schwefelkohlenstoffvergiftung.
    Monatsch. Psychiat. Neurol., 16:48.
Raneletti, A. (1931) Die berufliche Schwefelkohlenstoffvergiftung in Italien. *Arch. Gewerbepathol.
    Gewerbehyg.*, 2:664.
Rechenberg, H. K. von (1957) Schwefelkohlenstoffvergiftung und das sulfocarbonische vasculare
    Spätsyndrom. *Arch. Gewerbepathol. Gewerbehyg.*, 15:487.
Richter, R. (1945) Degeneration of Basal Ganglia from chronic CS₂ Poisoning in Monkeys. *J.
    Neuropathol. Exptl. Neurol.*, 4:324.
Roche, L., J. M. Robert and P. Paliard (1962) Intoxication par le Sulfate de Diméthyle. *Arch.
    Mal. Prof.*, 23:391.
Rossi, L. (1955) La Funzionalita renale nel Sulfocarbonismo cronico professionale. *Folia Med.*,
    38:557.
Rubin, H. H. and A. J. Arieff (1945) CS₂ and H₂S; Clinical Study of chronic low-grade Exposure.
    J. Ind. Hyg. Toxicol., 27:123.
Rubin, H. H., A. J. Arieff and F. W. Tauber (1950) CS₂ and H₂S: Follow-up clinical Study of low-
    grade Exposures. *Arch. Ind. Hlth.*, 2:529.
Ruikka, I. (1959) Postprandial Serum Turbidity in chronic CS₂ Poisoning. *Ann. Med. Intern. Fenn.*,
    48 (Suppl. 31) 1.
Saita, G. and L. Gattoni (1957) Il Processo emogoagulatorio del Solfocarbonismo cronico. *Med.
    Lavoro*, 48:229.
Sax, N. Irving (1957) *Dangerous Properties of Industrial Materials*. Reinhold, New York.
Scheel, L. D., R. G. Keenan, J. T. Mountain, J. Kopp, J. Holz and R. Killens. *XIIIth Internat.
    Congr. Occup. Health, New York.*
Schwartz, L., L. Tulipan an D. J. Birmingham (1957) *Occupational Diseases of the Skin*. 3rd. ed.
    Lea and Fibiger, Philadelphia.
Simon, K. H. (1961) Chronische Vergiftung durch Schwefelkohlenstoff. *Med. Monatschr.*, 16:810.
Smyth Jr., H. F., C. P. Carpenter and C. S. Weil (1951) Range Finding Toxicity Data, List IV.
    Arch. Ind. Hyg., 4:119.
Snapper, L. (1941) *Chinese Lessons to Western Medicine*. Interscience, New York.
Souček, B. (1960) Cited by Brieger (1961) Effect of CS₂ on the Level of Cholesterol and its Esters
    in the Blood Serum. *Pracov. Lek.*, 12:243.
Souček, B. and Z. Madlo (1956) Dithiocarbamincarbonsäuren als Abbauprodukte des Schwefel-
    kohlenstoffs. *Arch. Gewerbepathol. Gewerbehyg.*, 14:511.

Stokinger, H. E. (1963) The Metals. In: F. A. Patty (1963). *Industrial Hygiene and Toxicology*. Interscience, New York.

Stoughton, R. W. and B. H. Robbins (1936) Anaesthetic Properties of Tetrahydrofuran. *J. Pharmacol. Exptl. Therap.*, 58:171.

Strittmatter, C. F., T. Peters and R. W. McKee (1950) Metabolism of labelled CS_2 in Guinea pigs and Mice. *Arch. Ind. Hyg.*, 1:54.

Tara, S. (1959) À propos de Sulfate de Métyle. *Arch. Mal Prof.*, 16:368.

Tara, S., A. Cavigneaux and Y. Delplace (1954) Accidents oculaires par Sulfate de Méthyle. *Arch. Mal. Prof.*, 15:291.

Teisinger, J. and B. Souček (1949) *Sur l'Absorption et l'Élimination de Sulfure de Carbone chez l'Homme exposé et non exposé*. Proc. IXth Internat. Congr. Ind. Med., p. 198. John Wright & Sons, Bristol, 1949.

Terrien, F. (1920) Deux Cas d'Amblyopie de Sulfure de Carbone. *Paris Med.*, 35:317.

Tomassia, A. (1882) De l'Intoxication suraigüe par le Sulfure de Carbone. *Ann. Hyg. publ. Paris*, 3me Ser., 7:292.

Vigliani, E. C. (1946) l'Intossicazione cronica da Sulfuro da Carbonio. *Med. Lavoro*, 37:165.

Vigliani, E. C. (1954) CS_2 Poisoningin Viscose Rayon Factories. *Brit. J. Ind. Med.*, 11:235.

Vigliani, E. C. and C. L. Cazzullo (1950) Alterazione del Sistema nervosa centrale di Origine vascolare nel Solfocarbonismo. *Med. Lavoro*, 41:49.

Vigliani, E. C. and B. Pernis (1954) *Atti XI Congr. Internat. di Med. del Lavoro. Naples*. Vol. I, p.375.

Vigliani, E. C. and B. Pernis (1955) Klinische und experimentelle Untersuchungen über die durch Schwefelkohlenstoffebedingte Atherosclerosis. *Arch. Gewerbepathol. Gewerbehyg.*, 14:190.

Wachtel, C. (1920) Über die Wirkung ätzender Ester. *Zschr. Exptl. Pathol. Therap.*, 21:1.

Weber, S. (1902) Über die Giftigkeit der Schwefelsäure-dimethyl Esters. *Arch. Exptl. Pathol. Pharmakol.*, 47:113.

Weise, W. (1933) Magen-darm Erkrankungen durch chronische Schwefelkohlenstoffe und chronische Schwefelwasserstoffe Inhalation. *Arch. Gewerbepathol. Gewerbehyg.*, 4:219.

Weist, H. J. (1959) Schwefelkohlenstoffbestimmungen im Blut ohne und bei Schwefelkohlenstoff-Exposition. *Arch. Gewerbepathol. Gewerbehyg.*, 17:430.

Wiley, F. H., W. C. Hueper and W. F. and W. F. von Oettingen (1936) Toxic Effects of low Concentrations of CS_2. *J. Ind. Hyg. Toxicol.*, 18:733.

Williams, R. T. (1959) *Detoxication Mechanisms*. Chapman and Hall, London.

Zaharadnik, R., V. Mansfield and B. Souček (1955) Analytische Verwendung der Reaktion von Histamin und Histidin mit Schwefelkohlenstoff. *Pharmazie*, 10:364.

Zapp, J. A. Cited by Fairhall (1957) as a personal communication.

Zeglio, P. (1942) Su di una complessa Sindroma nervosa de Intossicazione Sulfocarbonica. *Med. Lavoro*, 33:121.

Zeglio, P. (1946) Sulla Prognosi delle Polynevrite Sulfocarbonio. *Med. Lavoro*, 37:288.

Addendum:

135. Dioxan

Synonym: diethylene dioxide

Structural formula: O⟨C—C⟩O / ⟨C—C⟩

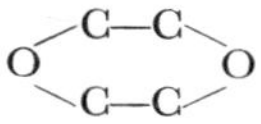

Molecular formula: $C_4H_8O_2$

Molecular weight: 88.10

Properties: a colourless liquid with an odour of Butyl Alcohol. Stable to light but forms an explosive peroxide in air especially in the presence of moisture.

> *boiling point:* 101.3
> *vapour pressure:* 37 mm Hg at 25 °C
> *vapour density (air = 1):* 3
> *specific gravity (liquid density):* 1.035
> *flash point:* 11 °C
> *conversion factors:* 1 p.p.m. = 3.6 mg/m³
> 1 mg/l = 278 p.p.m.
> *solubility:* miscible with water in all proportions; miscible with petroleum, aromatic hydrocarbons, castor and linseed oils and most organic solvents. Dissolves cellulose acetate and nitrate (water increases its solvent properties for these (Durrans, 1950)).
> *maximum allowable concentration:* 100 p.p.m. A.C.G.H.I., Elkins (1959) suggests 50 p.p.m.

ECONOMY, SOURCES AND USES

Production

By polymerising ethylene oxide with caustic soda, or by dehydrating ethylene glycol.

Industrial uses

As a solvent for lacquers, varnishes, paints, dyes, fats, waxes resins and plastics (polyvinyl polymers; Malten and Zielhuis, 1964). It is also used in the preparation of tissues for histology.

BIOCHEMISTRY

Estimation in the atmosphere

(1) By interferometer or combustible gas indicator, or possibly by spectrographic technique (Rowe, 1963).
(2) By reaction with tetranitromethane, with production of a bright yellow colour (Reid and Hoffman, 1929).

Metabolism

Except for the fact that dioxan can be absorbed by the skin in toxic amounts (Fairley *et al.* 1934) its actual metabolic process is uncertain. Fairley *et al.* suggested that it was converted to diglycolic and oxalic acids, but Wiley *et al.* (1938) found no more excretion of oxalic acid in the urine of dogs and rabbits fed repeatedly with dioxan than in that of control animals, in contrast to those fed ethylene glycol and ethylene glycol monoacetate. Von Oettingen and Jirouch (1931) had already suggested that the relatively low toxicity of dioxan in acute dosage compared with that of ethylene glycol was due to the rapid decomposition of dioxan in the organism.

TOXICOLOGY

The acute toxic effects of dioxan to animals by single dosage as described by various earlier authorities do not give a view of dioxan toxicity conformable with the fact that in 1933 five persons died, with severe kidney and liver damage, from an unusually heavy dosage. Among these earlier authorities Yant *et al.* (1930) found dioxan to have only a mild toxic effect, with adequate warning from its irritant properties, but the severe effects of the only industrial poisoning ever reported were confirmed in animals by De Navasquez in 1945.

Dioxan is an irritant of mucous membranes, especially of the nose and eyes and also of the gatric and pulmonary mucous membranes but not apparently of the skin. Human beings have been reported to suffer from irritation of the eyes, nose and throat on exposure to 300 p.p.m. (Silverman *et al.*, 1946).

A recent interesting experiment by Franceschini (1964) has led him to suggest that dioxan may have an *in vitro* effect similar to that of thalidomide on the growth of embryonic bone. He immersed the tibial buds of day-old chicks in a culture medium to which was added dioxan in a concentration of 4375. The appearances which developed were those of arrest of linear growth, nearly complete disappearance of the fundamental substance of cartilage, disappearance of the pre-existing structure, and practically complete arrest of mitotic activity.

Bibliography on p. 726

According to Wirth and Klimmer (1936) it can cause not only injury to the kidneys and liver of animals but also possible paralysis and damage to the blood-forming organs.

Toxicity to animals

(1) *Acute*

(a) *Lethal dose.* – *(i) Oral*, LD50, for mice, rats and guinea pigs, 5.66 g/kg, 5.17 g/kg and 3.90 g/kg respectively (Laug *at al.*, 1939). – *(ii) Subcutaneous* for mice, 10 ml/kg as compared with 2.5 ml/kg for ethylene glycol (Von Oettingen and Jirouch, 1931). – *(iii) Intravenous*, for rabbits, 1.5 ml/kg (De Navasquez, 1935). – *(iv) Inhalation*, for guinea pigs, 1000–3000 p.p.m. for 3 h or more (Yant, *et al.*, 1930); mice, 8000 p.p.m.; cats 10.900 p.p.m. (death sometimes delayed for several days), (Wirth and Klimmer, 1936); for mice, rats, guinea pigs and rabbits 4000–11000 p.p.m. (Lehmann and Flury, 1943).

(b) *Narcotic Dose.* – According to Knoefel (1935) dioxan, when given by intraperitoneal injection or stomach tube has a rather low narcotic effect, much lower than that of some formals and acetals.

(2) *Chronic*

By inhalation, for cats, rabbits and guinea pigs, a dose of 2700 p.p.m. daily for 8 h was followed by death of 7 out of 10 after 4–26 exposures, the remainder after 34; fatal uraemia resulted only after unexpectedly high administration (De Navasques, 1945). Fairley *et al.* (1934) reported 1000 and 5000 p.p.m. for 1½ h a day as giving a 'high mortality' due to lung injury, while Gross (1943) recorded no mortality in cats, rabbits and guinea pigs inhaling 1350 p.p.m. 8 h at a time up to 45 times. Acquired tolerance with repeated sublethal doses was observed by De Navasquez.

SYMPTOMS OF INTOXICATION

With oral administration, weakness, depression, incoordination and coma preceding death.

With intravenous injection, loss of weight, drowsiness and ataxia, polyuria followed by anuria and coma leading to death in 2–6 days (De Navasquez, 1935).

With inhalation, irritation of mucous membranes, squinting and lachrymation, emaciation and retching, delayed deaths usually due to pneumonia (Yant *et al.*, 1930). Cramps, narcosis, dyspnoea, sometimes convulsions, death due to respiratory failure (Fairley *et al.*, 1934).

CHANGES IN ORGANISM

The toxic effects of diozan are chiefly focussed on the *kidneys* and *liver* but in animals these lesions appear to be less marked with acute than with chronic poisoning, death – especially with inhalation – often resulting from injury to the lungs.

With intravenous injection, however, there appears to be a selective action on the *kidneys*, consisting, according to De Navasquez, of acute hydropic degeneration of the convoluted tubules, causing swelling and blockage of the tubules so that uraemia develops rapidly. With single inhalation of high concentration these lesions were not especially prominent in the investigation of Yant *et al.* but kidney damage was found in animals dying some days after exposure.

With repeated exposure to low concentrations over a long period Fairley *et al.* observed degeneration of the tubular epithelium, with congestion and haemorrhage, and following skin absorption, in one rabbit, severe necrosis of the kidney cortex. Changes in the *liver* varied following single oral administration from animal to animal, but with repeated dosage showde, accoding to Gross (1943) 'dropsical changes', while De Navasquez noted 'hydropic degeneration' in which the vacuoles were packed with granules of glycogen which he considered a manifestation of disturbed glycogen metabolism.

Gross also observed that even when death was due to lung injury following acute inhalation, damage to the liver, such as he described, was nearly always present.

The *lungs*, in the investigation of Yant *et al.*, showed hyperaemia in those animals subjected to 1000–3000 p.p.m., while those of Gross developed oedema and pneumonia with exposure to 4000–11000 p.p.m, and those of Fairley *et al.* lethal lung injury with 5000–10000 p.p.m.

The *brain* in the animals exposed to 1000–3000 p.p.m. showed congestion (Yant *et al.*).

Toxicity to human beings

There has been considerable discussion as to the warning properties of dioxan in concentrations liable to be harmful to exposed workers. Yant *et al.* stated that 1600 p.p.m. caused slight burning of the eyes with lachrymation, and 5550 p.p.m. a burning sensation in the throat. Fairley *et al.* reported in some subjects only a feeling of constriction in the throat, a transitory warmth in the chest and a tendency to more rapid respiration; all these sensations decreased with prolonged exposure. Silverman, Schulte and First (1946) on the other hand reported that 200 p.p.m. was the highest concentration which caused no discomfort. Since the irritation produced was only transitory, Rowe (1963) concludes that the warning properties of dioxan are completely inadequate to prevent exposure to toxic amounts.

The fatal cases of 1933

The symptoms complained of by the 5 men who died, and of others who recovered were in the opinion of most authorities due to a few acute exposures

Bibliography on p. 726

rather than to chronic poisoning. This view is borne out by the fact that the process, in which cellulose acetate silk yarn was treated with dioxan, had been in operation for more than a year with no symptoms of ill-health having been observed, and that an alteration in the experimental plant involving a higher exposure to dioxan had been installed only two months before symptoms occurred. These consisted of anorexia, nausea and vomiting, complained of not only by the men who died but also by some of their co-workers. No jaundice had been present, but in one (non-fatal) case the liver was palpable, with a positive indirect Van den Bergh reaction, and a trace of albumen and a few red corpuscles in the urine. Other workers also showed a trace of albuminuria and some leucocytosis.

In the 5 fatal cases the gastric symptoms were more severe and were associated with pain and tenderness in the abdomen and lumbar region, irritation of the upper respiratory passages, coughing, headache, drowsiness, vertigo, suppression of urine and coma, leading to death, within two weeks.

Post-mortem appearances (Barber, 1934) showed macroscopically enlargement of the kidneys with areas of haemorrhage on the suface, and an enlarged and pale liver not stained with bile. Microscopically, the kidneys showed necrosis of the outer part of the cortex, vascular in distribution and with haemorrhage at the edge of the necrotic zone. The liver also showed complete necrosis of the inner half or two-thirds of each lobule, but no fatty degeneration. In one case the lungs were oedematous. Three of the men showed a leucocytosis of 24000, 21400 and 38000 respectively, with neutrophilia.

The ultimate cause of death was attributed to haermorrhagic nephritis. The importance of early symptoms of gastric disturbances as an indication of liver involvement was later emphasised by Estler (1935), and Rowe (1963) again stresses the fact, obvious from this unfortunate accident, that dioxan does not possess warning properties adequate to prevent exposure dangerous to life.

REFERENCES

Barber, H. (1934) Haemorrhagic Nephritis and Necrosis of the Liver from Dioxan Poisoning, *Guy's Hosp. Rept.*, 84:267.
Durrans, T. (1950) *Solvents*, 6th ed., Chapman and Hall, London.
Elkins, H. B. (1959) *The Chemistry of Industrial Toxicology*, Wiley, New York.
Estler, W. (1935) Gewerbliche und experimentelle Vergiftungen mit Dioxan im Schrifftum, *Ärztl. Sachverstztng.*, 41:119.
Fairley, A., E. C. Linton and A. H. Ford Moore (1934) Toxicity to Animals of 1:4-Dioxan, *J. Hyg.* 34:486.
Franceschini, M. (1964) L'Azione del Diossano e della Talidomide sull'accrescimento in Coltura della tibia embrione di Pollo, *Sperimentale*, 114:117.
Gross, E. (1943) cited by Lehmann and Flury, 1943, *Toxicology and Hygiene of Industrial Solvents*, Wilkins and Wilkins, Baltimore.
Knoefel, R. K. (1935). Narcotic Potency of some Cyclic Acetals. *J. Pharmacol. Exptl. Therap.*, 53:440.
Laug, F. P., H. O. Calvery, H. J. Morris and Woodard G. (1939). The Toxicology of some Glycols and Derivatives. *J. Ind. Hyg. Toxicol.*, 21:173.

Malten, K. E. and R. L. Zielhuis (1964) *Industrial Toxicology and Dermatology in the Production and Processing of Plastics*, Elsevier, Amsterdam.

Navasquez, S. De (1935) Experimental tubular Necrosis of the Kidneys accompanied by Liver Changes due to Dioxan Poisoning, *J. Hyg.* 35:540.

Nelson, N. (1951) Solvent Toxicity with particular Reference to certain Octyl Alcohols, *Med. Bull.*, 11:226.

Oettingen, W. F. Von and E. H. Jirouch (1931) Pharmacology of Ethylene Glycol and some of its Derivatives. *J. Pharmacol. Exptl. Therap.*, 42:335.

Reid, E. W. and H. E. Hoffman (1929) 1-4 Dioxan, *Ind. Eng. Chem.*, 21:695.

Rowe, V. K. (1963) Derivatives of Glycols, in *Industrial Hygiene and Toxicology* (F. A. Patty, Ed.), vol. II, 2nd ed., Interscience Publishers.

Silverman, L., H. F. Schulte and W. E. First (1946) Further Studies on Sensory Response to certain Industrial Solvent Vapours, *J. Ind. Hyg. Toxicol.*, 28:262.

Wirth, W. and O. Klimmer (1936) Zur Toxikologie der organischen Lösungsmittel, 1:4-Dioxan. *Arch. Gewerbepath. Gewerbehyg.*, 7:192.

Wiley, F. H., W. C. Hueper, S. D. Bergen and F. R. Blood (1938) Formation of Oxalic Acid from Ethylene Glycol and related Solvents, *J. Ind. Hyg. Toxicol.*, 20:269.

Yant, W. P., H. H. Schrenk, C. P. Waite and F. A. Patty (1930) Acute Response of Guinea pigs to Vapors of some new commercial organic Compounds: Dioxan, *Publ. Hlth. Rept.*, Washington.

Subject Index

pseudocumene *(ctnd)*
    production and properties, 116
    toxicity to animals, 117
        to human beings, 118
    toxicology, 117
Pyranton A, see diacetone alcohol
pyridine, 304
    estimation in air, 305
    industrial uses, 304
    metabolism, 305
    production and properties, 304
    toxicity to animals, 306
        to human beings, 306, 307
    toxicology, 305

Rationite, see dimethyl sulphate

Schamberg's disease, 167
Sextate, see methyl hexalin acetate
Sextol, see methyl cyclohexanol; heptanol
S.G.O.T., 176–200
    estimation, 177
silicone oils, 691
silicium compounds, 691 ff
S.O.C.T., 200
Solactol, see ethyl lactate
Solvent GC, see ethylene glycol monoacetate
Solvulose, see ethylene glycol monoethyl ether
Striate syndrome in CS_2 poisoning, 709
styrene, 98
    estimation in air, 99
    industrial uses, 99
    metabolism, 99
    production and properties, 98
    toxicity to animals, 100
        to human beings, 101
    toxicology, 100
sulphite process, 105
sulphuric ether, see diethyl ether

1,1,2,2-tetrachloroethane, 220
    estimation in air, 221
    industrial uses, 221
    metabolism, 221
    production and properties, 220
    toxicity to animals, 222
        to human beings, 224–229
    treatment, 229
tetrachloroethylene, 213
    effect on blood alcohol, 215
    estimation in air, 214
    industrial uses, 213
    metabolism, 214
    production and properties, 213
    toxicity to animals, 215–217
        to human beings, 217–219

    toxicology, 215
tetrachloromethane, see carbon tetrachloride
tetraethoxysilane, see ethyl silicate
tetraethyl orthosilicate, see ethyl silicate
tetrahydrofurane, 700
    industrial uses, 700
    production and properties, 700
    toxicity to animals, 701
        to human beings, 701
    toxicology, 700
tetramethyl orthosilicate, see methylsilicate
tetrahydronaphthalene, see tetralin
Tetralex, see tetrachloroethylene
tetralin, 119
    estimation in air, 120
    industrial uses, 120
    metabolism, 120
    production and properties, 119
    toxicity to animals, 121
        to human beings, 123
    toxicology, 121
tetranitromethane, 297
thrombocytopenia, 35, 37
toluene, 66 ff
    benzene content, 66, 67, 75
    estimation in air, blood, tissues and urine, 67, 68
    industrial uses, 67
    production and properties, 66, 67
    metabolism, 68
    toxicity to animals, 69–72
        to human beings, 72–76
    toxicology, 68
transyl, 199
trichloracetic acid, 192, 193, 201, 222
trichlorethanol, 194
trichloroethane-1-1-1, 253
    estimation in air, 254
        in blood, tissues and urine, 255
    industrial uses, 254
    metabolism, 255
    production and properties, 253, 254
    toxicity to animals, 256
        to human beings, 257
    toxicology, 255
trichloroethane-1-1-2, 258
    estimation in air, blood and tissues, 258
    industrial uses, 258
    metabolism, 258
    production and properties, 258
    toxicity to animals, 259
    toxicology, 259
trichloroethylene, 189 ff
    action on blood alcohol, 196
    addiction to, 211
    estimation in air, 191